# TOOTH WEAR

## THE QUINTESSENTIAL CHALLENGE

# TOOTH WEAR

## THE QUINTESSENTIAL CHALLENGE

Debora R. Vilaboa
Beatriz R. Vilaboa
Jose Manuel Reuss
Debora Reuss

QUINTESSENCE PUBLISHING

Berlin | Chicago | Tokyo
Barcelona | London | Milan | Mexico City | Paris | Prague | Seoul | Warsaw
*Beijing | Istanbul | Sao Paulo | Zagreb*

One book, one tree: In support of reforestation worldwide and to address the climate crisis, for every book sold Quintessence Publishing will plant a tree (https://onetreeplanted.org/).

A CIP record for this book is available from the British Library.
ISBN: 978-1-78698-120-2

QUINTESSENCE PUBLISHING DEUTSCHLAND

Quintessenz Verlags-GmbH
Ifenpfad 2–4
12107 Berlin
Germany
www.quintessence-publishing.com

Quintessence Publishing Co Ltd
Grafton Road, New Malden
Surrey KT3 3AB
United Kingdom
www.quintessence-publishing.com



Editing: Quintessence Publishing Co, Inc, Batavia, IL, USA
Layout, Production and Reproduction: Quintessenz Verlags-GmbH, Berlin, Germany

Printed and bound in Croatia by Grafički zavod Hrvatske d.o.o.

## Table of Contents

# SECTION II. ASSESSING AND TREATING TOOTH WEAR 85

## CHAPTER 4. DIAGNOSIS AND TREATMENT PLANNING IN TOOTH WEAR 87



## CHAPTER 5. INCIPIENT TOOTH WEAR 129



## CHAPTER 6. MODERATE TOOTH WEAR: TREATMENT STRATEGIES 167



## CHAPTER 7. SEVERE TOOTH WEAR: TREATMENT STRATEGIES 215

# Foreword

## Why is Tooth Wear the Quintessential Challenge?

The Ancient Greeks believed a certain type of air could be found in the upper section of heaven, a type of air that was purer and more splendid than the air inhaled by mere mortals. This dazzling substance, or essence, inhaled by the Gods was known as ether.

Aristotle classified ether as the fifth natural element. To the four natural elements that had previously been identified by the Ionic philosophers—earth, water, air, and fire—Aristotle added a new, completely different element in his theory of nature.

When faced with the traditional four elements that made up the sublunar world, corruptible and subject to change—and given to imperfect, rectilinear movements—ether, the element that occupied the superlunary layers of the cosmos, the element from which the celestial spheres housing the planets and stars were made, was incorruptible, moving eternally and perfectly in circles, presenting characteristics that brought them closer to the divine.

Medieval philosophers gave ether the Latin name of "quintessence" for its aforementioned characteristic of being the fifth element that made up the Universe. The concept of quintessence gained significant importance in alchemy both in the Middle Ages and in the Early Modern Period.

In traditional alchemy, quintessence came to be identified as the Philosopher's Stone (elixir of life), an essence that could transform any metal into gold. Alchemists searched for quintessence on Earth, but, believing that they would find very limited quantities here given its celestial origins, they mainly tried to find a formula to obtain ether by combining the other elements.

They had hoped to use quintessence as medicine in the form of an elixir. Given the purity and the divine quality of quintessence, alchemists believed that by taking the elixir an individual would remain free of any type of impurity and sickness, and they would even become young again (rejuvenate). Quintessence began to be identified with a spiritual energy that could unite and dissolve the other four elements; the soul of the world. Paracelsus maintained that quintessence was the element that would bring new life to the body and the soul. Inspired by the archaic Pythagorean doctrine, alchemists considered quintessence to be the spark of the divine in the human, of the heavenly in the earthly, of the infinite in the finite.

In this book, the problems associated with tooth wear (TW) are approached from four different aspects, elements, or basic dimensions: physical, functional, psychologic, and social, to which is added a fifth dimension, fifth element, or fifth essence, so to speak. As with alchemy, the preservation of the teeth involves a series of elements and combining these in the best way possible to achieve quintessence.

The esthetic dimension could be considered as the fifth element of those contributing to dental well-being. Just as quintessence, or ether, was the purest natural element, or essence, for the ancient philosophers, the esthetic dimension is the purest element, or essence, when facing the challenge of TW.

As the essence of the alchemists was centered around an element that offered the perfect combination of the other elements, it is important to clarify that we consider here a wider sense of the concept of esthetics, in its Greek meaning. In this way, we understand esthetics in its deepest and most profound state.

Esthetics is connected to feelings and how those feelings are perceived: the outside world, the world we see, what we hear, what we taste, what we smell, and what we touch. While esthetics can be approached according to the relationship each individual has with the world around them, it can also be approached according to the relationship each one of us has with others. Esthetics is the domain of the senses and perception. It encapsulates both the perception we have of others and the perception others have of us, and in turn the perception that we have of the perception that others have of us.

The teeth occupy a fundamental position in personal esthetics; the mouth is one of the principal and primary ways we present ourselves: a personal cover letter. Dental esthetics are a fundamental pillar for self-esteem and an individual's confidence; therefore, through our mouth, teeth, and smile we are able to communicate a lot about ourselves, our personality, and our moods. The perception others have of us is very much related to the appearance of the mouth and teeth.

How do others perceive me? What image do I present of myself? Do I give off a youthful image, do I come across as a healthy person, confident in myself, and what in turn is of interest to others?

The response to these questions involves the teeth and the mouth as fundamental components. A person with a deteriorated mouth seems aged, in a bad state of health, and is going to feel as though others see them in this way too. Therefore, people may feel their self-esteem is undermined, and this in turn projects an even more deteriorated self-image; it is a vicious circle.

Think on this deterioration, of how it is perceived by others and how it is going to continue, affecting the different areas of the mouth in an itinerant, constant, and progressive way. This thought will lead you to be aware of your finiteness and that the Universe, with its huge regions where the ether dwells, will continue its course without you being able to do anything to prevent it. The divine quintessence in its eternal and perfect movement is unconnected to this suffering.

Alberto Álvarez Fernández
Spanish philosopher and economist, childhood friend of the authors

## Foreword

Drs Debora and Beatriz Vilaboa have a passion for dentistry that has pushed them to search for better ways to deliver treatment while respecting the benefits of tooth preservation. Their enthusiasm for and dedication to this work is transmitted to their students and their team. In this book, they now share their vision with a wider audience.

After medical and dental school, Drs Vilaboa wanted to address the need for dental restoration with a legitimate desire to improve smiles, and they pioneered with other colleagues in esthetic dentistry. They believed in restoring worn dentitions and anterior guidance with porcelain laminate veneers and worked to overcome the general reluctance toward adhesive restorations in a time when traditional prosthodontics seemed preferable.

They have always described their career as a "journey," and I have been honored to count myself as a companion on that journey. Not only have they attended every continuing education seminar and congress that I have organized, but I was proud to mentor them as they became active members of the European Academy of Esthetic Dentistry and have remained an active part of their family since then. I had the pleasure of knowing their father and mother and brilliant brother Jorge. In addition, the parallelism between Debora's and my family has been a matter of joy for all of us, and in both families, the next generation (Jose Manuel and Alfonso, through surgical and restorative disciplines and Debora and Jaime as orthodontists) has also chosen to devote their lives to dentistry. The torch is being passed on.

The Vilaboa family is one of business talent. Their group practice is well structured and patient centered and a source of inspiration to us. It has flourished because they understood how a multidisciplinary approach and the fluent use of the newest digital tools could enhance the patient experience and the treatment processes.

Inside this book, readers will find an integrative and multidisciplinary approach to tooth wear, which covers surgery, implants, orthodontics, and restorations (both direct and indirect), with the goal of improving oral health and achieving esthetic dentistry. In addition, the economic burden of tooth wear is softened with well-supported protocols that help make treatment accessible in all cases.

Overall, this is a comprehensive book for tooth wear that is easy to read and that effectively compiles all clinical aspects—from the concept and diagnosis to treatment and communication. Enjoy the reading and we will continue to meet along the journey.

Professor Jaime A. Gil
President International Federation of Esthetic Dentistry (IFED)

# Preface

The appetite for new restorative paths continues apace. At the same time, the digital evolution of the dental industry continues to thrive, with unprecedented possibilities for a more precise and predictable outcome.

This may well be a pivotal moment for the practice of dentistry with the advent of full digital workflows and the intermediate traditional-digital hybrid to suit all practitioners.

Whether the dental practitioner is a digital flow purist or a believer in traditional chairside dentistry, the patient always remains analog, reminding us that the mouth truly is a live test bench with the patient headlined for comfort, well-being, and a pleasing result.

As in any other field, flexible and prepared human power leads to productivity and efficiency improvement.

Sticking strictly to only one flow, be it CAD/CAM or manual, may be holding the overall process back from time-saving and precise outcomes both in the diagnostic and restorative phases.

The approach of treating only to repair diseased tissue associated with lesions may prove a limited perspective, while the trend to treat in a primarily esthetically driven way may leave the patient unprotected as a concomitant shift in lifestyle can be devastating in already demineralized tissue.

Perhaps one can be tempted by a self-content attitude, delivering restorations in the same manner as with any other dental condition. But in doing this there is not much space to ask oneself why. Why has this happened? Why has the patient lost the protection of saliva? Why are the lesions different in every patient, and even within the same mouth? Why is there no pain? Why is there no space? Why is the patient oblivious of so much tooth structure loss? Why are we more prepared to choose our preferred treatment option? Why are we doing that? Why is it necessary? Why should the patient with TW have the same regular checkups as other patients?

In asking yourself why, you will serve the patient better, as many procedures that initially would have been deemed necessary will probably be left out after questioning whether the principles of maximum tooth preservation are still present, making the overall treatment more accessible and acceptable for the patient. Nonetheless there should be general rules or protocols as in any other field of medicine, as any decision will have an impact not only on the treatment outcome but on the overall tooth survival.

Artificial intelligence and facial and surface recognition will most probably deliver treatment tools unimaginable today.

The recognition that preventing TW and intercepting further TSL may be less hazardous than imitating nature has made a quantum leap in recent years. All disciplines of modern dentistry and medicine, when focused on early detection and minor intervention, may demonstrate a shortcut to flatten the TW curve.

When reading this book, the authors hope you have a feeling of a déjà vu, as this is intended to be a reader-friendly compilation of observation, study, and clinical work that surely you too have experienced. If so, we hope it inspires clinicians who wish to treat TW patients.

Embark, and enjoy your journey¡

## Dedicated to

Our families with love.

My son, José Manuel, whom I admire.
My daughter, Débora, who fills my life with joy.
With gratitude to both of them for following in my professional steps.
Laura, who has enriched our family.
Manuel, a source of joy and strength.
My husband, José, who always believed in me.

Diego, the sunshine of my life.
My husband, Jesus, for thinking I am the one.

Our brother George, the leader of our family; Marta, the love of his life; Clara, the new orthodontist in our family; Bea; and Paula.

In loving memory of Manuel and Pilar, our parents whose love inspired us all.
Débora and Beatriz R. Vilaboa

Manu, you are my world. My mother Débora and my aunt Beatriz, my role models.
My father, the most positive person I have ever met. My brother, the best working partner I could ever have.

The women in my family, Patricia, Marta and Eva for their generous and incondiotional support. To Manuel and Jose for your love to Manu and me.
Clara, Beatriz, Paula and Diego we have grown together with an unbreakable bond.
S. Ochandiano, D. Martin, M. Pulido, B. Mateo, E. McLaren, R. Romano, De Rossa and D. de Franco, my true inspiration.
Débora Reuss

Laura, my love, my everything.
My mother and father, sister, and aunt, for their endless love and support.
My mentors, Drs Martínez Corriá, Gil, and Moy. Your input in my professional life is priceless.
José M. Reuss

## Thank you

This is a dedication to those who have accompanied us throughout our professional and personal lives. Thank you to our patients for blessing us with their confidence.

Thank you to our team for believing in our project. Thank you to Drs Mercedes Pulido, Borja Mateo, Amparo Llorente, and Maria Araujo; we have sailed many seas. Thank you to Dr Marta Lago; your father would be proud of you. Thank you to Drs Veronica Rubio, Laura Peix, Cristina Fernandez, Jaime Fernandez, and Beatriz de Lujan for enriching our restorative mission. Thank you, Julia, Veronica, Adina, Juana, Sandra and Marisa. We need you so much. Thank you, Angel, Karmel, and Andrea, you landed in the middle of the storm. Thank you, Carmen Fernandez and Jess Ride-Out, continuing our writing during the weekends was easier with your help. Thank you Silvia Muriel, you have been an asset.

Thank you to Laura Cifuentes; we knew from the beginning we were in good hands. Thank you, Rocio Perez Durias, you inspire us. Thank you, Paloma, for taking the torch. Thank you Marc Romea for the support and input.

Thank you to Elena Perez, you said you would do it, and you did it. Thank you for being with us. By the way, yes, you are kidnapped and the ransom payment will be high.

Thank you to Carlos Barja, Gonzalo Medina, Santiago Dalmau, and your team. Thank you to Stefano and Fernando Tonarelli; God bless our lecture in Warsaw. Thank you to the Rutten brothers. Thank you to Javier Rubio and to Arturo Calvo.

Thank you to our family from the European Academy of Esthetic Dentistry for your friendship and support.

Thank you to Jaime Gil for your lifelong mentorship. Thank you to our colleagues from BQDC. You are the best.

Thank you to Alberto Alvarez for your reflections. Thank you to Gonzalo Rada for your drawings. Thank you to Ines Castellanos for your lifestyle photography.

Thank you to the Haase family. You are not just our editors; you are much more than that.

Débora and Beatriz R. Vilaboa,
Jose Manuel and Débora Reuss

## Authors

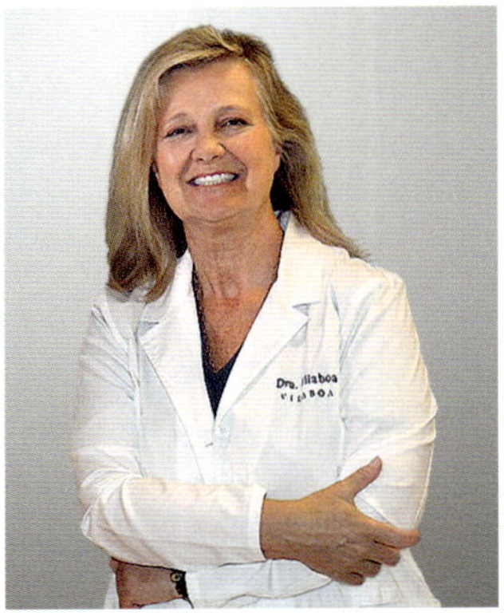

### DEBORA R. VILABOA

Dr Debora R. Vilaboa graduated from the Complutense University Faculty of Medicine and Surgery in Madrid. The same year, she was accepted at the Seville School of Dentistry, where she obtained her dental degree. Later on she chose to attend the Advanced Pediactric Dentistry Program at the University of Southern California in Los Angeles.

After establishing the Vilaboa Clinic in 1987, she found that some cases could not be explained by caries nor periodontal disease and began gathering data. She lectured on tooth wear as early as 1992, both in Spain and the United States. Understanding how to approach the treatment of young children helped Dr Deborah Vilaboa in her work with tooth wear patients, many of whom had a fear of dentistry. As a pioneer in the field of porcelain laminate veneers, she treated such cases with a novel adhesive concept.

Dr Debora Vilaboa soon became a member of the Spanish Society of Stomatological Prosthetics (SEPES) and the Spanish Society of Periodontology (SEPA). Her passion for treating patients and continuing education was rewarded in becoming an active member of the European Academy of Esthetic Dentistry (EAED). She was then able to pursue her restorative and prosthodontic interests, thanks to a truly collaborative and generous exchange of knowledge among the active members that is still a driving force for the team at Vilaboa Clinic. She is also an active member of the Italian Academy of Esthetic Dentistry (IAED).

Dr Debora Vilaboa was invited by the San Pablo CEU University to create an undergraduate Esthetic Dentistry Department that she co-directs with her sister, Dr Beatriz Vilaboa. She lectures worldwide in esthetic dentistry, with a focus on tooth wear. She was a contributor to Esthetics in Dentistry (Quintessence, 2016). Given her medical background, Dr Deboarh Vilaboa is devoted to understanding and treating conditions arising from medical and oral imbalances, and through her research, she has obtained several patents related to her work. She is an active member of the American Academy of Oral Medicine (AAOM), a fellow member of the International College of Dentists (ICD), and an academic at the Pierre Fauchard Academy.

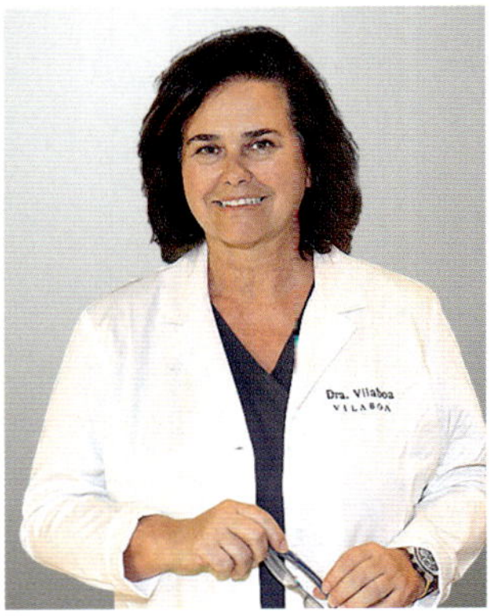

### BEATRIZ R. VILABOA

Dr Beatriz R. Vilaboa received her degree in medicine and surgery with honours from the Complutense University of Madrid from which she also attained her specialty in stomatology. She joined Clinica Vilaboa in Madrid soon after her sister Dr Debora R. Vilboa founded it in 1987. She enjoys her private practice at the Vilaboa Clinic, dedicated to esthetic and restorative dentistry.Her devotion to treating patients using the most conservative approach possible motivated her to embrace the adhesive-additive concept to provide solutions to the tooth wear patient. Her interest in tooth wear culminated with a PhD from San Pablo CEU University Faculty of Medicine in Madrid, where she is now Co-Director of the undergraduate Esthetic Dentistry department. Dr Beatriz Vilboa's passion for teaching is also evident in the many courses that she and her sister have given over the last 30 years.

Dr. Beatriz Vilaboa has the honour of being an active member of the European Academy of Esthetic Dentistry (EAED) and the Italian Academy of Esthetic Dentistry (IAED). She is also founding member of the International Academy of Adhesion (IAA). Her desire to better help patients suffering from cancer and other major medical conditions pushed her to become a member of the American Academy of Oral Medicine (AAOM). She is also a member of the Spanish Society of Stomatological Prosthetics (SEPES) and Spanish Society of Periodontology (SEPA), as well as a fellow member of the International College of Dentists (ICD) and an academic from the Pierre Fauchard Academy. She lectures worldwide on esthetic and restorative dentistry and especially on tooth wear.

Dr Beatriz Vilaboa treasures friendship with colleagues worldwide and believes that the common passion for dentistry goes beyond borders.

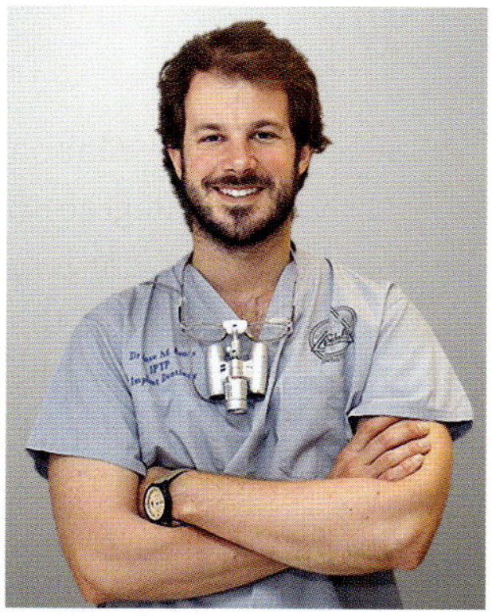

## JOSE MANUEL REUSS

Dr Jose Manuel Reuss graduated in dentistry from the University Complutense of Madrid, where he also obtained a Master's Degree of Science. As a postgraduate in surgical implant dentistry at the University of California at Los Angeles, he was a recipient of a grant from the American Academy of Implant Dentistry for preclinical and clinical research. During his postgraduate research, he focused on bone regeneration with growth factor technologies.

Dr Jose Manual Reuss's clinical background both in implant surgery and prosthodontics has led him to develop a facially guided restoration concept. In particular, severe tooth wear or highly dysfunctional cases can benefit from the combination of digital protocols and a more traditional classical workflow. His current clinical and research foci relie on the integration of facial scanners into guided surgery systems, restorative protocols, and clinician-technician communication.

As an affiliate member of the European Academy of Esthetics Dentistry, he is an enthusiast of multidisciplinary thinking and is therefore also a member of the Spanish Society of Prosthodontics (SEPES), the Spanish Society of Periodontics (SEPA), the Academy of Osseointegration (AO), and the European Academy of Osseointegration (EAO).

Dr Jose Manuel Reuss is a Collaborating Professor in the Postgraduate Prosthodontics Department in the field of implant and restorative dentistry at the University Complutense of Madrid, the University of Leon, and at the Esthetic Dentistry Department at the University San Pablo CEU of Madrid. His current focus of research is digital implant dentistry and severe tooth wear with the aim to optimize diagnostic and treatment phases and engage the working team in research. His goal to simplify the communication between the team members of an integrated multifaceted treatment plan challenges Dr Reuss almost as much as his passion for sports in his personal life.

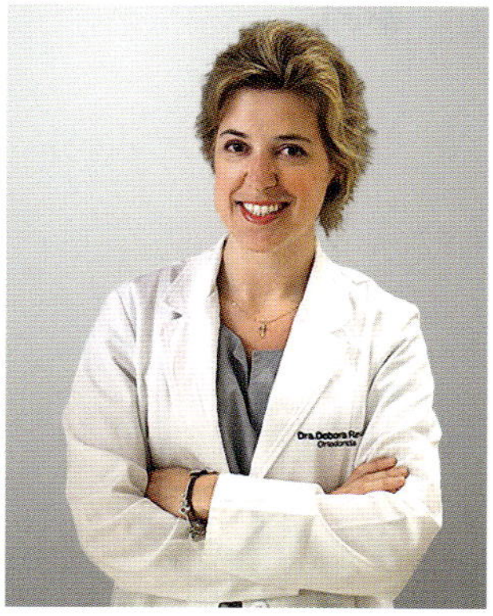

## DEBORA REUSS

Dr Debora Reuss obtained her Master's Degree in Orthodontics at the European University of Madrid, 4 years after graduating as a dentist from San Pablo CEU University of Madrid. Having completed several postgraduate specialty courses (including Damon self-ligating and Invisalign systems), she joined the Spanish Orthodontics Society (SEDO) and the Spanish Society of Aligners (SEDA). As a Member of the American Association of Orthodontics (AAO), she is a firm believer in facial- and profile-guided orthodontics.

Dr Reuss trained in occlusion at the Pankey Institute of Miami and believes that a classical concept of occlusion must be a driving force in treating orthodontic patients.

Her passion for treating patients within a multidisciplinary approach has inspired her to attend continuing education courses on occlusion, restorative, and prosthodontic topics and is the reason behind her affiliation with the Spanish Society of Stomatological Prosthetics (SEPES) as well as the reason why she became affiliate member of the European Academy of Esthetic Dentistry (EAED) and the Italian Academy of Esthetic Dentistry (IAED). Dr Reuss teaches at the Esthetic Dentistry Department at San Pablo CEU University of Madrid.

Multidisciplinary thinking led her to join the Vilaboa Team in Madrid to help treat tooth wear patients with a minimally invasive philosophy to prevent further wear and to ensure conservative performance of the required restorations. An education in three-dimensional thinking as an orthodontist is key in leading the tooth wear team to a facially guided restoration as an architect of the oral complex.

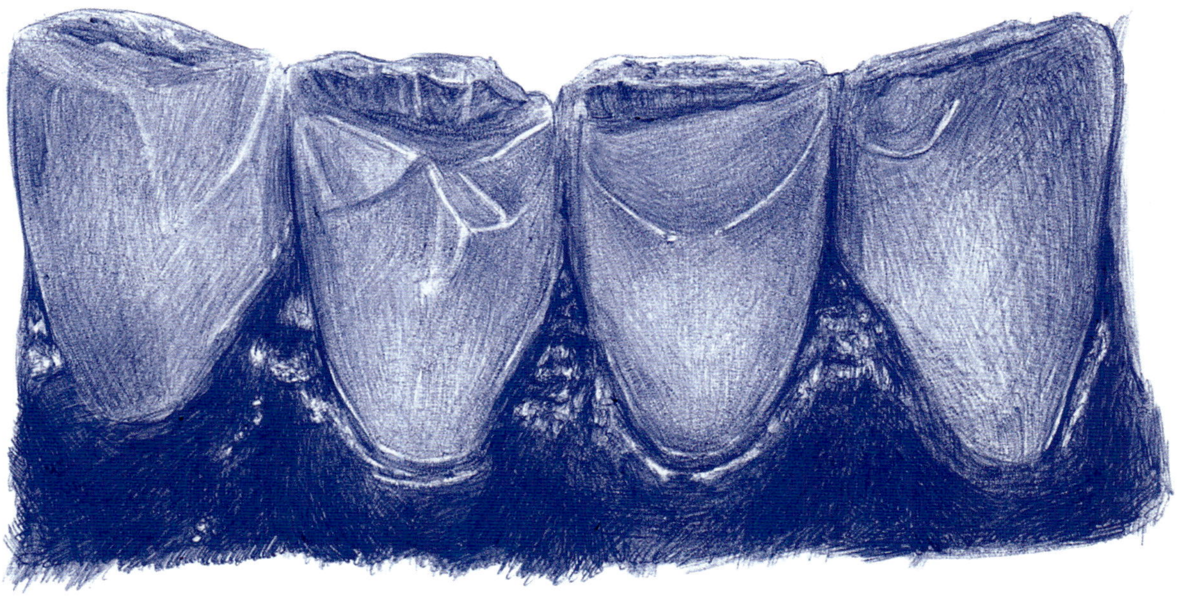

*Teeth talk; you just need to watch.*

# SECTION I UNDERSTANDING TOOTH WEAR

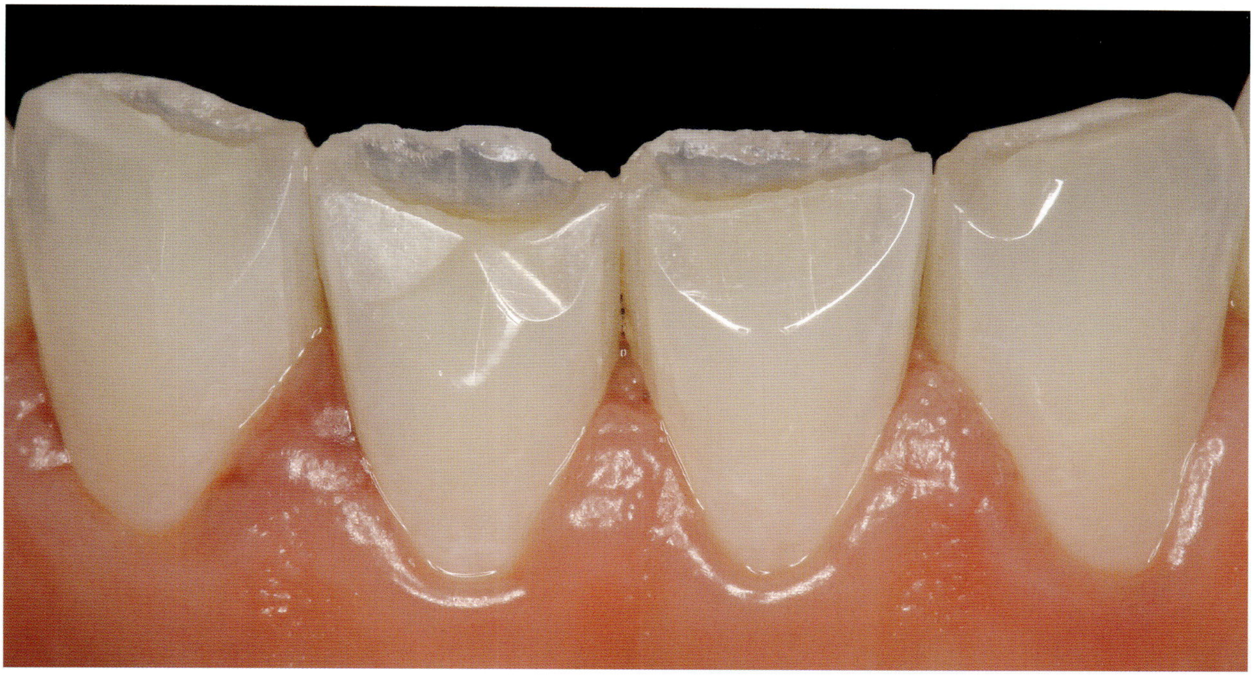

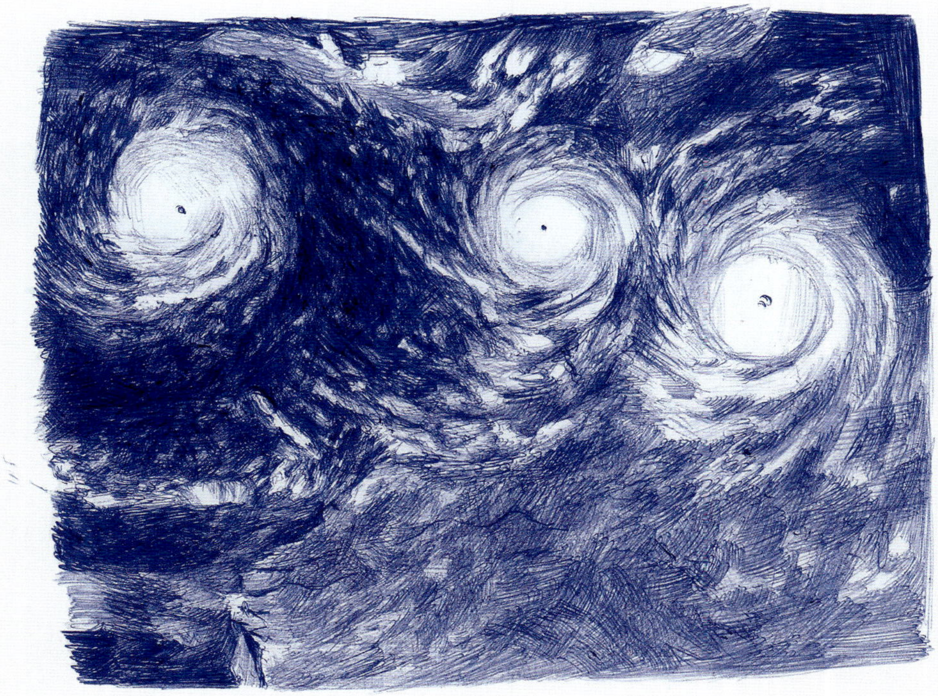

*The Perfect Storm: A critical or disastrous situation created by a powerful concurrence of factors.*

—definition from the Merriam-Webster dictionary

CHAPTER 1

# TOOTH WEAR: A MAJOR HEALTH ISSUE

Tooth wear (TW) understood as non-carious surface loss is damage to teeth—independent of trauma or bacteria and not explainable by the patient's age—that can compromise tooth survival.

TW may well be one of the biggest challenges posed to both the dental professional and the patient today.

Progressive, irreversible, multifactorial, and insidious in nature, it ideally requires a comprehensive approach and a trained team with the ability to recognize TW at its earliest onset and establish preventive measures and a patient-centered treatment path.

Conversely, a wait-and-see attitude is not desirable as wear progression may prove devastating even in young dentitions over a short period of time. The course and cycle of TW is closely interrelated with general health conditions and lifestyle, with a documented negative impact in four dimensions: physically, functionally, psychologically, and socially.

Yet there is a fifth dimension when facing the challenge of TW connected to feelings, well-being, self-esteem, and self-image.

Understanding TW, finding better treatments for our patients, and contributing to a flattening of the TW curve is a team task.

## 1. The Global Burden of Tooth Wear

Over the last decades, TW has trespassed beyond the boundaries of anthropology, gradually invading the pages of peer-reviewed journals, congresses and webinars of the restorative and prosthodontics fields of dentistry.

Traditionally, the wearing of the dentition has been considered a consequence of aging. Even though TW can occur at any stage of life, it is in adulthood and beyond where TW is most prevalent. The world is seeing an unprecedented growth in its aging population throughout all countries and regions, an effect of globalization. It is only a matter of time before this growing group of patients with worn dentitions will include everyone of us, if it has not already. While longevity is a success story, not preparing protocols and services according to growing needs will negatively impact our practices in the long run and may exclude wide sectors of our society from the benefits of the aftermath of development and well-being.

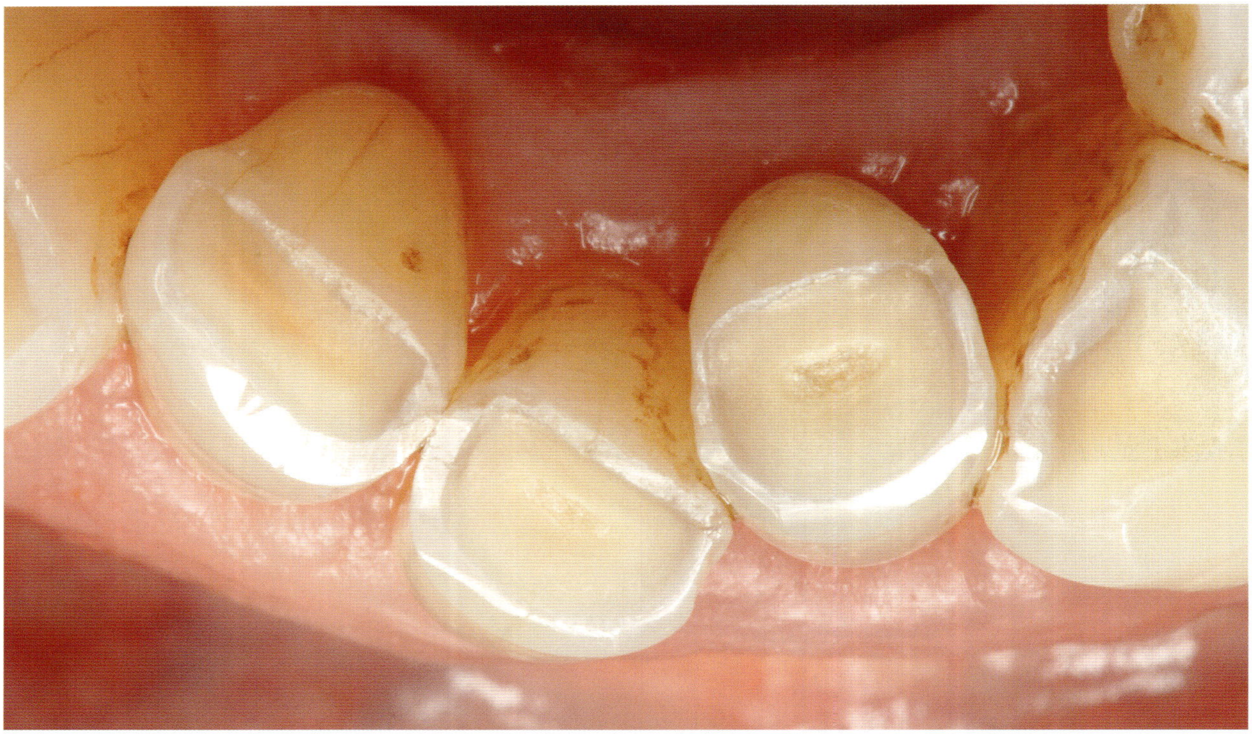

**Fig 1-1** This image shows that worn enamel caused by grinding or tooth clenching can facilitate further tooth loss with the onset of acidic attack. This 62-year-old male patient was diagnosed with GERD at the age of 60. The acidic attack onset will meet with an already worn, flattened tooth that lacks enamel protection and is therefore more susceptible to erosion.

Life expectancy has also been stated to be responsible for the deterioration of the dentition, as well as other aspects of the oral cavity such as salivary function. Other parameters like general health and lifestyle of the individual are key to oral health and a well-maintained tooth structure. Today oral health is regarded as an integral part of general health, especially after multiple studies have linked oral health to major health conditions (Fig 1-1).

TW is undoubtedly a challenge for the dental profession in the current decade.

Commonly undiagnosed and unfortunately underestimated during the initial stages, TW, when left untreated, leads to anatomical loss of valuable tooth structure, increased permeability of pathogens, functional impairment, psychologic impact, social disability, and esthetic changes. Pain, high risk of tooth fracture, and eventually premature tooth loss will follow long-term untreated severe TW.

TW is also responsible for facial and dentoalveolar compensation that is unfortunately unable to overcome the bone consequences of premature tooth loss.

TW is common in patients throughout the world, in some cases associated with habits like acidic diets. Strikingly, young adults and even children may experience TW to a noticeable amount by the time they are diagnosed. It is often asymptomatic for many years until an issue such as a fracture, restoration failure, or abscess brings the patient to the office (Fig 1-2).

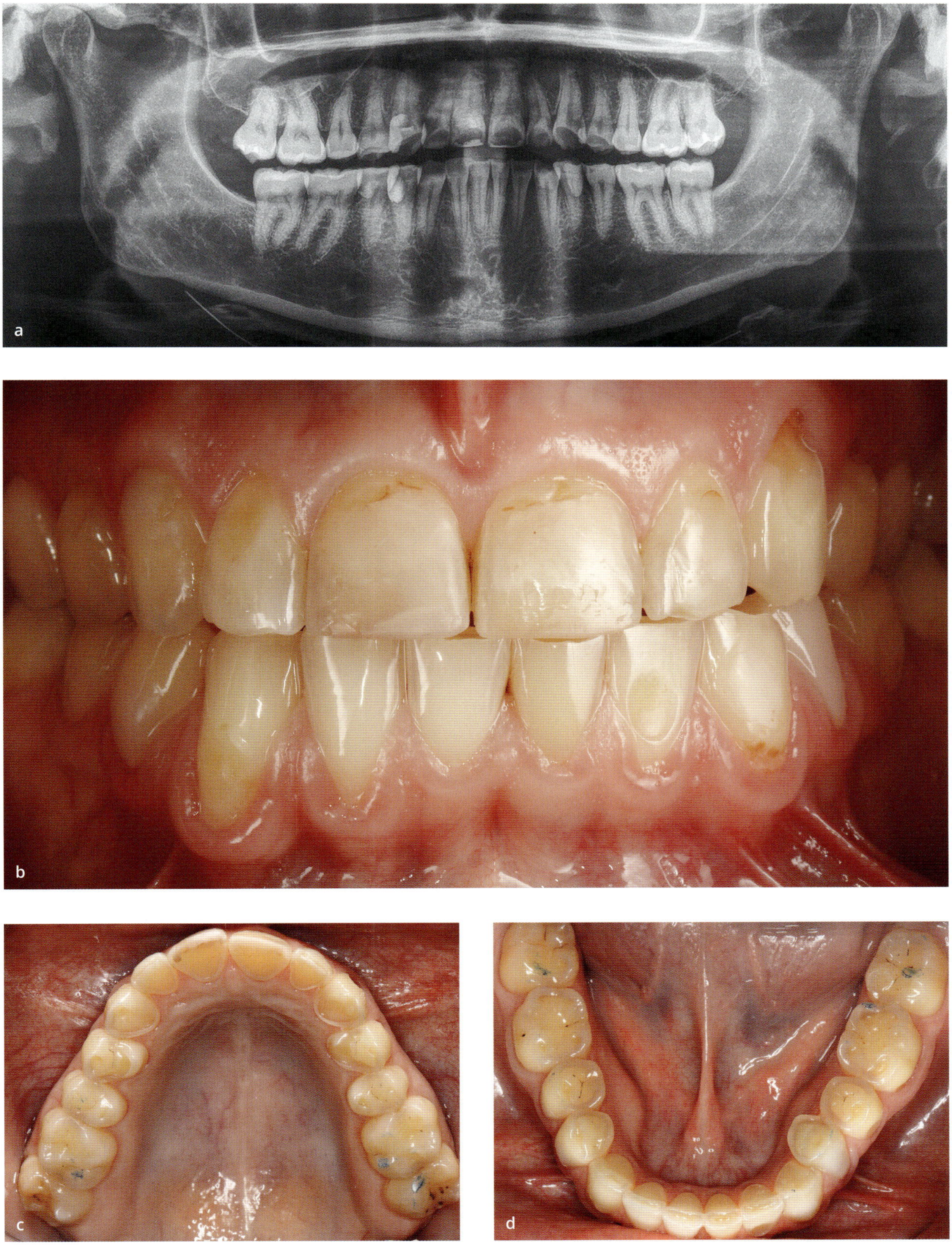

**Fig 1-2** The radiographic exam of this young adult revealed both low incidence of caries and periodontal compromise (a). Single tooth–oriented treatments have not been able to prevent TW from progressing. Hard tissue loss is seen in the form of disappearance of occlusal and facial anatomy and topography of cusps and occlusal fossae. Note the remaining composite restorations resisting erosive attack. Photos were taken before any hygiene and prophylaxis was performed, and the low presence of biofilm is noticeable (b to d). (See more on this case in chapter 7.)

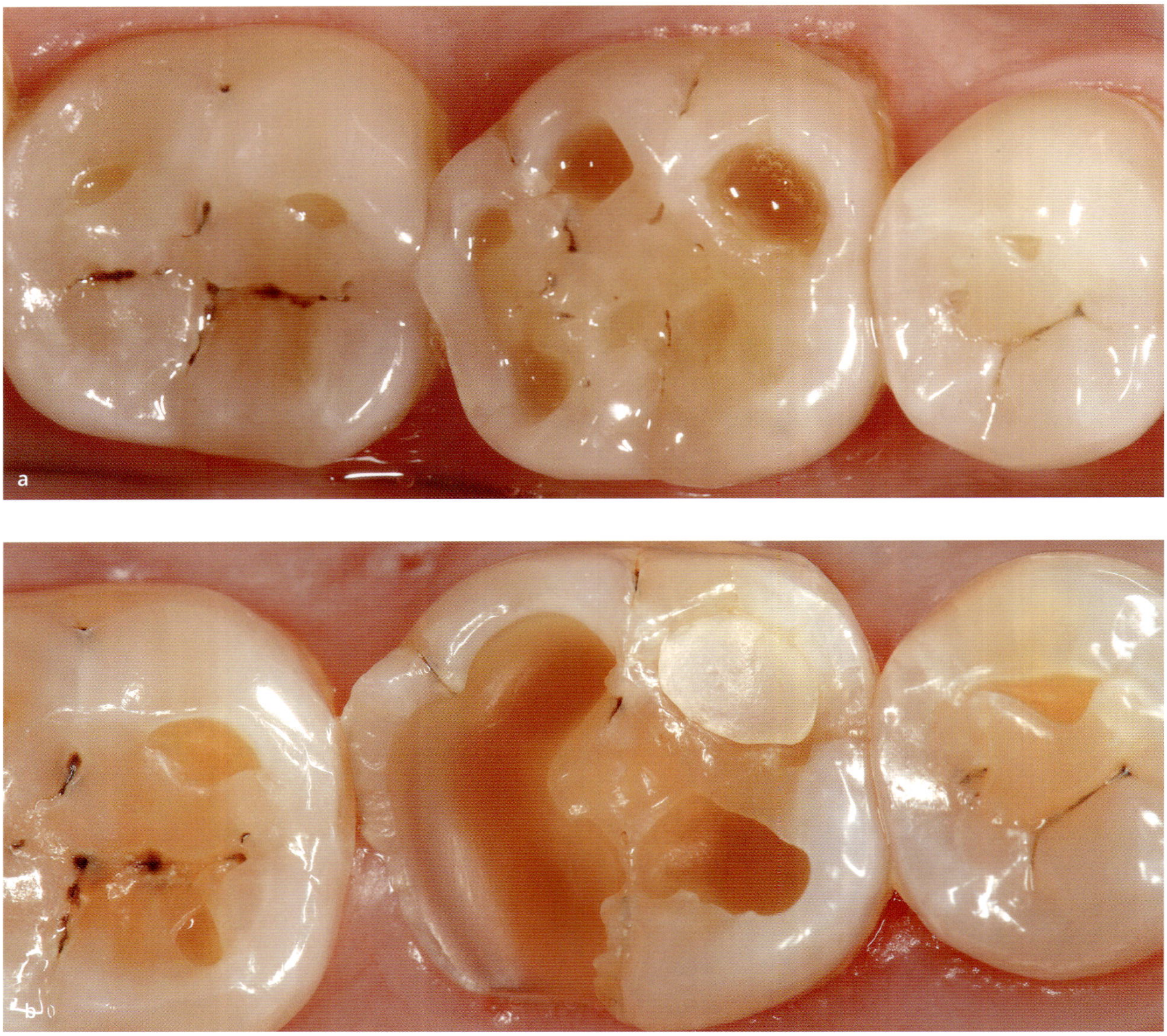

**Fig 1-3** A 55-year-old male patient with exposed dentin as a result of prolonged exposure to an acidic environment. Patient was free of symptoms despite the obvious erosive lesions (a). Progression of tooth structure loss of untreated lesions over an 8-year time period (b).

The wait-and-see approach can have unprecedented consequences as TW is multifactorial, cyclic, and progressive. Even in the absence of the original etiologic factor, it can lead to further tooth loss in the original site of TW or distant sites of the mouth (Fig 1-3).

In the 2020s, TW is defined by irreversible tooth surface loss (TSL) affecting either enamel or enamel and dentin by factors different to the ones responsible for caries or trauma.[1] This loss of tooth structure comprises damage to the macro and micro aspects of teeth. The different clinical presentations include attrition, abrasion, abfraction, and erosion, or a combination of all of these.

The increasing number of papers on TW and erosion serve as evidence of the exponential growth of awareness of dental practitioners and researchers regarding this topic. This comes as no surprise since both the occurrence and severity of TW has been growing rapidly over recent decades.

Furthermore, escalating occurrence in the young population today predicts an avalanche of worn dentitions, dramatically changing the scenario to one in which dentists will have to perform and deliver restorations susceptible to more failure[2] (Fig 1-4).

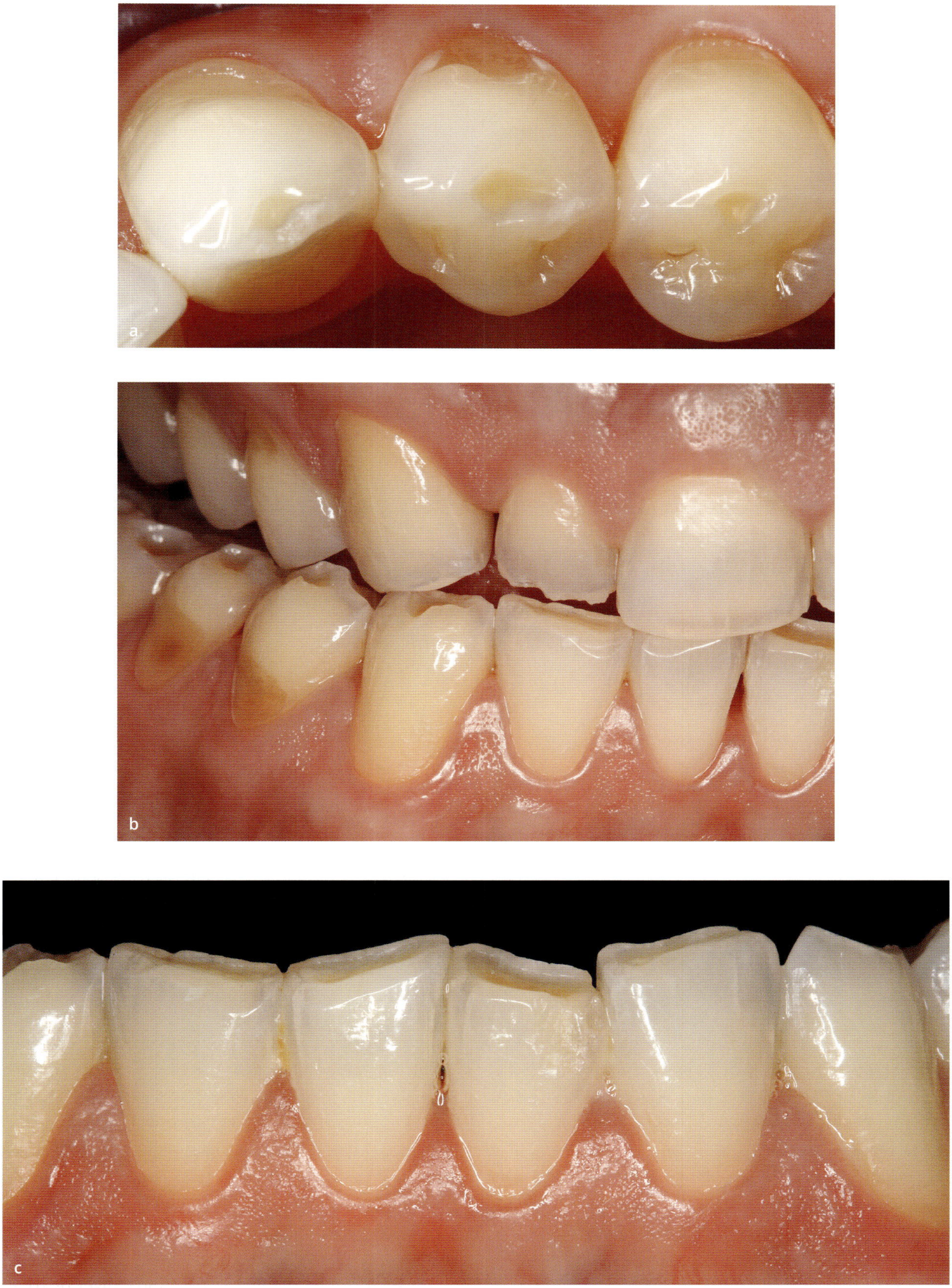

**Fig 1-4** Multifactorial TW in a 38-year-old male patient. Note distinctive vestibular defects in relation to a combination of abrasion, erosion, and abfraction, together with generalized manifest erosive damage (a). Capricious occlusal anatomy evocative of an erosive skyline landscape (b). Roller coaster incisal profile (c).

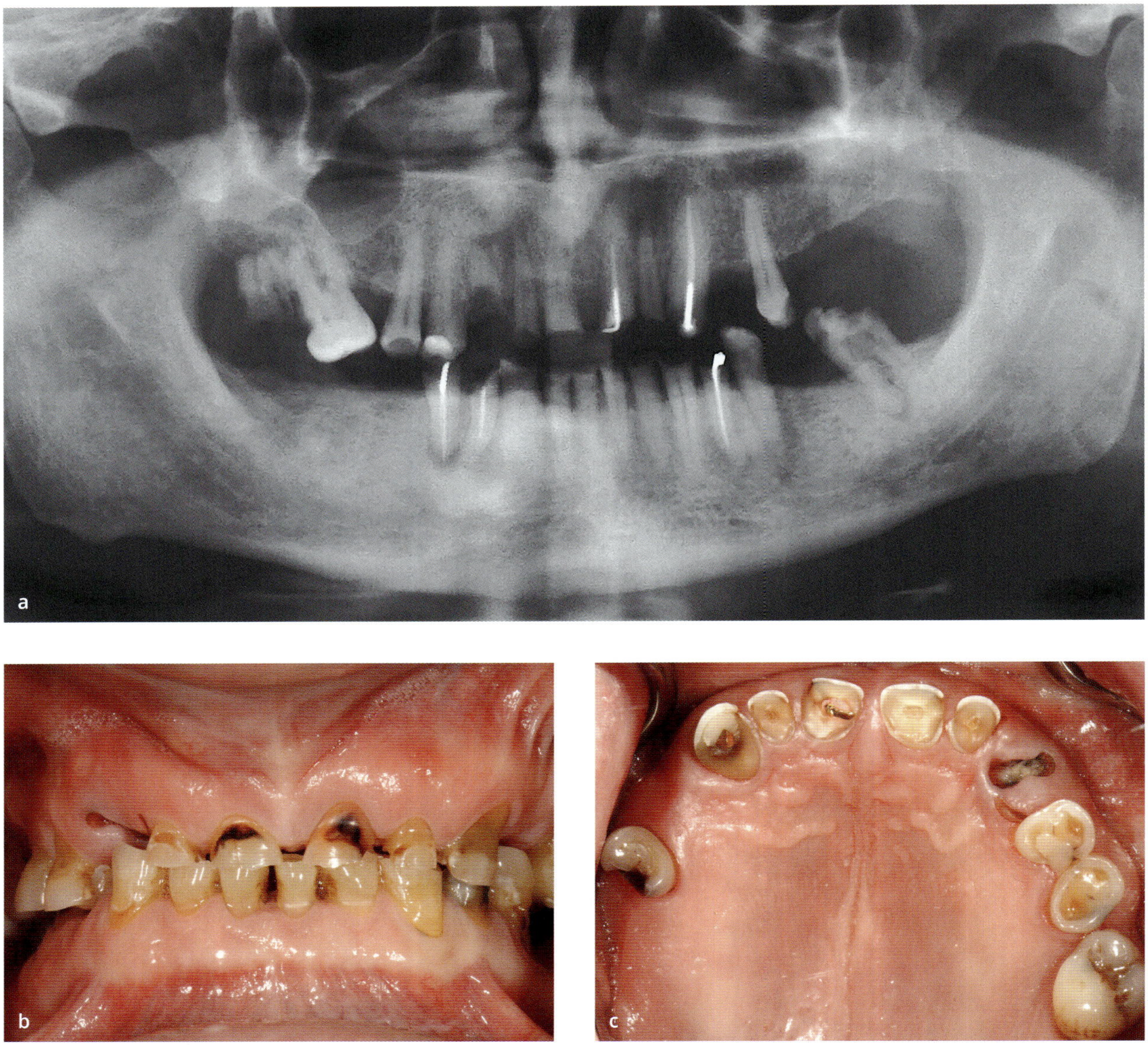

**Fig 1-5** Note in the panoramic radiograph periapical lesions in relation with extreme TW (a). A 68-year-old male patient with multifactorial TW lesions such as attrition, abrasion, abfraction, and erosion (b). Most of the enamel and dentin is gone, exposing pulp chambers and root canal filling materials with severe TW and premature tooth loss (c).

Moreover, the geriatric challenge for dental medicine associated with a still-lengthening life expectancy comes from the fact that preventive strategies in the adult, plus better hygiene and nutrition, as well as preventive and treatment strategies of comorbidities of dental diseases (eg, caries and diabetes, periodontitis and cardiovascular conditions), have provided the opportunity for more people to keep their teeth even in the later decades of their life.

Some authors have anticipated that edentulism will be present in only 2.6% of people by 2050, mostly in the oldest and poorest demographic groups[3] (Fig 1-5).

On the other hand, the emerging number of people diagnosed and treated for cancer, and very recently those with secondary effects of the COVID-19 virus, pose a challenge as erosion will be present in dentitions even in the absence of high acidic affluence. Polypharmacy, chemotherapy, and noncommunicable general health conditions will course with salivary gland dysfunction, be it hyposalivation or alteration of the composition of saliva, a hidden cause and potentiator of TW, as will be discussed in chapter 2.

Dental professionals will have to do a quantum leap in their understanding of TW and have a cascade of

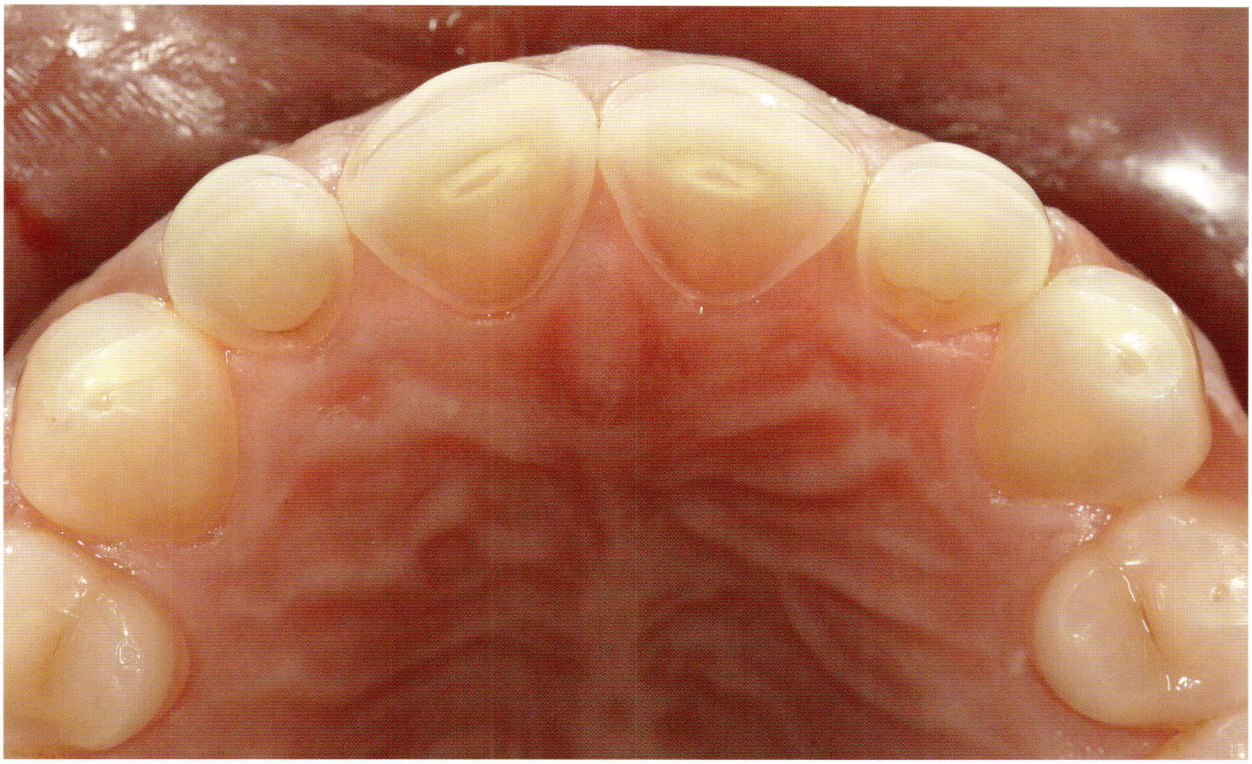

**Fig 1-6** Erosive wear in a 27-year-old woman with noticeable absence of bacterial plaque and distinctive perimolysis pattern with exposed dentin and intact enamel at the gingival margin. Generalized loss of palatal anatomy leads to breakage of incisal edges and crown shortening. (See more on this case in chapter 7.)

possible treatment strategies to be able to care for their patients in this prospective future (Fig 1-6).

While caries and periodontal diseases are plaque-related conditions, TW is independent of the level of plaque accumulation. In fact, caries and erosion cannot happen simultaneously on the same tooth surface at the same time.[4]

While innate defense mechanisms against caries are multiple and effective in healthy patients to contain progression of or even revert the lesion, erosion and attrition—and the combination of both—are progressive and do not encounter a remineralizing parallelism.

Plaque-removing strategies and fluoride together with hygiene measures can change the course of carious disease. Unfortunately, such preventive measures do not stop TW.[5]

Caries is a classic condition that is easily recognized and managed by dentists and their teams when compared to TW. The decline in caries incidence and rate of progression in some countries has shifted caries intervention toward a less invasive approach.

However, the type of restorative approach is far more dependent on the professional ability and background of the dentist than on the disease of the patient. In fact, both the treatment strategies and the diagnosis vary widely between dentists who do not make an individual diagnosis and evaluation but rather respond automatically towards caries.[6]

Many factors have been accounted for in the variability of treatment decisions between dentists when confronting caries. These include dentist education, oral hygiene status, financial considerations, workload, number of years in practice, school attended, and the dentist's feeling on the speed of progression of the lesion, all of them leading to false-positive and false-negative interventions.[7]

The decisions on why, how, and when to intervene on a tooth are going to affect its life cycle and survival as well as the oral status of the patient.

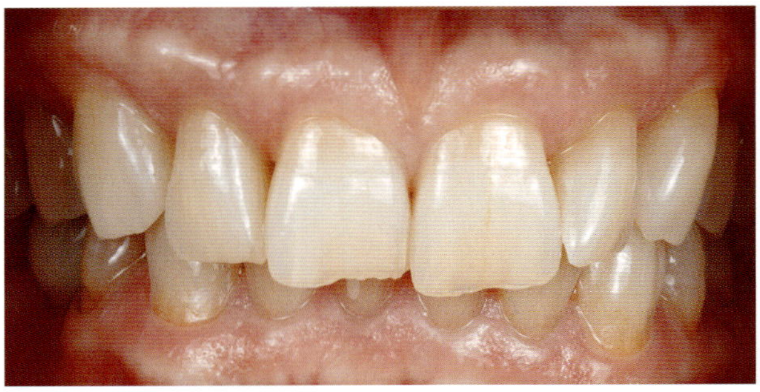

**Fig 1-7** Note incisal edge wear in a 62-year-old man associated with a long-standing malocclusion in an otherwise healthy and functioning mouth. (See more on this case in chapter 8.)

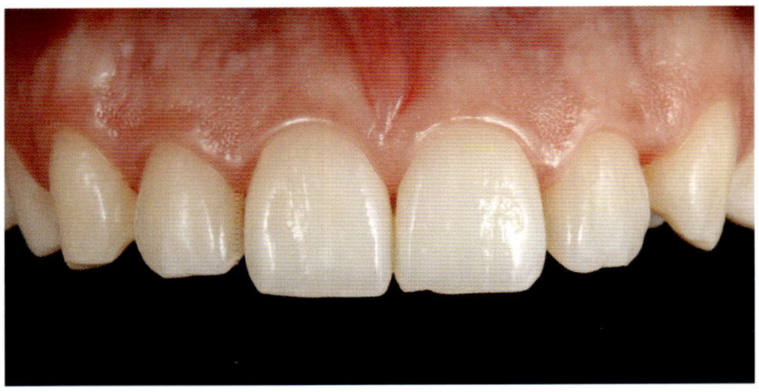

**Fig 1-8** Teenager with incipient TW affecting incisor edges and canine cusps due to a parafunctional habit (lip biting). (See more on this case in chapter 5.)

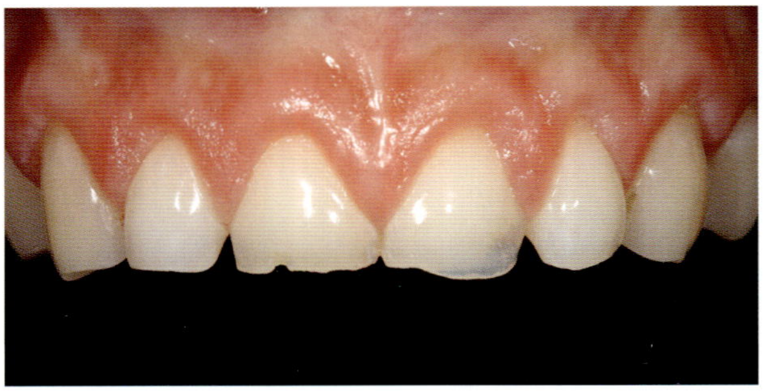

**Fig 1-9** Erosive damage in a young female patient. Incisal wear due to palatal erosion. Note translucency due to palatal structure loss. (See more on this case in chapter 7.)

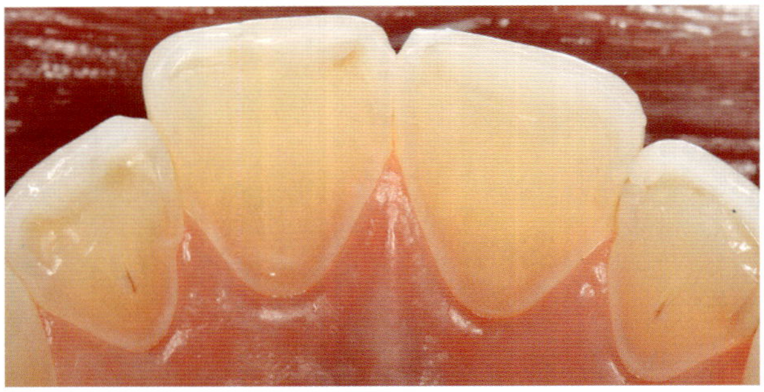

**Fig 1-10** Acid erosion dissolution of tooth structure in a young woman. Note the characteristic remaining enamel halo at the gingival margin.

## 2. Physiologic Versus Pathologic Wear

Experts agree upon the fact that a certain degree of TW is physiologic with the passing of the time. However, excessive or premature wear cannot be related to age. In other words, premature TW that occurs in the younger patient cannot be attributed to the patient's age.

Notwithstanding the above, the acceptance of a normal amount of TW should be taken into consideration relative to the patient's age. For example, incisal edge wear in the absence of other findings like insufficient guidance protection in a 62-year-old patient is reasonably compatible with good oral health and may only need consideration from an esthetic point of view (Fig 1-7).

Conversely, in a teenager, incisal or canine cusp wear should raise concerns as parafunctional habits may lead to exponential damage in future years. The insidious character of TW causes a subtle change in the anatomy that goes unnoticed to the untrained eye (Fig 1-8).

Despite the existing debate around the definitions and terminology in the universe of TW, there seems to be agreement that while attrition or abrasion to a certain extent can be physiologic, erosive damage should always be considered to be pathologic (Figs 1-9 and 1-10).

## 3. Anthropologic and Contemporary Tooth Wear

The story of human evolution, where we come from and who we are, has been explained through morphologic study and more recently with the aid of the genome of fragmented human fossils. The anthropologic study of the human dentition, more than any other part of the body, has contributed to our knowledge about our primitive ancestors.

Attrition and abrasion have existed since the beginning of humanity. Teeth were utilized as tools to soften, blend, and tear raw materials like animal skins, branches, and hunting devices.

Interestingly, in specimens from our ancestors dating back to the early medieval ages, erosion seems almost nonexistent (Figs 1-11 and 1-12). Similarly, anthropologists are not familiar with the emerging phenomenon of erosion, as no signs of erosion are seen in prehistorical fossils.

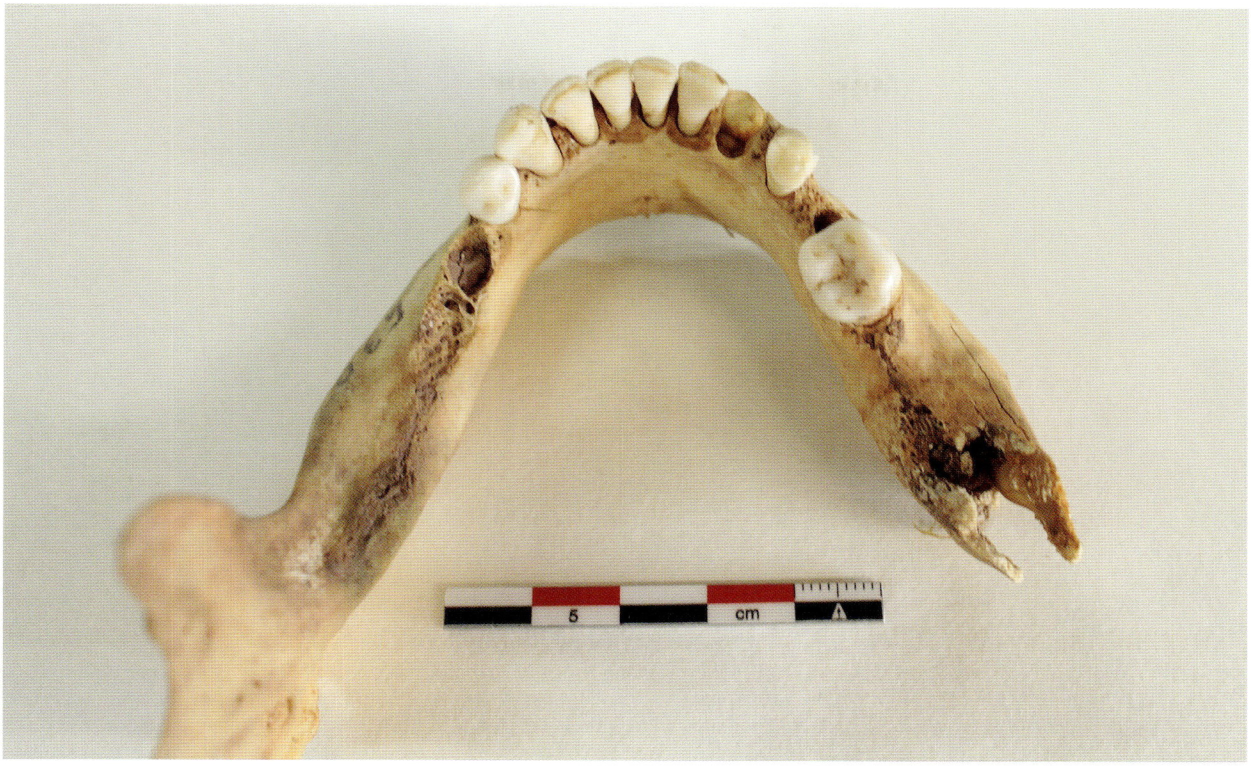

**Fig 1-11** Attrition and abrasion signs in this specimen from the Middle Ages before the advent of the modern "erosive era." (Courtesy of the Anthropological Collection of the Museum of the School of Legal Medicine at Complutense University of Madrid.)

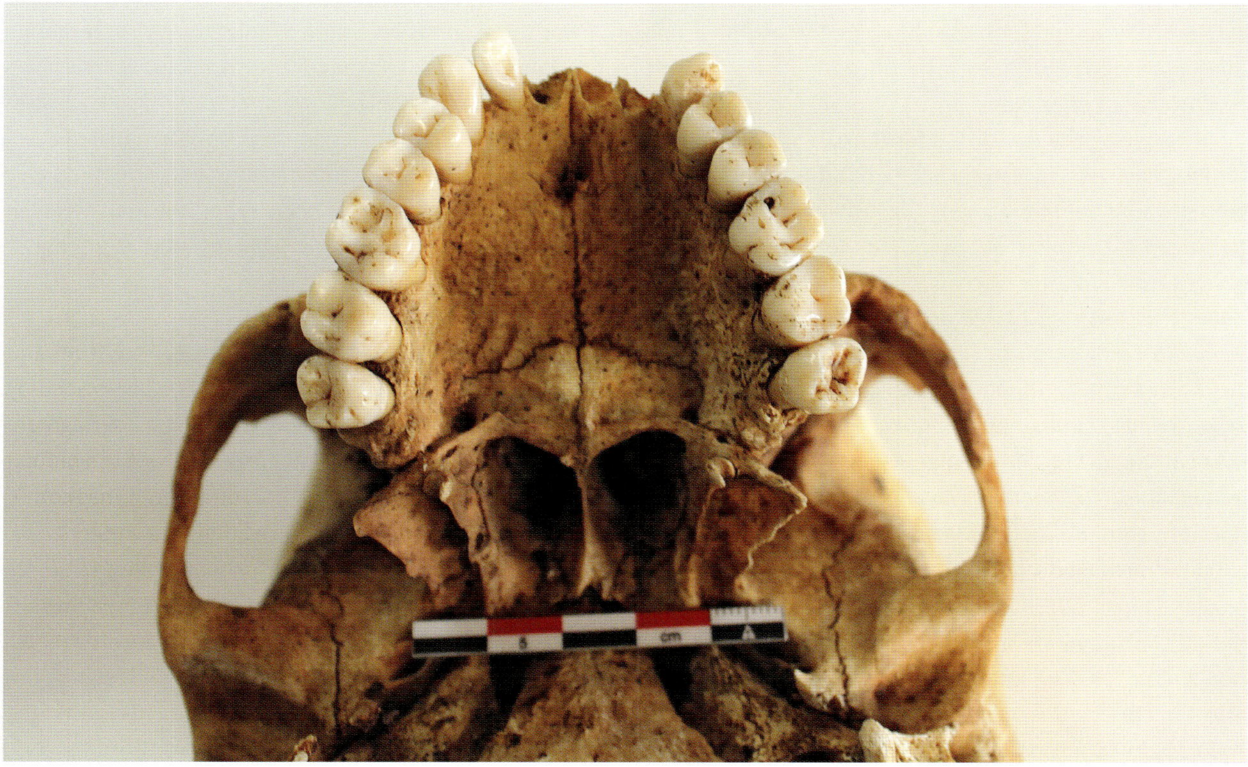

**Fig 1-12** Note the caries- and erosion-free dentition despite the primitive oral hygiene regimen in the Middle Ages. The absence of fast food or cariogenic drinks and the presence of a local, non-industrialized diet explain the lack of caries and erosion signs. Harsh and coarse food ingredients such as in hunted meat and/or raw vegetables and grasses support the attrition signs. (Courtesy of the Anthropological Collection of the Museum of the School of Legal Medicine at the Complutense University of Madrid.)

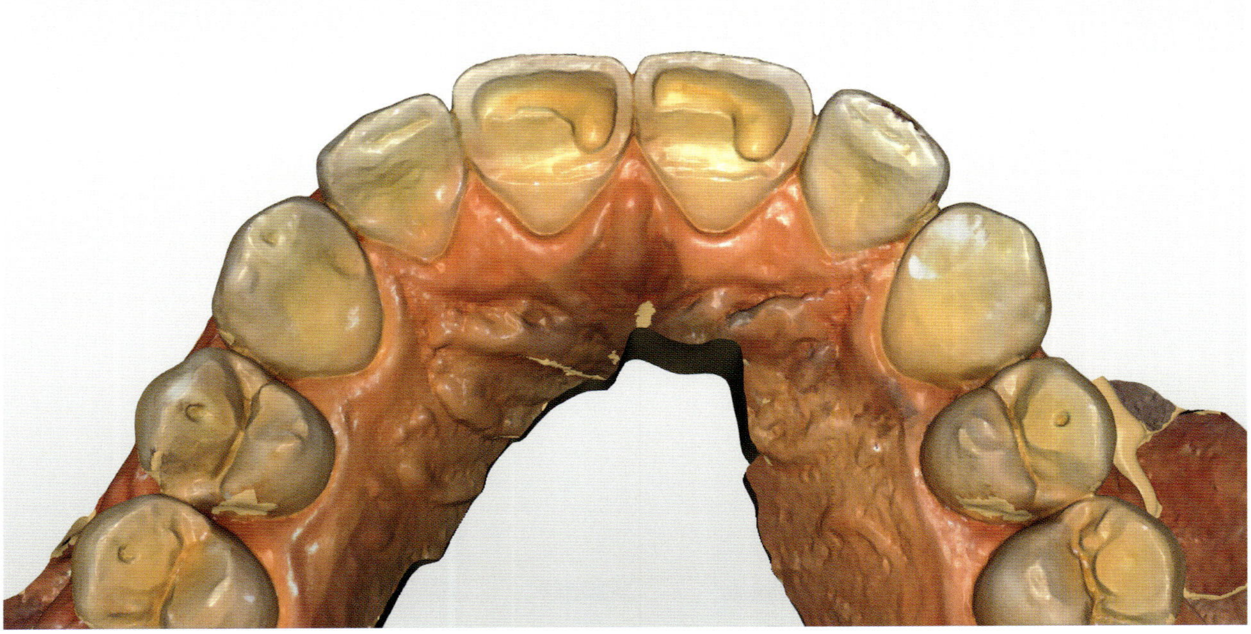

**Fig 1-13** The accuracy that photography and new technologies provide today, together with the increasing understanding of TW, enables a better differentiation of the mechanisms behind TW. However, the concomitant and alternant course of the different origins of TW pose challenges, both to the patient and the dental team, in the everyday practice.

Biologic anthropology considers that human functional evolutionary adaptation starts in climate and environmental changes that in turn dictate the form, size, and characteristics of humans.

The concept "form follows function," originally coined for industrial design, can be applied to the adaptation of teeth throughout human evolution. When humans of the *Homo* genus started to eat fruits and meat and later were able to cook with the discovery of fire, teeth proved unnecessarily wide and large and consequently started to evolve to a smaller size.

The canine of hominids diverged in form from the ape's, losing prominence in the arch. By the time the humans of the *Homo* genus settled down, their canines were essentially like ours today, drawing a slightly curved line in harmony with the row formed by the incisors.

The increased thickness of the human enamel appears to be an adaptation to a longer life expectancy of humans, who benefit from a reservoir of wear-resistant, non-shedding tissue for the years to come.[8]

Rapidly occurring extensive wear in the short life span of prehistoric humans of the *Australopithecus* genus found in specimens of South African fossils are a manifestation of very abrasive diets in otherwise caries-free and erosion-free individuals, as acid erosion is an unseen phenomenon until modern times.[9] For many decades, anthropologists did not distinguish between the three major terms *abrasion*, *attrition*, and *erosion*, even though erosion was almost absent in anthropologic libraries borrowing the term from geologists.

It is only recently that dentistry has differentiated clearly between these three mechanisms that affect modern dentition. Nevertheless, complexity lies ahead as they can be overlapping, subsequent, or concomitant[10] (Fig 1-13).

## 4. Prevalence of Tooth Wear

Several difficulties lay behind the ample variation of results when assessing TW prevalence. First was the lack of a universally accepted case definition. Second was the difficulty in accepting a unified TW index. When using the TW term and its different subcategories, some authors refer to TW as a synonym to erosion, whereas others clearly separate erosion and TW into different categories.

Lifestyle and contemporary habits have created the actual TSL scenario (Fig 1-14).

Double-digit figures of the prevalence of TW, ranging from 70% in primary dentition in German children[11-13] to 78% in the same age group of Australian children,[14] reveal a reason to worry.

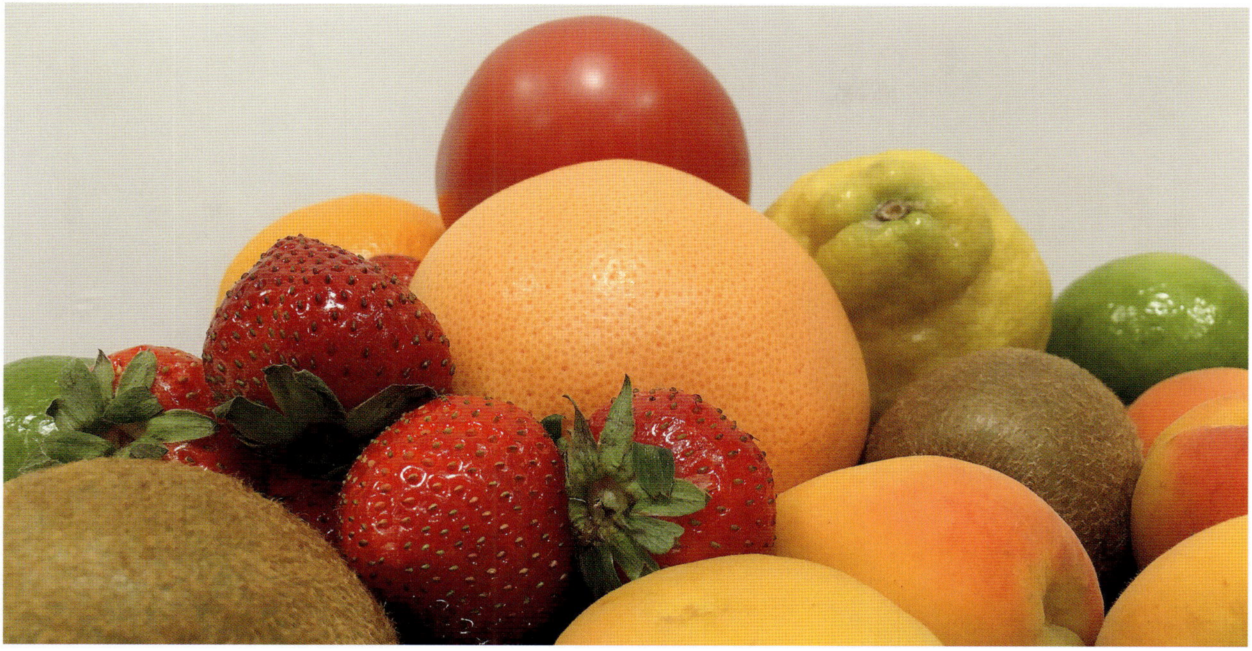

**Fig 1-14** Lifestyle and dietary habits with acidic fruits and beverages are behind many cases of TW in young patients today.

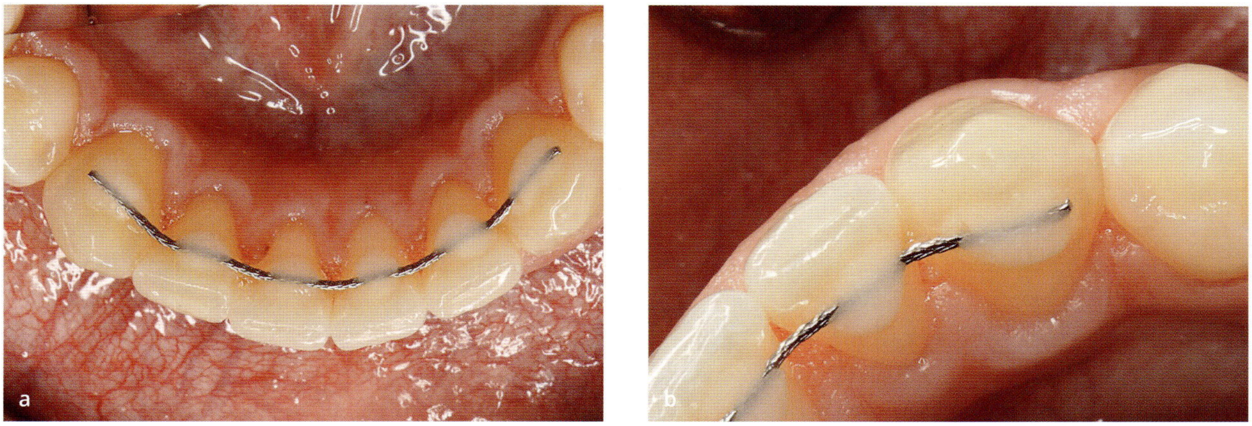

**Fig 1-15** Incipient TW in an adolescent clinically diagnosed during a checkup for hygiene and prophylaxis with a hygienist (a). Detail of flattening from incipient TW lesions affecting incisal edges as well as canine cusps (b).

Prevalence of TW in permanent dentition ranges from 8% to 31% in 14-year-old children in the United Kingdom, while other teenager populations show an overall prevalence of 10% to 90%[15,16] (Fig 1-15).

Although epidemiologic studies have predominantly studied children and the younger population, research has shown a high incidence of TW in adults that may affect up to 77% of their anterior teeth.[17] Sex distribution has shown a significantly higher occurrence of TW in males with ratios such as 2.3:1[18] and 1.7:1.[19]

Lifestyle, dietary habits, and stress, together with higher masticatory forces, may explain the higher occurrence in men. Severity of wear has also been found to be higher in men than in women.[20]

An exception is TW found predominantly in women suffering from eating disorders.

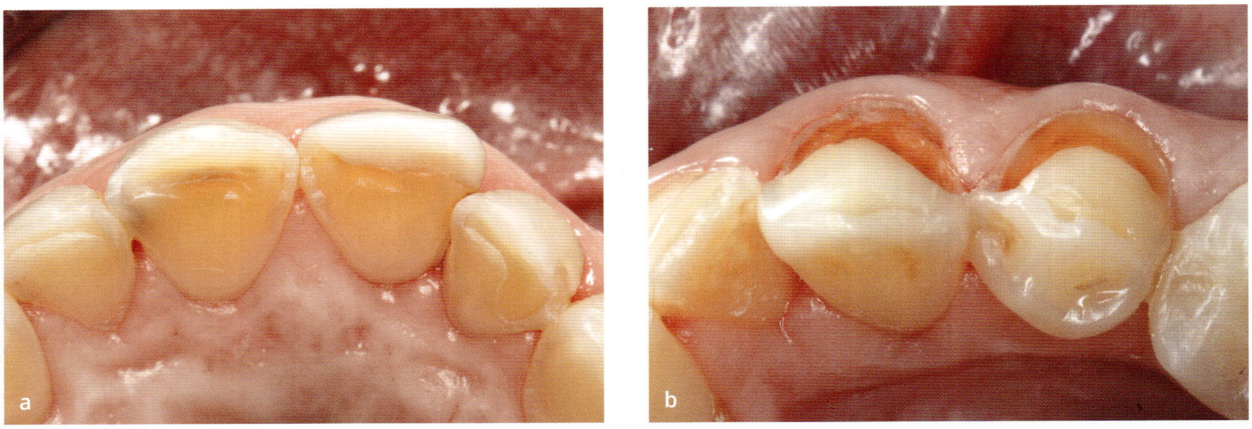


**Fig 1-16** Erosive wear with enamel dissolution in a male patient in his 60s with chronic unspecific digestive complaints compatible with the presence of gastric reflux and an active social life (a and b).

## 5. Tooth Wear and General Health

The modern concept of general health is inseparable from oral health. TW when left untreated evolves into an oral condition that impacts negatively on quality of life. TW is commonly present in cases of premature tooth loss.

Failure to detect moderate to severe cases of TW and treat them with restorative, noninvasive approaches, leaves the patient and the dentist victims of repeated tooth-oriented treatments that unfortunately will not change the evolution of TW.

In order to understand comorbidity of TW, it should be taken into consideration that the oral cavity is part of both the digestive and respiratory tracts (Fig 1-16). Therefore, any condition that affects the respiratory apparatus may cause damage in the oral cavity and vice versa. Pneumonia, pulmonary fibrosis, and asthma can be triggered or caused by poor oral hygiene, a shift in the oral microbiome, or a definite oral dysbiosis. This has been acknowledged recently as the *oral-lung axis.*[20]

Conversely, patients with mouth breathing, obstructive sleep apnea (OSA), pulmonary insufficiency, chronic obstructive pulmonary disease, or pulmonary fibrosis and patients on an oxygen regimen exhibit varying grades of TW.

Similarly, patients with gastroesophageal reflux disease (GERD) have a higher incidence of dental erosion with a reciprocal negative effect. It has been found that patients with GERD have a low salivary flow.[21] In another study by Correa et al, while there was no significant difference between patients with GERD and a control group when it came to salivary flow, the results showed a significant difference in the salivary buffering capacity, with it being lower in the GERD group[22] (Fig 1-17).

On the other hand, patients with worn dentitions and impaired mastication are at higher risk of esophageal and gastric disease, which can be the origin of the TW, and in a vicious cycle the worn dentition can aggravate and perpetuate the digestive problems (Fig 1-18).

Saliva is the most important biologic factor affecting the progression of dental erosion.[23] Medication-induced salivary gland dysfunction (MISGD), specifically a decreased salivary flow or a change in the salivary composition, is a common comorbidity of many conditions and diseases and their associated medication. In the 2014 World Workshop on Oral Medicine, clear conclusions arose identifying the strong connection between medication and xerostomia, with xerostomia occurring in almost 50% of patients taking antihypertensives. This percentage increased to 71% in patients taking antidepressants.[24] Intake of prescribed medications follows a growing pattern as stated by the data collected by health organizations such as the Center for Disease Control in the United States.

Another growing group of patients in whom premature, devasting TW can be seen is in those suffering from eating disorders. The prevalence of bulimia nervosa in young women reaches 5%, while anorexia, with an onset during early adolescence, has a prevalence of 2%.[25,26]

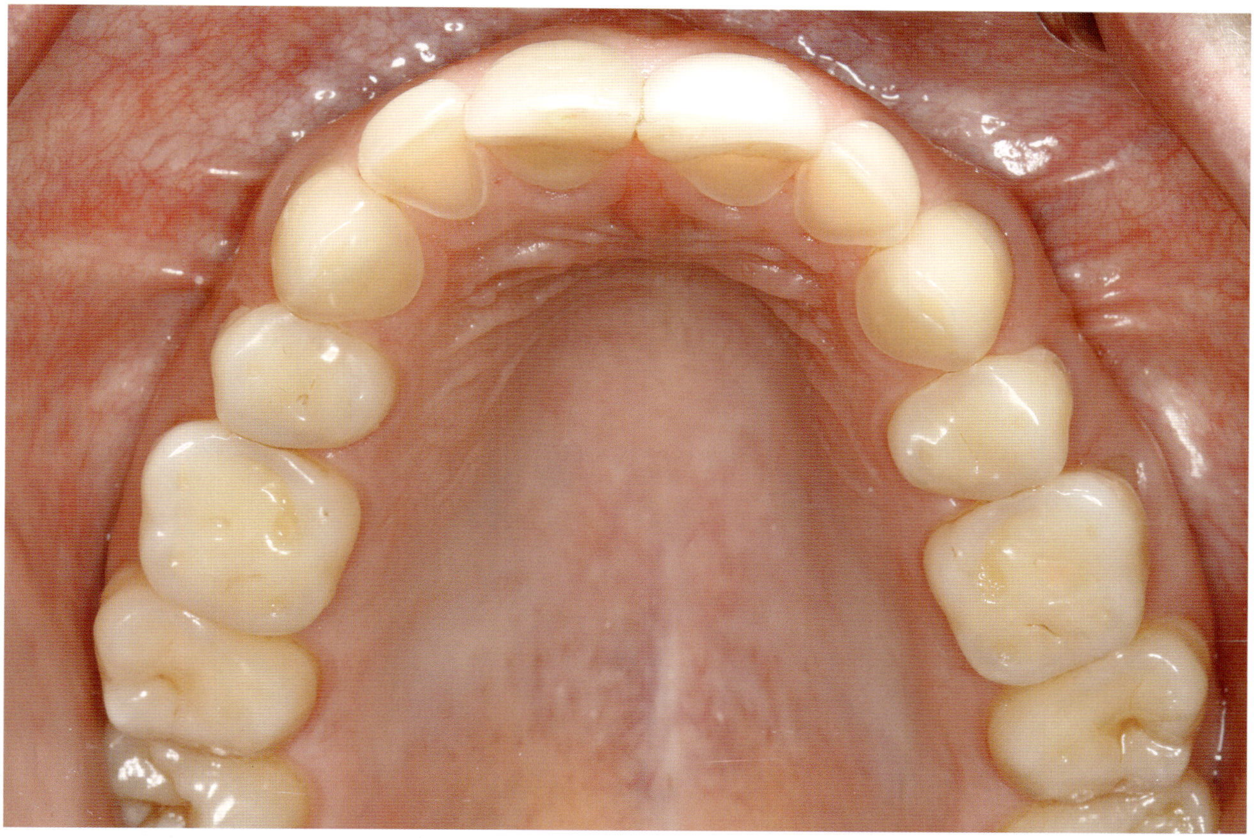

**Fig 1-17** A 21-year-old male patient with generalized TW that has eliminated anatomical and morphologic features. The "cleansing effect" of acids removes all biofilm and impedes the adhesion of the acquired pellicle with the result of an immaculate mouth that should not hinder the diagnosis of premature wear. A presumptive silent reflux diagnosis needs to be confirmed in this very young adult.

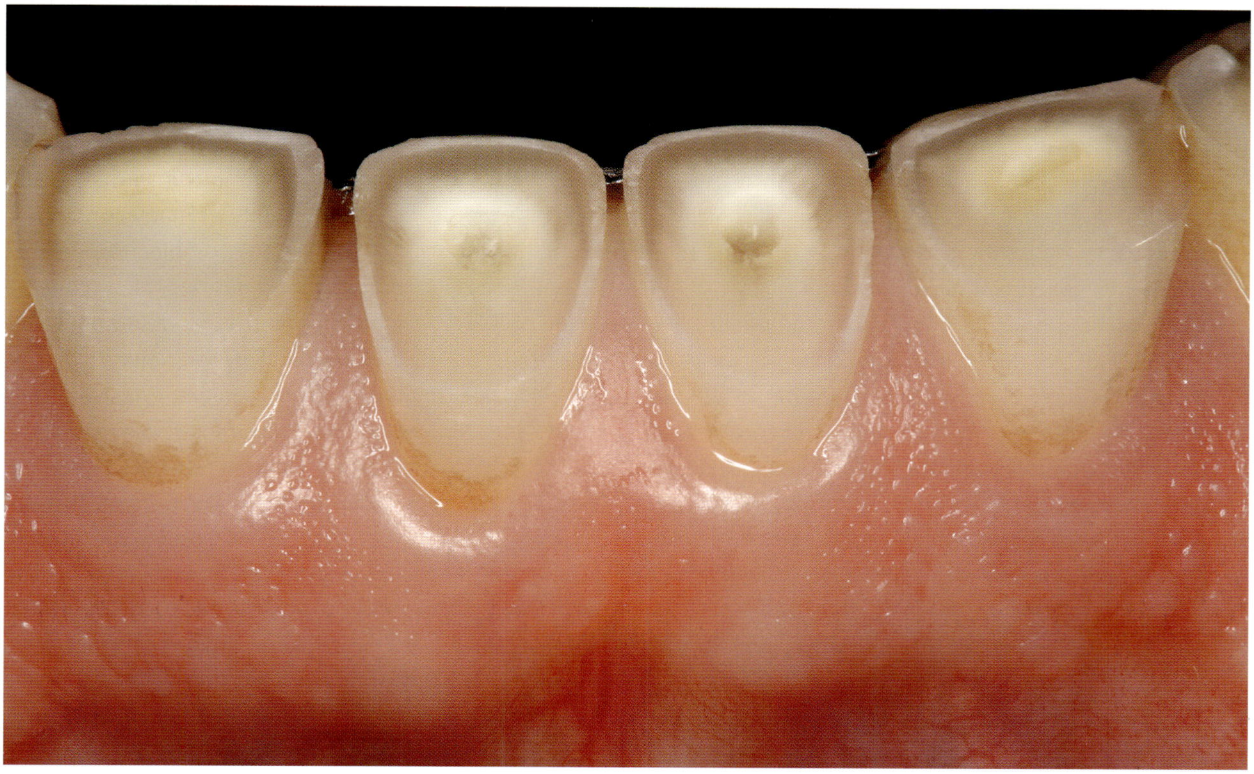

**Fig 1-18** A 40-year-old male patient with severe wear nearing pulp exposure.

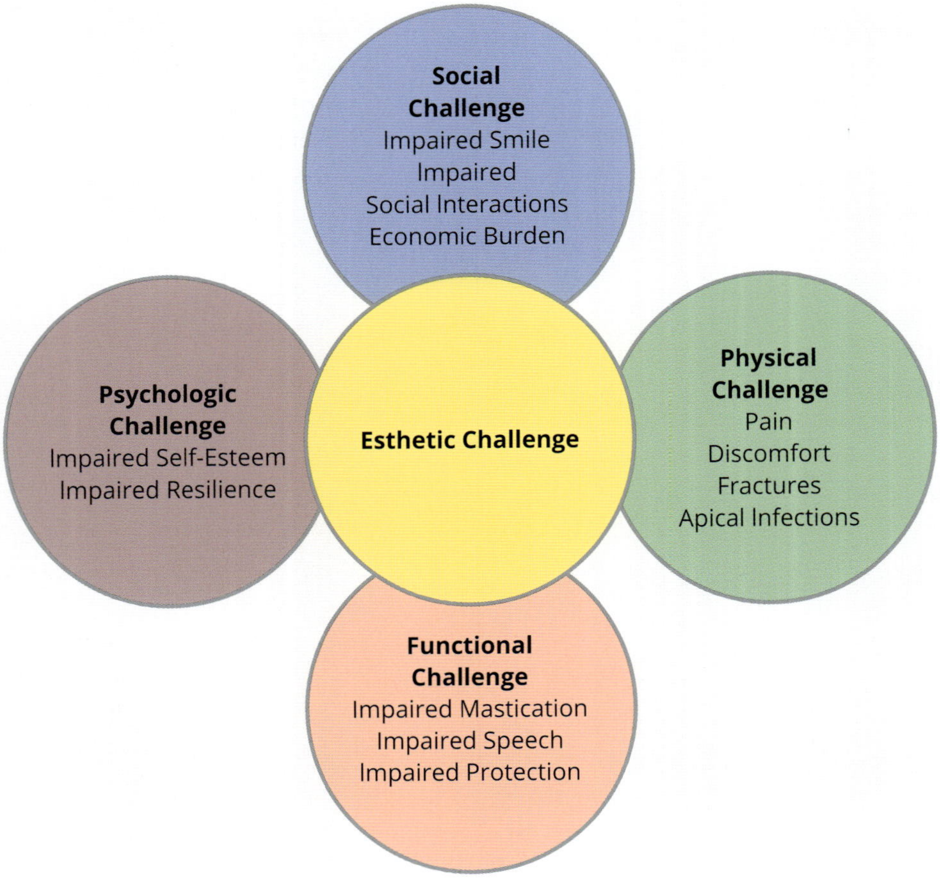


**Fig 1-19** Tooth wear as the quintessential challenge. As explained in the front pages of this book, treating the worn dentition is the quintessential challenge to the dentist as the patient's functional, biologic, psychologic, social, and esthetic disability calls for immediate action.

## 6. The Quintessential Challenge of Tooth Wear

TW has implications for the patient in all aspects physical, functional, psychologic, social, and esthetic.

The TW treatment team should shift from restorative thinking to tooth structure thinking and spare no occasion to educate the patient in line with structure-preserving strategies. The challenge is larger today as more people remain active for longer periods of life, and the evidence is strong showing that TW, as a threat to oral health, will impact all aspects of well-being—physical, psychologic, and social—throughout a lifetime[27,28] (Fig 1-19).

All attempts to safe and effectively improve hyposalivation will provide better chances for our TW patients.

Another aspect that should not be overlooked is the significant expense that repetitions of restorations incur for a patient. Controlling the overall cost of the patient's present treatment and most importantly considering right from the start the expenditure that will be needed in the future should be part of the treatment strategy.

3D technologies were first marketed as a promise to render high-end restorations to more people at reasonable cost. Unfortunately, the trend is to make things more expensive and not more affordable.

The challenge remains in the hands and mind of the dentist, who needs to apply practical and accessible protocols in order to serve the goal of saving resources for the patient and to bring the treatment closer to the patient.

TW affects all spatial dimensions and planes of the dentition. 3D tools and 3D workflow when used in a patient-centered modus operandi may be of great help, even if it requires a jump from digital to analog domains to serve patients better. This aspect, described in this book as "hop-on, hop-off" from digital to analog and vice versa is further explained in chapter 4.

## 7. The Economy of Tooth Wear: The TW Curve Shape

The social science of economics explains through graphs and curves not only principles but also trends.

The COVID-19 sanitary crisis has increased the interest and the knowledge of the general population in terms of understanding how the economy will recover from the COVID-19 impact. Digitalization together with education and a sustainable economy are three of the recommended measures to recover and stabilize a system.

In the same manner as economists represent the market's health drop in a crisis by a downward chart, TW and its impact in oral health can follow a downhill course, implying a progressive decrease in oral and general health. How and when we intervene as a TW treatment team, depending on the treatment type and timing, will mark the recovery pattern and the future resilience to relapse.

As in economics, digitalization, sustainable treatments, and patient education in healthy lifestyle choices are key to managing TW in a dental practice, as there is no single factor that can reduce the challenge of TW both to the dentist and to the patient.

Eventually there will be recessions, some exogenous and some intrinsic, both in economics and in health that cannot be avoided nor prevented.

In times of repeatable relapses or recessions, easy-to-implement noninvasive interventions have proven effective for dealing with TW in a clinical environment.

### V-Shape Recovery

This is the ideal recovery shape and the most optimistic one. The V-shape recovery curve implies a fast and effective recovery (Fig 1-20).

Once the treatment and preventive measures have been applied, no lasting TW sequelae will impact negatively on the health of the patient.

Chances to achieve V-shape recovery are higher in cases where TW is detected, intercepted, and treated in its incipient/moderate stages. Implementing preventive measures is key to long-term recovery (Fig 1-21).

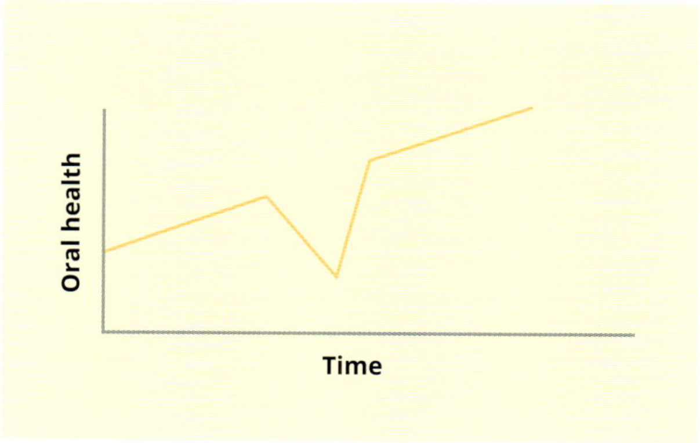


**Fig 1-20** V-shape recovery.

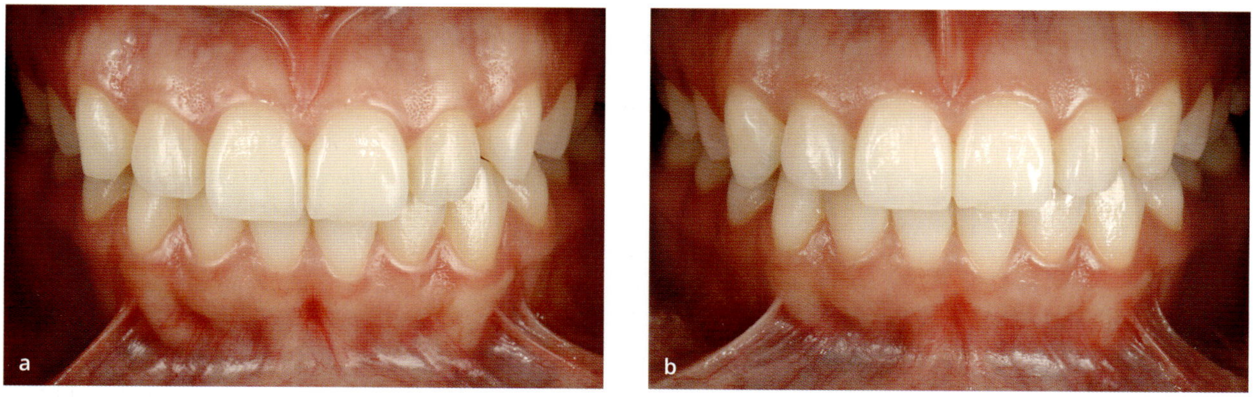


**Fig 1-21** Early treatment enables interception of TW damage provided the patient receives correct coaching regarding lifestyle habits (lip biting in this particular case). For the patient to remain free of further damage, patient-dentist communication is indispensable (a and b). (See more on this case in chapter 5).

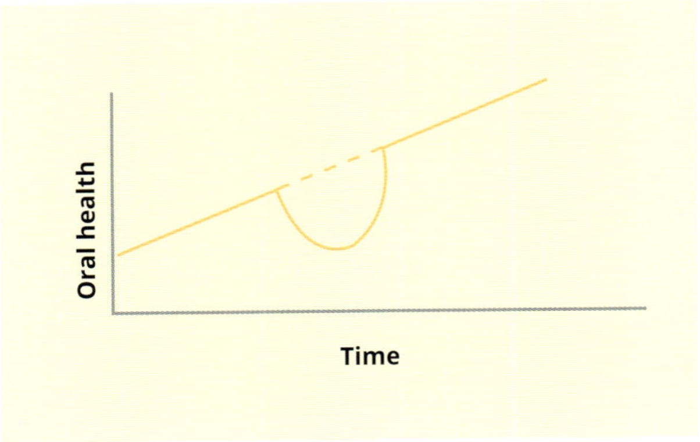


**Fig 1-22** U-shape recovery.

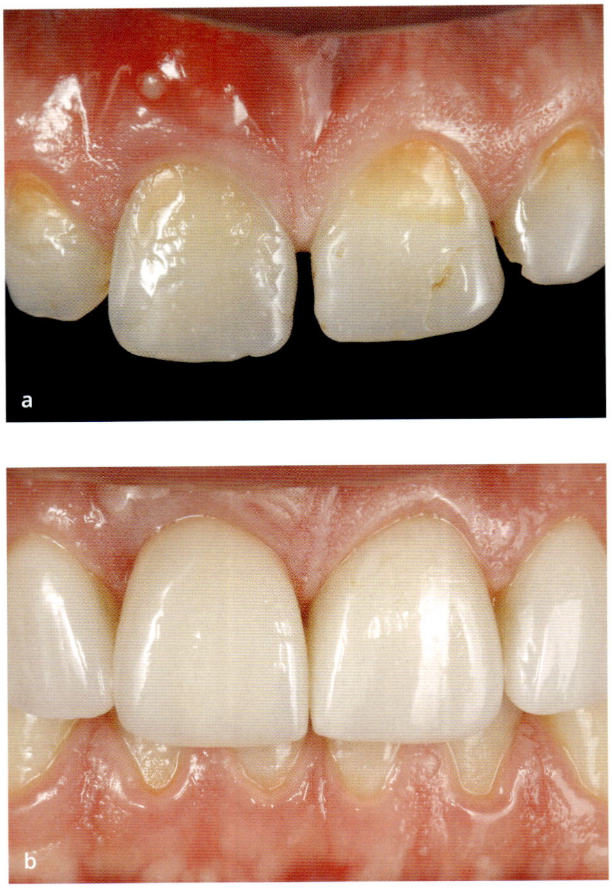


**Fig 1-23** Severe TW has destroyed all the occlusal anatomy and enamel barrier on this patient with a hopeless tooth due to extensive TW. Patient commitment is mandatory to recover and maintain the restored health (a and b). (See more on this case in chapter 9.)

## U-Shape Recovery

Patients who draw a U-shape curve in their recovery pattern sustain lower oral health for a variable period of time (Fig 1-22).

This is normally the case in severe cases that require sustained patient commitment as well as a coordinated multidisciplinary treatment approach. Patients can lose their motivation as they lose sight of "the light at the end of the tunnel." A U-shape recovery is sometimes unavoidable such as with implant or orthodontic therapy, which take time and have a complex provisionalization period and compromised occlusal support in the worst scenarios. It should be anticipated that patients can also lose their confidence in the professional team taking care of them. Furthermore, a concomitant challenge may appear (such as a new medical condition) that impedes a total recovery (Fig 1-23).

## W-Shape Recovery

The W-shape curve has also been described in economy as a "double dip" (Fig 1-24).

This is the case where the patient has an initial good and effective recovery but before regaining health, relapses into another downturn or even drops out of treatment, which might endanger a good and prompt outcome. In these cases, a reevaluation should be done, and a new treatment should be discussed (Fig 1-25).

## K-Shape Recovery

This happens when part of the team performs well but in an isolated manner. Despite the fact that part of the treatment plan can be a success for a certain amount of time, the overall success is challenged as there is no true multidisciplinary approach (Fig 1-26).

In such cases, the generalized TW will progress and endanger the apparently successful part of the treatment, bringing back the patient to the original status (Fig 1-27).

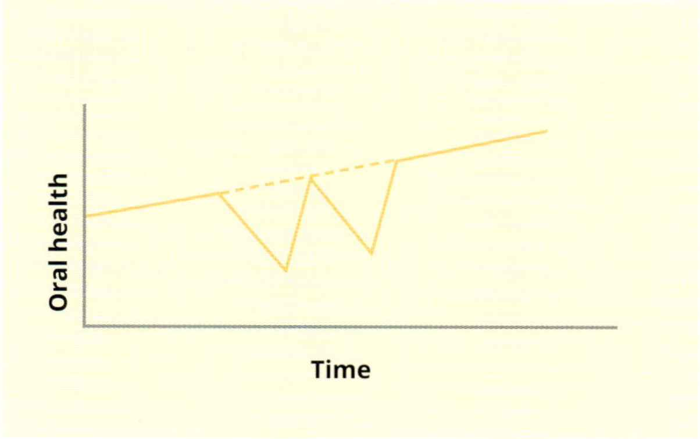


Fig 1-24 W-shape recovery.

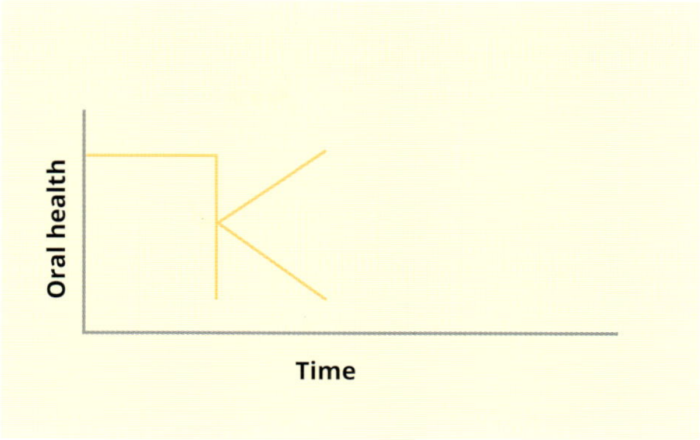


Fig 1-26 K-shape recovery.

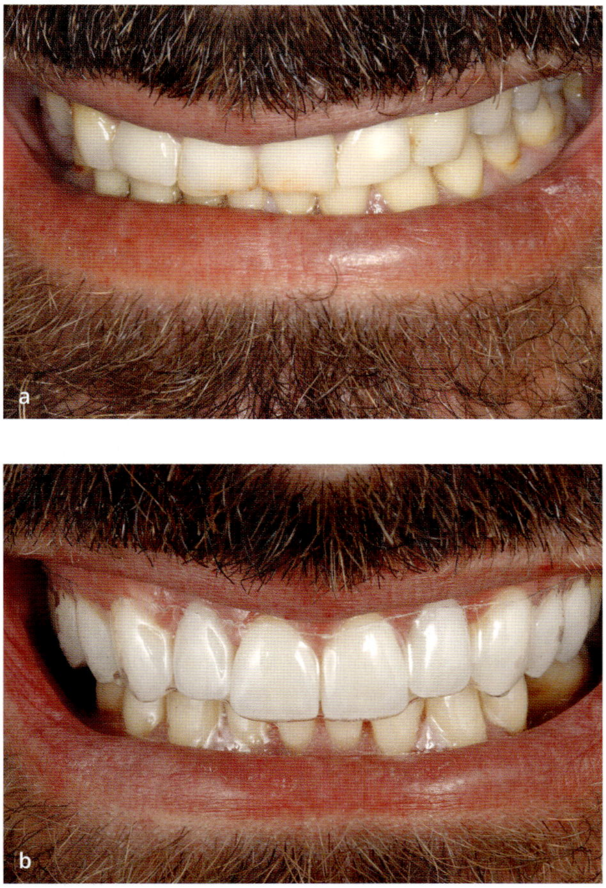

Fig 1-25 Tobacco-related complications arose in the surgical phase, with the onset of a new surgical procedure and a demotivation process that represented a risk for the final outcome. Empathizing with the patient while reemphasizing the general treatment goal is usually helpful to regain patient's trust (a and b).

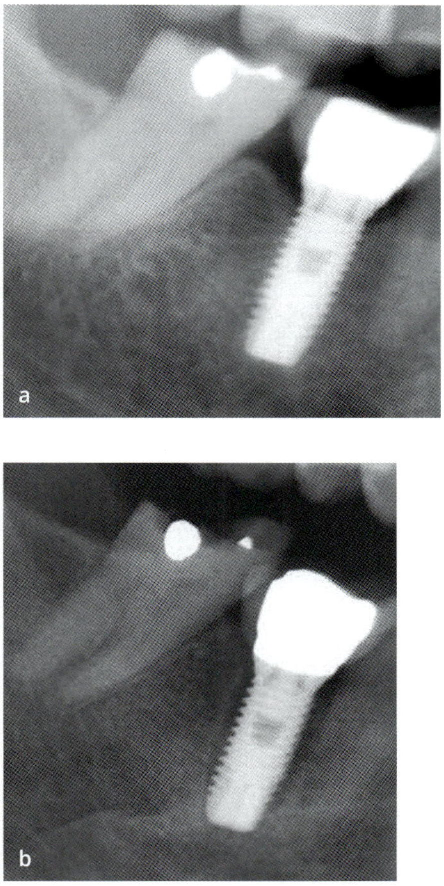

Fig 1-27 Even though excellent osseointegration was achieved, the underestimation of the overall TSL led to occlusal implant overload and implant failure. See the loss of tooth structure in the interval between the radiographs. Erosion eliminated the occlusal support of adjacent and contralateral teeth. The occlusal porcelain of the screw-retained implant crown had suffered from occlusal prematurities with repeated chipping and screw dislodgment, signs that had alerted the dentist to the issue. In this case the patient rejected any TW restorative treatment, resulting in progression to implant loss (a and b). (See more on this case in chapter 9.)

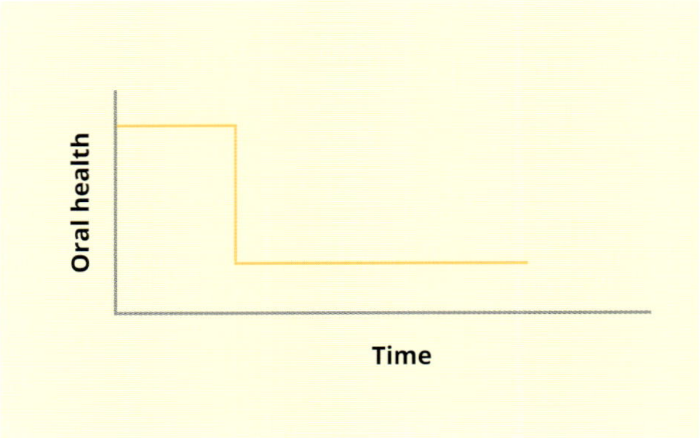


**Fig 1-28** L- shape recovery.

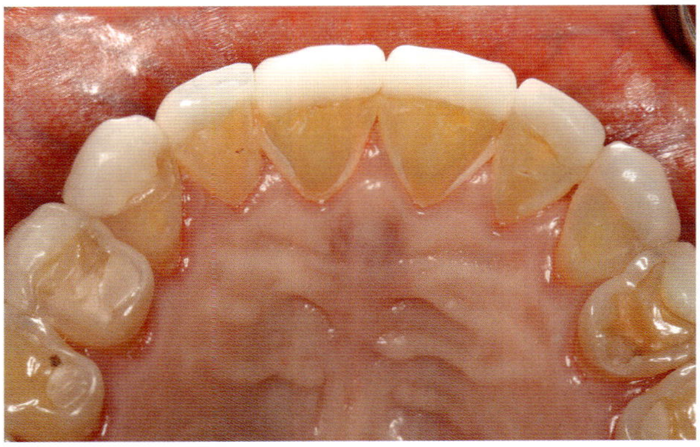

**Fig 1-29** Buccal restorations of anterior teeth performed decades ago were not able to free the patient from the TW cycle that continued to challenge tooth structure. Facially driven 3D-planned orthodontic treatment will in many cases provide the required space to allocate palatal restorations with no further tooth reduction.

## L-Shape Recovery

This is the least desirable scenario (Fig 1-28).

Patient lacks motivation to undergo the treatment and to further follow preventive measures, or the dental team lacks the required experience to effectively treat the TW condition that is negatively impacting the patient's oral and general health. This also occurs when patients are treated "one tooth at a time" without a general concept and protocol and a comprehensive diagnosis and treatment plan to address TW.

Years ago, when TW was far from being understood, it was not unusual to find patients that had been treated exclusively on the labial aspect of the anterior teeth, taking only the esthetic appearance into consideration. An example would be patients seriously affected by medical conditions producing acid erosion (eg, eating disorders, GERD) with extensive dissolution of the palatal aspect of maxillary teeth that were only treated with direct or indirect labial restorations of the maxillary anterior teeth. Even though those patients were satisfied with the treatment, the TW damage continued to advance with devastating effects over the years (Fig1-29).

# 8. The Geography of Tooth Wear

Tooth wear is found today throughout the world and linked mainly to lifestyle and contemporary dietary habits. Globalization is like a tsunami, diluting traditional idiosyncratic culinary patterns and leaving teeth buffeted by a merciless acidic challenge.

A review coming from Freiburg University in 2017 shows a large variation in global prevalence of erosion ranging from 0% to 100%. The lack of homogeneous study design and the fact that data are only available from certain countries, with close to zero information from the continents of Africa, South America, Asia, and many countries from southeastern Europe, explain this huge variation. As per the aforementioned review, estimating the global prevalence is complex as comparison between local studies is a complicated task due to the variation of study designs[29] (Table 1-1).

This review points out differences in data between the primary and permanent dentition.[29] For the ease of the reading, data of erosive TW both in children and adults have been summarized in Table 1-2.

The effects of characteristic, proprietary habits in certain cultures such as drinking vinegar beverages along with the use of komesu (fermented rice vinegar) and kurosu (unpolished rice vinegar) in Japan have turned out to be mild in comparison to the worldwide expansion of branded carbonated soft drinks that are cited as predominant risk factors in most of the epidemiologic studies regarding erosion prevalence and etiology.[30] The use of fermented and acidic food and drink in diets seems to be increasing, with the potential to change the oral microbiome in the same manner as a cariogenic diet changes the oral microbiota to acid-resistant and acid-generating bacteria such as *Streptococcus mutans*. The shift of the microbiota to a population of acidic bacteria that are adapted to an acidic environment and are themselves a source of acetic metabolites may have unprecedented consequences.[31]

**Table 1-1** Global mean erosion prevalence as per the review by Schlueter and Luka.[29]

| | |
|---|---|
| Global mean erosion prevalence | 1%–100% |
| Global mean erosion prevalence in primary teeth | 30%–50% |
| Global mean erosion prevalence in permanent teeth | 20%–45% |

**Table 1-2** Prevalence of erosion in children and adults in various countries.

| | CHILDREN | ADULTS |
|---|---|---|
| Australia | 0%–33% | |
| Brazil | 1%–62% | |
| China | 6%–15% | 44% |
| Denmark | | 2% |
| Finland | | 18%–75% |
| France | | 26% |
| Germany | 32%–71% | 24%–40% |
| Great Britain | 28%–50% | 3%–100% |
| India | 29% | |
| Israel | | 37%–62% |
| Italy | | 21% |
| Japan | | 26% |
| Norway | | 20%–38% |
| Saudi Arabia | 31% | 28% |
| Switzerland | 100% | 8%–82% |
| USA | | 25% |

Globalized communications that favor rapid transmission of lifestyle attitudes and dietary habits lay behind the increase in erosion prevalence documented over the last decades in many countries throughout the world.

In countries like Japan, even though not many epidemiologic studies have analyzed the effect of the traditional Japanese dietary pattern versus more international foods, interesting data show how adherence to a traditional Japanese diet was associated with a decrease in diastolic and systolic blood pressure both in men and women.

The positive effect of the traditional Japanese diet should be further studied, but results so far show a beneficial link with protection from noncommunicable diseases such as cardiovascular disease and hypertension.[32]

Several studies from Japan show 25% of adults presenting erosive wear. Dietary habits were mainly behind this double-digit figure. Acidic juices are to be blamed in young patients, while acidic fruits are the culprit in older patients.[33]

Age-specific dietary habits were found among adults in Tokyo suffering from erosive wear. Greater soda and sports drink consumption was linked to increased incidence of erosive wear in adults independently of their age.[34]

Accordingly, age, acidic beverages, xerostomia, and brushing habits have been shown to be behind the erosive wear found in Beijing adults.[35,36]

Moving from Asia to North America, prevalence of erosive wear in Mexico was 31.7% in a study in which high intake of carbonated drinks and xerostomia were found to be determinantal risk factors. Mexican children consume 27.8% of their energy from caloric beverages, whole milk, fruit juice with sugar, and carbonated and noncarbonated sugared beverages. In addition to the increasing erosion figures, a great concern regarding obesity is arising in Mexico.[37]

Regarding Russia, there is a huge deviation in erosion prevalence among the population in different regions of Russia. In most regions the prevalence is low (from 1% to 6%); however, in some regions it can reach up to 50%.[38]

Erosion prevalence of 17.4% found in Cuban children in a study performed in the year 2000 was linked to consumption of oranges. The specific political circumstances in Cuba at the time of the study, with Cuba isolated from the rest of the world, may explain why erosion in children was not due to carbonated soda drinks but to citrus fruits instead.[39]

An erosion prevalence map unites data from the aforementioned research and review studies[29,38,39] (Fig 1-30).

The role of hyposalivation in TW will be described in chapter 2. Nevertheless, its significance is so high when confronting TW that a map of xerostomia prevalence, as per a systematic review from 2018, is shown in this chapter[40] (Fig 1-31).

| | EROSION PREVALENCE | | EROSION PREVALENCE |
|---|---|---|---|
| Australia | 0%–33% | Italy | 21% |
| Brazil | 1%–62% | Japan | 26% |
| China | 6%–89% | Malaysia | 68% |
| Colombia | 53% | Mexico | 17%–32% |
| Cuba | 17.4% | Norway | 59% |
| Denmark | 2%–14% | Poland | 42% |
| Finland | 18%–75% | Russia | 1%–50% |
| France | 26%–57% | Saudi Arabia | 28%–31% |
| Germany | 14%–72% | Spain | 26% |
| Great Britain | 3%–100% | Sweden | 16% |
| Greece | 52%–79% | Switzerland | 8%–28% |
| Iceland | 0%–31% | Switzerland | 100% |
| India | 9%–29% | Turkey | 28%–53% |
| Ireland | 47% | Uruguay | 53% |
| Israel | 37-62% | USA | 25% |

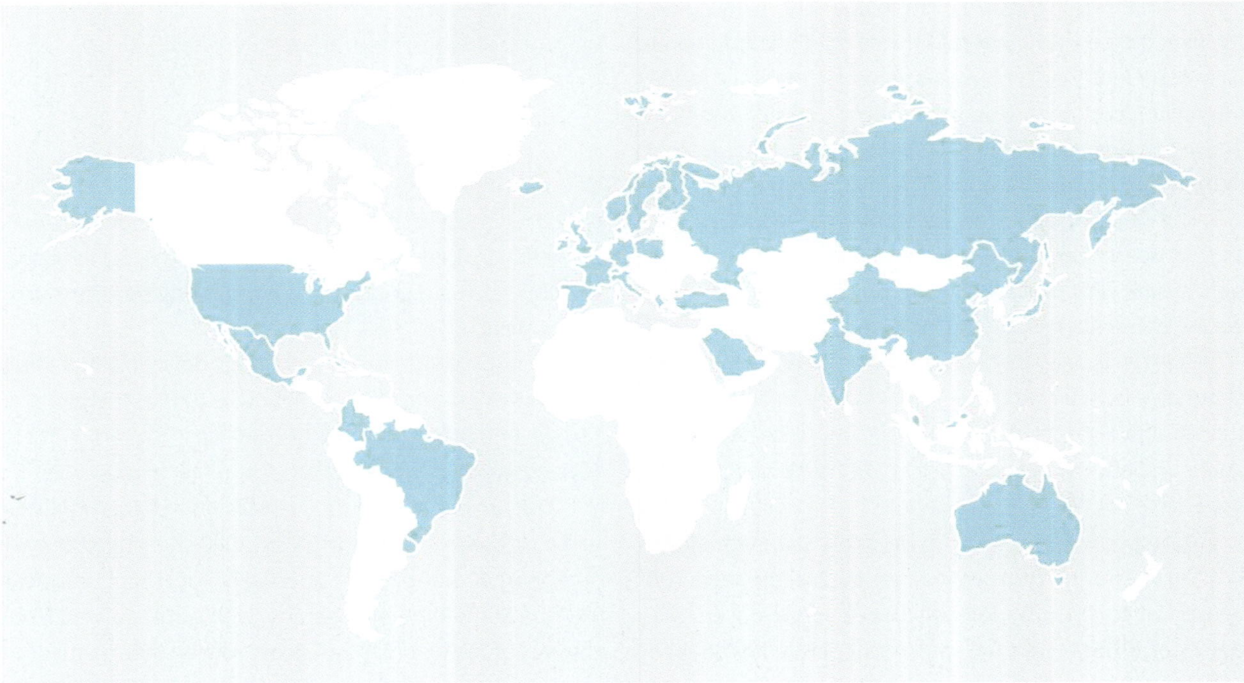

**Fig 1-30** World tooth erosion map, modified from Schlueter and Lucca.[29] Marked in blue are geographic areas with significant documented data from erosion prevalence in children and adults.

| | XEROSTOMIA PREVALENCE | | XEROSTOMIA PREVALENCE |
|---|---|---|---|
| Australia | 10.0% | Japan | 17.6% / 10.2% |
| Australia | 20.5% | Japan | 34.8% |
| Brazil | 11.0% | Korea | 25.8% |
| Canada | 29.5% | Mexico | 45.1% |
| Denmark | 29% | New Zealand | 13.1% |
| England | 17.2% / 15% | Norway | 29.6% |
| Finland | 11.7% / 46,7% | Spain | 13% |
| Finland | 30.8% /40.3%/ 15.9% | Sweden | 27.7% |
| Finland | 46% | Sweden | 35% |
| Germany | 0.1% | Sweden | 37.4% / 57.5% / 62.3% |
| Israel | 37.7% | USA | 35.3% |
| Japan | 16.2% | USA | 39% |

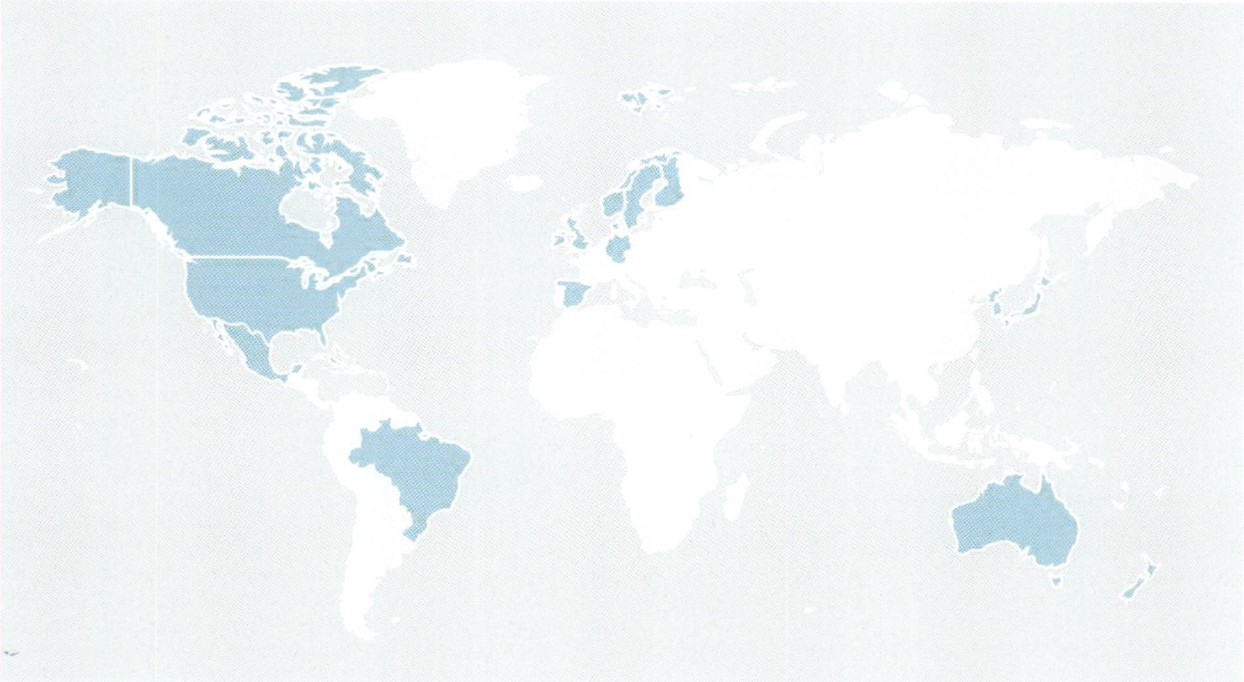

**Fig 1-31** World xerostomia map. Marked in blue are geographic localizations with significant documented data on xerostomia prevalence.

## 9. Key Points

- Progressive, irreversible and multifactorial, TW requires a comprehensive approach and a trained team to provide early diagnosis, preventive measures, and a patient-centered treatment path.
- TW is linked to lifestyle and general health conditions.
- Attrition and abrasion may, to a certain extent, be considered physiologic: erosion should always be regarded as pathologic.
- The estimated global prevalence of erosion has a huge variation, ranging from 0% to 100%.
- Sex distribution has shown a higher presentation in males.
- Ideal recovery from a TW impact requires patient re-education, a comprehensive treatment approach, a trained team, and ideally an early diagnosis that favors a conservative treatment modality.

## References


1. Loomans B, Opdam N, Attin T, et al. Severe tooth wear: European consensus statement on management guidelines. J Adhes Dent 2017;19(2):111–119.
2. Stoichkov B, Kirov D. Analysis of the causes of dental implant fracture: A retrospective clinical study. Quintessence Int 2018;49:279–286.
3. Slade GD, Akinkugbe AA, Sanders AE. Projections of U.S. edentulism prevalence following 5 decades of decline. J Dent Res 2014;93:959–965.
4. Lussi A. Dental erosion clinical diagnosis and case history taking. Eur J Oral Sci 1996;104(2 [Pt 2]):191–198.
5. Larsen MJ, Richards A. Fluoride is unable to reduce dental erosion from soft drinks. Caries Res 2002;36(1):75–80.
6. Bader JD, Shugars DA. What do we know about how dentists make caries-related treatment decisions? Community Dent Oral Epidemiol 1997;25(1):97–103.
7. Jobim Jardim J, Henz S, Barbachan E Silva B. Restorative treatment decisions in posterior teeth: A systematic review. Oral Health Prev Dent 2017;15(2):107–115.
8. Larsen CS. A Companion to Biological Anthropology. Chichester, UK: Wiley-Blackwell, 2010.
9. Sperber GH. Dental wear: Attrition, erosion, and abrasion—A palaeo-odontological approach. Dent J (Basel) 2017;5(2):19.
10. Ungar PS. Teeth: A Very Short Introduction. 2014: Oxford: Oxford UP, 2014.
11. Ganss C, Klimek J, Giese K. Dental erosion in children and adolescents—A cross-sectional and longitudinal investigation using study models. Community Dent Oral Epidemiol 2001;29:264–271.
12. Wiegand A, Müller J, Werner C, Attin T. Prevalence of erosive tooth wear and associated risk factors in 2-7-year-old German kindergarten children. Oral Dis 2006;12(2):117–124.
13. Smithers G, Gregory JR, Bates CJ, Prentice A, Jackson LV, Wenlock R. The National Diet and Nutrition Survey: Young people aged 4–18 years. Nutr Bull 2000;25(2):105–111.
14. Kazoullis S, Seow WK, Holcombe T, Newman B, Ford D. Common dental conditions associated with dental erosion in schoolchildren in Australia. Pediatr Dent 2007;29(1):33–39.
15. Mouatt RB. Children's dental health in the United Kingdom 1983—A review. Health Bull (Edinb) 1986;44:283–285.
16. Al-Majed I, Maguire A, Murray JJ. Risk factors for dental erosion in 5-6 year old and 12-14 year old boys in Saudi Arabia. Community Dent Oral Epidemiol 2002;30(1):38–46.
17. El Wazani B, Dodd MN, Milosevic A. The signs and symptoms of tooth wear in a referred group of patients. Br Dent J 2012;213(6):E10.
18. Rees JS, Thomas M, Naik P. A prospective study of the prevalence of periapical pathology in severely worn teeth. Dent Update 2011;38(1):24–26,28–29.
19. Banks I. No man's land: Men, illness, and the NHS. BMJ 2001;323(7320):1058–1060.
20. Gaeckle NT, Pragman AA, Pendleton KM, Baldomero AK, Criner GJ. The oral-lung axis: The impact of oral health on lung health. Respir Care 2020;65:1211–1220.
21. Yoshikawa H, Furuta K, Ueno M, et al. Oral symptoms including dental erosion in gastroesophageal reflux disease are associated with decreased salivary flow volume and swallowing function. J Gastroenterol 2012;47:412–420.
22. Correa MC, Lerco MM, Cunha Mde L, Henry MA. Salivary parameters and teeth erosions in patients with gastroesophageal reflux disease. Arq Gastroenterol 2012;49:214–218.
23. Buzalaf MA, Hannas AR, Kato MT. Saliva and dental erosion. J Appl Oral Sci 2012;20:493–502.
24. Villa A, Wolff A, Aframian D, et al. World Workshop on Oral Medicine VI: A systematic review of medication-induced salivary gland dysfunction: Prevalence, diagnosis, and treatment. Clin Oral Investig 2015;19:1563–1580.
25. Cooper PJ, Charnock DJ, Taylor MJ. The prevalence of bulimia nervosa. A replication study. Br J Psychiatry 1987;151:684–686.
26. Milosevic A, Slade PD. The orodental status of anorexics and bulimics. Br Dent J 1989;167(2):66–70.
27. Vaupel JW. Biodemography of human ageing. Nature 2010;464(7288):536–542.
28. Inglehart MR, Bagramian R. Oral Health–Related Quality of Life. Chicago: Quintessence, 2002.
29. Schlueter N, Luka B. Erosive tooth wear–A review on global prevalence and on its prevalence in risk groups. Br Dental J 2018;224(5):364–370.
30. Nanda K, Taniguchi M, Ujike S, et al. Characterization of acetic acid bacteria in traditional acetic acid fermentation of rice vinegar (komesu) and unpolished rice vinegar (kurosu) produced in Japan. Appl Environ Microbiol 2001;67:986–990.
31. Gullo M, Caggia C, De Vero L, Giudici P. Characterization of acetic acid bacteria in „traditional balsamic vinegar". Int J Food Microbiol 2006;106(2):209–212.
32. Niu K, Momma H, Kobayashi Y, et al. The traditional Japanese dietary pattern and longitudinal changes in cardiovascular disease risk factors in apparently healthy Japanese adults. Eur J Nutr 2016;55(1):267–279.
33. Kitasako Y, Sasaki Y, Takagaki T, Sadr A, Tagami J. Age-specific prevalence of erosive tooth wear by acidic diet and gastroesophageal reflux in Japan. J Dent 2015;43:418–423.
34. Kitasako Y, Sasaki Y, Takagaki T, Sadr A, Tagami J. Erosive tooth wear among different tooth types and surfaces in Japanese adults 15 to 89 years old. Oral Health Prev Dent 2017;15:357–364.
35. Sun K, Wang W, Wang X, Shi X, Si Y, Zheng S. Tooth wear: A cross-sectional investigation of the prevalence and risk factors in Beijing, China. BDJ Open 2017;3(1):16012.
36. Zhang J, Du Y, Wei Z, Tai B, Jiang H, Du M. The prevalence and risk indicators of tooth wear in 12- and 15-year-old adolescents in Central China. BMC Oral Health 2015;15(1):120.
37. González-Aragón Pineda ÁE, Borges-Yáñez SA, Lussi A, Irigoyen-Camacho ME, Angeles Medina F. Prevalence of erosive tooth wear and associated factors in a group of Mexican adolescents. J Am Dent Assoc 2016;147(2):92–97.
38. Kuzmina E, Janushevich C, Kuzmina I. The Prevalence of oral diseases among the Russian population. NOHS 2019. Moscow, 2019, pp 302
39. Künzel W, Cruz MS, Fischer T. Dental erosion in Cuban children associated with excessive consumption of oranges. Eur J Oral Sci 2000;108(2):104–109.
40. Agostini BA, Cericato GO, Silveira ERD, et al. How common is dry mouth? Systematic review and meta-regression analysis of prevalence estimates. Braz Dent J 2018;29:606–618.

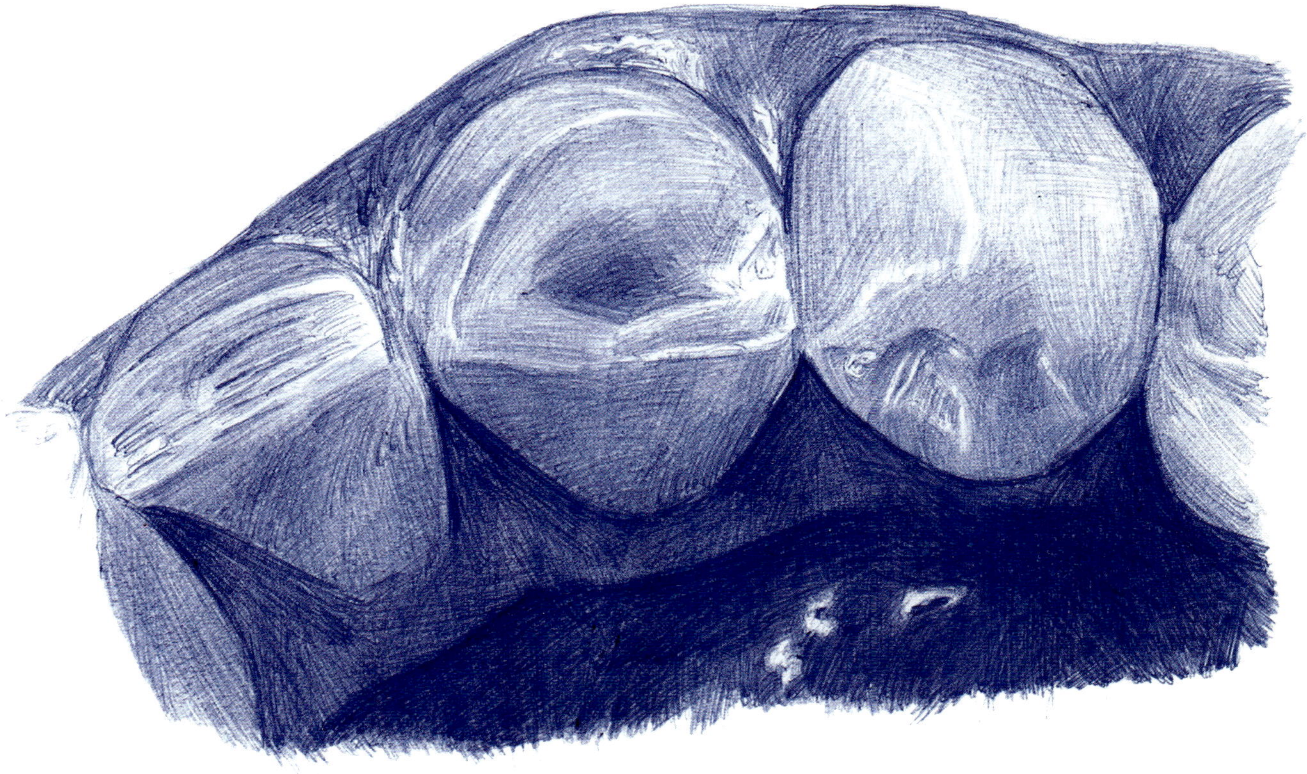

*When the well's dry, we know the worth of water.*

—Benjamin Franklin, American statesman, co-father of the US Declaration of Independence

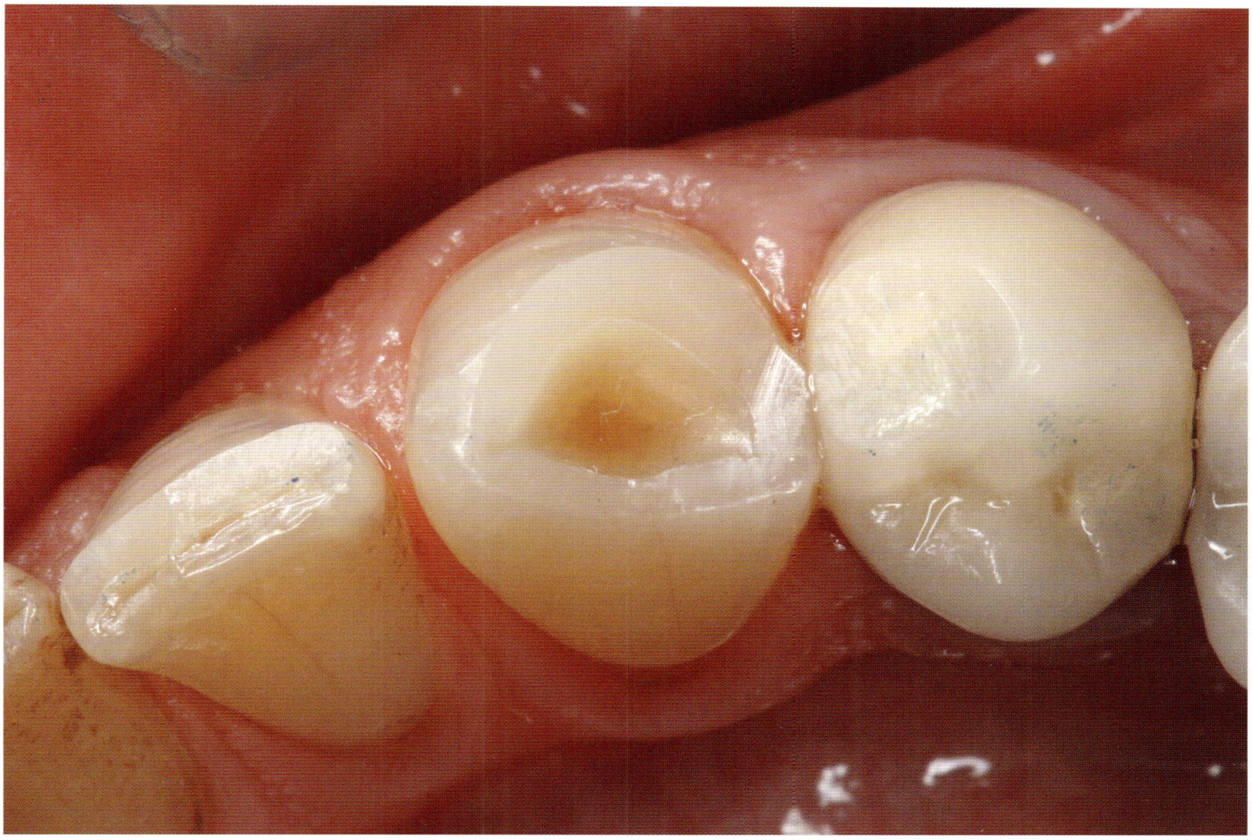

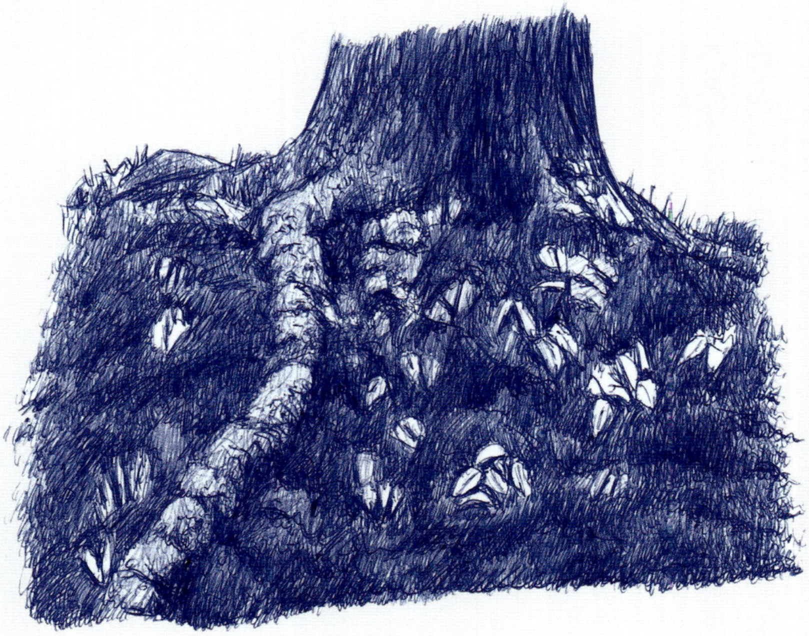

*When one tugs at a single thing in nature, he finds it attached to the rest of the world.*

—John Muir, naturalist and explorer

CHAPTER 2

# TOOTH WEAR AND SALIVA: THE FIRST LINE OF DEFENSE

The human body is a perfect machine. Everything in the human body has a function and interacts in multiple ways that are not yet fully understood.

According to today's research, saliva, classically described as a food bolus facilitator, has unprecedented vital functions such as regulating hypertension, the cardiovascular nitric-oxide mechanism (NO pathway), and obesity; protecting oral tissues; and providing hydration and fluidification.

In fact, saliva is critical to the preservation and maintenance of all oral tissues, providing an appropriate physicochemical environment.

To restorative dentists, saliva could seem outside the scope of their concern. However, it is essential to understand why teeth dissolve and which conditions will render teeth more susceptible to erosive attack in order to provide patients with effective treatments and preventive measures.

Saliva, described today as the curator of oral health, explains the relationship between the different tissues in the mouth and the connections between tooth wear and general health and opens a window of opportunity for implementing preventive measures in vulnerable patients to stop tooth wear and maintain tooth structure.

## 1. The Oral–General Health Connection

The oral cavity is the entry to the body for pathogens and noxious agents that may change the oral microflora and environment, causing oral dysbiosis; it is the atrium to numerous essential conditions.

The mouth is part of the gastrointestinal and airway apparatus, meaning it has many common features with other digestive and respiratory organs, such as the mucosa, but with the unusual component of hard tissue, ie, teeth (Fig 2-1).

Oral care and oral health are integral components of general health. Loss of teeth and poor oral care are significant indicators of poor general health. Scientific literature proves that a reduced number of teeth, as well as inadequate prosthodontic treatment, are directly associated with a poorer quality of life.[1] Interestingly, in a study undertaken in North Carolina, individuals under 65 years of age who had never visited a dentist were less likely to have lost 6 teeth or more. The explanation for this may be that either these individuals were too young or had simply taken good care of their teeth.[2] Implicit in the conclusions and results of this and other behavioral risk factor studies

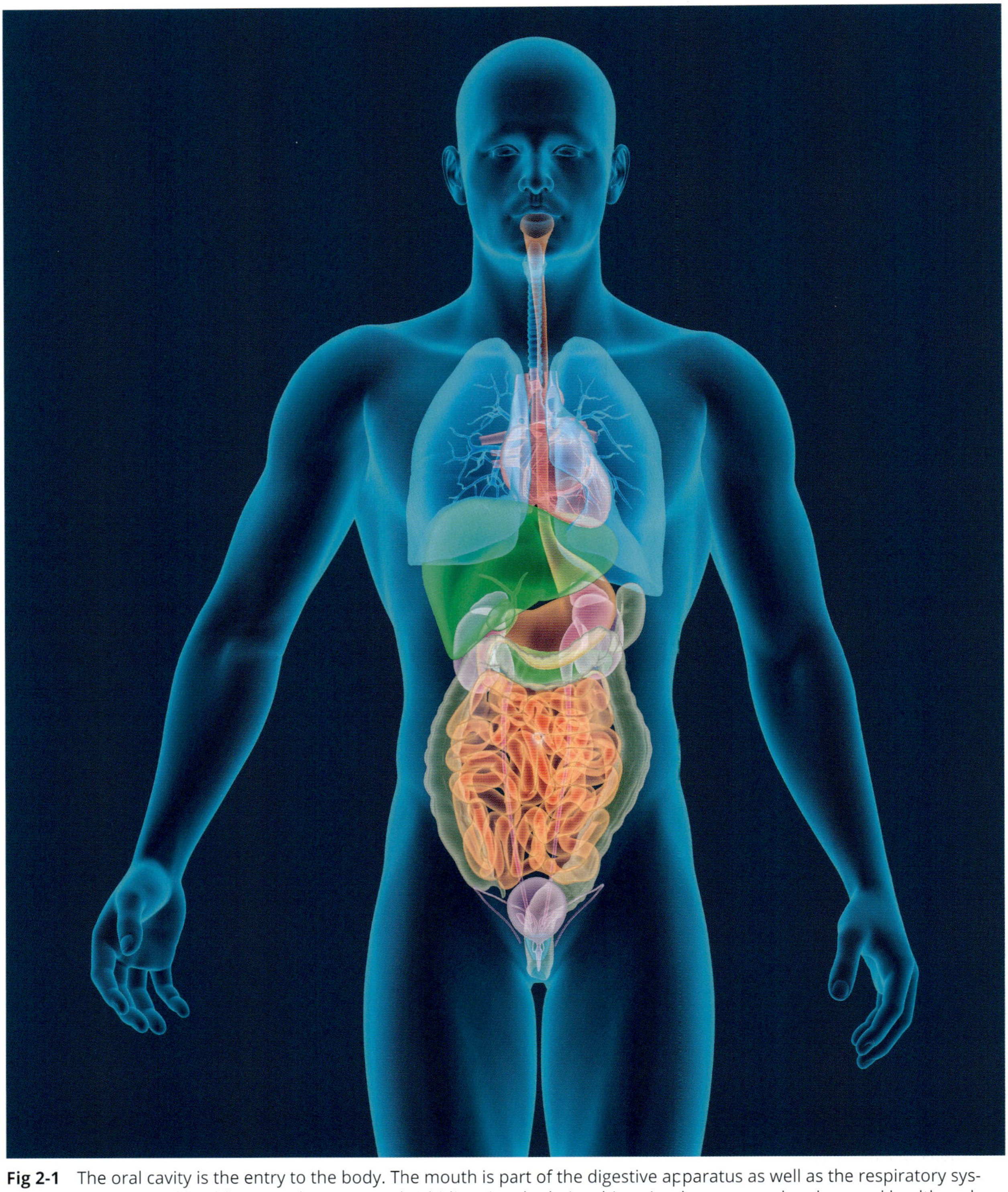

**Fig 2-1** The oral cavity is the entry to the body. The mouth is part of the digestive apparatus as well as the respiratory system. Oral and general health cannot be separated. A bidirectional relationship exists between oral and general health and oral and general disease.

is the importance of oral care by means of oral hygiene in attaining and maintaining good general health.[3–6]

The mouth is connected to other parts of the body. There is an enormous research interest that transcends dental and gingival physiology. This is described in an emerging body of evidence, leading to manifold newly described oral-body axes, including the oral-gut,[7,8] oral-lung,[9] oral-brain,[10] oral-joint,[11] oral-heart,[12] oral-liver,[13] oral-breast,[14] and oral-gut-skin axes,[15] to name some of the most representative studies.

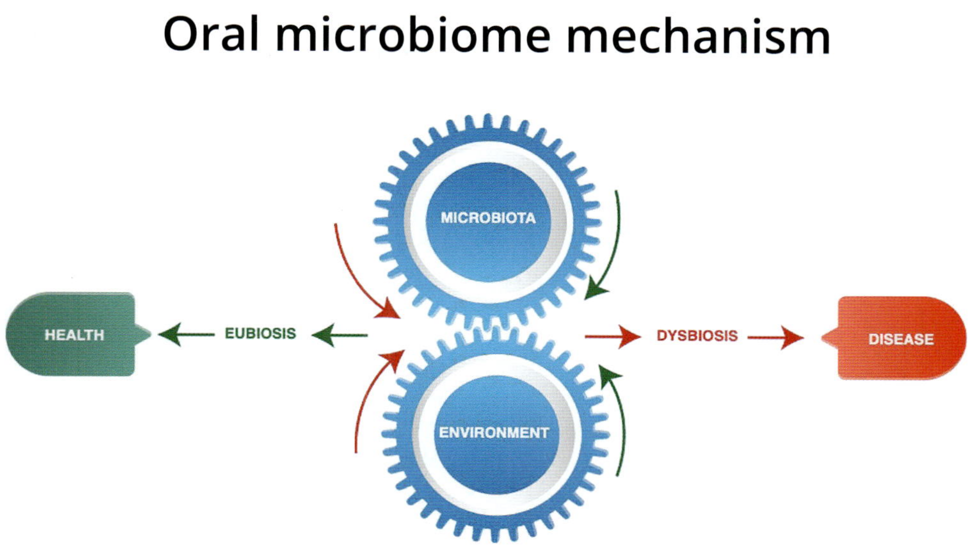


**Fig 2-2** The balance between health and disease is mediated by the interrelationship of the microbiota and the environment, able to convert eubiosis (health) into dysbiosis (disease) and vice versa. Dysbiosis refers to a state of the microbiome of any area of the body, including mucosal (eg, oral, respiratory) or skin surfaces, in which the normal diversity or function of the ecologic network is disrupted, even if such dysbiosis does not result in a detectable decrease in health. Dysbiosis may be due to a decrease in diversity; the overgrowth of one or more pathogens or pathobionts, able to cause disease only when certain genetic or environmental conditions are present in a patient; or the shift to an ecologic network that no longer provides a beneficial function to the host and therefore no longer promotes health. Dysbiosis may be induced by illness (eg, diabetes, cancer), treatment (eg, radiation), an agent (eg, an antibiotic reducing commensal flora), or other environmental factors.

## 2. Saliva and the Oral Microbiome: Defenders of Oral and General Health

Up until recently, removing dental plaque has been the fundamental measure used to prevent oral diseases. On the other hand, it seems that the oral microbiome and saliva may regulate the virulence of certain key pathogens like *Porphyromonas gingivalis*, which may change the environment and start a microbial shift, leading to dysbiosis and inflammation-mediated periodontal disease and eventually disease beyond the area of the oral cavity.[16] Today, the understanding of how the human microbiome and saliva are responsible for oral and general health is one of the most relevant topics for researchers and is filling the front pages of mass media[17] (Fig 2-2).

One thing remains unchanged; the homeostasis of the oral cavity is maintained by saliva, essential for a balanced and symbiotic relationship between human microbiome and the host. Saliva is key to oral and oropharyngeal health and therefore to general health. Saliva's outstanding physiologic properties constitute the first line of defense of the oral cavity against pathogens as well as chemical and physical challenges.

Microbiome and microbiota are sometimes used as synonyms. *Microbiota* means the set of microorganisms comprising bacteria, fungi, archaea, viruses, and parasites that live in or on our body, while *microbiome* is a wider term that refers to the whole habitat, including not only microorganisms but also their genes, metabolites, and ecosystem. This invisible-to-the-eye architectural 3D structure relies on an extracellular matrix that serves as a physicochemical scaffold for the biofilms and is key to the onset of dysbiosis and the recovery of health (eubiosis). This scaffold not only has chemical properties but also physically contributes to the shape of this universe, providing protection from environmental offenses such as changes in humidity, pH shifts, temperature oscillation, antiseptics, antibacterial agents, and stress, among others.

Saliva is fundamental for eubiosis (Figs 2-3 and 2-4).

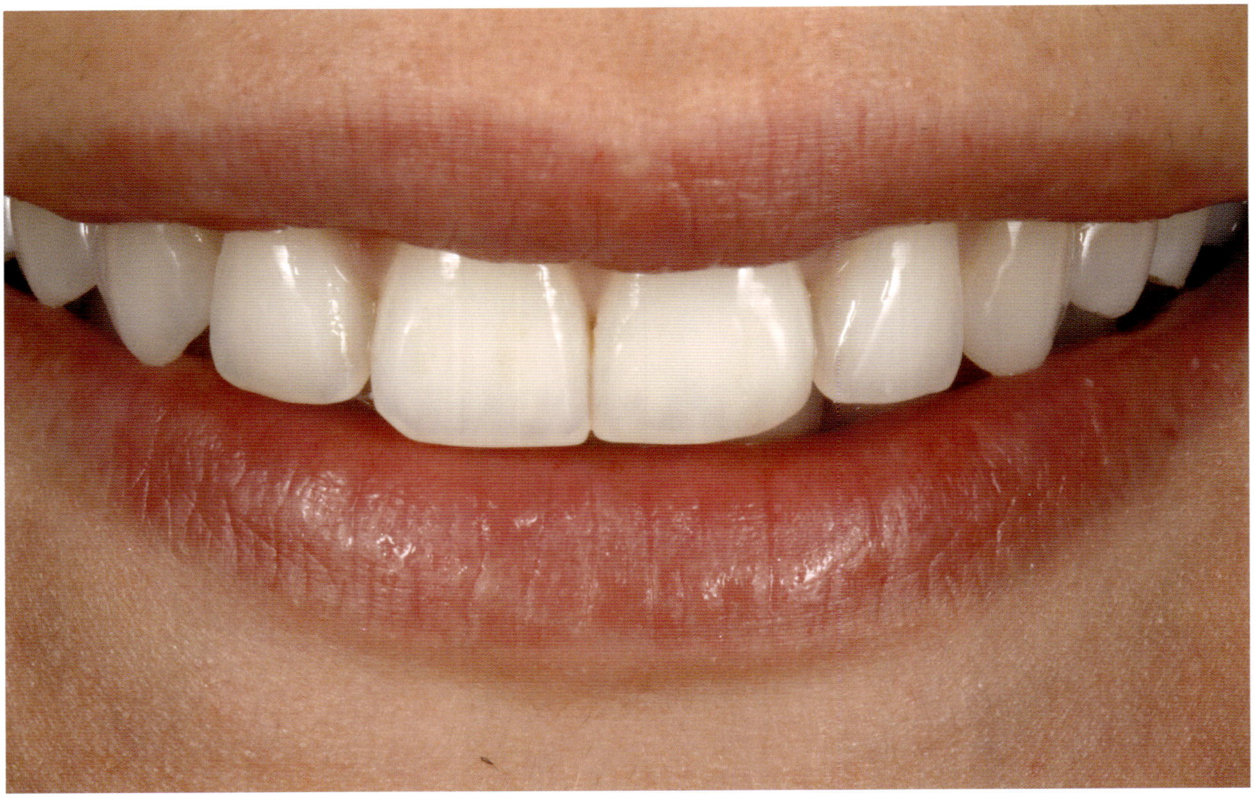

**Fig 2-3** Saliva protects the human microbiome and the teeth from erosion and caries, while simultaneously safeguarding the integrity of the mucosal barrier in both the digestive and respiratory systems. A healthy mouth helps prevent numerous conditions and/or diseases, both communicable and noncommunicable.

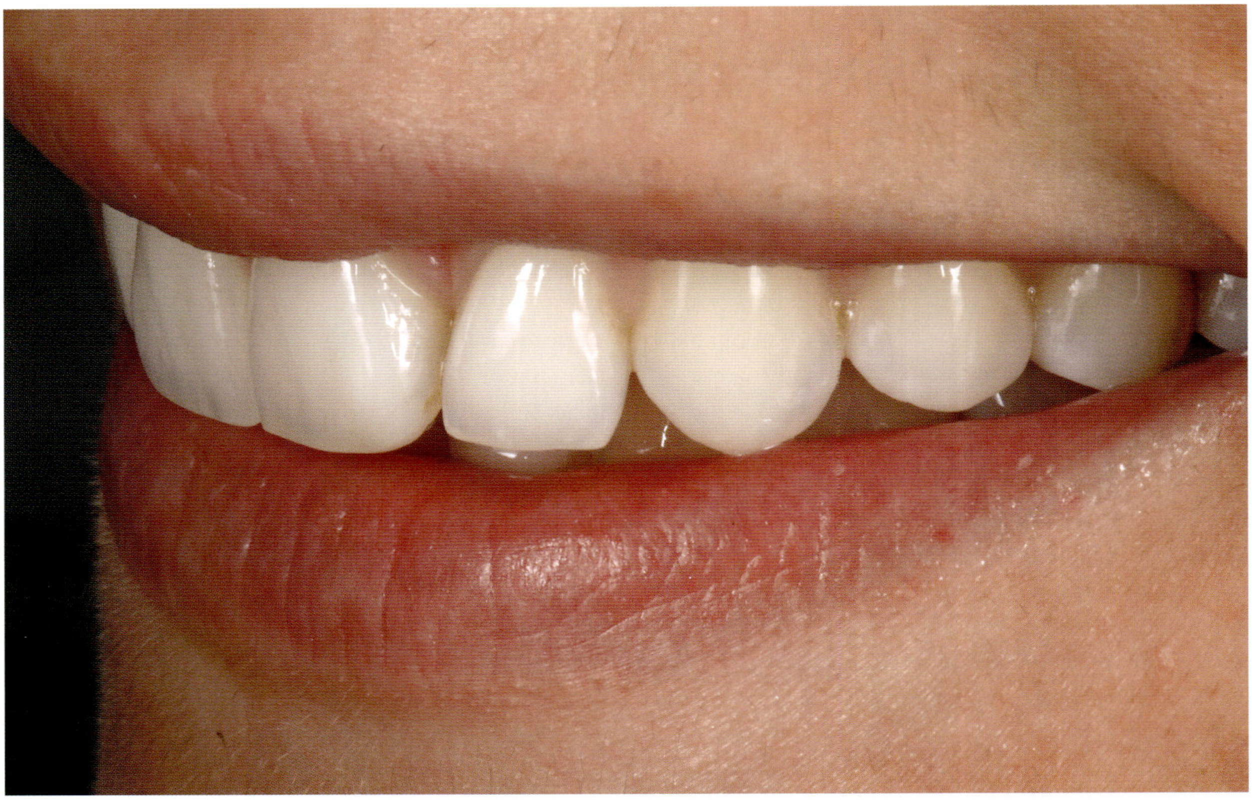

**Fig 2-4** A sufficient salivary flow is indispensable for oral homeostasis. In cases of hyposalivation a cascade of dysbiosis will disrupt the oral balance.

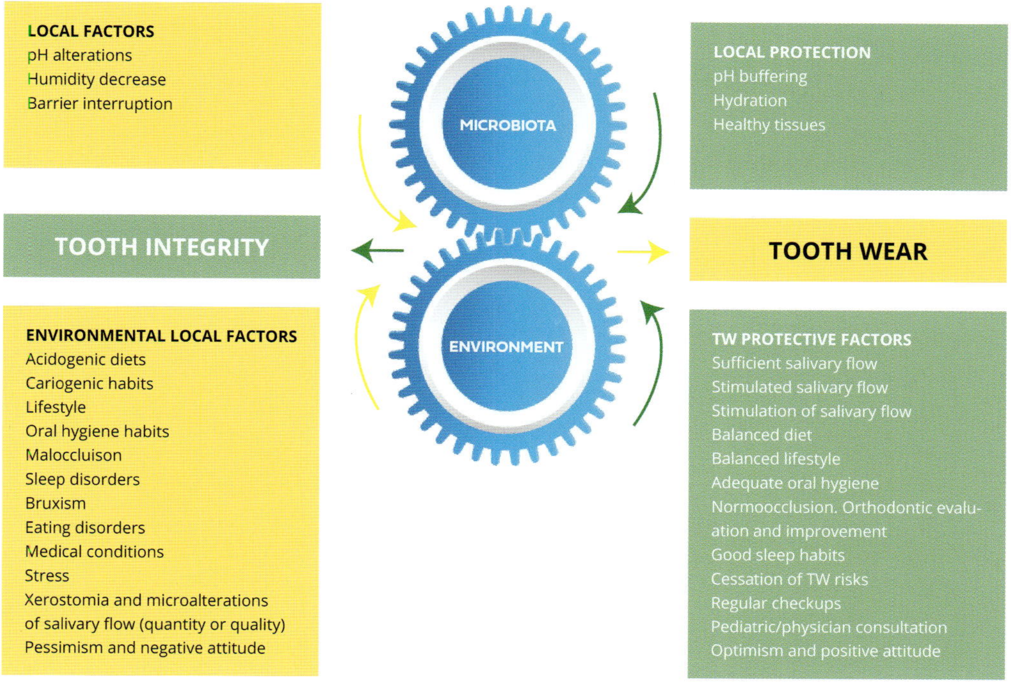


**Fig 2-5** The vicious circle of dysbiosis associated with TW illustrates the interrelationship between tooth integrity and tooth wear as a result of the fine tuning between a shift in microbiota (individually composed acquired pellicle) and an environmental shift (eg, inflammation, acidification, antibacterial agents). The more TW and tooth structure loss, the bigger the challenge to the oral microbiota, which find flatter and altered dental surfaces to which to attach. In advanced cases of TW, loss of interproximal areas follows the disappearance of all occlusal surfaces with the loss of specific microbiota habitats. Finally, mastication is impaired, with a shift toward a softer diet and further loss of teeth and more profound oral dysbiosis.

## 3. Saliva, the Oral Microbiome, and Tooth Wear

Recent research in the oral cavity is consistent with the finding that oral dysbiosis and a dysbiotic biofilm is behind common highly prevalent diseases like caries and periodontitis. Teeth have their own microbiome that protects them from challenges via symbiosis. At the same time, teeth themselves, when healthy, are a barrier to the maxillary bones from the moment they penetrate the oral mucosa during eruption. When eventually a tooth is lost, mucosa takes its place and closes the gap because the barrier function is mandatory for human survival. Both the tooth and its microbiome are in different compartments, physicochemically attached to one another, and the integrity of both compartments is mandatory for health and the barrier function. When the microbiome is damaged, the separation and integrity of both compartments is lost or disrupted, and a new dysbiotic relationship between the host and the microbiome leads to a nonsymbiotic inflammatory condition (periodontitis) and/or increased tooth permeability (hypersensitivity, demineralization, and loss of tooth structure). Tooth surfaces are protected against acids by proteins, enzymes, lipids, and carbohydrates, among others. When the eubiotic microbiome is lost, disrupted, or damaged, the barrier of the tooth is lost. Hypersensitivity, demineralization, caries, and tooth wear either of physical, chemical, or mixed origin occur (ie, bruxism, erosion, abfraction, or attrition). The disrupted microbiome barrier stops acting as a lipophilic shield, and teeth start to dissolve in the acidic or extremely acidic media. Every mouth is different. The mineral content of teeth and the thickness of the enamel also vary between individuals. In vitro research conditions have ignored the living microbes, their ecosystem, and saliva (microbiome) that may well be the major reservoir of minerals, water, peptides, and proprietary metabolism that stop and prevent the human teeth from dissolving. When teeth are physically ground and worn down, the habitat is changed as the initially hidden dentin emerges, providing an altered support for the microbiome that causes dysbiosis. Once this is established, the microbiome loses its attachment surface with the progression of TW; therefore, as TW increases, protection from the microbiome decreases[18] (Fig 2-5).

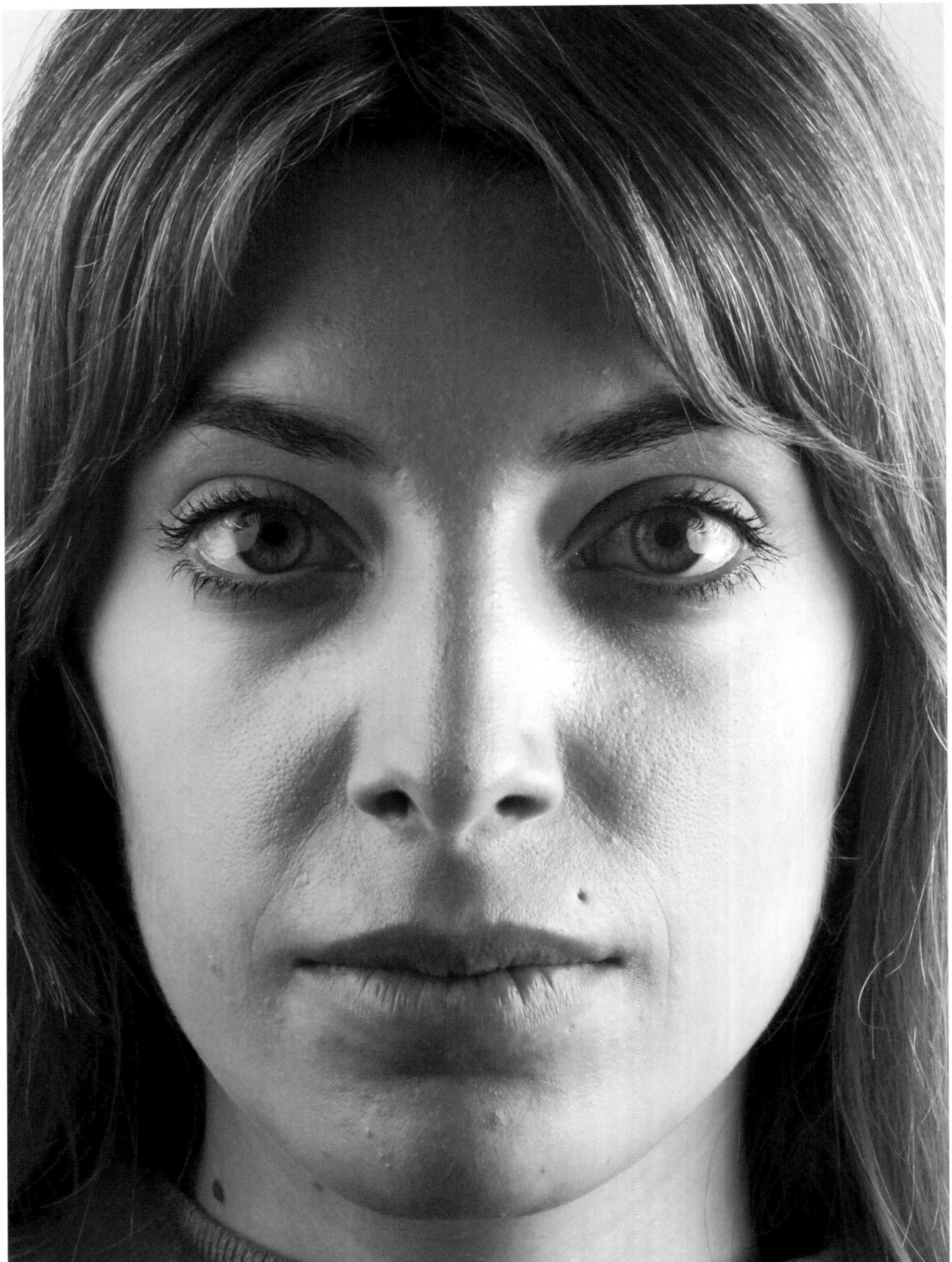

**Fig 2-6** The smile is a unique human feature, a communication tool with powerful implications. The smile is connected with central neurologic functions and is a reflection of the psychologic characteristics of the person. Billions of neurons and myocytes otherwise at rest are activated before smiling.

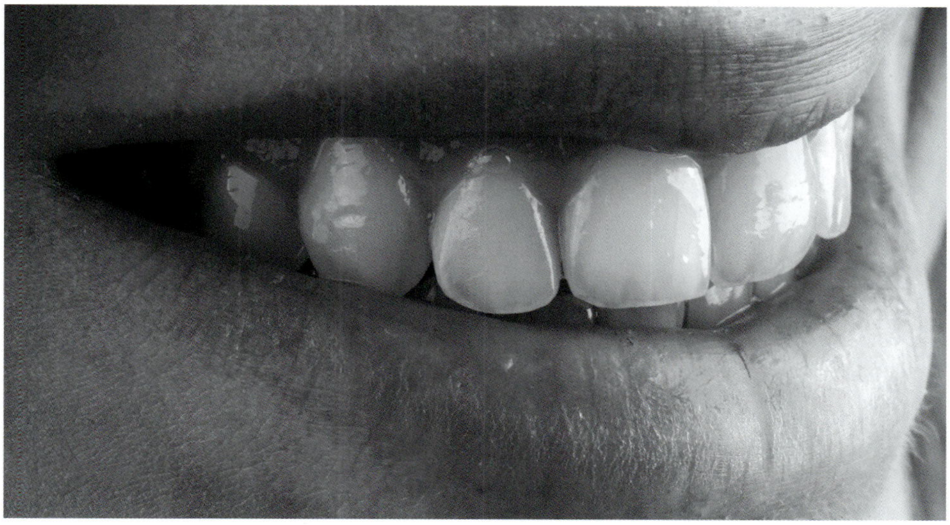

**Fig 2-7** The abundance of saliva in a healthy young female maintains oral equilibrium.

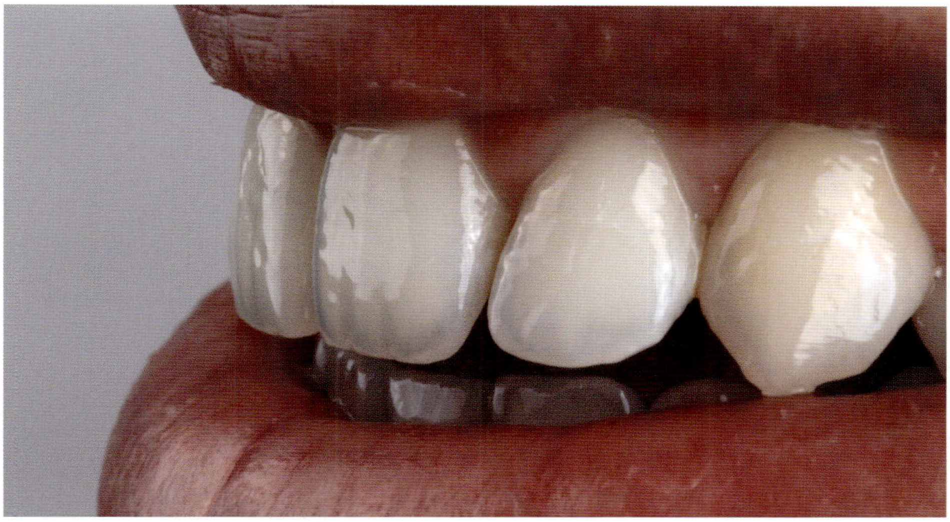

**Fig 2-8** Mountains, cathedrals, stones, and dissolve in water. Teeth would also if it were not for saliva. Saliva plays a key role in assuring the existence of the unique enamel topography, microhardness, and optical properties.

Saliva is a unique biologic exocrine fluid that plays a critical role in the preservation of oropharyngeal health. Saliva protects teeth from erosion and caries while simultaneously safeguarding mucosa from the disruption and the intrusion of pathogens. Saliva has been called the "microbial curator" and "gatekeeper of the oral cavity" as a result of the important role it plays in defending the body from the intrusion of microbes.[19] The ultimate role of saliva is defensive, against either pathogens or acids, a defense that may be neither effective nor sufficient if the threat is considerable or sustained. In patients with salivary gland disruption, which can be understood to be either an altered salivary composition or a diminution of salivary flow, hyposalivation, xerostomia, or dry mouth syndrome, the defensive capacity will be lower. In conditions where salivary flow is diminished or the composition of saliva is altered, there is a microbial shift and/or an environmental change leading to an increased risk of caries, erosion, tooth wear, gingivitis, and respiratory infections.[20] In otherwise healthy individuals, dental caries usually takes years to develop. However, this is not the case in individuals with chronic low salivary flow disturbance, in whom it can happen over the course of months. This is the case with diabetes patients reported to have decreased salivary flow and a change in salivary composition, which leads to a higher risk of caries as well as periodontal and other bacterial infections.[21,22]

When saliva is altered or missing, the aspect of the teeth changes, and this has an impact on the smile (Figs 2-6 to 2-10).

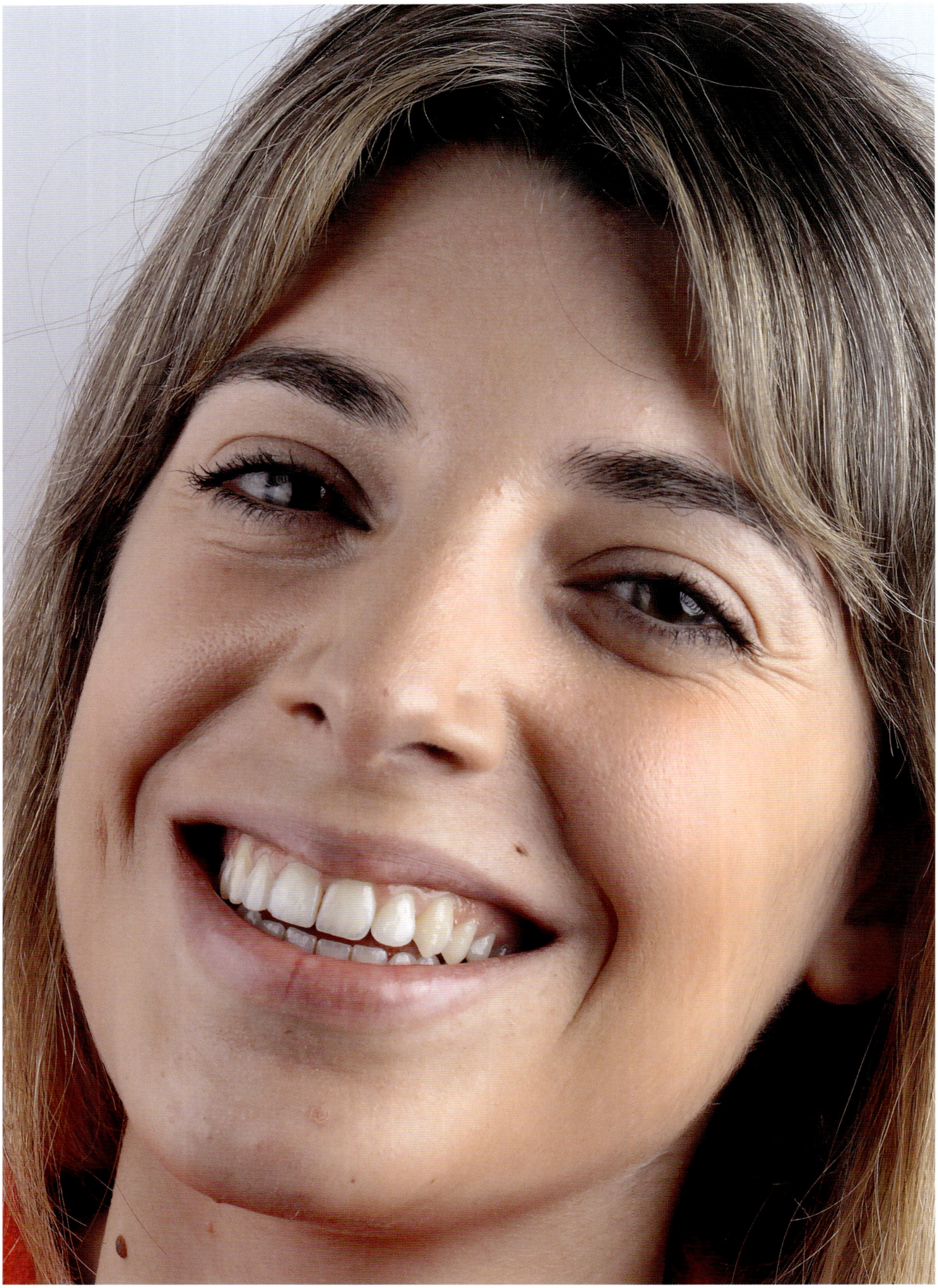

**Fig 2-9** The role of the smile and its self-perceived attractiveness are able to sculpt personality traits.

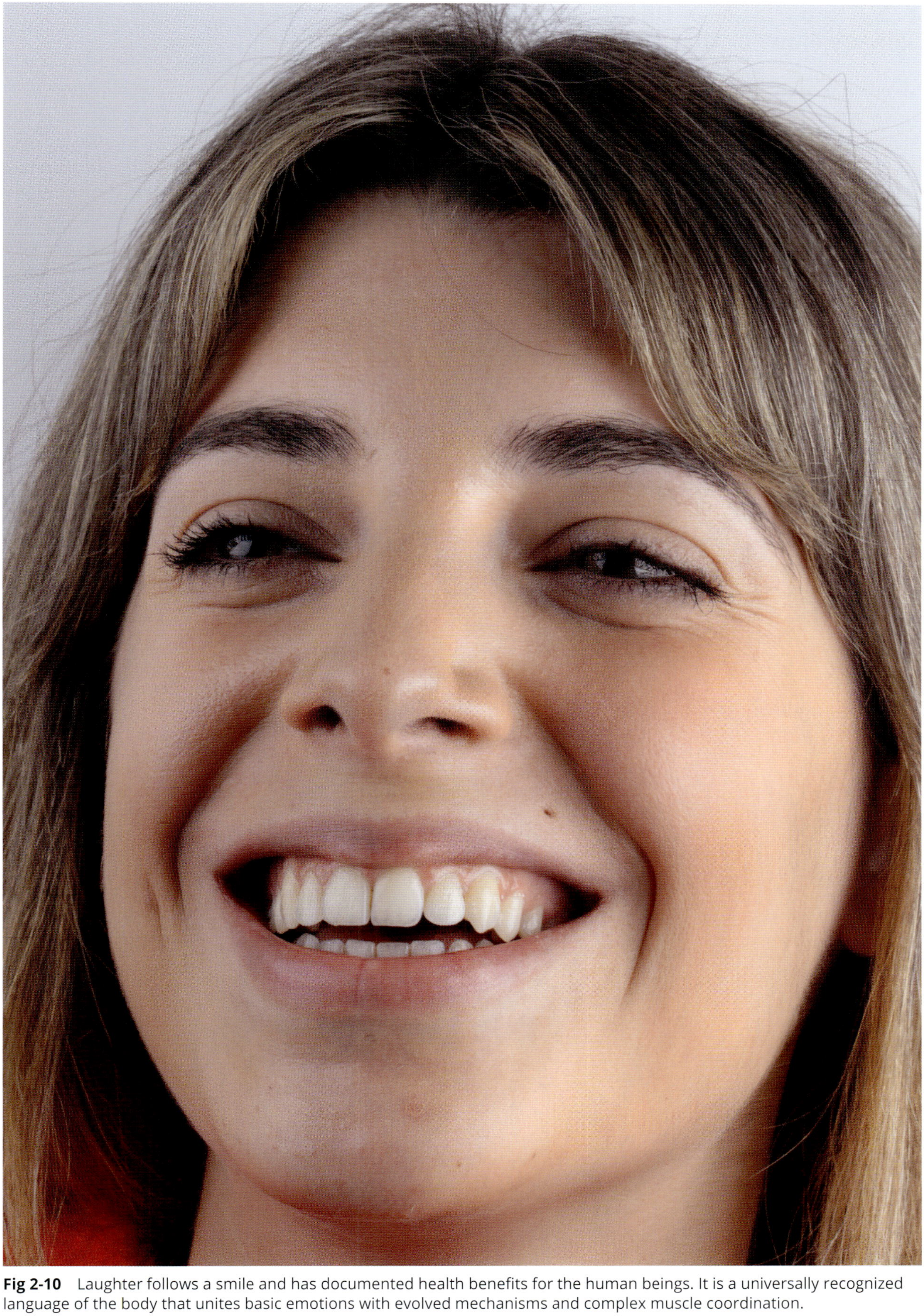

**Fig 2-10** Laughter follows a smile and has documented health benefits for the human beings. It is a universally recognized language of the body that unites basic emotions with evolved mechanisms and complex muscle coordination.

## 4. The Importance of Unstimulated Salivary Flow for the TW Patient

Saliva is not an ultrafiltrate of plasma. Total saliva produced daily varies from 0.6 to 1.5 L, with 20% coming from major salivary glands (parotids), 65% from submandibular glands, 8% from sublingual glands, and less than 10% from minor glands. There are two kinds of saliva in terms of origin. The first, originating in the major glands, is called stimulated salivary flow (SSF) and is secreted mainly after stimuli like chewing, taste and olfactory. The second is called unstimulated salivary flow (USF), also known as resting saliva, and is produced in minor glands scattered mostly throughout cheeks, lower lip, palate, and pharynx. Paradoxically, the secretion from minor salivary glands (USF) is more important in terms of its protective components, namely proteins, calcium, and phosphates, which are indispensable for the mineral homeostasis of the teeth. The proteins in saliva, together with the mineral ions, are the agents of USF protection against erosion (Fig 2-11).

While these two distinct flows (USF and SSF) vary in volume, origin, composition, and function, one system usually stimulates the other, and therefore separation of the two flows cannot be absolute. Thus, we arrive at the term *whole salivary flow*. In fact, both types of salivary flow, unstimulated and stimulated, work redundantly. An example of this is the three major systems that contribute to the buffer capacity of saliva: bicarbonate excreted by SSF, phosphate, and proteins, the latter two pertaining to the USF; all of them work differently but coordinately in a healthy individual to protect teeth from acidic challenges, whether bacterial or nonbacterial. Moreover, saliva's hypotonicity (99% is water) is essential for taste, known to additionally stimulate saliva production, creating a positive feedback loop for more saliva secretion and increased tooth and mucosa protection (Fig 2-12).

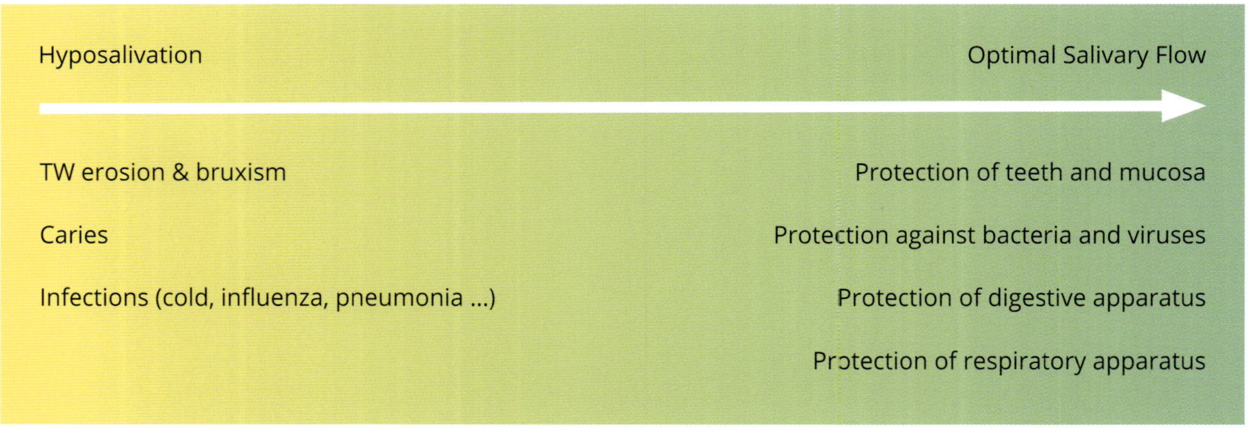


**Fig 2-11** Hyposalivation versus optimal salivary flow. Schematic representation of salivary flow volume and its consequences.

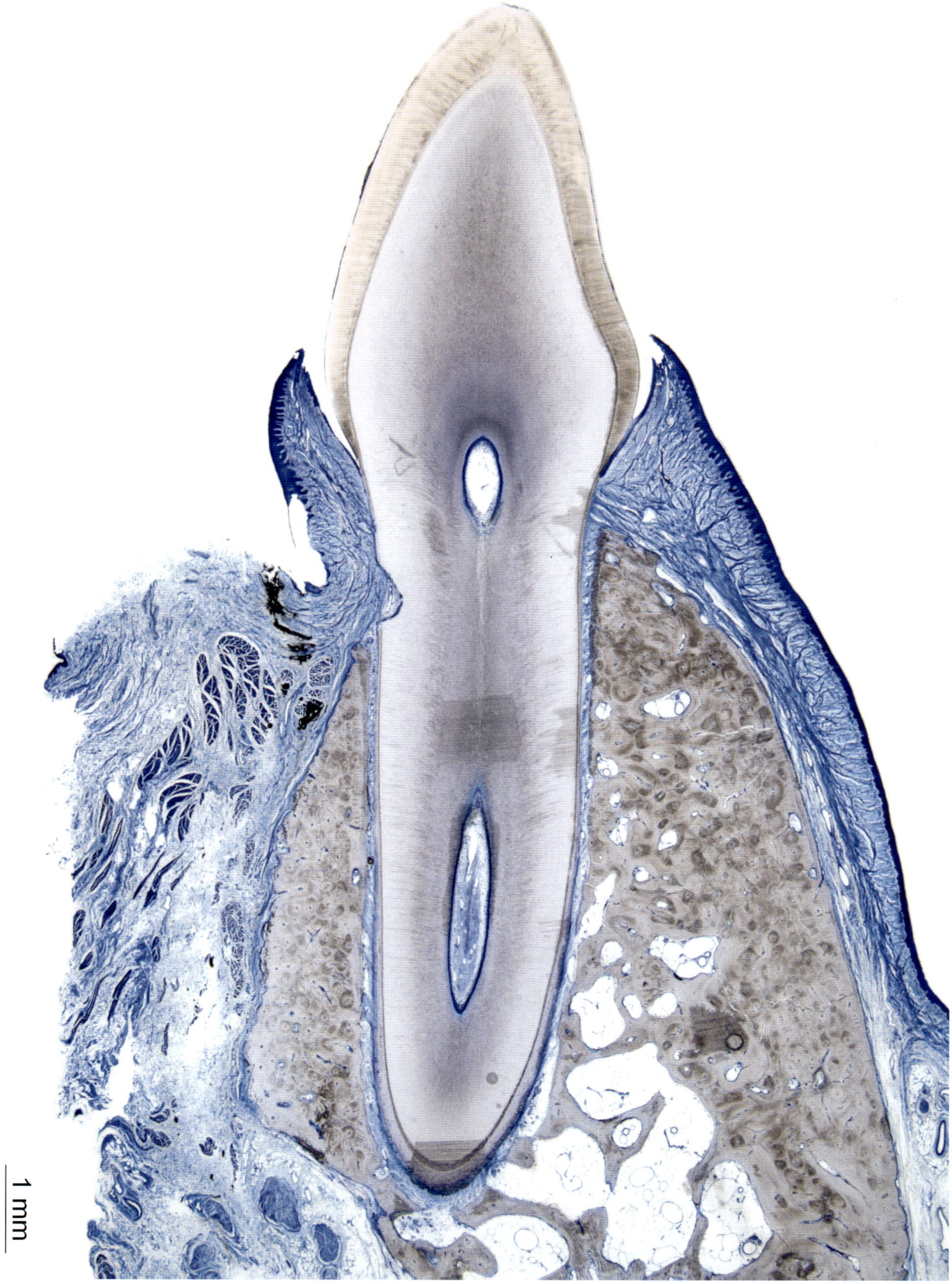


**Fig 2-12** Despite the fact that enamel is the hardest tissue of the body, it performs as a semipermeable membrane, allowing the passage of certain molecules. Formed mainly by inorganic content in the form of hydroxyapatite, its beauty relies upon its translucent characteristics. Saliva is key in providing enamel protection.

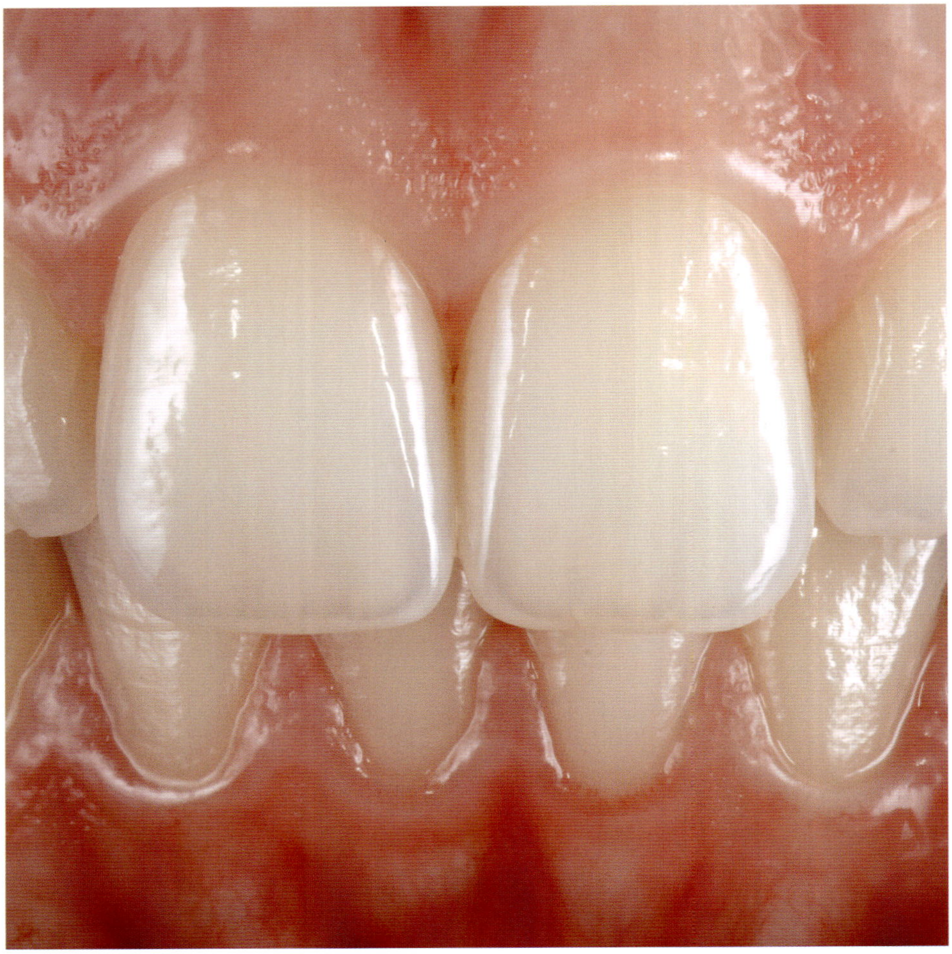

**Fig 2-13** The amount of saliva, oral health, and general health are intrinsically interrelated. Saliva maintains the healthy teeth, gingiva, and mucosa of an 18-year-old patient. When saliva is altered or diminished, the esthetic appearance and functional performance of the smile and dentition are in danger.

## 5. Saliva and Erosion

Saliva plays a fundamental role in enamel and dentin homeostasis. Saliva dilutes acids, oxidants, and noxious substances (Fig 2-13).

Salivary clearance of acids and other dangerous agents through swallowing, together with food, microbes, cells, and debris, is directly parallel to the amount of saliva. On the other hand, acid stimulates saliva, and saliva contains bicarbonate that buffers oral pH. Unstimulated saliva contains calcium and phosphate, therefore providing a supersaturated milieu that enables mineral gain by the tooth. Natural saliva has other specific functions linked mainly to USF against acid, as it forms a glycoproteic physicochemical protective layer attached to enamel and dentin surfaces. This hydrogel-like coating is permeable for mineral deposition whilst at the same time being an active barrier against acid. The amount of minerals, ions, or proteins is directly correlated to the amount of flow.

Conversely, a decreased salivary flow rate, especially USF, is associated not only with fewer defensive-type glycoproteins, enzymes, and immunoglobulins, but also with a low pH of saliva and decreased buffering capacity. It has been shown that a low salivary flow rate and low buffering capacity are strongly associated with dental erosion, even in children.[23] A review of dental erosion indicates that it may affect children at a rate ranging from 10% to 80%.[24] Erosion affects all ages and has a progressive course (Fig 2-14).

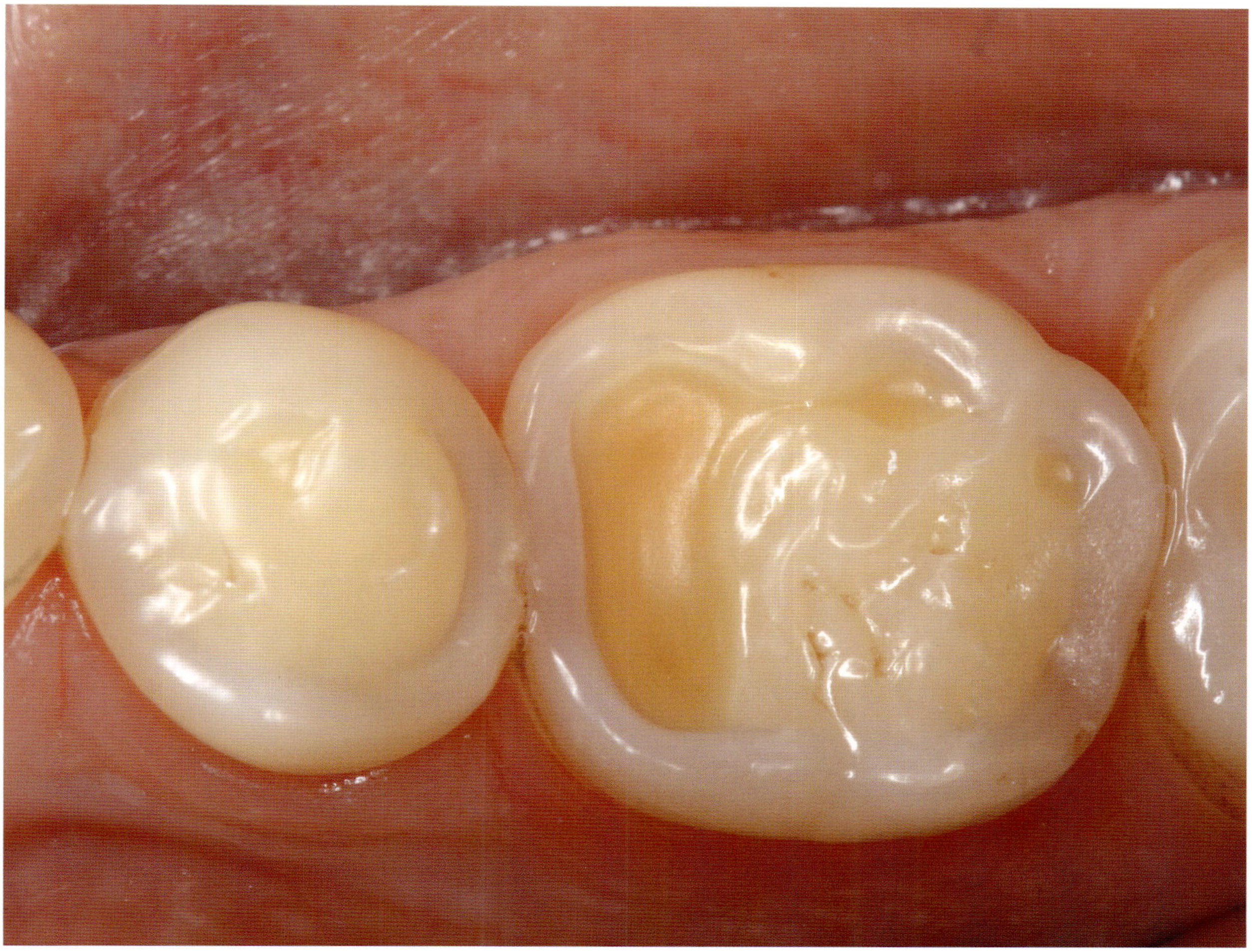

**Fig 2-14** Severe erosive lesions in an 18-year-old male patient with asthma showing enamel loss and dentin exposure. The patient had been on beta-2 agonists that have been reported to cause xerostomia. Additionally, bronchodilators reportedly provoke relaxation of the esophageal sphincter, which may explain the appearance of GERD in this young group of patients. Moreover, low pH aerosols contribute to severe TW, which might be difficult to understand without considering the micro-mechanisms by which saliva and strong, sustained acidic challenge are implicated. Characteristic erosive lesions with enamel halo surrounding the teeth can be observed. First molars often exhibit more profound erosive damage when compared to the surrounding teeth, giving an indirect date of an early-age erosive challenge.

In the case shown in Fig 2-15, a dysbiotic environment caused by tobacco, stress, and anxiety has facilitated erosive TW and atypical caries associated with severe hyposalivation. Special attention should be given to patients diagnosed with noncommunicable diseases such as cancer, diabetes, and psychologic disorders. Palatal enamel dissolution is leading to dentin exposure in this young female patient in her early 20s with a history of intense and long-standing stress, tobacco use, and anxiety (Fig 2-15a).

The buccal aspects of the mandibular incisors look as if they have been affected by incisal wear (Fig 2-15b). When looking from an occlusal angle, rampant atypical caries is seen in a location where caries is seldom found. Under normal conditions, salivary flow ejected from the sublingual glands onto the lingual and incisal aspect of the mandibular incisors, together with the cleansing movement from the tongue, provides extraordinary caries protection. Thus, the appearance of caries in such a location can only be understood when taking into consideration the stress and associated medication-related hyposalivation, also linked to erosive signs throughout the dentition (Fig 2-15c). Palatal partial indirect restorations, in this case feldspathic porcelain, were delivered, providing protection from the ongoing uncontrolled erosive challenge (Fig 2-15d).

Erosion can be neither inhibited nor prevented totally with the use of fluorides in typical daily dosages; there is an increasing demand for identifying chemical agents or components that might have anti-erosive potential or

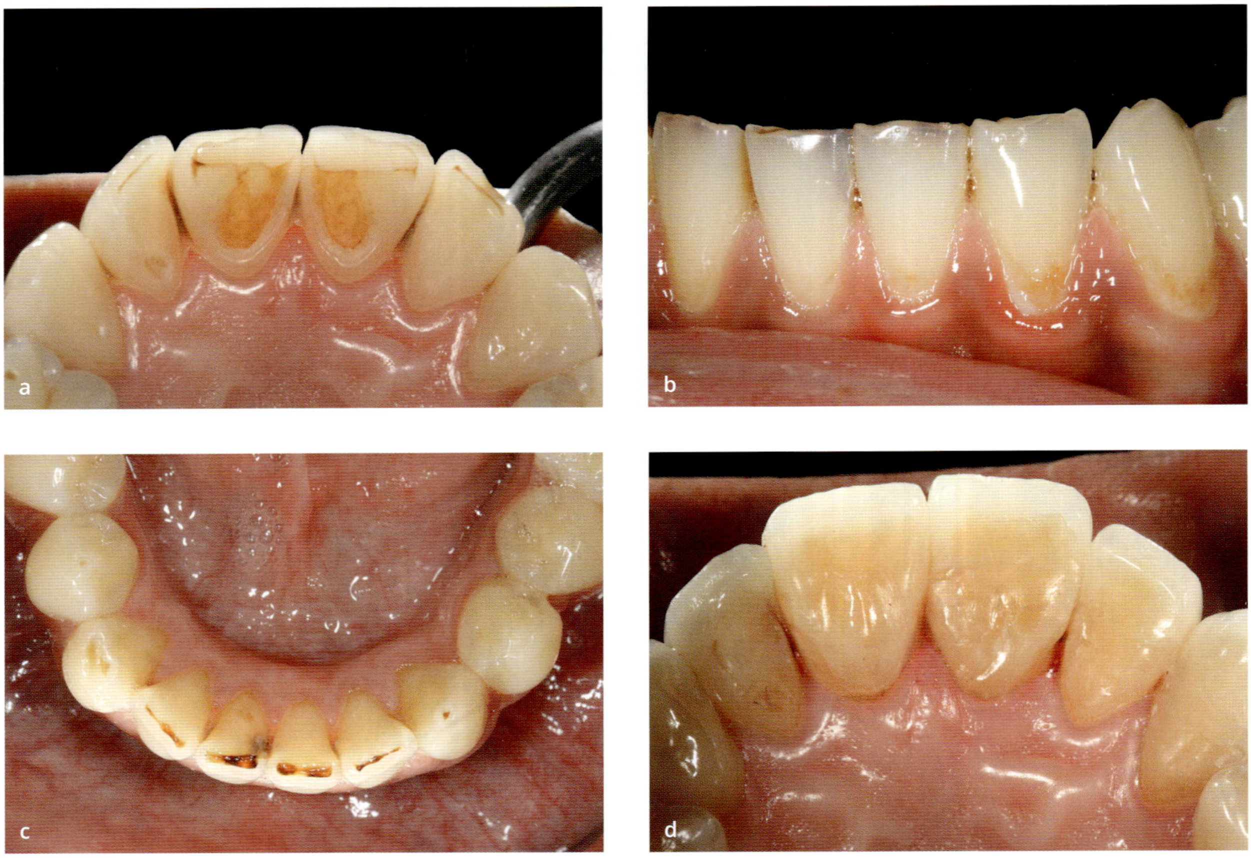


**Fig 2-15** While TW is described as nonbacterial TSL, the role of microbiome, microbiota, and the environment in the protection of the teeth is of paramount importance (a to d).

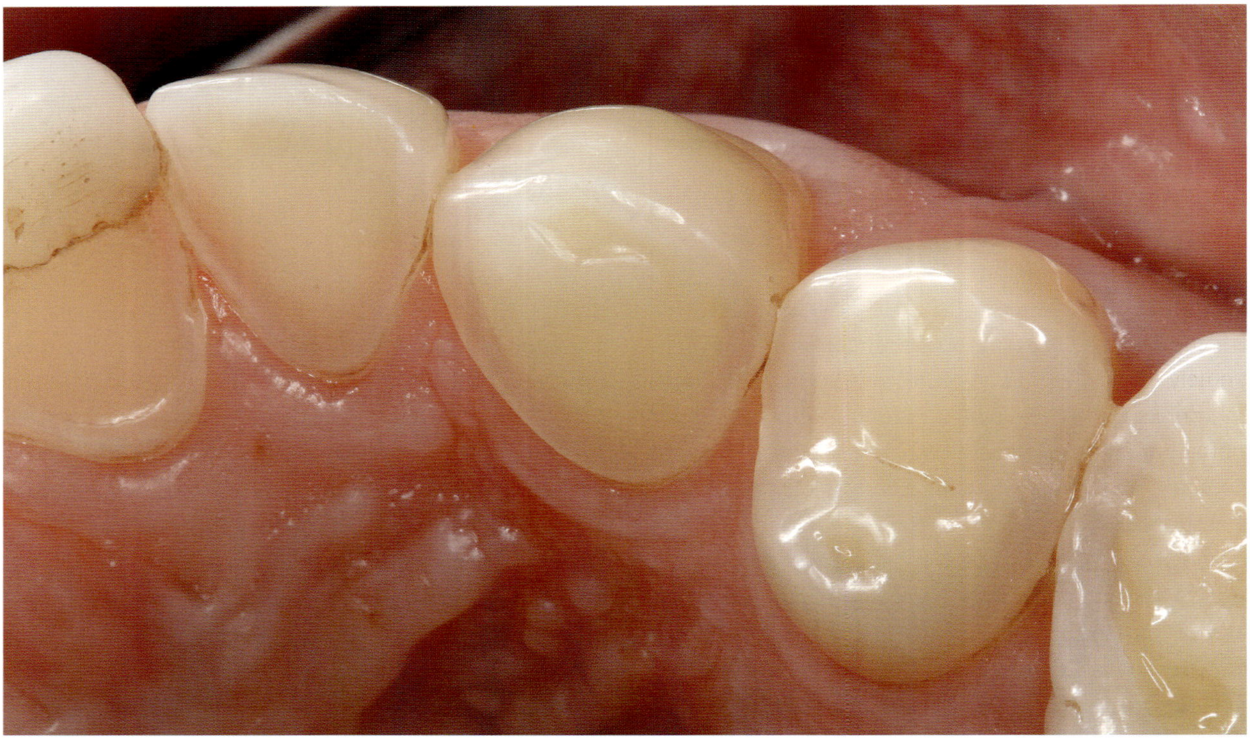

**Fig 2-16** Palatal surface of maxillary incisors and canine showing dissolution of enamel surface due to acid impact in a very young male patient who declares that compulsive intake of soda drinks is the only possible risk factor of erosion. See how the enamel margin is maintained at the gingival margin, probably due to the protective effect of the crevicular fluid and proteins.

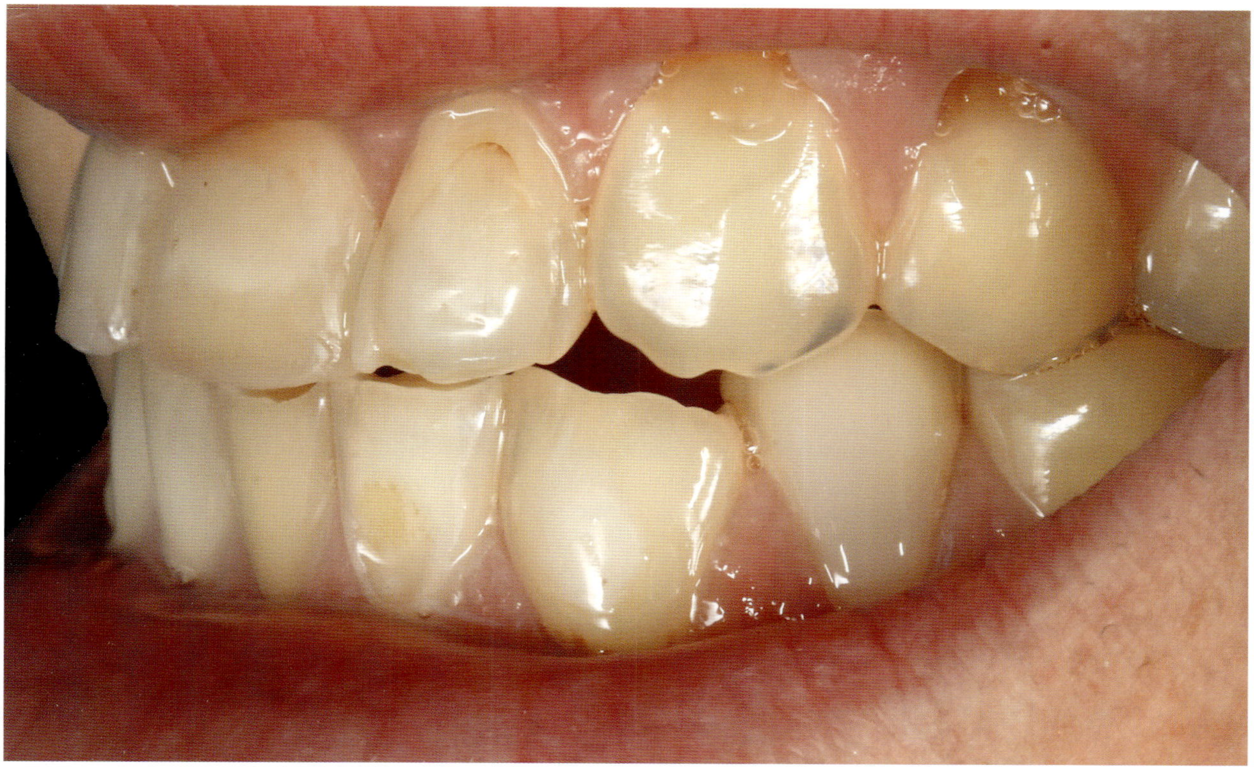

**Fig 2-17** Lifestyle and so-called healthy diets are related to the increase of erosive TW in developed countries. Citrus fruits and soda drinks, when in excess, may have a destructive impact on the tooth surface. It is of paramount importance that the general practitioner and the TW team are aware of the hidden mechanisms behind TW as all involved in the management of these conditions need to consider a potentiation of natural salivary flow as fluoride alone seems to have a rather grim future in terms of defending against TW.

increase the anti-erosive potential of oral hygiene products, especially in patients suffering from dry mouth or from very acidic challenges. Most soft drinks on the US market have a pH equal to or lower than 3 (erosive or extremely erosive), leading to an exponential increase in enamel loss with a pH nearing 2 (Fig 2-16). Moreover, authors like Larsen have shown that fluoride is unable to reduce erosion from soft drinks. Fluoride, and its combinations in concentrations with non-toxicologic side effects, seems unable to reduce erosive lesions. In extremely acidic erosive environments like those found in soft drinks, with a pH around 3 or lower, fluoride seems ineffective even in concentrations of 20 ppm.[25]

For all these reasons, there is a general consensus that stimulating salivary flow, increasing both quality and quantity of saliva and its buffer capacity, plays an important role in preventing and minimizing the effects of erosion on enamel and dentin wear. As the number of proteins and amount of minerals excreted to the mouth increase in the same proportion as USF, evidence supports that a direct impact can be expected in defensive and anti-erosive capacity, and thus, all efforts should be made to increase salivary flow.[26]

## 6. The Critical pH

Contrary to what was accepted at the beginning of the 21st century, there is no fixed pH beyond which enamel dissolves.[27] The initial reference of a critical pH of 5.5 was soon obsolete as such a critical number depends on the acidity of the solution to which teeth are exposed, the acidity of dental plaque, the amount of minerals both in the solution and the teeth, and the number of proteins that bind minerals to the acquired dental pellicle. Other variables to be considered are time, circadian rhythm and its relationship with the salivary challenge (acid at night will be devastating to teeth as there is no saliva in the mouth), and type of diet (Fig 2-17).

Teeth will dissolve in any solution that does not contain calcium and phosphate, including water, even though water is neutral with a pH of 7. The fact that USF is supersaturated in these two ions prevents teeth from dissolving in the presence of saliva at least until the critical pH is reached. The confluence of other variables like amount of salivary flow and mineral saturation of saliva explains why some teeth will resist better than others. When USF is diminished, the amount of calcium and phosphate ions

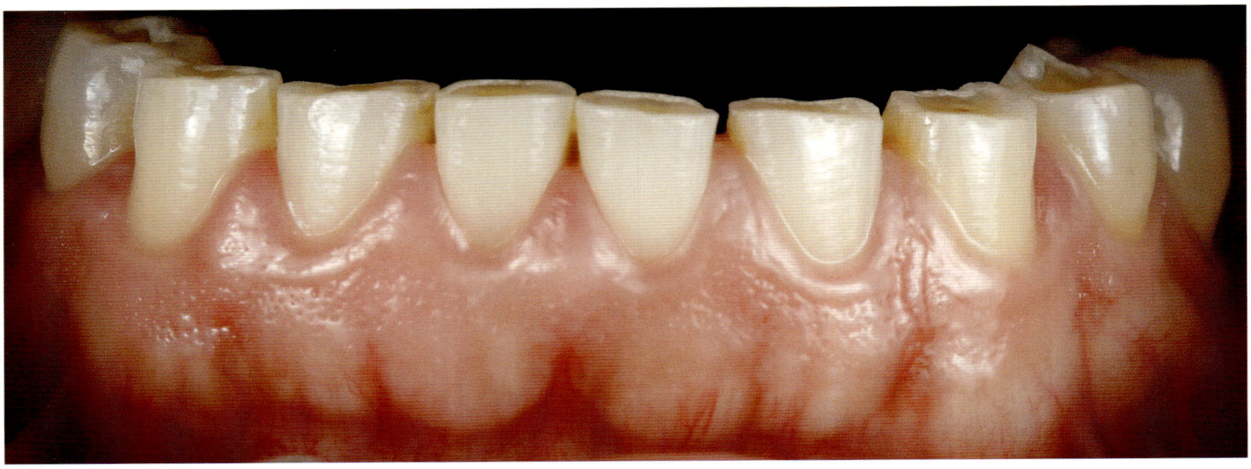

**Fig 2-18** Mandibular arch of a 40-year-old high-powered businessman, whose partner in life reports a lot of "noise" during the night. He has had a stressful life with a very demanding job and poor sleep for the last 15 years.

is also lower, and the critical pH for teeth to demineralize does not need to be as low as pH 5.1 to be harmful[27] (see Fig 2-17).

In other words, when USF is decreased or altered, a critical pH as close to neutrality as 6.5 may cause enamel loss. A decreased salivary flow rate, especially USF, is associated with a low pH of saliva and decreased buffering capacity. Recently, a pioneer study found that an increased number of salivary proteins in the acquired enamel pellicle might be protecting some patients affected by GERD who incomprehensibly had no erosion of their teeth.[28]

As aforementioned, the fundamental role of fluoride in caries prevention should not be taken for granted in managing tooth erosion.[29] In view of the abundant research, promoting the natural protection from saliva seems, alternatively, a wise approach.

## 7. Bruxism and Saliva

Individual personality traits with high self-demand are determinant factors that contribute to the appearance of nonfunctional (parafunctional) movements of the mandible with or without audible sound during the day or the night (Fig 2-18).

Certain authors have found signs of wear in bruxists, while others do not see such a determinant relationship. Hyposalivation or decreased saliva quality that serves poorly both as lubricant and protection from erosion may well explain these discrepancies.[30–35] Furthermore, the aforementioned authors have found that TW is not a reliable predictor of bruxism and conclude that if attrition lesions are seen in bruxism, it may well be because of the coexistence of acid tooth structure softening that facilitates a higher susceptibility to the parafunctional bruxist condition.[32]

The causes of sleep bruxism (SB) cannot be understood by single risk factors. Stressful lifestyles and anxiety are accounted as risk factors for SB. In adults, bruxism has proven to have a multifactorial origin, including alcohol, caffeine, smoking, insomnia, OSA, central neurologic disorders, and genetic-familial factors.

Bruxism has two circadian manifestations; it can appear during the night as SB or during wakefulness. The first is far more damaging to tooth structure as the saliva protection is scarce during the night.

The well-known saliva stimulation cycle is predominantly based in the mouth, pharynx, and esophagus and is switched on by peripheral sensory signals from taste and mechanoreceptors that are triggered by food and mastication. This process also involves higher brain centers and salivary centers of nuclei in the medulla. During sleep, oromotor activities such as phasic and tonic muscle movements may well be providing the fundamental lubrication for the oral cavity in the absence of mastication. The dryness of the oroesophageal tissues may act as a critical limit that stimulates the oromotor activity, causing the masticatory system to stimulate saliva secretion to lubricate the oral cavity. The precise mechanism is yet to be well understood.[36] The body of evidence is not yet sufficient to establish that SB is secondary to nighttime oral dryness. The cofactors of sleep disorders, OSA, xerostomia, and SB appear in an increasing number of studies. The cause and the consequence are not yet clear.

## 8. Improving Salivation: The Invisible Guard

Salivary gland hypofunction (SGH), otherwise referred to as hyposalivation or xerostomia/dry mouth disrupts the normal homeostasis of the oral cavity and alters the physicochemical balance between the teeth and the environment, leading to TSL and TW. It is the main kind of salivary gland dysfunction (SGD).

SGD is caused primarily by medications. In the extensive systematic review led by Harvard University for the World Workshop on Oral Medicine on the epidemiology of hyposalivation, the rate of the condition was found to be as high as 25% in medicated 32-year-olds, with 50% of adults taking antihypertensives and 70% of patients on antidepressants.[37–39]

A number of questionnaires have been proposed to determine the presence of SGD (hyposalivation and xerostomia). The simplest but most applicable in busy general practices like dental offices correlates well with major salivary gland output and consists of asking the following questions:

- Does the amount of saliva in your mouth seem to be too little, too much, or you do not notice it?
- Do you have any difficulty swallowing?
- Does your mouth feel dry when eating a meal?
- Do you sip liquids to aid in swallowing dry food?

A positive answer to all four was found to be associated with salivary gland hypofunction.[40]

The Fox questionnaire is short both for the patient and the investigator and may be employed effortlessly in the dental clinic when screening for TW-associated conditions.

Therapeutic strategies toward improving saliva flow and composition are good hydration, humidifiers, avoidance of irritating dentifrices and foods, and use of sugar-free chewing gums and saliva stimulants.

The important side effects of systemic sialagogues in patients with cardiac, respiratory, and ophthalmologic conditions as well as uncontrolled hypertension make them impractical for the dental professional. It is in the oral stimulation of saliva where the TW team should take a step forward.

Saliva stimulants based on acids such as malic or hyaluronic acid, among others, have been reported to potentially lead to enamel erosion, a critical issue in the TW population. Acidic preparations should not be prescribed to dentate patients, in whom hyposalivation implies an added risk for dental caries.[41]

Mucin-based spray showed controversial results with little evidence that the saliva substitute was more effective than placebo.[42]

Topical dry-mouth products containing olive oil, betaine, and xylitol have been found to be safe and effective in reducing xerostomia and increasing salivary flow in polymedicated patients.[43] This same composition was studied in a proof-of-principle study and found to offer protection against enamel and dentin erosion, even in the presence of severe erosive conditions. Even though this is an in vitro result, the authors state that it could be speculated that the protective effect might be more enhanced under less severe erosive conditions. Such conditions are present with the in vivo saliva potentiating effect that the previous clinical trial demonstrated. The synergistic potential anti-erosive and saliva-stimulant effect of this composition may be able to help prevent TSL in patients with TW at initial stages or during erosive cycles. In this same proof-of-principle study published in *Acta Odontologica Scandinavica*, the aforementioned composition was confronted with an acidic fluoridated solution that showed even higher protection against erosion due to, in view of the authors, its lower pH value. (The lower the pH, the higher the amount of fluoride dissociated available.) However, as the authors of the study state, it has to be taken into consideration that the acidic mouthrinse might induce an increase in mineral loss not suitable for patients suffering from hyposalivation and exhibiting initial lesions.[44]

A topical saliva stimulant should be free of side effects, both local (erosion derived from acidic and acid-containing formulations or caries from sugar-containing formulations) and systemic, while being able to increase the quantity and hence the quality of saliva, as has been highlighted.

The growing prevalence of hyposalivation certainly poses a challenge and may well be behind the increasing incidence of TW in first-world countries today.

## 9. Key Points

- Saliva is critical to the preservation and maintenance of all oral tissues.
- Saliva is described as the curator of oral health.
- Saliva and the oral microbiome are natural defenders of oral and general health.
- Oral dysbiosis is behind common and prevalent oral diseases. Teeth have their own microbiome that protects them from challenges.
- Once teeth are worn down the habitat is changed, with impaired support for the microbiome, and dysbiosis may appear.
- There is no standard critical pH at which enamel dissolves. Other factors such as the presence of saliva and the amount of minerals influence this measure.
- Safe and effective saliva stimulation is fundamental in the TW patient.

## References


1. Brennan DS, Spencer AJ, Roberts-Thomson KF. Tooth loss, chewing ability and quality of life. Qual Life Res 2008;17(2):227–235.
2. Imai S, Mansfield CJ. Oral health in North Carolina: Relationship with general health and behavioral risk factors. N C Med J 2015;76(3):142–147.
3. Brennan DS, Mittinty MM, Jamieson L. Psychosocial factors and self-reported transitions in oral and general health. Eur J Oral Sci 2019;127:241–247.
4. Brennan DS, Spencer AJ, Roberts-Thomson KF. Socioeconomic and psychosocial associations with oral health impact and general health. Community Dent Oral Epidemiol 2019;47(1):32–39.
5. Keuskamp D, Amarasena N, Balasubramanian M, Brennan DS. General health, wellbeing and oral health of patients older than 75 years attending health assessments. Aust J Prim Health 2018;24(2):177–182.
6. Brennan DS, Singh KA. General health and oral health self-ratings, and impact of oral problems among older adults. Eur J Oral Sci 2011;119:469–473.
7. Lira-Junior R, Boström EA. Oral-gut connection: One step closer to an integrated view of the gastrointestinal tract? Mucosal Immunol 2018;11(2):316–318.
8. du Teil Espina M, Gabarrini G, Harmsen HJM, Westra J, van Winkelhoff AJ, van Dijl JM. Talk to your gut: The oral-gut microbiome axis and its immunomodulatory role in the etiology of rheumatoid arthritis. FEMS Microbiol Rev 2019;43(1):1–18.
9. Gaeckle NT, Pragman AA, Pendleton KM, Baldomero AK, Criner GJ. The oral-lung axis: The impact of oral health on lung health. Respir Care 2020;65:1211–1220.
10. Bowe W, Patel NB, Logan AC. Acne vulgaris, probiotics and the gut-brain-skin axis: From anecdote to translational medicine. Benef Microbes 2014;5(2):185–199.
11. Lorenzo D, GianVincenzo Z, Carlo Luca R, et al. Oral-gut microbiota and arthritis: Is there an evidence-based axis? J Clin Med 2019;8(10).
12. Forkosh E, Ilan Y. The heart-gut axis: New target for atherosclerosis and congestive heart failure therapy. Open Heart 2019;6(1):e000993.
13. Acharya C, Sahingur SE, Bajaj JS. Microbiota, cirrhosis, and the emerging oral-gut-liver axis. JCI Insight 2017;2(19):e94416.
14. Amodio J, Palioto DB, Carrara HH, et al. Oral health after breast cancer treatment in postmenopausal women. Clinics (Sao Paulo) 2014;69:706–708.
15. Szántó M, Dózsa A, Antal D, Szabó K, Kemény L, Bai P. Targeting the gut-skin axis—Probiotics as new tools for skin disorder management? Exp Dermatol 2019;28:1210–1218.
16. Yamashita Y, Takeshita T. The oral microbiome and human health. J Oral Sci 2017;59(2):201–206.
17. Davis N. The human microbiome: Why our microbes could be key to our health. The Guardian 26 Mar 2018. https://www.theguardian.com/news/2018/mar/26/the-human-microbiome-why-our-microbes-could-be-key-to-our-health. Accessed 13 Jan 2022.
18. Hannig CM, Hannig M, Attin T. Enzymes in the acquired enamel pellicle. Eur J Oral Sci 2005;113(1):2–13.
19. Vila T, Rizk AM, Sultan AS, Jabra-Rizk MA. The power of saliva: Antimicrobial and beyond. PLoS Pathog, 2019;15(11):e1008058.
20. Dawes C, Pedersen AM, Villa A, et al. The functions of human saliva: A review sponsored by the World Workshop on Oral Medicine VI. Arch Oral Biol 2015;60(6):863–874.
21. Ferizi L, Dragidella F, Spahiu L, Begzati A, Kotori V. The influence of type 1 diabetes mellitus on dental caries and salivary composition. Int J Dent 2018;2018:5780916.
22. Amerongen AV, Veerman EC. Saliva—The defender of the oral cavity. Oral Dis 2002;8(1):12–22.
23. O'Sullivan EA, Curzon ME. Salivary factors affecting dental erosion in children. Caries Res 2000;34(1):82–87.
24. Reddy A, Norris DF, Momeni SS, Waldo B, Ruby JD. The pH of beverages in the United States. J Am Dent Assoc 2016;147:255–263.
25. Larsen MJ, Richards A. Fluoride is unable to reduce dental erosion from soft drinks. Caries Res 2002;36(1):75–80.
26. Villa A, Wolff A, Narayana N, et al. World Workshop on Oral Medicine VI: A systematic review of medication-induced salivary gland dysfunction. Oral Dis 2016;22:365–382.
27. Dawes C. What is the critical pH and why does a tooth dissolve in acid? J Can Dent Assoc 2003;69:722–724.
28. Martini T, Rios D, Cassiano LPS, et al. Proteomics of acquired pellicle in gastroesophageal reflux disease patients with or without erosive tooth wear. J Dent 2019;81:64–69.
29. Lussi A, Carvalho TS. The future of fluorides and other protective agents in erosion prevention. Caries Res 2015;49(Suppl 1):18–29.
30. Johansson A, Fareed K, Omar R. Analysis of possible factors influencing the occurrence of occlusal tooth wear in a young Saudi population. Acta Odontol Scand 1991;49(3):139–145.
31. Xhonga FA. Bruxism and its effect on the teeth. J Oral Rehabil 1977;4(1):65–76.
32. Khan F, Young WG, Daley TJ. Dental erosion and bruxism. A tooth wear analysis from south east Queensland. Aust Dent J 1998;43(2):117–127.
33. Fyhn AA. Why the Norwegian Nurses' Association says 'no' to nursing assistants in operating rooms. Interview by Bjorn Arild Ostby [in Norwegian]. Sykepleien 1988;76(1):20–22,24–25.
34. John MT, Frank H, Lobbezoo F, Drangsholt M, Dette KE. No association between incisal tooth wear and temporomandibular disorders. J Prosthet Dent 2002;87(2):197–203.
35. Abe S, Yamaguchi T, Rompré PH, De Grandmont P, Chen YJ, Lavigne GJ. Tooth wear in young subjects: A discriminator between sleep bruxers and controls? Int J Prosthodont 2009;22:342–350.
36. Thie NM, Kato T, Bader G, Montplaisir JY, Lavigne GJ. The significance of saliva during sleep and the relevance of oromotor movements. Sleep Med Rev 2002;6(3):213–227.
37. Murray Thomson W, Poulton R, Mark Broadbent J, Al-Kubaisy S. Xerostomia and medications among 32-year-olds. Acta Odontol Scand 2006;64:249–254.
38. Hasan SS, Keong SC, Choong CL, et al. Patient-reported adverse drug reactions and drug-drug interactions: A cross-sectional study on Malaysian HIV/AIDS patients. Med Princ Pract 2011;20(3):265–270.
39. Nonzee V, Manopatanakul S, Khovidhunkit SO. Xerostomia, hyposalivation and oral microbiota in patients using antihypertensive medications. J Med Assoc Thai 2012;95(1):96–104.
40. Fox PC, Busch KA, Baum BJ. Subjective reports of xerostomia and objective measures of salivary gland performance. J Am Dent Assoc 1987;115:581–584.
41. Villa A, Wolff A, Aframian D, et al. World Workshop on Oral Medicine VI: A systematic review of medication-induced salivary gland dysfunction: Prevalence, diagnosis, and treatment. Clin Oral Investig 2015;19:1563–1580.
42. Furness S, Worthington HV, Bryan G, Birchenough S, McMillan R. Interventions for the management of dry mouth: Topical therapies. Cochrane Database Syst Rev 2011;(12):CD008934.
43. Ship JA, McCutcheon JA, Spivakovsky S, Kerr AR. Safety and effectiveness of topical dry mouth products containing olive oil, betaine, and xylitol in reducing xerostomia for polypharmacy-induced dry mouth. J Oral Rehabil 2007;34:724–732.
44. Meyer-Lueckel H, Schulte-Mönting J, Kielbassa AM. The effect of commercially available saliva substitutes on predemineralized bovine dentin in vitro. Oral Dis 2002;8(4):192–198.

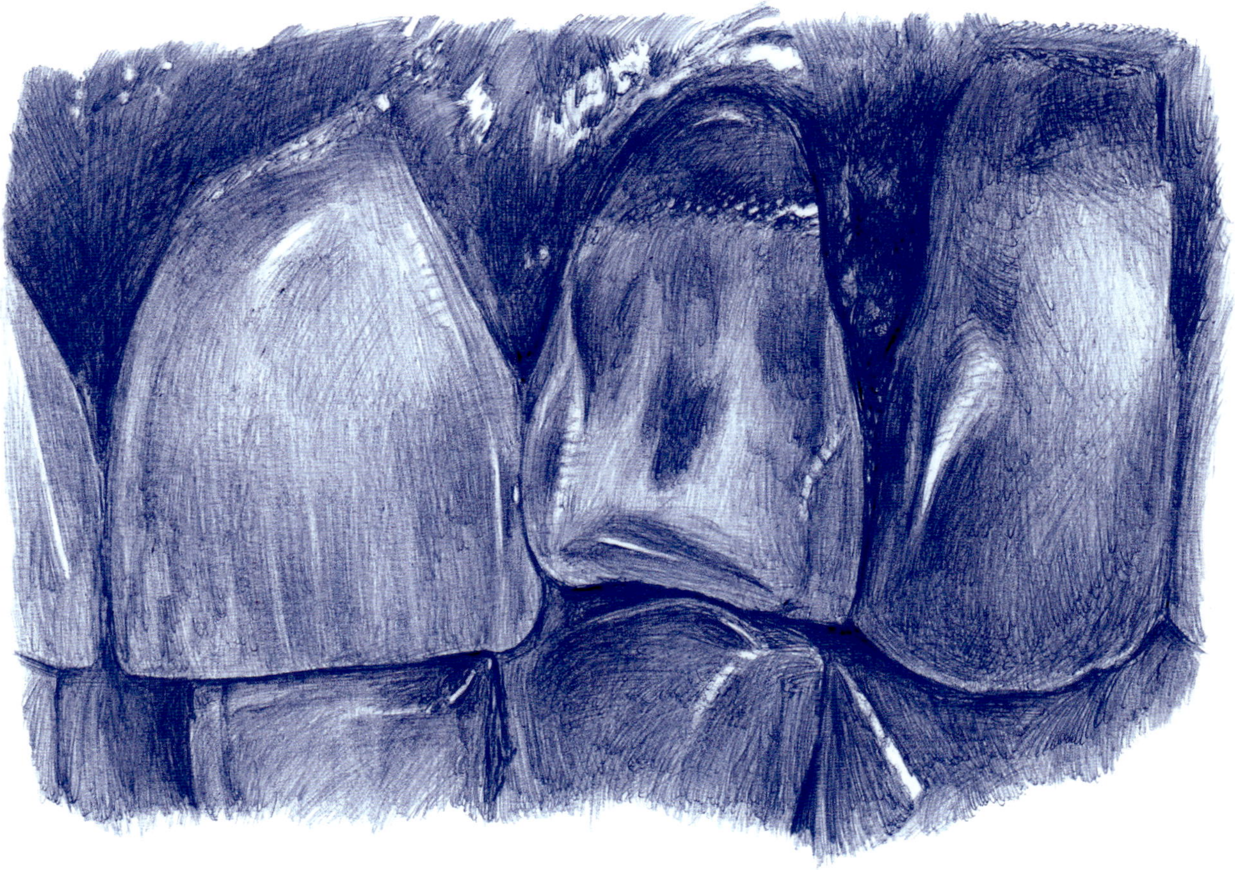

*He who has a why can endure any how.*

—Friedrich Nietzsche, German philosopher

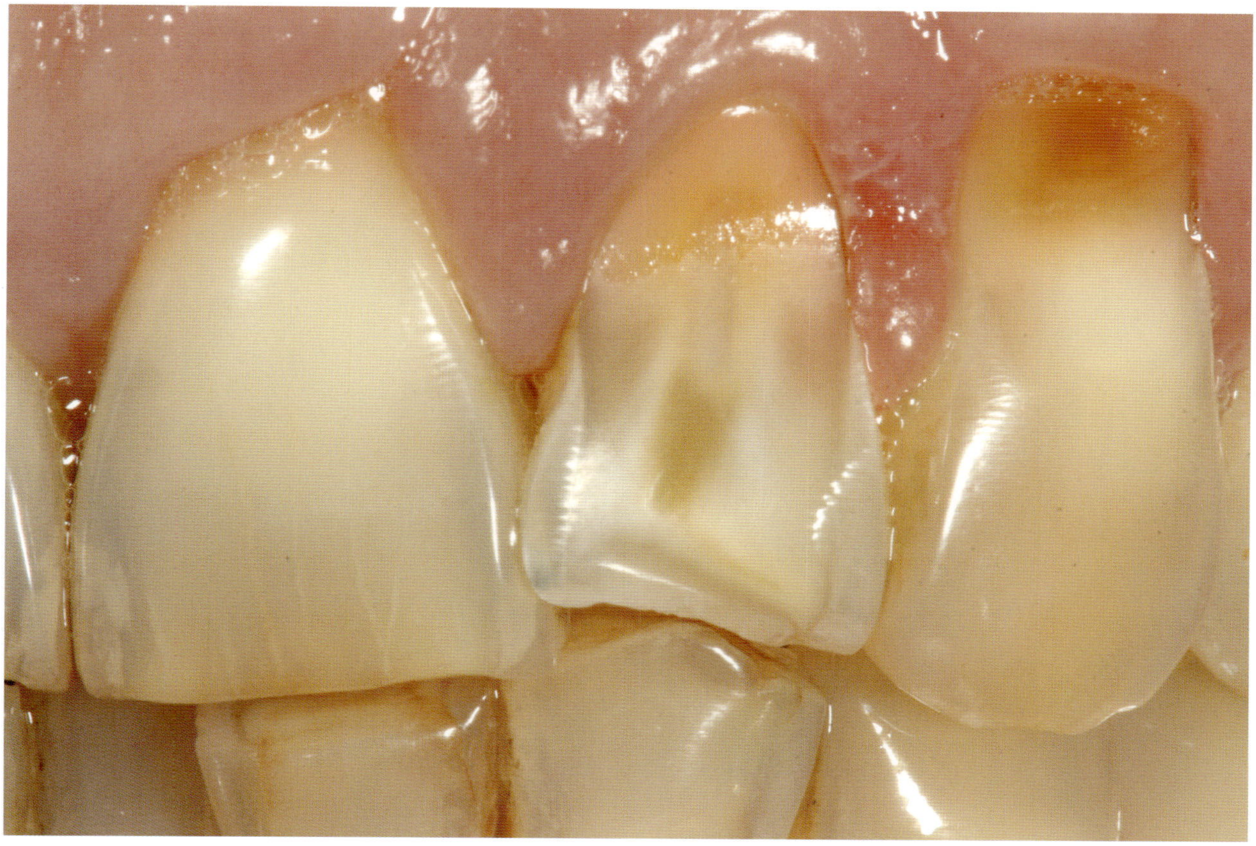

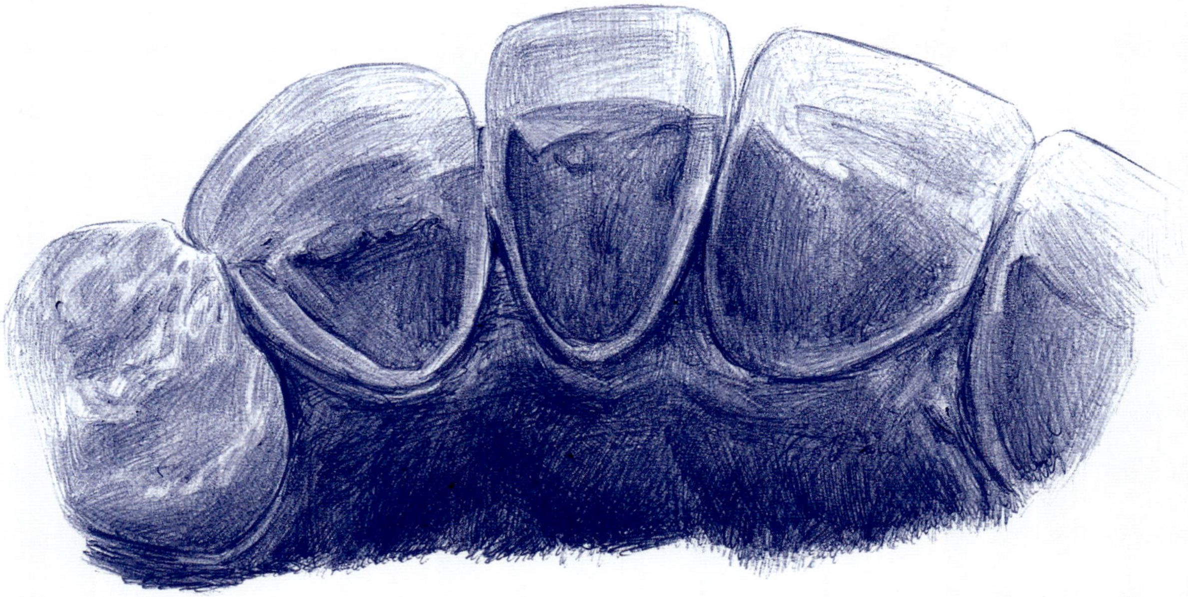

*The man who views the world at fifty the same as he did at twenty has wasted thirty years of his life.*

—Muhammad Ali, American professional boxer, activist, and philanthropist

CHAPTER 3

# ETIOLOGY AND TYPES OF TOOTH WEAR

In order to understand TW, it is essential to identify and differentiate between the distinct types of TW. Many attempts have been made to clearly classify TW, which is also described as non-carious tooth surface loss (NCTSL) or tooth surface loss (TSL).

The increased prevalence of TW and its irreversible damage is a reason for concern, and no delay in its understanding by the general practitioner is acceptable. A broad constellation of risk factors has been linked to TW. Moreover, as mentioned in the previous chapter, hyposalivation is an underlying and potentiating factor that may explain cases in which TW and its origins are beyond the frontiers of understanding.

The challenge is significant if we take into consideration that the etiology is, in the vast majority of cases, multifactorial and manifests itself in multiple and insidious ways.

## 1. Tooth Wear: Classical Nomenclature

Teeth are considered mechanical tools for food mastication. The anatomy of a tooth is directly linked to its efficiency.[1] Information about lifestyle is intrinsically linked to the appearance of the individual's teeth.[2]

Based on evidence provided by Van't Spijker et al in 2009, it is generally agreed that a loss of 28 to 30 μm per year should be considered physiologic and part of the aging process as long as it is not in excess of 1 mm as the patient enters their sixth decade (middle age).[3] Pathologic wear compromises tooth survival and is not associated with aging.

Looking back at the literature, publications on TW classification date as far back as 1946 to 1947.[4,5]

The difficulty remains in the fact that TW is modulated by the impact of several risk factors; thus, without the study of the medical history of the patients and the analysis of their lifestyle and nutritional habits, the precise origin of TW cannot be diagnosed.[6,7] In other words, the members of the TW team need to ask themselves repeatedly: why?

TW is a noncommunicable condition where the etiologic factors are interconnected (Fig 3-1).

The common classical terminology is therefore not able to comprehensively explain the wear mechanism. Recently, Grippo encouraged the introduction of the term *biocorrosion* as a substitute for the traditional term *erosion* in 21st century dental glossaries. Biocorrosion is understood as the chemical, biochemical, and electromechanical action on teeth, produced either by endogenous or exogenous acidic and proteolytic degradation of enamel and dentin, as well as the piezoelectric/electromechanical action on the collagen in dentin.[8]

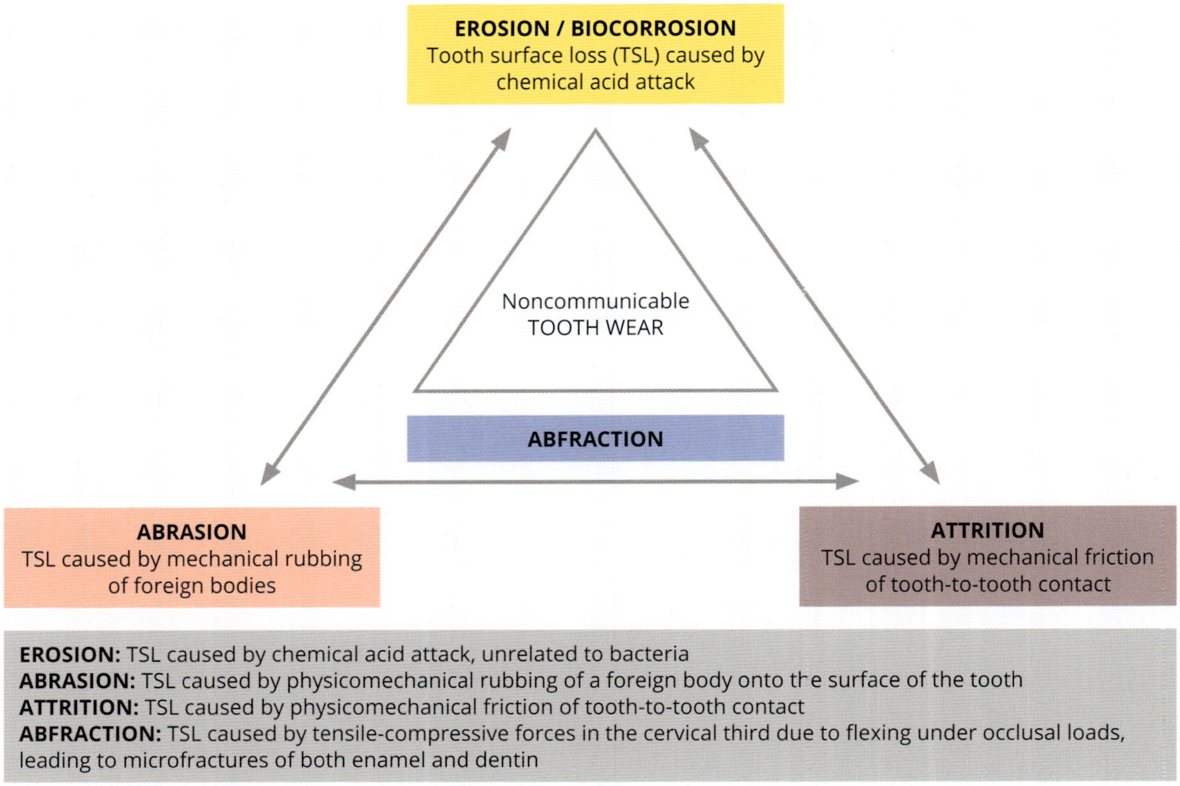


**Fig 3-1** The interrelated etiologic factors of TW, a noncommunicable disease.

## 2. The Etiology of Tooth Wear

Increased longevity, parallel to a decreased rate of tooth loss, is behind the rise of the so-called physiologic TW. The prevalence of TW is on the rise, with one in every four adults suffering from the condition.

Despite the clear origin-differentiated description of TW types, clinically TW is far from being exclusively related to a unique causation, be it erosion, abrasion, attrition, or abfraction. In most cases, it is the result of a concomitant action from a combination of several, or all, of the aforementioned processes (Figs 3-2 to 3-7).

Simultaneous erosion and abrasion showed a 50% increase in wear rate compared with alternating erosion and abrasion.[9] Furthermore, an in vitro research study proved that, in the absence of an acidic milieu, to eliminate 1 mm of enamel would take 2,500 years using only a toothbrush and 100 years when combining toothpaste and a toothbrush; surprisingly, 2 years would be a sufficient amount of time if the mouth had been exposed to acid prior to using the toothpaste and toothbrush.[10,11]

### The Link Between TW and Lifestyle: TW and Diet

General and oral health may be positively or negatively impacted by lifestyle, nutrition, and behavioral factors.

TW, a noncommunicable condition, is closely connected to modern life, as is the case with other conditions such as diabetes, obesity, hypertension, and cancer.

Human health is the result of the interrelationship of nutritional, socioeconomic and cultural factors, and genetics, with all of them being determined and even modified by environmental conditions.[12] The human microbiome with its thin, flexible line between eubiosis and dysbiosis also plays a fundamental role.

Good oral and general health should be able to provide well-being. Human bodies are near-perfect machines that need a balance of nutrients as well as good sleep and regular exercise, which will also help maintain a positive mental attitude to better endure life's challenges. When this balanced lifestyle is impaired, oral health and tooth structure are endangered[13,14] (Table 3-1).

| | | |
|---|---|---|
| **EROSION / BIOCORROSION** (Chemical acid wear) | ← Extrinsic acid | Diet (fruit juices, soda drinks, vinegar, acidic diets) |
| | ← Intrinsic acid | Gastroesophageal reflux |
| | | Eating disorders |
| **ABRASION** (Mechanical wear by foreign bodies) | | Abrasive toothbrushing |
| | | Abrasive toothpastes |
| | | Abrasive foods |
| | | Effect of dental appliances |
| **ATTRITION** (Mechanical wear by own teeth) | | Bruxism |
| **ABFRACTION** (TSL from load stress) | | Excessive functional load |
| | | Eccentric loading |
| | | Diminished occlusal support |

**Fig 3-2** Schematic classical TW etiology chart.

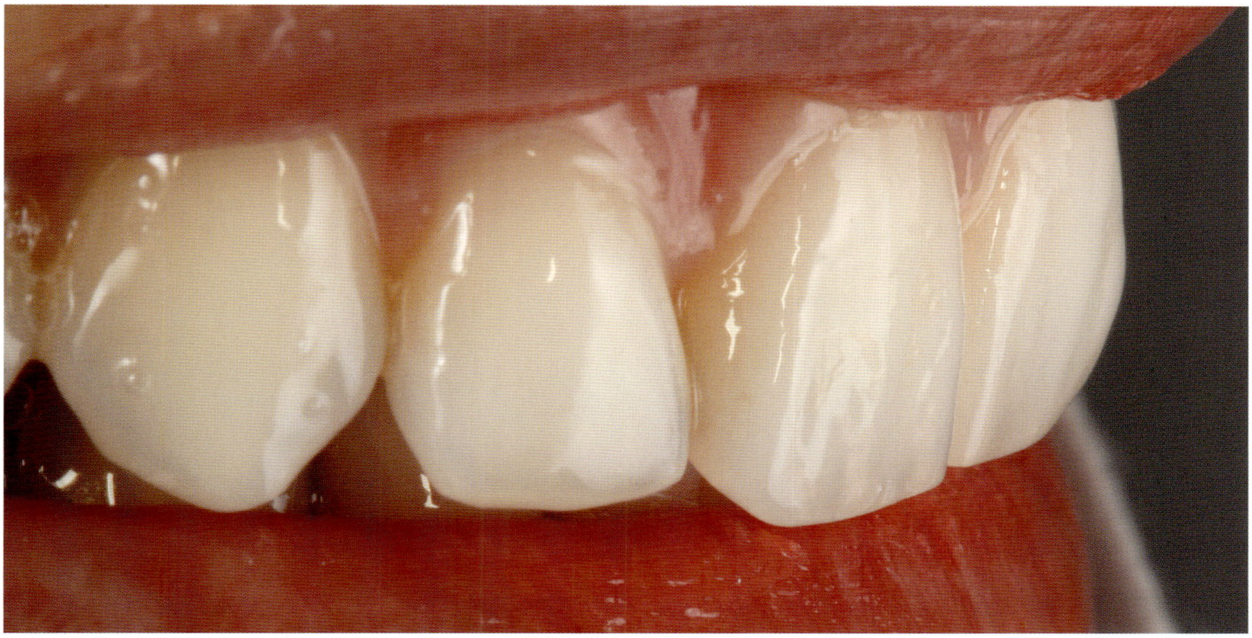

**Fig 3-3** Sound enamel is rich in anatomical and textural details. Known to be translucent, it offers to the eye a rainbow of subtleties and shades that escapes on many occasions not only the expert's eye but also the computerized artificial intelligence. Healthy enamel is very hard; however, when acid attack softens the enamel, it becomes highly susceptible to the concomitant action of abrasion, attrition, or both.

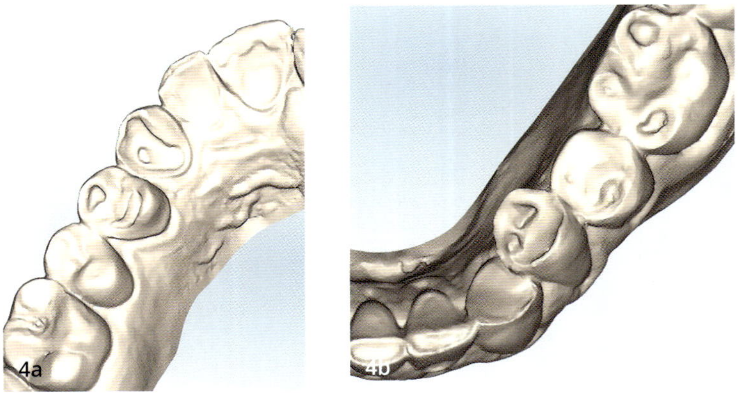


**Fig 3-4** Acid literally erases the palatal structure of anterior teeth, leading in many occasions to pulp exposure. A delay in taking action will impede a conservative approach. Volcano like occlusal lesions associated with erosive challenges will evolve into a total disappearance of anatomy. Partial STL images originating from an intraoral scanning record show destructive blurring and flattening of occlusal anatomy (a and b).

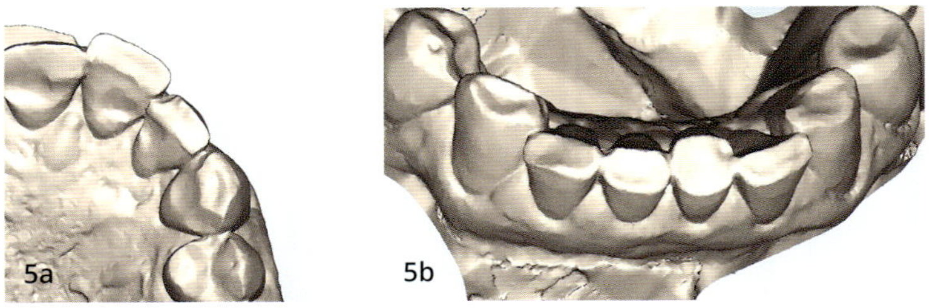


**Fig 3-5** Attrition is frequently identified by flat, sharp, shiny surfaces that perfectly match antagonist teeth. Clinically, initial signs may be the appearance of a wear facet on a canine tip or an incisal edge. It is not infrequent to detect it in the anterior region of the mouth. Loss of incisal anatomy can already be seen in children. Incisal edges present themselves more as tables than edges. The role of previous erosion defended by certain authors as mandatory in order for attrition wear to occur is not easily deducted without the patient's history (a and b).

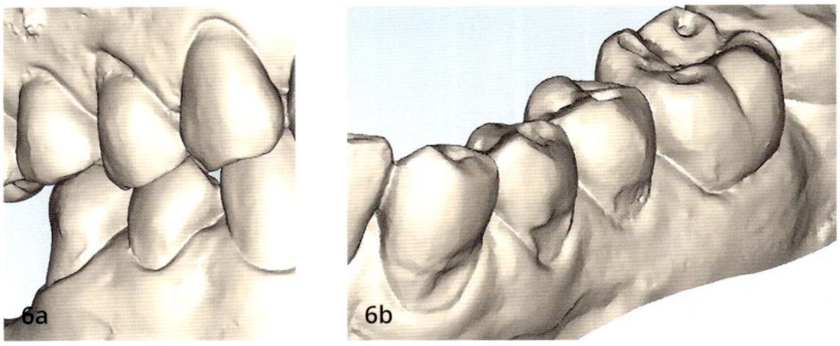


**Fig 3-6** Frequently found in routine practice, wear lesions localized at the gingival third of the teeth are described as non-carious cervical lesions (NCCLs). Traditionally thought to be caused by abrasion challenges, such as inadequate toothbrushing, erosive attack, or flexural-overloading forces, today the body of opinion agrees upon the fact that this type of lesion is due to multiple etiologic factors. The huge variety of morphology and clinical presentations is in relation to the multifactorial impacts that take part in the development of such lesions (a and b).

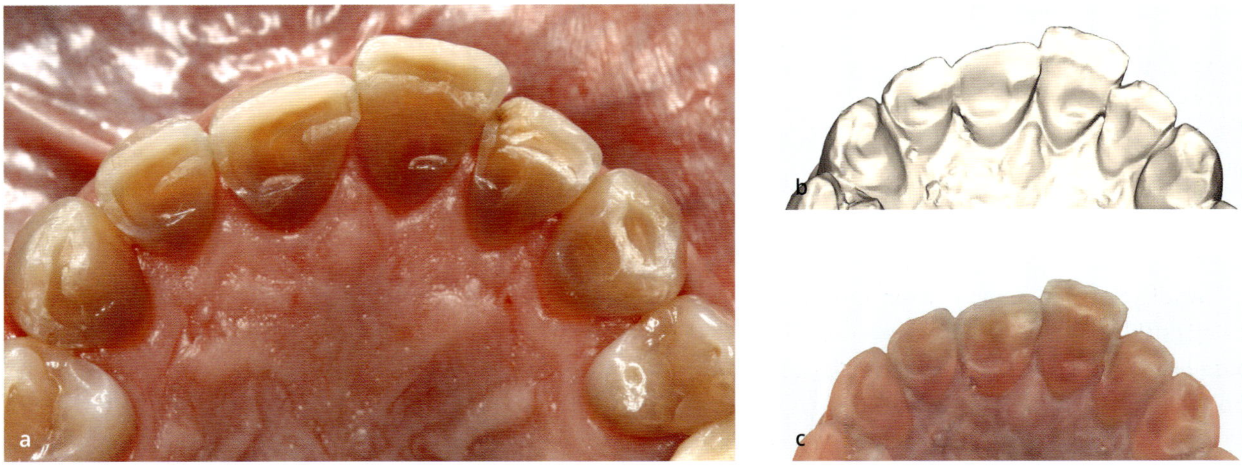


**Fig 3-7** Digital recording of the maxillary arch of a male patient in his 5th decade of life. Concomitant erosion and attrition have drawn different wear patterns in which half of the anterior region of the mouth is affected by acid, thus creating a thin knife-edge incisal anatomy, while the other half, cut down by attrition forces, shows a broad occlusal table-like incisal edge. Erosion has most probably weakened the enamel shield because of the low pH, facilitating the destruction of enamel originated by tooth grinding. The asymmetric erosive pattern is compatible with the patient's medical history of GERD and the fact that he usually sleeps on his right side (a to c).

**Table 3-1** Lifestyle and tooth wear.

| | |
|---|---|
| **BALANCED DIET**<br>■ Water, proteins, fat, minerals, carbohydrates, vitamins | **UNBALANCED DIET**<br>■ Excess of acids, vegetarian-fruitarian diets, fasting<br>■ Overweight<br>■ Food intolerances |
| **NON-EROSIVE DRINKS, PROTECTIVE FOODS**<br>■ Water, milk, cheese, yogurt | **EROSIVE DRINKS, FOODS**<br>■ Soda drinks, fruit juices, herbal teas, vinegar, lemon |
| **REGULAR SUSTAINABLE EXERCISE**<br>■ Medium workout or team sports | **EXCESSIVE INTENSE SPORTS**<br>■ Extreme consumption of acidic sports drinks, dehydration<br>■ Indoor extensive swimming |
| **EQUILIBRATED NON-STRESSFUL LIFE**<br>■ Good balance of personal/professional life. | **STRESSFUL LIFE**<br>■ Hyperconnectivity, on-the-go diets, overuse of information technology (lack of sleep, consumption of soda drinks)<br>■ Parafunctional habits such as fingernail biting, lip biting, pen biting, etc<br>■ Intake of xerostomia-causing medication |
| **GOOD ORAL HYGIENE HABITS**<br>■ Medium-soft toothbrushes<br>■ Low-abrasiveness toothpastes<br>■ Oral hygiene regimen to stimulate saliva | **QUICK-HARSH ORAL HYGIENE HABITS**<br>■ Coarse toothbrushes<br>■ Abrasive toothpastes<br>■ High-speed ultrasonic-electric-toothbrushes |
| **GOOD SLEEP**<br>■ Average 7 to 8 hours every 24 hours | **POOR SLEEP**<br>■ Stress, intake of sleeping pills, bruxism, snoring, sleep apnea<br>■ pH drop during mouth breathing at night, oromotor abrupt muscle activity while awakening |
| **POSITIVE MENTAL ATTITUDE**<br>■ Promotes social life and optimism | **NEGATIVE MENTAL ATTITUDE**<br>■ Anxiety, depression, stress, abuse of medicaments, intake of xerostomia-causing medication, pessimism |
| **OVERALL GOOD GENERAL HEALTH**<br>■ Regular visits to the GP or specialist<br>■ Continuity of care | **MEDICAL CONDITIONS**<br>■ GERD, eating disorders, psychologic disorders, sleep disorders, Sjögren syndrome, salivary gland dysfunction, diabetes, high blood pressure, cerebral palsy, Down syndrome, asthma, allergies<br>■ Attention deficit and hyperactivity disorder (ADHD) Intake of medication |
| | **ADDICTIONS AND DRUG ABUSERS**<br>■ Caffeine or cola dependence<br>■ Alcohol, tobacco, drug (cocaine, ecstasy) abuse |
| **NORMAL SALIVA FLOW**<br>■ Good salivary function and enjoyment of tastes | **HYPOSALIVATION**<br>■ Polymedication<br>■ Stress, anxiety<br>■ Medical conditions<br>■ Congenital conditions |

Acidic diets have been linked to erosive wear. So-called healthy diets may include an excess of fruit or fruit-based beverages that increase the likelihood of suffering from TW (Fig 3-8).

Vegetarian-fruitarian or fasting diets have shown to enhance TW erosive risk as much as unbalanced diets that lead to obesity and increased body mass index (BMI).[15,16]

Traditionally, the classification of TW causes has been organized into distinct, watertight compartments corresponding to their relationship to abrasion, attrition, erosion, or abfraction mechanisms. Today, we know that many of the TW risk factors may be able to induce several types of TW; a micromolecular imbalance due to hyposalivation may be behind them. As an example, let's consider sleep disorders, in which TW may be related to the attrition mechanism in night bruxism but also connected to erosion, which is enhanced by a pH drop during the night and a lack of effective saliva protection during sleeping hours. In fact, modern lifestyle is a perfect storm for TW development (Figs 3-9 and 3-10).

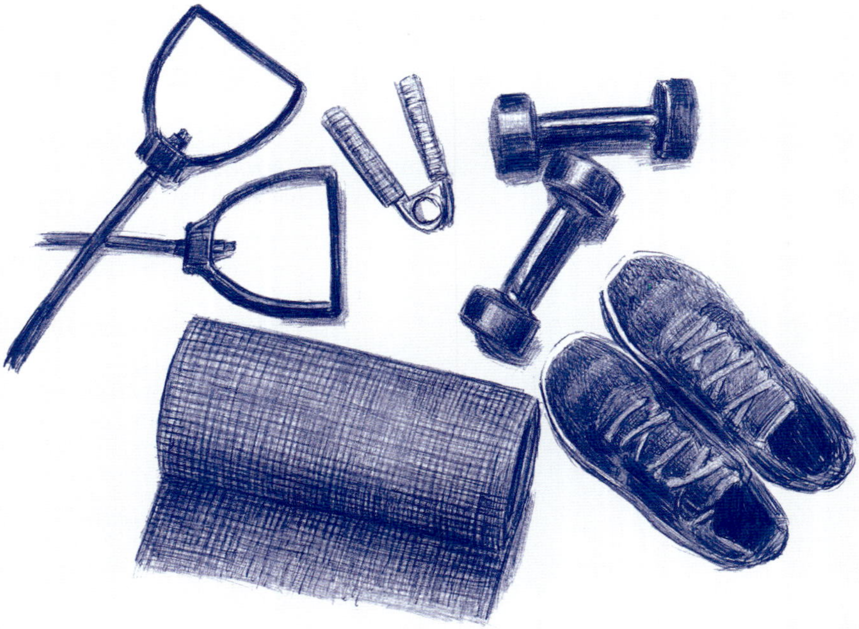

**Fig 3-8** There is sometimes a fine line between what is good for you and what could potentially be detrimental to one's health. Extensive sports, dehydration, and acidic sport drinks may pose a real danger to tooth structure.

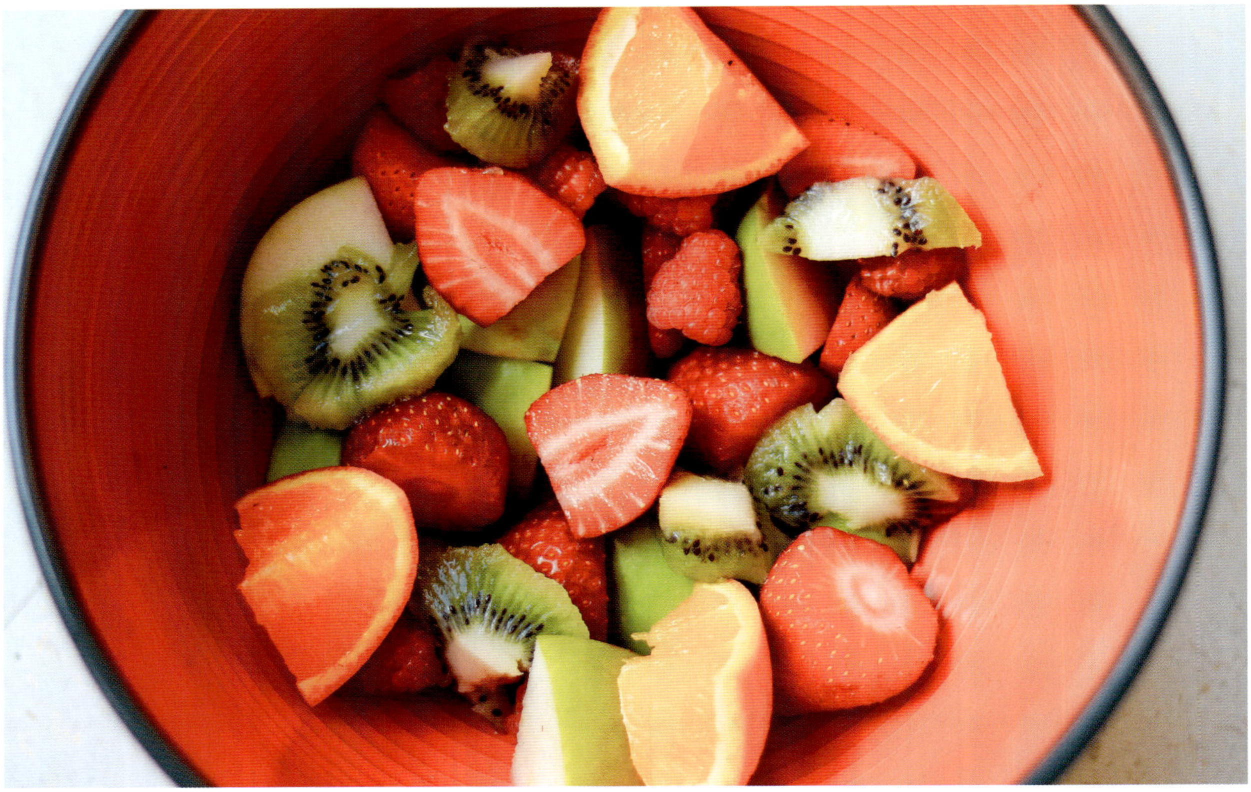

**Fig 3-9** Eating and lifestyle patterns during childhood will in many cases continue during adulthood. Stress, fast food habits, and unbalanced diets are transmitted to children at home. A significant increase in consumption of soft drinks and fruit juices is perceived in everyday life. Children walk home after school connected by phones or tablets while eating industrialized snacks and acidic fruit juices or carbonated drinks. When confronting TW in children, specific anatomical considerations must be taken into account, as well as the fact that noninvasive long-lasting restorations will be desirable. Moreover, efforts in education, coaching, and prevention should not be underestimated in terms of increasing the chances the child will not become a TW patient in adulthood.

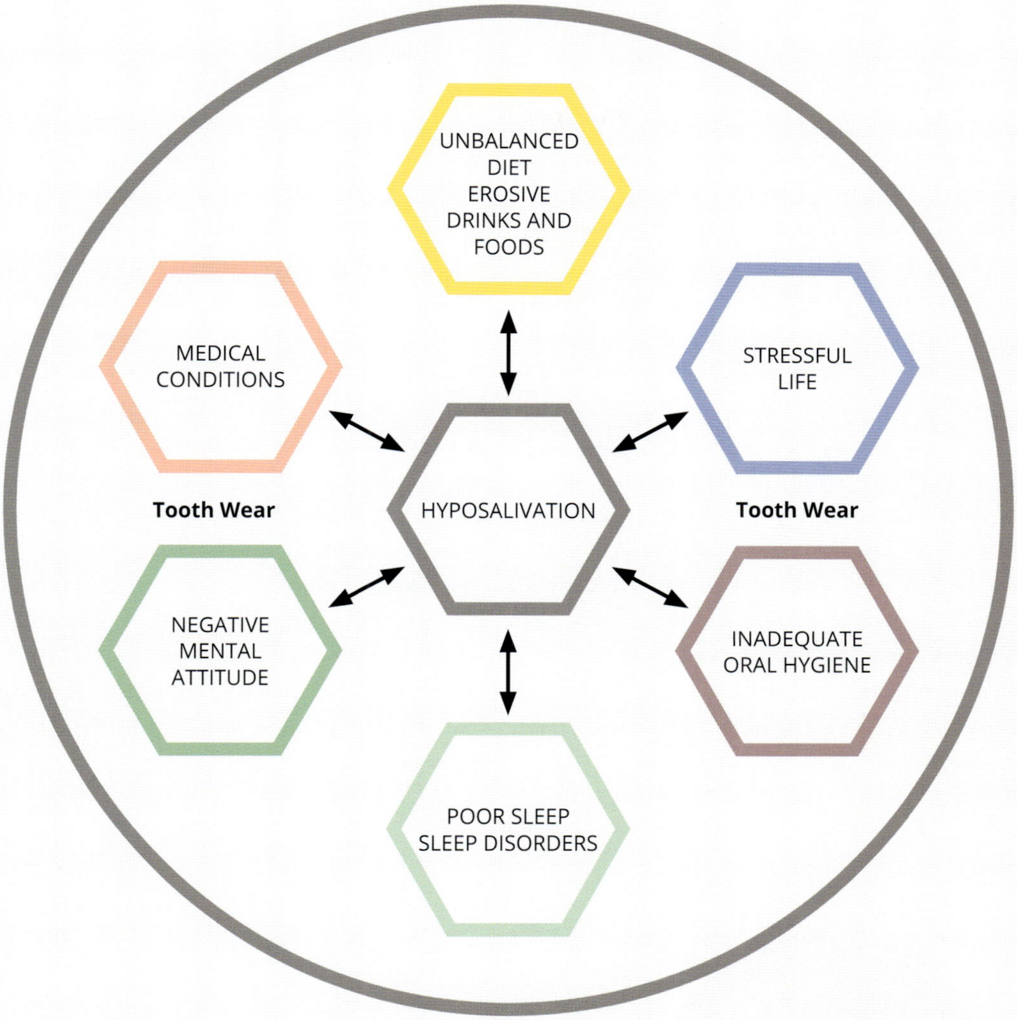


**Fig 3-10** Lifestyle hyposalivation and TW. Lifestyle refers to activities, habits and behaviors that conform everyday life. Modern lifestyle has certainly meant many advantages for modern men however contemporary lifestyle patterns are also a challenge to health. Lifestyle modification may prove very beneficial for human health. Hyperconnectivity and stress on a non-stop basis, unbalanced diets (even if the so called "healthy diets"), sleep alteration all create a good breeding ground for medical conditions, not to underestimate the need of medication for health impairment that accompanies the longer life expectancy that is enjoyed nowadays. Behind all the above mentioned, saliva disturbances will soon appear and prove to work as a TW potentiator.

## 3. Tooth Wear and the Pediatric Patient

TW is a common condition in pediatric dentistry. Although erosion is by far the most prevalent type of TW in children, it is not uncommon to find it with coexisting attrition or abrasion.

Erosion prevalence data has been profusely documented in the pediatric population with ample variation. The results show reason for concern.[17]

A survey of the diet and nutrition of young people aged 4–18 years living in private households in the UK in the late 1990s found a 65% erosion prevalence in the primary dentition and a 61% prevalence in permanent teeth in 7- to 10-year-olds, a 52% prevalence in 11- to 14-year-olds, and a 65% prevalence in 15- to 18-year-olds.[18] Ganss and collaborators found a 70.6% erosion prevalence in the primary dentition and an 11.6% prevalence in the permanent dentition in children in Germany.[19] McGuire et al found a 45.9% erosion prevalence in US teenagers in 2009.[20]

The primary dentition is more prone to complications associated with erosion and TW when compared with the permanent dentition. Dentin is affected sooner due to the enamel being thinner in children. Lower unstimulated salivary flow, which leads to a lower buffering capacity, as well as decreased enamel microhardness are determinant in rapid progression.[21]

High caries risk in children as well as hypoplastic defects can be indicators of TW in the coming years.[22]

### Erosive Wear in Children

Research shows that the prevalence of erosive TW in children and adolescents has grown unabated from the end of 20th century to the present day. The overall erosive prevalence in permanent teeth in children and adolescents is approximately 30%. A 32% prevalence of erosion has also been documented in primary teeth.[23,24]

Studies of the primary dentition have found that dentin exposure related to TW increases with age.[25,26]

High consumption of soft drinks is related to erosive damage in children, as well as the drinking method, with extended retention time in the oral cavity before swallowing (Fig 3-11). Frequency of consumption and duration should also be taken into consideration. Other habits such as acidic fruit intake or industrial fruit beverages have been shown to have a deleterious effect. Children should not go to bed with drinking bottles containing acidic beverages; the erosive potential is much higher at bedtime when no saliva protection is in place.

Mouth breathing and upper respiratory conditions such as asthma or allergies, together with intake of medication, are associated with erosive tooth wear in children and adolescents[21] (Fig 3-12).

Liquid or effervescent medication formulations are high in acidic content in order to provide an attractive flavor for children, posing an extra erosive challenge. Furthermore, an acidic composition is required to obtain drug dispersion in liquid forms, multiplying the damage.[27]

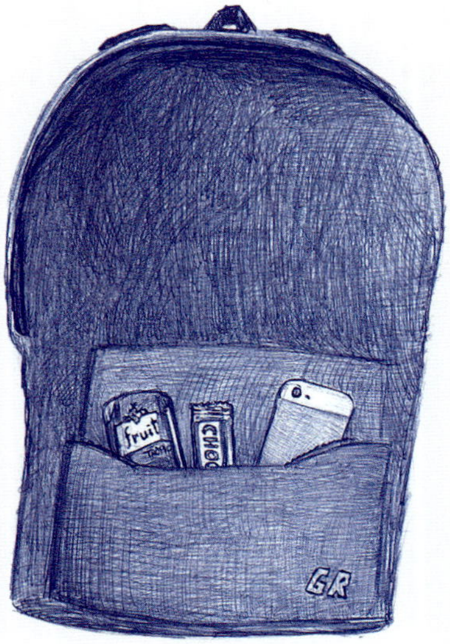


**Fig 3-11** Carbonated soda drinks, industrialized fruit juices, and candies have invaded dietary patterns in children. Lifestyle coaching needs to be implemented early in children with a high incidence of caries because an uncontrolled cariogenic diet will increase the chances of developing erosive wear with the passing of the years.

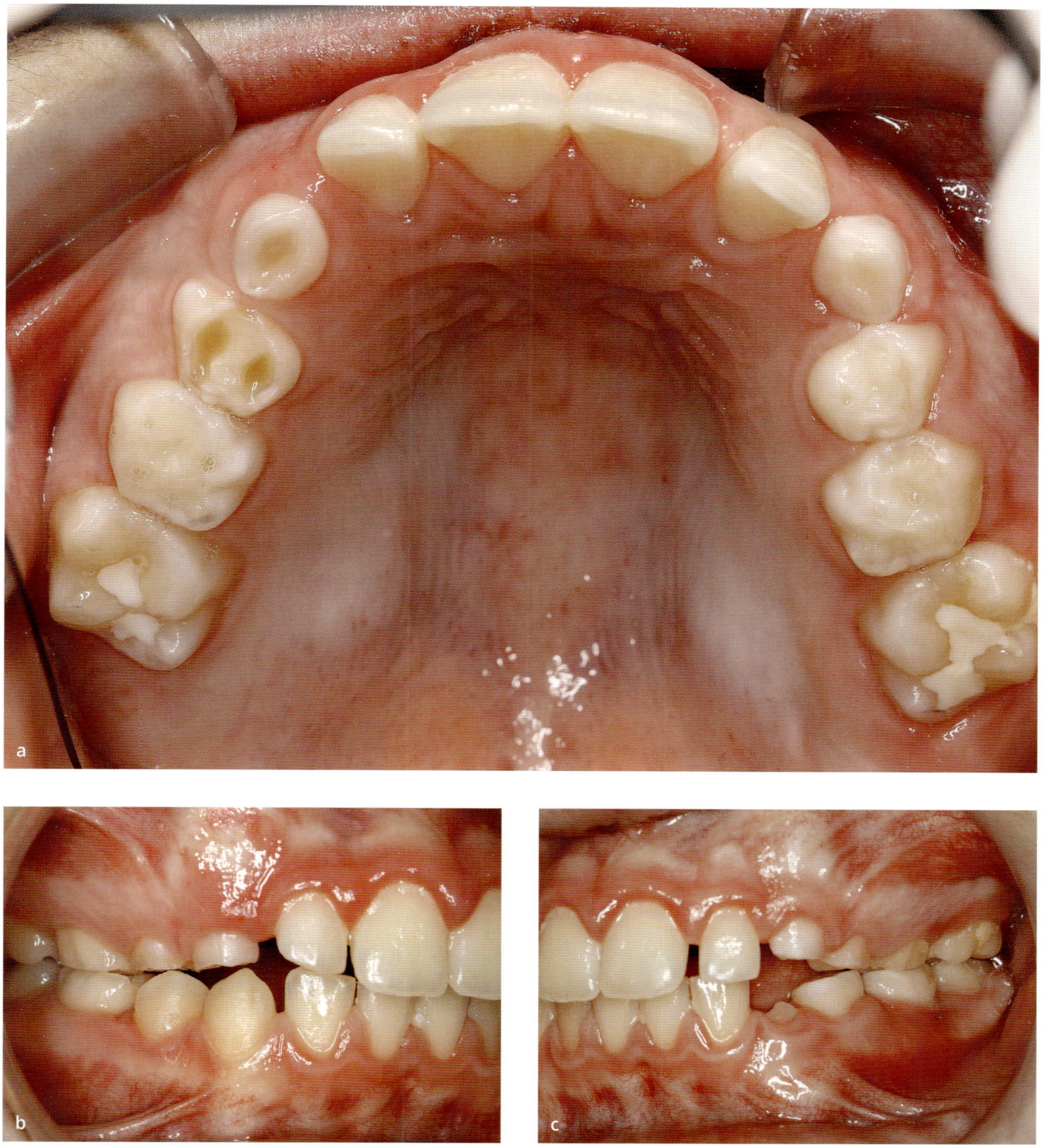


**Fig 3-12** A young child with upper respiratory difficulties has a secondary mouth breathing pattern with associated increased plaque and gingivitis. The long-standing poor sleep hygiene with snoring and night awakening since preschool age has deprived the oral cavity of the innate protection and cleansing of natural saliva. The erosive potential of these conditions is present in the mixed dentition and will eventually damage permanent teeth if they are not addressed (a to c).

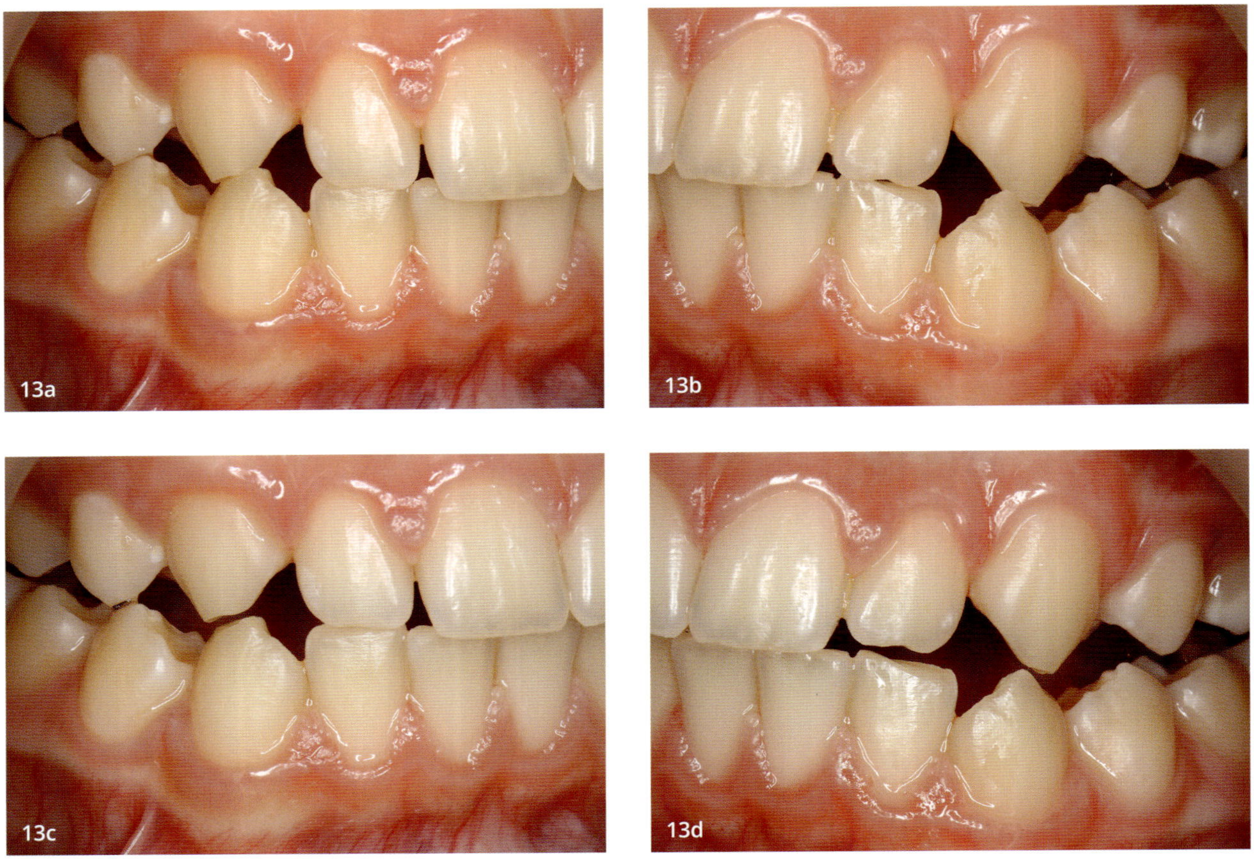


**Figs 3-13 and 3-14** Incipient lesions of attrition localized at the tip of the canines of two brothers in their early teens. Tooth grinding at night and a familial history of bruxism support the presumptive diagnose of SB. Note the coexisting erosive lesion in mandibular right premolars and damage also in mandibular incisors (3-13a to 3-13d). Traumatic tooth structure loss can be seen in the maxillary incisors of the older brother that should not be confused with TW (3-14). Occlusal views show overall good oral health apart from the incipient wear (3-14c and 3-14d). It is important to differentiate TW lesions from the existing iatrogenic vestibular damage due to mechanical grinding produced when the orthodontist removed the brackets. The final image shows incisal traumatic lesions restored as well as restored attrition lesion at the tip of the canine. For the sake of preserving as much tooth structure as possible, vestibular iatrogenic enamel defects will only be monitored (3-14h).

## Attrition in Children

The International Classification of Sleep Disorders published by the American Academy of Sleep Medicine describes sleep bruxism (SB) as an oral parafunction that originates grinding or clenching of the teeth during sleep associated with notorious sleep arousal activity.[28]

Bruxism, diurnal or nocturnal, may also produce rhythmic movements of the jaw that may produce occlusal trauma.[29]

It is highly common (86%) that adults who declare being bruxers have also been bruxers during childhood[30] (Figs 3-13 and 3-14).

SB seems to be multifactorial, with both environmental and genetic factors possibly involved. Increased anxiety can be found in children suffering from SB when compared with the normal pediatric population.

A familial predisposition has been documented, though no clear genetic code has been described.[31] Social/environmental inputs are crucial as was proven in the twin study from Finland.[31–32]

## TW and Down Syndrome

The impact of periodontitis and caries has been documented in patients with Down syndrome. Moreover, the literature shows that TW is significantly more frequent in children with Down syndrome than in children without it. A multifunctional origin has been found with the coexistence of attrition and erosion.[33,34]

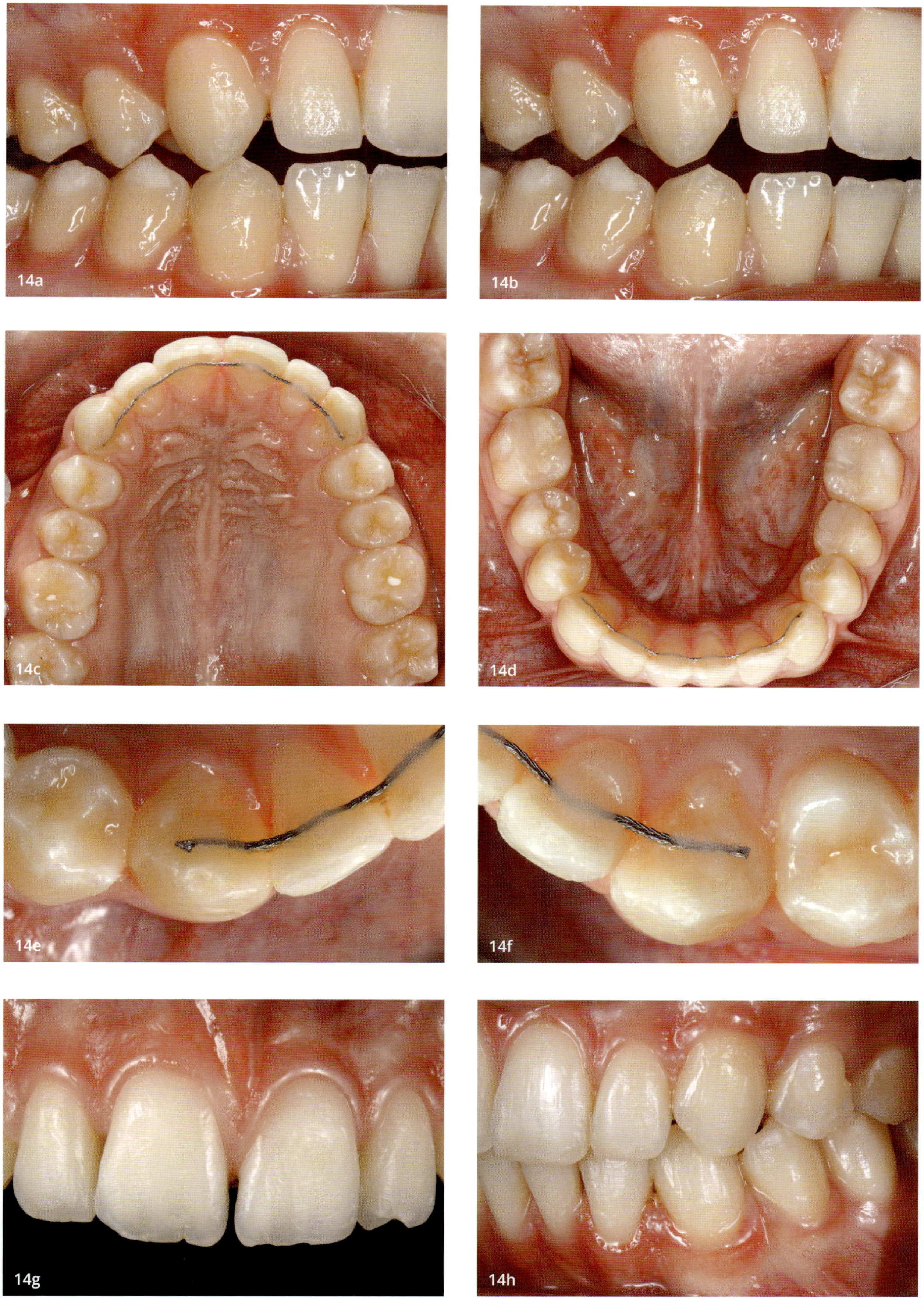
14a
14b
14c
14d
14e
14f
14g
14h

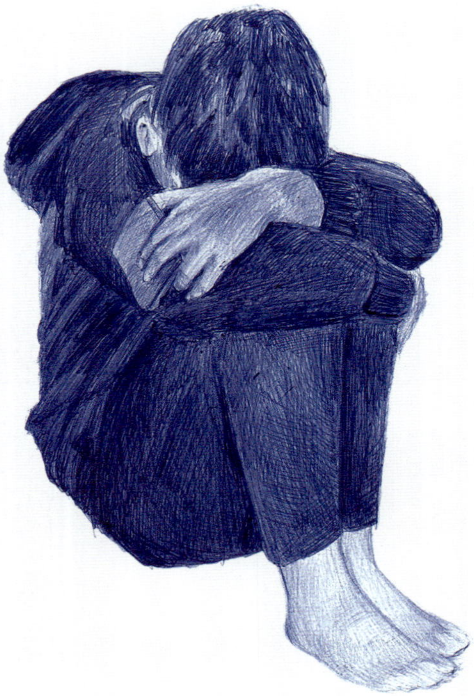

**Fig 3-15** Bullying is an intentional, long-lasting psychologic or physical attack with an imbalance of power between the bully (perpetrator) and the bullied child (victim). Bullying is on the rise and negatively impacts the physical and mental health not only of the perpetrators and victims but others in their environment.

## TW and Prader-Willi Syndrome

Neonatal hypotonia, endocrine disturbances, hyperphagia, intellectual developmental disorder, oral abnormalities, and a cohort of other signs and conditions constitute the genetic disorder known as Prader-Willi syndrome, in which severe TW is a significant problem.

Studies have shown a high incidence of GERD in Prader-Willi individuals, probably in relation to their overweight status. Routine screening for salivary characteristics, TW, and GERD should be implemented in patients with Prader-Willi Syndrome.[35,36]

## TW and ADHD

Between 3% and 7% of school-age children suffer from attention deficit hyperactivity disorder (ADHD). Studies consistently have found lower unstimulated salivary flow in children with ADHD, with or without pharmacologic treatment.[37,38]

The impact of long-term psychostimulant drugs prescribed to ADHD children include a significant subjective dry mouth feeling as well as very low salivary flow.[39]

Psychostimulant medication offers an improvement of anxiety symptoms in children with ADHD that may very well be related to a better control of ADHD symptoms.[40]

When pre-existing emotional symptoms that can lead to social or academic complications require additional medications such as antidepressants, the risk of decreasing salivary flow and an increased risk of TW must be anticipated.[41]

Several authors have found a significant increase of bruxism in ADHD children versus non-ADHD children.[42,43]

## TW and Bullying

Children who have been bullied remain at risk of poor health even decades after exposure. Psychologic distress remains an issue in adults who have been bullied as children.[44]

Bullying has been considered an adverse childhood experience (ACE) determinant in the development of psychologic and physical disturbances that can, however, be mitigated or controlled by self-esteem promotion[45] (Fig 3-15). Research has demonstrated the complex effects of stress on disease susceptibility and even immunologic distortions.[46]

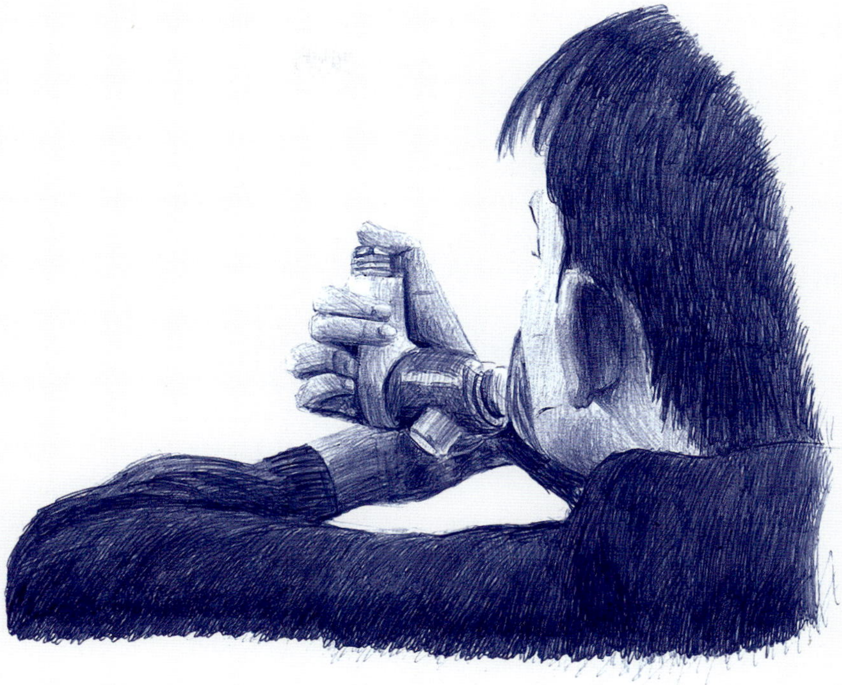

**Fig 3-16** Concomitant gastroesophageal reflux disease (GERD) in asthmatic patients may occur, aggravating the erosion risk, probably due to distension of the gastroesophageal sphincter in relation to chronic use of bronchodilators.

Studies have linked bullying with sleep disorders, poor sleep quality, and even sleep deprivation in children and adolescents.[47,48] Bullying has also been linked to nutritional disorders. Obese and overweight children are at higher risk of being bullied.[49] On the other hand, bullying perpetrators have been proven to have a poor-quality diet that may be linked to impaired oral health.[50]

Finally, being bullied during childhood has been related to the development of psychosomatic conditions. Irritable bowel disease is common in children exposed to stressful events. Irritable bowel disease is commonly accompanied by diarrhea that could eventually drive to secondary lactose deficiency, nausea, and vomiting.[51–54]

As per all of the above and the evidence that links TW with stress, anxiety, sleep disorders, unbalanced diet, obesity, and gastrointestinal disturbances, bullying in childhood should be further studied as a risk factor for TW in childhood, and bullied children should be examined for signs of TW.

## TW and Asthma

Asthma is a chronic inflammatory condition of the airway with airflow obstruction. Treatment includes bronchodilators, corticosteroids, and anticholinergic drugs, frequently in the form of nebulizers or inhalers (Fig 3-16).

Asthma, and long-term medication for asthma control, have been positively associated with TW.[55] Asthma medication may cause erosive damage through a double mechanism: the low pH in aerosols and the fact that beta-2 agonists such as terbutaline or salbutamol may produce xerostomia. Effects from gastric acids in the oral cavity have also been proven in asthmatic patients through a relaxation of the esophageal sphincter produced by bronchodilators. This mechanism could be the reason behind the development of GERD in asthmatic children.[56]

## TW and Type 1 Diabetes

Patients with diabetes suffer from reduced salivary flow rates that can be related to diabetic neuropathy or to disturbances in glycemic control. Saliva is essential in protecting against TW (erosion or attrition); therefore, patients with type 1 diabetes are at risk of developing TW at an early age.[57,58]

## 4. Tooth Wear in Adolescents and Adult Patients

### TW and Eating Disorders: Bulimia Nervosa

Erosion affects 20% of patients with anorexia nervosa and more than 90% of patients suffering from bulimia nervosa. Bulimia is characterized by episodes of binge eating followed by purges, which are normally produced through self-induced vomiting, strict dieting, intense physical activity, or use of diuretics and laxatives. Anorexia nervosa is characterized by a distorted perception of weight, overwhelming fear of gaining weight, and a very low body weight, usually attained through severe self-restriction of food (Fig 3-17).

Eating disorders (EDs) can be life threatening, and the dental practitioner, together with the dental team, may be able to detect its early signs. The psychologic management is complex and exceeds the dentist's capacity. When the patient does not openly disclose the ED, the family should be informed so that specialized support is given by an ED psychologic/psychiatric unit. Forcing the patient into admitting ED behavior could put the doctor-patient relationship at risk and may lead to the patient missing future appointments. In fact, experts advise not to inquire or discuss ED openly unless a safe environment has been created to gain patient confidence.[59]

Research has shown that dental erosion in bulimic patients is not linearly linked to frequency and duration of vomiting.[60] However, dental erosion risk and damage is higher in patients that vomit.[61] In fact, pathologic wear is more frequent after 1,100 vomiting episodes.[62] Such physical stress on the salivary glands may result in alterations in salivary secretion and viscosity. The parotid serous secretion is reduced, while an overcompensation of mucin is secreted from submandibular, sublingual, and minor salivary gland, thus producing a more viscous saliva. This is in line with the parotid bilateral enlargement that has been seen in bulimic patients in relation to histopathologic changes from serous parotid acini after vomiting episodes. Caloric restriction has also been proven in laboratory animals to reduce salivary flow while producing an enlargement of the parotids[63,64] (Fig 3-18).

Differences in dental erosion in bulimic patients may also relate to the individual's susceptibility and to enamel mineralization and enamel microhardness[65,66] (Figs 3-19 to 3-23).

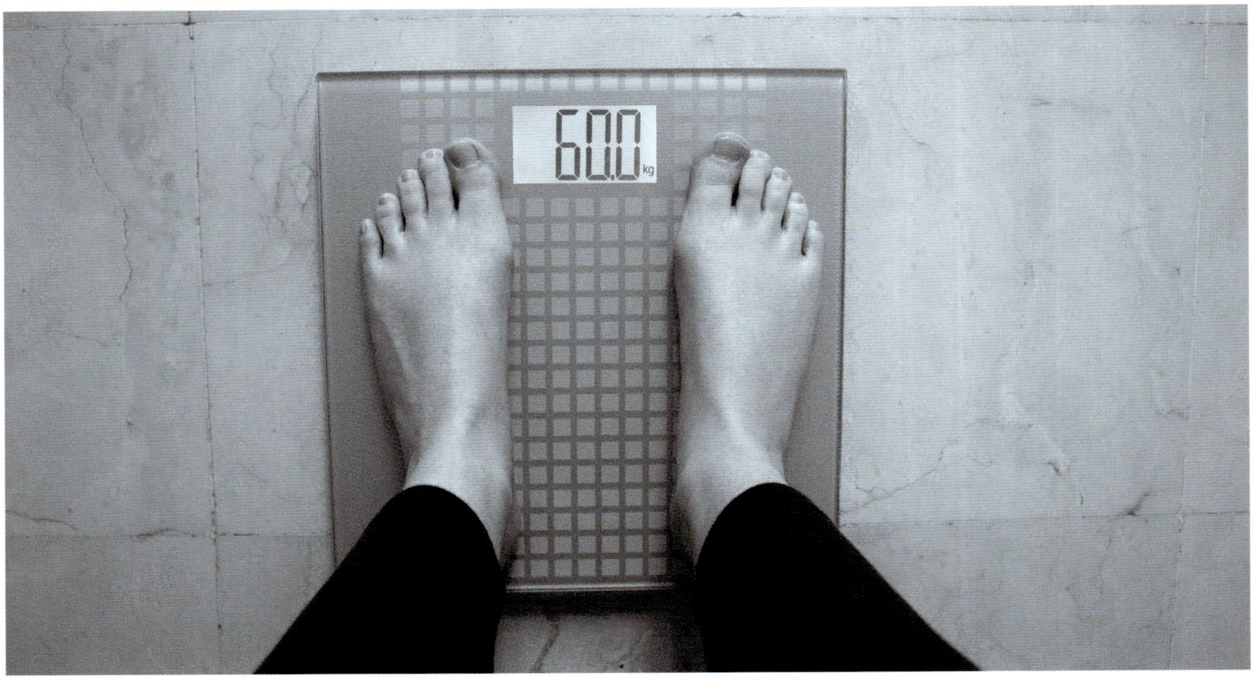


**Fig 3-17** EDs involve a pathologic relationship with food and a pathologic obsession about weight control. Social and even familial pressure to be thin and cultural preferences are certainly significant in the development of ED; however, only a given percentage of individuals exposed to the aforementioned pressures develop such a disorder. Thus it is clear that other factors are also implicated in their causation.

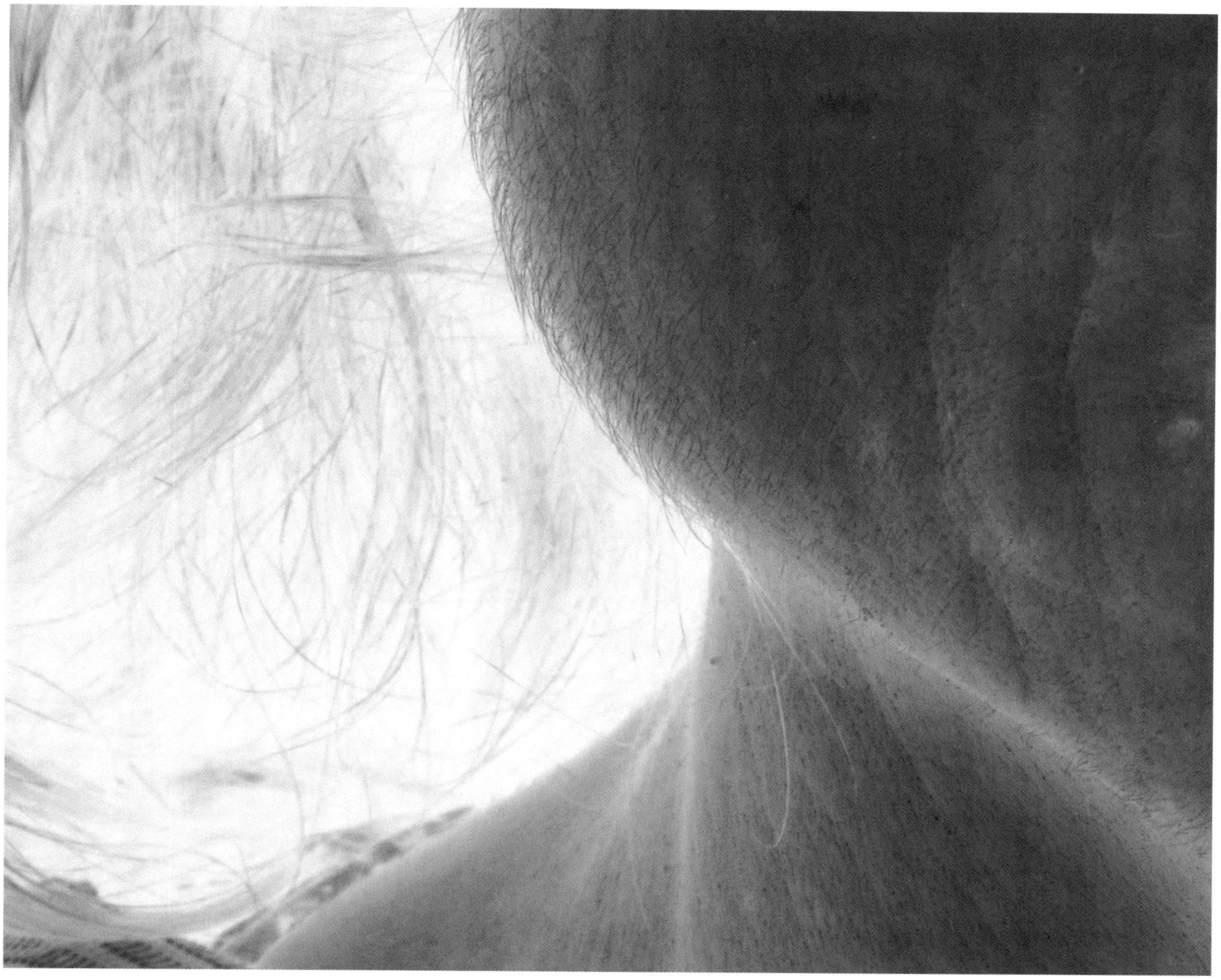

**Fig 3-18** Parotid bilateral enlargement is a facial sign that may serve as an indicator of repetitive vomiting episodes in patients that may not be ready to openly declare this condition. The prevalence of EDs is very high, especially in developed, industrialized countries. With the highest rates of morbidity and mortality among mental disorders in youngsters, EDs are a serious condition.

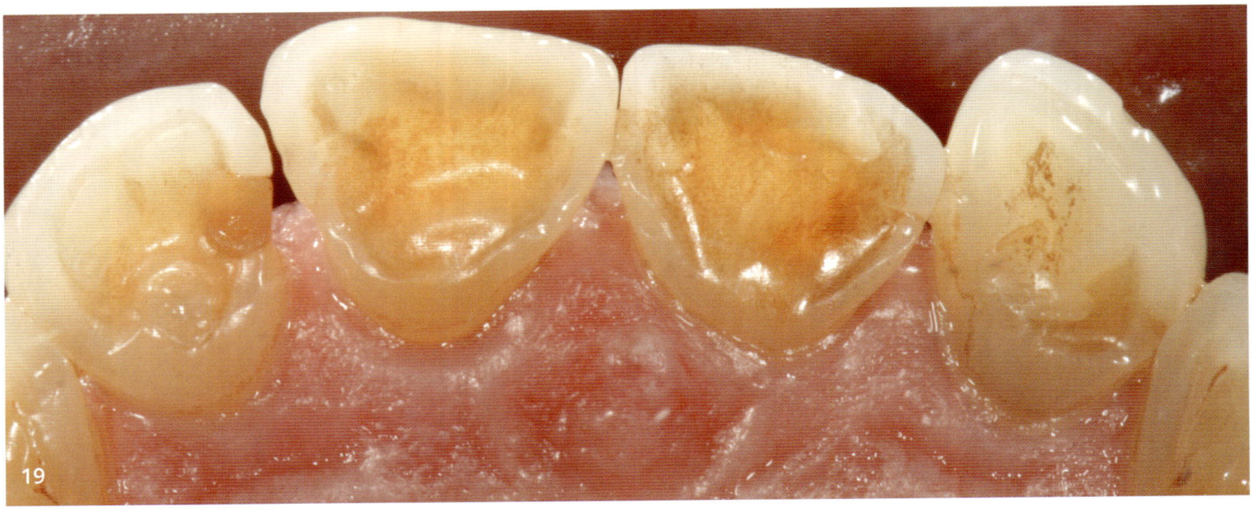
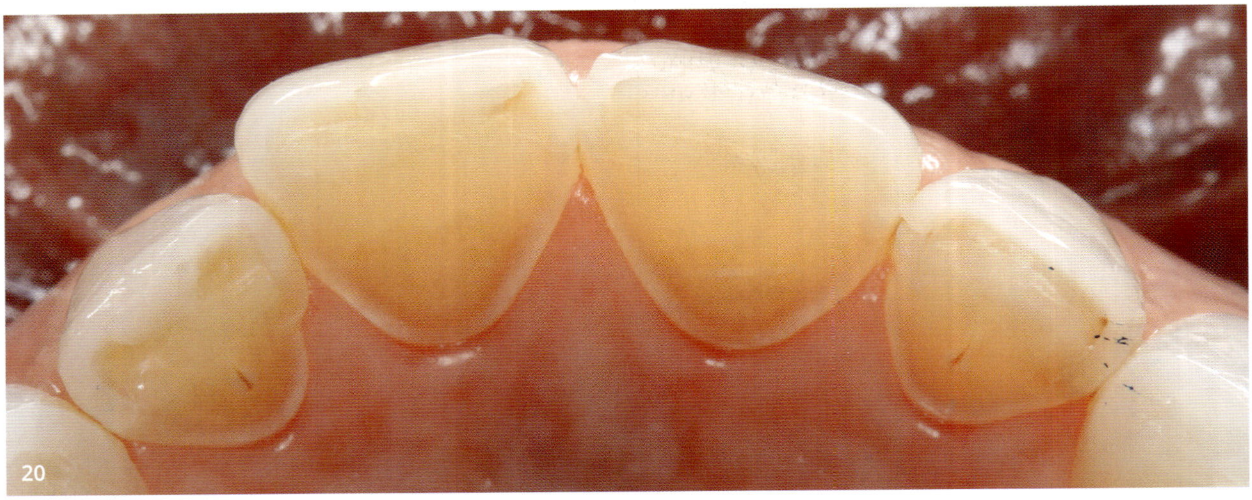
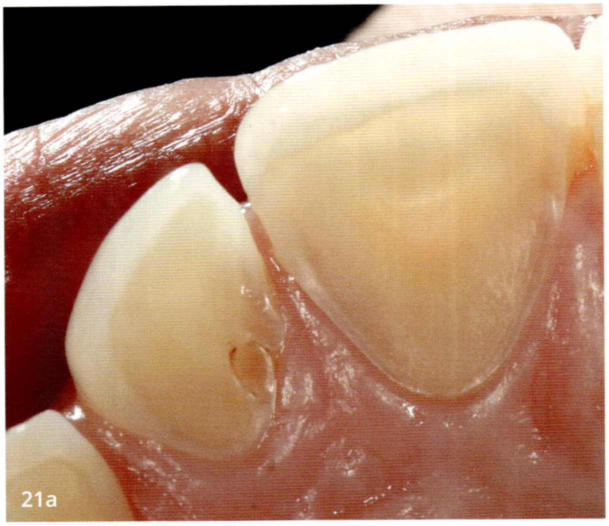
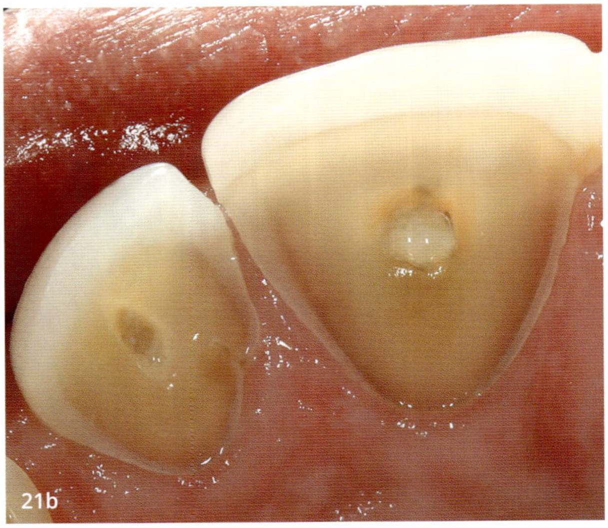

**Figs 3-19 to 3-21** A look at the palatal surface of the maxillary incisors can provide invaluable information for establishing the diagnosis of a TW patient. Internal sources of acid are normally accompanied by erosion of palatal tooth structure. With vomiting behavior, it is frequent to detect severe erosion of the palatal aspect of the central and lateral incisors, while erosion of the canines can be significantly lower as the tongue protects them during vomiting (3-19 and 3-20). Moreover, immediate toothbrushing in order to eliminate the taste and smell from gastric juices can accelerate TW. Dentin hypersensitivity is highly common when rapidly progressing palatal erosion has reached the proximity of the pulp. Patients at that point can require endodontic treatment. Early intervention may save not only overall tooth structure but also pulp vitality (3-21a and 3-21b).

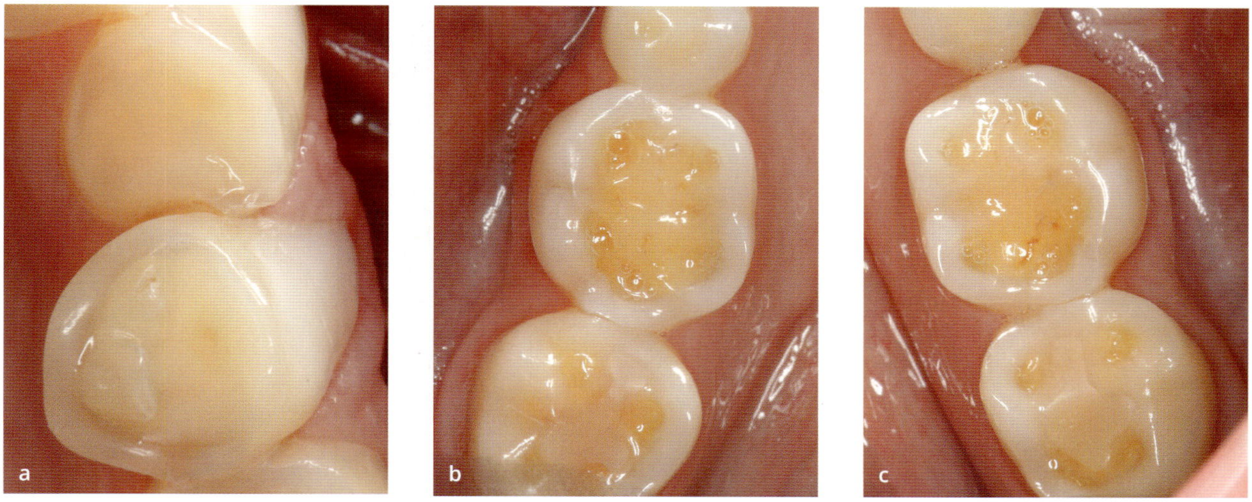

**Fig 3-22** EDs can create a devastating oral condition in very young patients. Many are the dilemmas with the patient with an ED. Should the dentist communicate to the family the etiologic suspicion? Should the dentist perform a restorative treatment before trying to implement a lifestyle coaching protocol? Taking into consideration that EDs represent a complex psychiatric disease, the role of the dental team seems relegated to providing the restorative treatment that protects and rehabilitates the dentition, even if the patient remains in the cycle of the eating disorder (a to c).

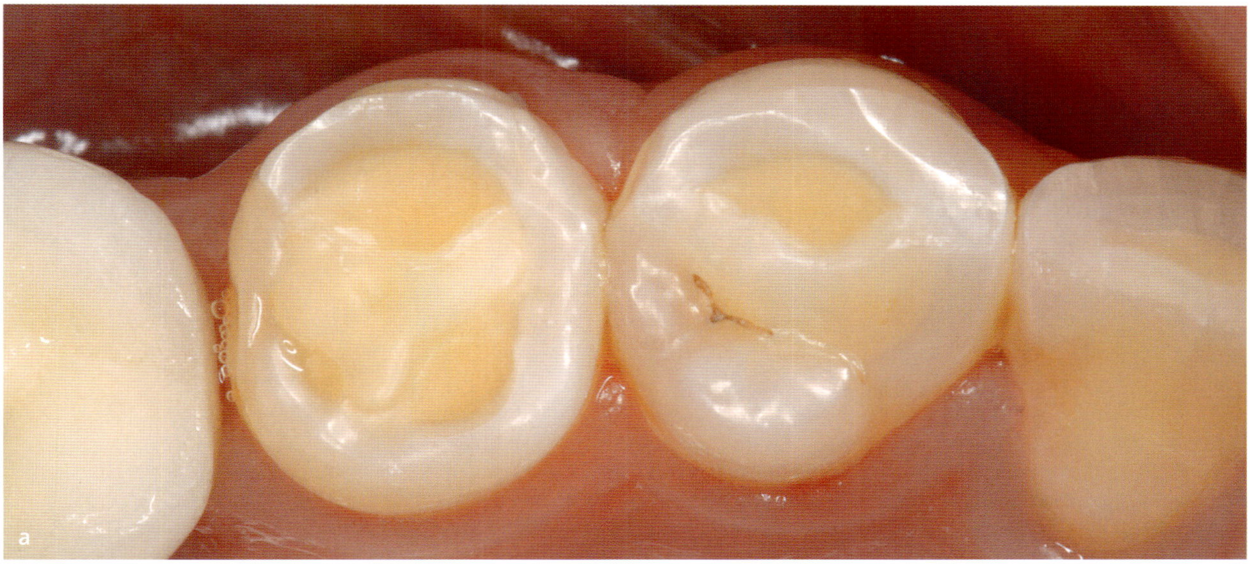

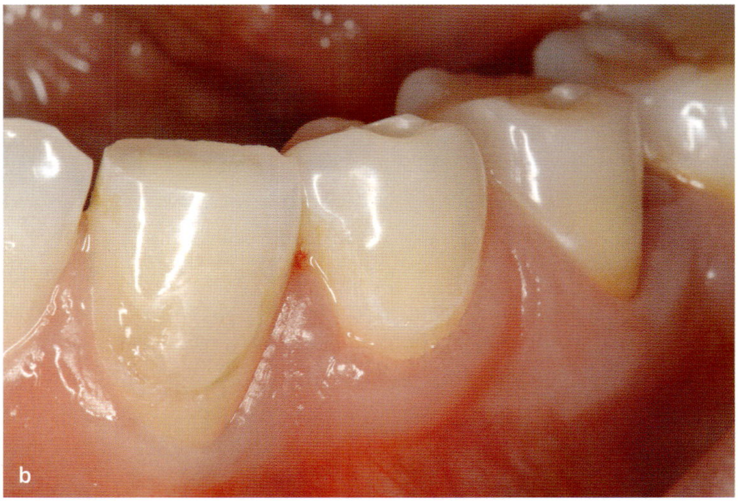

**Fig 3-23** In spite of the chemical cleansing effect from the acidic atmosphere in patients with EDs, it is clinically not uncommon to find a dysbiosis, recognized in this case by gingival inflammation. These soft tissue disorders associated with acidic challenges have recently been documented with high significance in GERD patients. (For more information, read the section below on TW and GERD.)

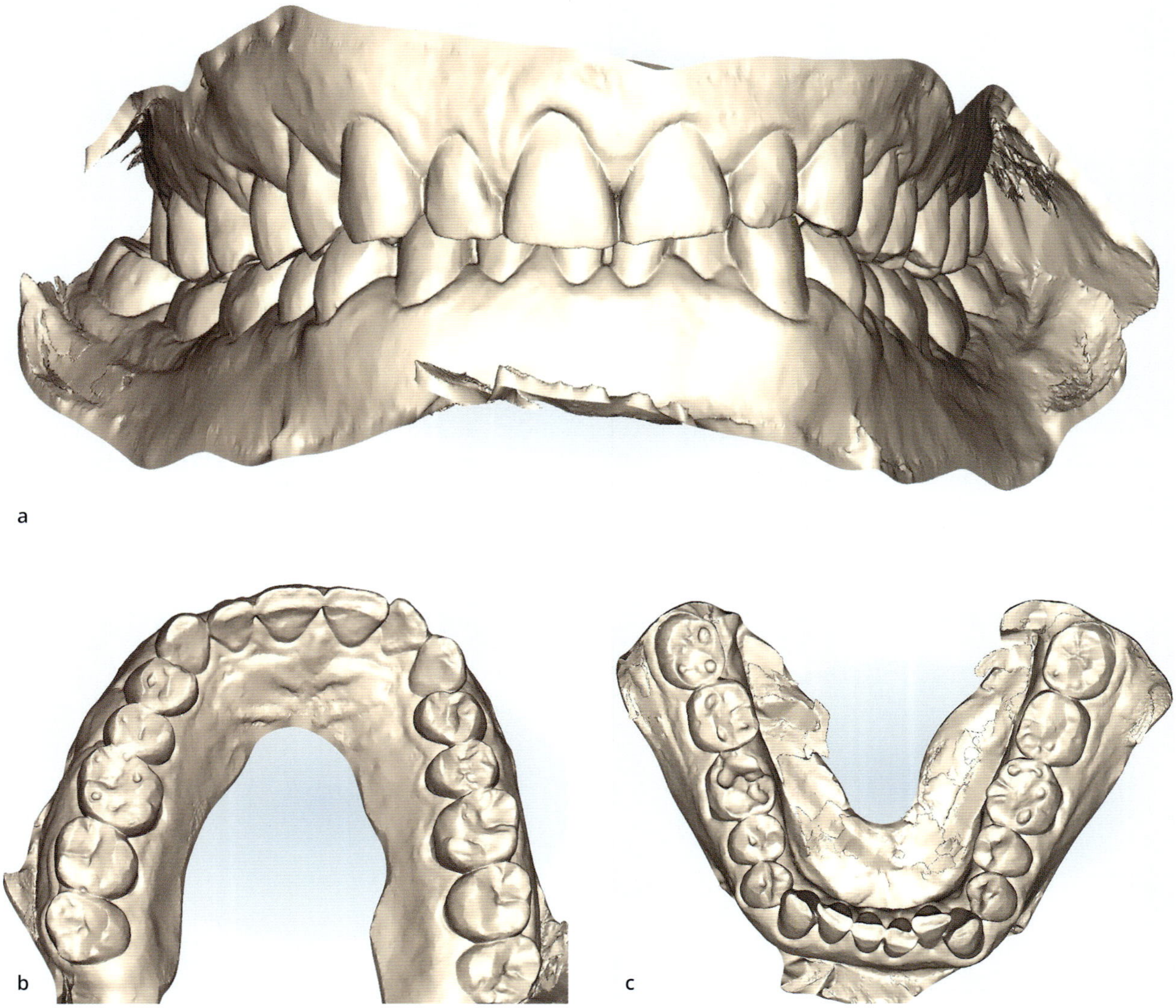

a

b

c

**Fig 3-24** The severity of the erosive damage due to acid attack in GERD is related not only to the duration and intensity of the pathology, but also to the existence or not of proper defensive saliva. Tooth loss is more notorious in the mandible in this adult confronted with GERD for the last 10 years. When confronting acid erosion from an internal origin (eg, GERD, EDs), it is mandatory to explore the "inside" of the mouth, as initially erosive damage will predominantly occur there (a to c).

## TW and Obesity

Obesity is known to alter multiple organs, including the salivary glands. The correlation between toothbrushing, oral health, quality of life, and noncommunicable and communicable diseases has already been described.[67] If TW is to be considered a noncommunicable disease or condition, all means of implementing correct and positive oral and general health behaviors, such as maintaining a healthy weight, may be a protection against TW. Recent data points out the changes in the oral microbiome in patients who are obese.[68]

## TW and GERD

Healthy individuals may experience gastroesophageal reflux (GER), a physiologic retrograde transit of gastric acid into the esophagus. This physiologic reflux usually happens after meals.[69]

However, GER can progress into gastroesophageal reflux disease (GERD), a condition known to affect the patient's quality of life and that can produce esophageal and extra-esophageal complications.

The esophagus is a 25-cm muscular tube with two natural anti-reflux barriers, the lower esophageal

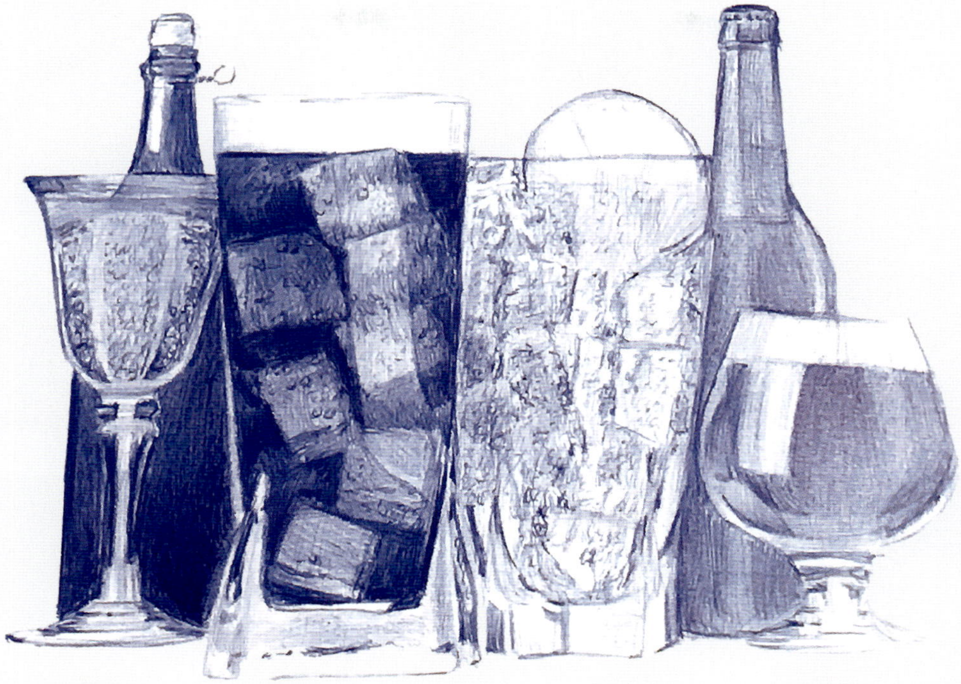

**Fig 3-25** GERD is commonly produced by a transitory relaxation of the LOS or excessive intra-abdominal pressure. Alcohol, amongst others, may create a LOS incompetence that produces GERD.

sphincter (LOS) at the gastroesophageal junction and the upper esophagus sphincter (UOS).

The main function of the UOS is to stop the flow of acid reflux or gastric content into the airway, while the main role of the LOS is to prevent the flow of gastric content or acid reflux into the esophagus. The LOS is not a strong sphincter[70] (Fig 3-24).

The gastroesophageal junction is of high significance as it is a site where premalignant changes may occur, creating the so-called Barret esophagus, a strong risk factor for esophageal adenocarcinoma. Although the possibility for a GERD patient to develop Barret esophagus is low, an increasing tendency has been documented.[71]

Risk factors for GERD are alcohol, nicotine, hiatal hernia, pregnancy, obesity, or heavy meals that increase intra-abdominal pressure and can create sphincter incompetence[72] (Fig 3-25).

Obstructive sleep apnea has also been linked to nocturnal reflux.[73,74] GERD can happen both day or night.[75] In fact, nocturnal GERD has been classified as a sleep disorder[76]; it occurs more commonly during the first hours of sleep.[77]

Esophagus manifestations of GERD are heartburn, regurgitation, epigastric pain, and dysphagia. Extra-esophageal effects are also common, such as chest pain, asthma, chronic coughing, and chronic hoarseness as well as a sensation of having a persistent ball in the throat called "globus."[78-81] Oral manifestations such as tooth erosion, halitosis, or mucositis are also frequent[82,83] (Fig 3-26).

Recent research has demonstrated the relationship between GERD and soft tissue disorders in a parallel proportion to the association between GERD and erosion.[84] Clinical experience shows that gingival inflammation is commonly associated with acidic erosive challenges, in particular papillae inflammation, thus supporting the nascent concept of gingival erosion. ED challenges in the presence of repeated vomiting courses with papillary and periodontal inflammation in the palatal aspect along with a lack of plaque accumulation because of the acid wash.

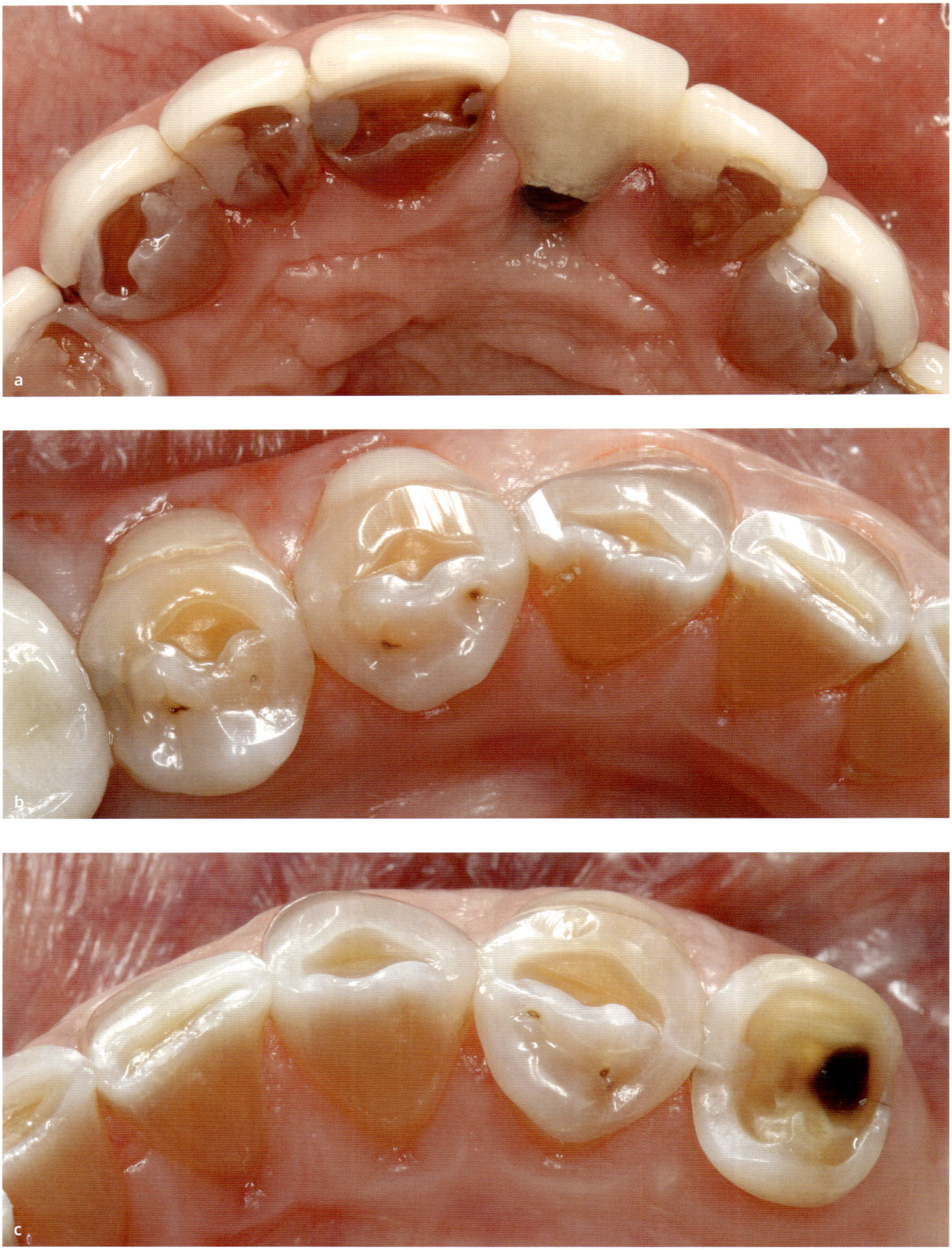


**Fig 3-26** The most commonly found erosion pattern when gastric acid is involved starts with the initial loss of enamel at the palatal surfaces of the maxillary incisors, followed by enamel loss from the palatal surfaces and cusps of molars and premolars. Note how insufficient treatment was performed more than a decade ago, addressing exclusively the esthetic concerns of the patient and overlooking the internal acid damage, leaving the patient helpless in confronting ongoing acidic attack on the palatal surfaces of the maxillary anterior teeth. Attrition wear facets can also be seen in this patient (a to c).

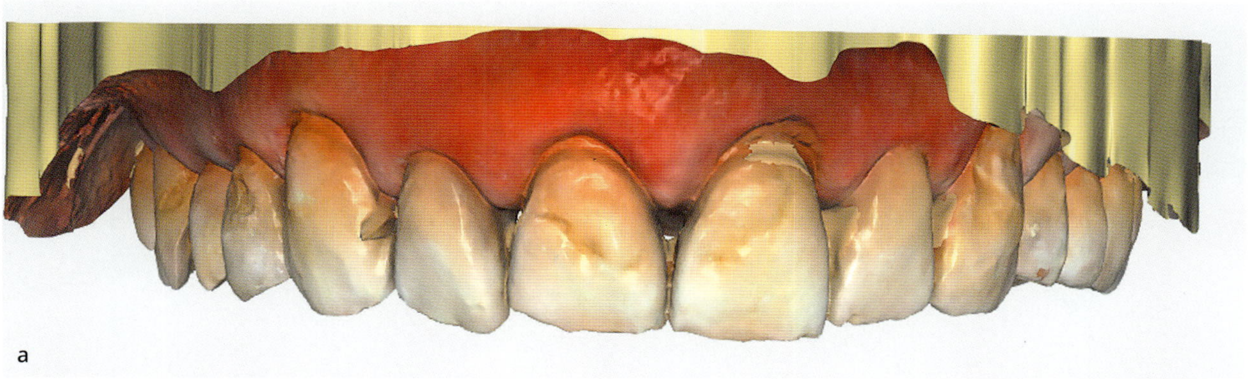
a

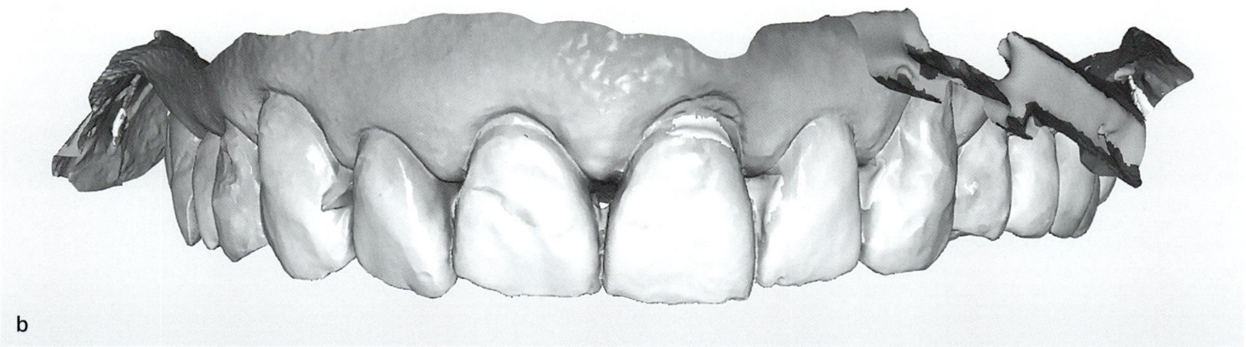
b

**Fig 3-27** Long-lasting GERD damage also reaches the vestibular aspects of the dentition. These images were created with an intraoral iTero scanner (Align Technology) and STL conversion. Tooth damage after long-term exposure to gastric secretion progresses in the following manner: initially the tooth salivary pellicle is lost, and later demineralization starts whenever the pH drops during GERD episodes.

Dental professionals may well be the first to do a GERD diagnosis, especially in so-called silent refluxers.

It is not infrequent in GERD patients to find widespread erosion that affects the occlusal surfaces of the molars and vestibular surfaces of all teeth[85–87] (Fig 3-27).

Intrinsic acid has a pH around 1.2, which is clearly under the traditional so-called critical pH of 5.5, below which dissolution of the enamel will take place.[88]

Even though saliva does have a protective role against gastric acid challenge, the interaction and concurrence between fluids and the surface tension will make it possible for acid to displace saliva and acquired biofilm from the teeth. This will create a situation where components coming from enamel demineralization will disappear from the environment, not allowing its reincorporation into the enamel (remineralization) when oral pH rises to its normal level; thus remineralization is clearly impeded[89] (Fig 3-28).

## TW and COVID-19

COVID-19, declared a pandemic by the World Health Organization (WHO) at the beginning of 2020 and caused by SARS-CoV-2 of the coronavirus family, has been a great challenge to global health and to economy worldwide. Recent research has been published that proves the association between periodontitis and severity of COVID-19 infection.[90] Further research is needed to determine how

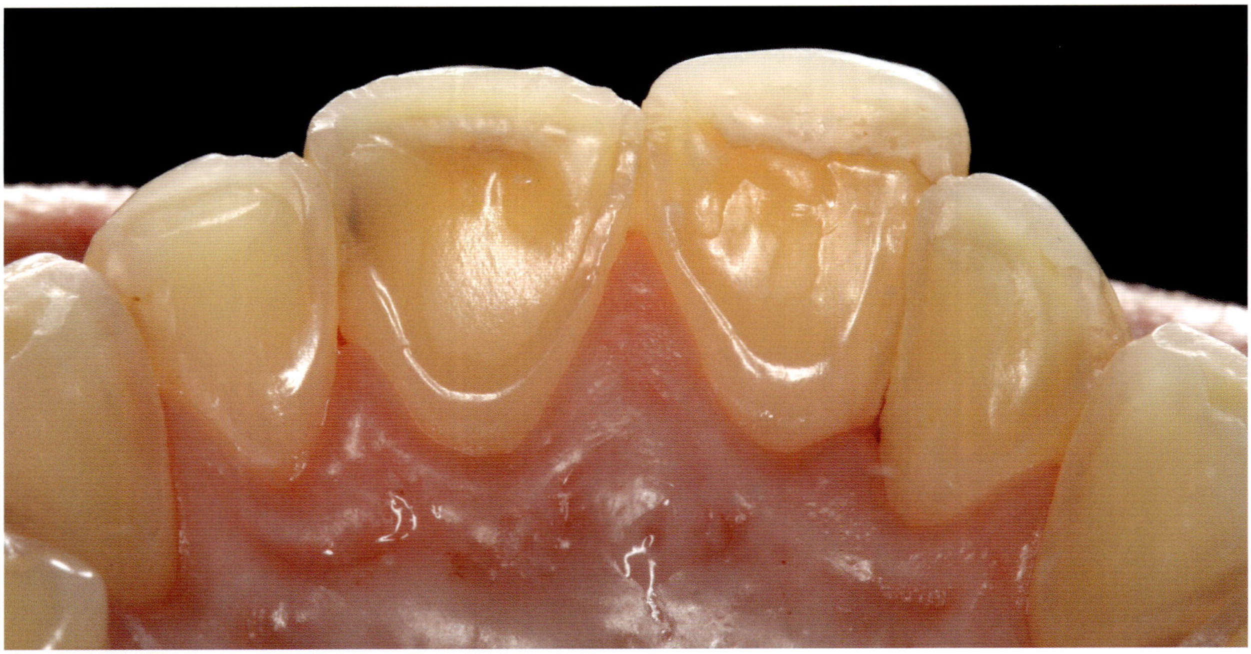

**Fig 3-28** Digestive disorders with no specific diagnosis have been suffered by the patient for years. Palatal TSL is not the only erosive damage in this patient.

other oral conditions, such as xerostomia, may well be determinant risk factors for COVID-19. Iwabuchi and coworkers already showed how hyposalivation increased the risk of acute respiratory infections such as influenza or the common cold.[91]

In line with all this, a bidirectional dynamic between COVID-19 and oral conditions is seen.

Stress, medication, increased access to cariogenic food while in confinement, rebounds of EDs, dehydration due to sustained use of protective masks, and hyposalivation in relation to the aforementioned, amongst other factors, are behind the rise of oral conditions detected not only in COVID-19 patients but also in the overall general population. Psychologic/emotional sequelae may well be long lasting not only for COVID-19 patients but also for the rest of the population. Antidepressant prescriptions have increased during the pandemic,[92] and the impact of loneliness, stress, and anxiety should not be overlooked.

COVID-19 has also affected sleep and diet quality. Alcohol intake has grown during the pandemic. Both conditions, sleep and diet, are related to saliva balance or imbalance.[93] Recent information outlines how low humidity negatively impacts the immune system when fighting respiratory viral infections.[94,95]

Anosmia, ageusia, and dental pain have been documented in relation to the COVID-19 pandemic.[96,97]

As per the previously described scenario, an increase in TW prevalence is to be expected in association with the COVID-19 pandemic (Fig 3-29).

## TW and Medication

Longer life expectancy is correlated with polypharmacy, which may produce secondary effects that can impact the salivary glands. Adverse effects on salivary glands may be salivary gland dysfunction (SGD), salivary gland hypofunction (SGH), xerostomia (subjective feeling of dry mouth), or subjective or objective sialorrhea (too much saliva).

Medication, especially with anticholinergic activity against µ3 muscarinic receptors is certainly one of the major causes behind xerostomia.

Patients under xerogenic medication are likely to experience a subjective dry-mouth feeling and sensation of having too little saliva in the mouth. Recent research has shown that current use of xerogenic medication is already positively linked to the presence of TW.[98] Patients should be instructed on how to recognize oral dryness as a predictor of TW.[98]

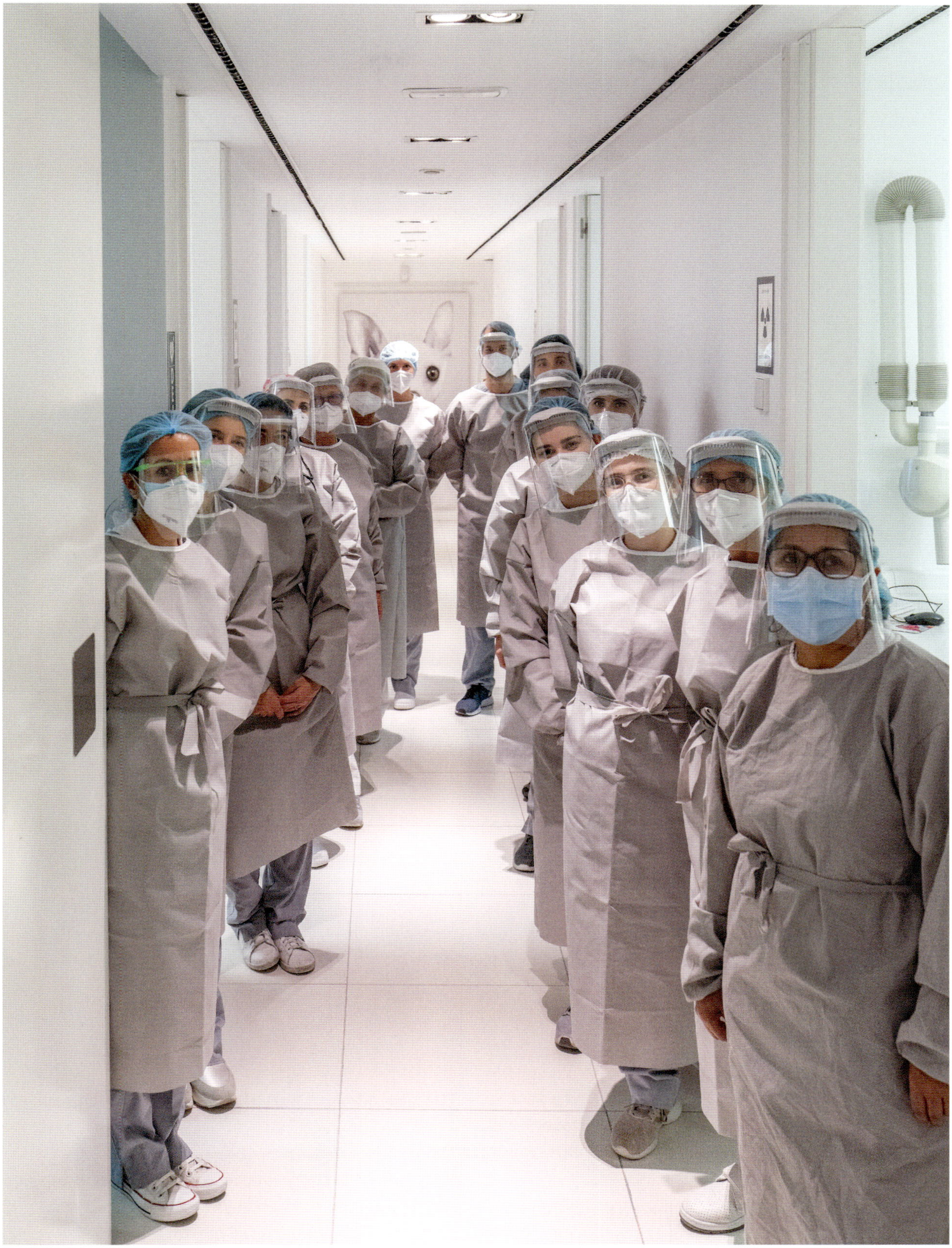

**Fig 3-29** After the initial months of the pandemic, scientists and researchers verified the relevance of the oral cavity not only in terms of the contagion and transmission of the virus, but also in the oral manifestations and sequelae of COVID-19 infection and, more recently, in the fact that oral disease may work as a potentiator for COVID-19. The oral cavity has therefore proven to be determinant both in the transmission of and the defense against COVID-19. The effort performed by dentists in infection control and COVID-19 prevention has enabled them to enjoy a very low intra–dental practice transmission rate.

**Table 3-2** Examples of medications reported to induce xerostomia or salivary gland hypofunction. Modified from Wolff et al.[101]

| | |
|---|---|
| Anti-emetics and anti-nauseants | Anti-emetics |
| Anti-obesity preparations, excluding diet products | Centrally acting anti-obesity products |
| | Serotonin-noradrenaline-dopamine reuptake inhibitor |
| Drugs for functional GI disorders | Synthetic anticholinergics, quaternary compounds |
| Agents acting on the renin-angiotensin system | ACE inhibitors |
| Antihypertensive | Imidazoline receptor agonists |
| | Methyldopa |
| Beta-blocking agents | Beta-blocking agents, non-selective |
| | Beta-blocking agents, selective |
| Calcium channel blockers | Dihydropyridine derivatives |
| | Phenylalkylamine derivatives |
| Cardiac therapy | Class I-b antiarrhythmics |
| Diuretics | Sulfonamides, plain |
| | Thiazides, plain |
| | Vasopressin antagonists |
| Urology | Drugs for urinary frequency and incontinence |
| | Alpha-adrenoreceptor antagonists |
| Antineoplastic agents | Monoclonal antibodies |
| Drugs for treatment of bone diseases | Bisphosphonates |
| Analgesics | Natural opium alkaloids |
| | Oripavine derivatives |
| | Other anti-migraine preparations |
| | Phenylpiperidine derivatives |
| Antiepileptics | Fatty acid derivatives |
| | Other anti-epileptics |
| Anti-Parkinson drugs, psycholeptics | Benzodiazepine derivations (anxiolytics) |
| | Benzodiazepine-related drugs |
| | Dopamine agonists Lithium |
| | Other anti-psychotics |
| | Other hypnotics and sedatives |
| Other nervous system drugs, psychoanaleptics | Drugs used in nicotine dependence |
| | Drugs used in alcohol dependence |
| | Other anti-depressants |
| | Non-selective monoamine reuptake inhibitors |
| | Selective serotonin reuptake inhibitors |
| Nasal preparations | Anti-allergic agents, excluding corticosteroids |
| Drugs for obstructive airway diseases | Anticholinergics |
| Antihistamines for systemic use | Amino alkyl ethers |
| | Other antihistamines for systemic use |
| | Piperazine derivations |
| Ophthalmologic drugs | Anticholinergics |
| | Sympathomimetics in glaucoma therapy |

Changing the formulation, number of medications, or the dosage could help reduce the TW risk associated with such drugs.[99,100] Communication with the physician is therefore essential.

The number of xerostomia-inducing drugs is extensive. Therefore, the population is exposed to a significant risk of TW when receiving a prescription. Table 3-2 presents a list of medications reported to induce xerostomia with high or moderate evidence, modified from Wolff et al.[101]

## TW and Sleep Disorders

### TW and sleep apnea

Sleep is a crucial physiologic function. Changes in sleep patterns will be followed by impaired levels of health, while good-quality sleep will enhance overall well-being. Sleep is essential for "recharging the batteries" expended during the day.

Sleep disorders are known to produce oral manifestations, including TW. The role of the dentist in

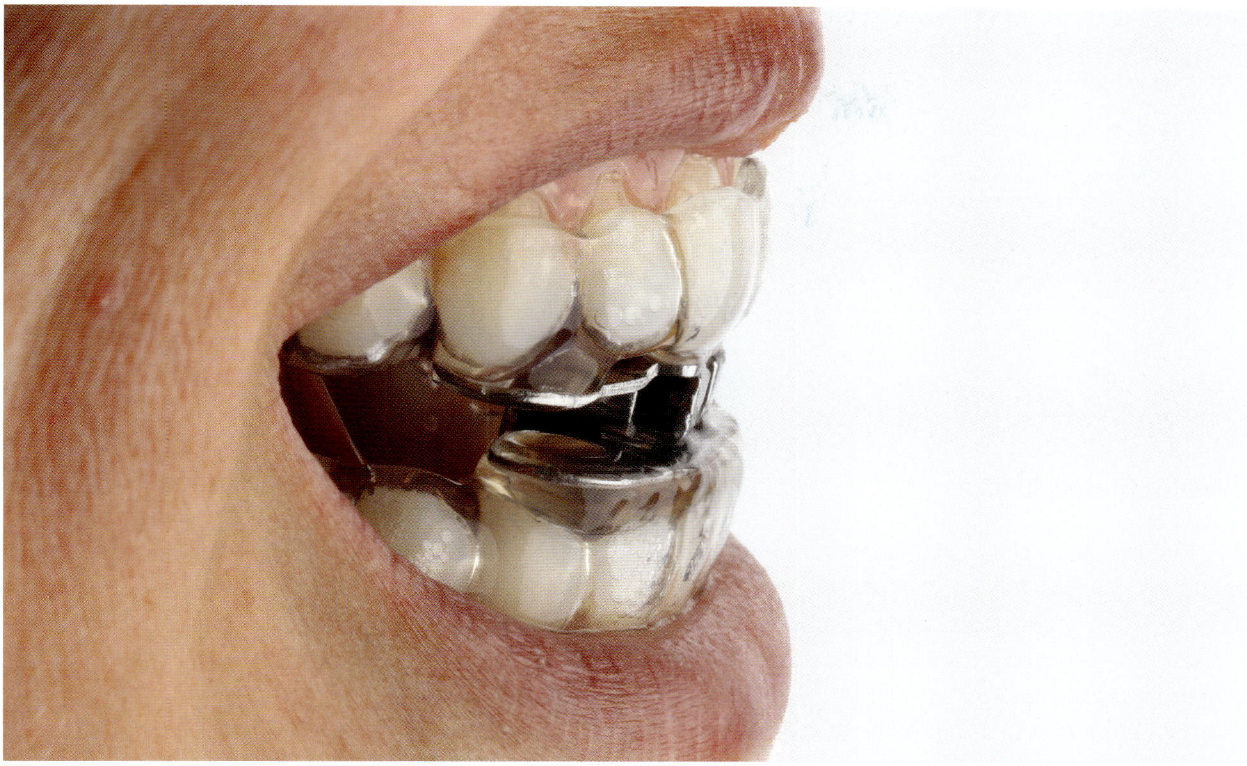

**Fig 3-30** Even sleep disorders considered to be minor, such as mouth breathing, can put the patient at risk of erosion. Sleep disorders are frequently underestimated by the dental team as the reason behind TW. Very low salivary production during the night leaves oral tissues helpless to face the low pH that challenges tooth structure during sleep hours. The use of mandibular advancement appliances for OSA and other sleep disorders may increase the overall TW risk for OSA patients through several mechanisms such as increased dehydration and erosion.

diagnosing and treating sleep disorders is important. Preventing the oral consequences of sleep disorders is in the dentist's hands. In fact, recently Lobbezoo et al coined the term *dental sleep medicine*,[102] while Lavigne and collaborators published the book *Sleep Medicine for Dentists*.[103] The increase of caries, periodontal disease, and TW with sleep disorders has been documented. Xerostomia, lifestyle, and increased release of inflammatory cytokines have been included in the complex mechanism of the abovementioned conditions. Circadian intraoral pH variation and oral microbiome alterations have also been implicated in oral-related sleep disorder consequences.[103]

Among sleep disorders, obstructive sleep apnea (OSA) plays a principal role. It is characterized by the complete or partial collapse of the upper airway during sleep. Prevalence of OSA is increasing and is estimated to affect between 9% and 38% of the general population.[104]

A recent study found a positive correlation between not only OSA and TW but also the severity of OSA and the severity of TW[105] (Fig 3-30).

In 2002, Lavigne et al in Montreal already hypothesized that salivary lubrication was necessary to protect tissue integrity during sleep. Furthermore, they outlined a scheme to highlight the influences contributing to TW in sleep disorders. Low salivary flow while sleeping, anxiety, snoring, increased tooth grinding, and preexisting poor enamel were considered determinant factors in producing excessive TW in sleep disorders.[106]

**Table 3-3** BEWE 0–3 erosive scale.

| | |
|---|---|
| 0 | No erosive wear. |
| 1 | Minimal damage restricted to enamel. |
| 2 | More extensive damage that may involve dentin but not affecting more than 50% of surface area. |
| 3 | Tooth loss affecting more than 50% of surface area and dentin exposure. |

**Table 3-4** Final BEWE index.

| | |
|---|---|
| < 2 | No risk |
| 3–8 | Low risk |
| 9–13 | Medium risk |
| > 14 | High risk |

## TW and Malocclusion

An existing body of opinion states that TW in malocclusion should not be considered pathologic but rather seen as a consequence of the given interocclusal dynamics.[107,108] Orthodontic correction of malocclusions can avoid oral consequences such as TW.

The TW pattern found in different types of malocclusions is characteristic of each malocclusion. Class II division 2, for example, shows marked wear on the labial surfaces of the mandibular incisors.

However, malocclusion risk factors such as mouth breathing may lead to a large variety of occlusal findings.[109] TW related to malocclusion is further described in chapter 8.

# 5. Tooth Wear Indices

Significant efforts are being made by international consensus groups, TW experts, and health and dental organizations to spread the word about the relevance of TW in oral health in the 21st century.[110,111]

Most of the indices that are used today have been inspired by Eccles (1979)[112] and Smith and Knight (1984).[113]

The index described by Smith and Knight is intended to measure TW no matter the etiology. Smith and Knight proposed dividing the teeth into four sections: buccal, palatal, cervical, and occlusal/incisal. Values are scored from 0 (no loss of tooth structure) to 4 (complete disappearance of enamel with pulp exposure). The values are then compared to the maximum level of acceptable TW, determined by the age of the patient. For example, Smith and Knight established the acceptable level of wear in a patient under the age of 25 to be zero. In this way, the Smith and Knight index is not ideal when measuring TW in the infant population. Subsequently, Ganss et al proposed a modification to the Smith and Knight index.[6]

In 2008, Bartlett, Ganss, and Lussi published a new scoring system for scientific and clinical needs regarding erosion wear named BEWE (Basic Erosive Wear Examination),[114] a four-point scale (0–3) that allows erosion assessment (Table 3-3).

The BEWE index rates the degree of erosive wear on all surfaces of all the teeth in a sextant. However, only the highest score is considered. An overall risk value (BEWE index) emerges by adding up the highest scores from all sextants (Table 3-4).

Other attempts have been made to detect and measure TW. The use of long-term monitoring of study models has proven effective when measuring TW progression. In this way, Bartlett found an apparent lack of progression in a group of selected patients utilizing longitudinal study of stone models. The lack of progression was attributed to the phasic, cyclic personality of TW as well as to the positive effect of preventive measures in certain patients.[115]

Photography is also an efficient tool not only to detect but also to monitor TW evolution. However, today's digital era offers the invaluable ability to superimpose 3D intraoral scanning, which enables TW lesions to be clearly detected. Monitoring TW evolution in untreated patients as well as the survival of TW restorations provides the dentist with optimal control. Tools such as TimeLapse from iTero and OraCheck from Primescan (Dentsply Sirona) provide excellent data (Fig 3-31).

The ample variation in TW prevalence studies may well reflect the complex task of describing and choosing a unified TW index. The variation in scale, choice of teeth, assessment, and other parameters make the actual data difficult to compare. Still, the challenge exists as to finding a simplified index that is easily applicable in everyday practice.

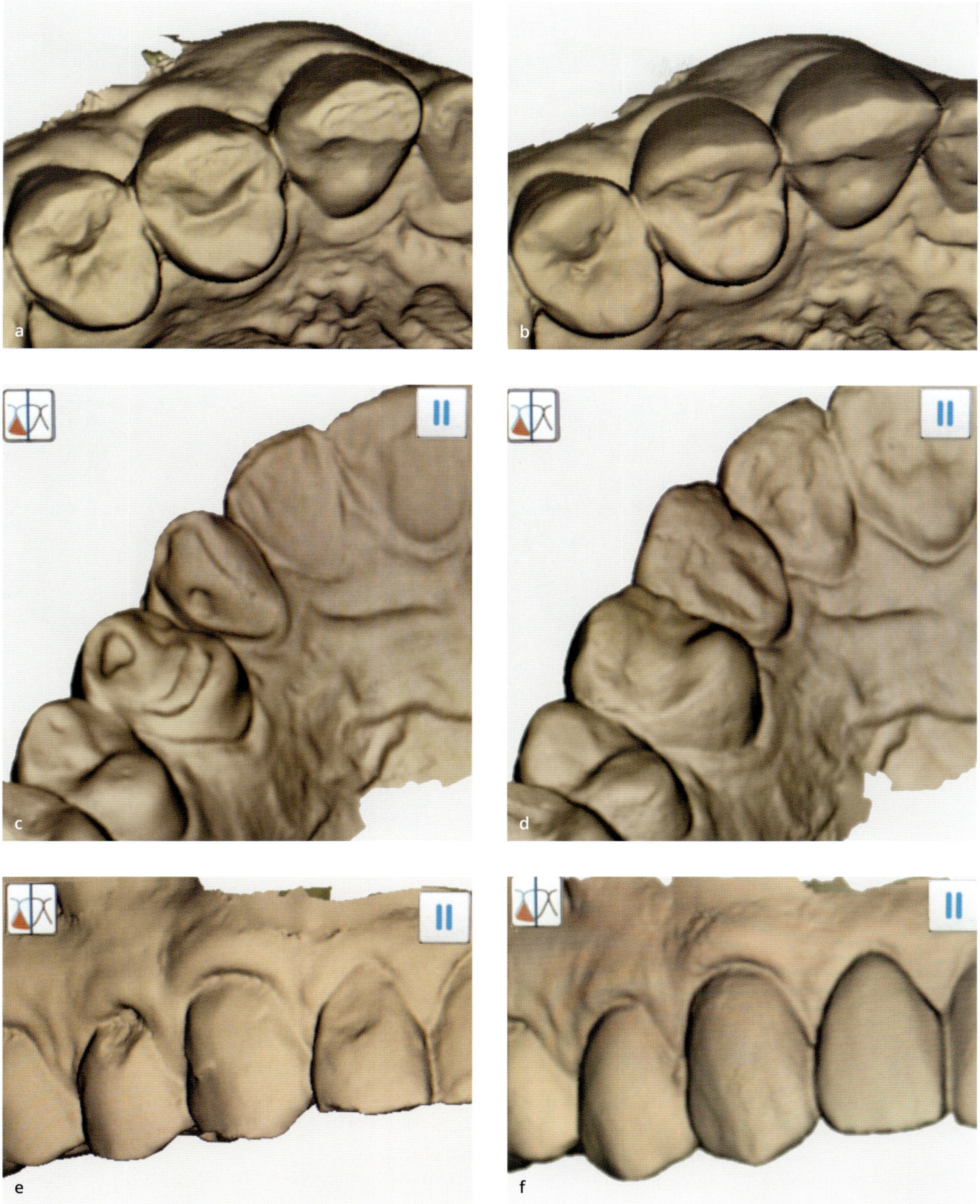


**Fig 3-31** Partial STL images originating from an iTero intraoral scanning record and TimeLapse program show the increment provided by restorations in a TW patient. Alternatively, this TimeLapse program can be used to monitor wear in a patient who chooses to delay treatment, to determine stability of a baseline situation, or to assess the outcome of restorative treatment. Primescan and OraCheck provide parallel information *(continued next page)*.

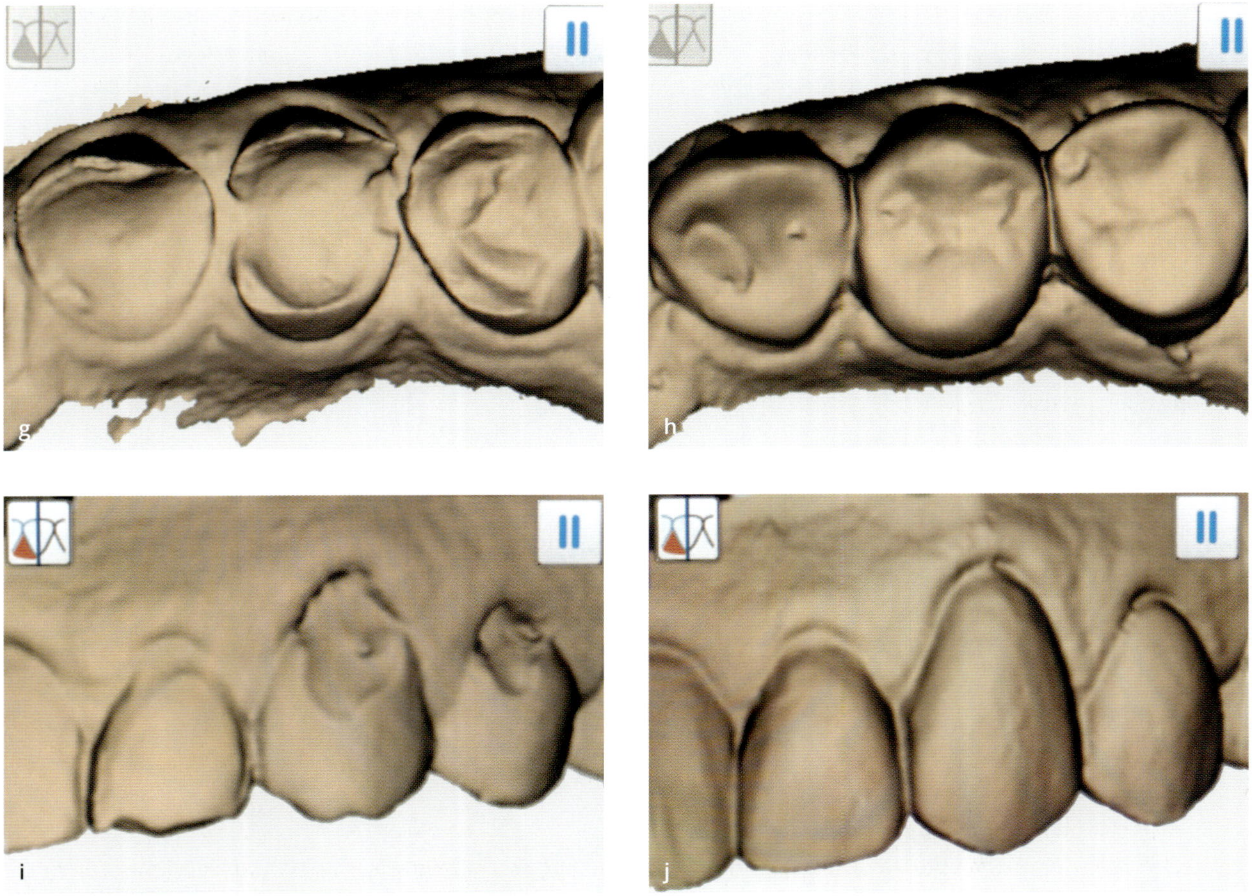


**Fig 3-31** *(continued)*

## 6. Following Tooth Wear Clues: Lifestyle and Health TW Questionnaire

Establishing a particular etiologic factor in a TW patient is a complex task. However, knowing and understanding the causes, even if overlapping, will help the dentist to provide better preventive treatment approaches.

The use of self-assessment questionnaires has been proven to be efficient and effective not only in helping to determine the causes of the condition but also in detecting populations at risk of a given oral disease or condition.

Self-assessment questionnaires have been successfully used in a wide variety of medical domains and have helped reinforce the significance of quality of life.[114] Standardization and validation of such questionnaires will enable their use not only in research and epidemiology but also in everyday clinical practice. The proposed Lifestyle and Health TW Questionnaire (see appendix 1) combines the input from previously existing questionnaires that enable, for example, identification of patients suffering from xerostomia and hyposalivation.[116,117]

## 7. Key Points

- TW is in the vast majority of cases multifactorial.
- A loss of 28 to 30 μm tooth structure per year is agreed to be part of the physiologic aging process.
- The TW umbrella includes tooth damage originated by erosion, abrasion, attrition, and abfraction. Superimposed erosion may skyrocket tooth loss.
- TW is a noncommunicable oral condition linked to lifestyle, nutritional and behavioral factors, and general health.
- Hyposalivation acts a TW potentiator.
- Children suffer from both erosion and attrition. Dietary habits such as intake of acidic soda drinks are behind the escalating figures of erosive TW in children.
- Medical conditions such as eating disorders, gastroesophageal reflux, obesity, medication intake, or sleep disorders are directly linked to TW.
- Significant efforts are being made to introduce TW management in everyday practice. The Basic Erosive Wear Examination (BEWE) provides a good tool for TW management.
- A Wear Easy Clinical Classification (WECC), subdivided into incipient, moderate, and severe wear is proposed by the authors as a simplified index for the dentist (see chapter 4).
- A Wear Aggravation Severity Scale (WASS) is hereby also proposed, as TW is a dynamic and many times chronic condition that has to be watched over time (see chapter 4).

## References


1. Lucas PW. Dental Functional Morphology: How Teeth Work. Cambridge: Cambridge UP, 2004.
2. Kullmer O, Benazzi S, Fiorenza L, Schulz D, Bacso S, Winzen O. Technical note: Occlusal fingerprint analysis: Quantification of tooth wear pattern. Am J Phys Anthropol 2009;139:600–605.
3. Van't Spijker A, Rodriguez JM, Kreulen CM, Bronkhorst EM, Bartlett DW, Creugers NH. Prevalence of tooth wear in adults. Int J Prosthodont 2009;22(1):35–42.
4. Robinson HB. A clinic on the differential diagnosis of oral lesions. Am J Orthod 1946;32:729–762.
5. Stafne EC, Lovestedt SA. Dissolution of tooth substance by lemon juice, acid beverages and acids from some other sources. J Am Dent Assoc 1947;34:586–592.
6. Ganss C, Young A, Lussi A. Tooth wear and erosion: Methodological issues in epidemiological and public health research and the future research agenda. Community Dent Health 2011;28(3):191–195.
7. Fares J, Shirodaria S, Chiu K, Ahmad N, Sherriff M, Bartlett D. A new index of tooth wear. Reproducibility and application to a sample of 18- to 30-year-old university students. Caries Res 2009;43(2):119–125.
8. Grippo JO. Biocorrosion vs. erosion: The 21st century and a time to change. Compend Contin Educ Dent 2012;33(2):e33–e37.
9. Eisenburger M, Shellis RP, Addy M. Comparative study of wear of enamel induced by alternating and simultaneous combinations of abrasion and erosion in vitro. Caries Res 2003;37:450–455.
10. Addy M, Shellis RP. Interaction between attrition, abrasion and erosion in tooth wear. Monogr Oral Sci 2006;20:17–31.
11. Addy M, Hunter ML.Can tooth brushing damage your health? Effects on oral and dental tissues. Int Dent J 2003;53(Suppl 3):177–186.
12. Curtis T, Kvernmo S, Bjerregaard P. Changing living conditions, life style and health. Int J Circumpolar Health 2005;64(5):442–450.
13. Young WG. The oral medicine of tooth wear. Aust Dent J 2001;46(4):236–250.
14. Su JM, Tsamtsouris A, Laskou M. Gastroesophageal reflux in children with cerebral palsy and its relationship to erosion of primary and permanent teeth. J Mass Dent Soc 2003;52(2):20–24.
15. Staufenbiel I, Adam K, Deac A, Geurtsen W, Günay H. Influence of fruit consumption and fluoride application on the prevalence of caries and erosion in vegetarians—A controlled clinical trial. Eur J Clin Nutr 2015;69:1156–1160.
16. Kamal Y, O'Toole S, Bernabé E. Obesity and tooth wear among American adults: The role of sugar-sweetened acidic drinks. Clin Oral Investig 2020;24:1379–1385.
17. Linnett V, Seow WK. Dental erosion in children: A literature review. Pediatr Dent 2001;23(1):37–43.
18. Smithers G, Gregory JR, Bates CJ, Prentice A, Jackson LV, Wenlock R. The National Diet and Nutrition Survey: Young people aged 4–18 years. Nutr Bull 2000;25(2):105–111.
19. Ganss C, Klimek J, Giese K. Dental erosion in children and adolescents—A cross-sectional and longitudinal investigation using study models. Community Dent Oral Epidemiol 2001;29(4):264–271.
20. McGuire J, Szabo A, Jackson S, Bradley TG, Okunseri C. Erosive tooth wear among children in the United States: Relationship to race/ethnicity and obesity. Int J Paediatr Dent 2009;19(2):91–98.
21. Johansson AK, Sorvari R, Birkhed D, Meurman JH. Dental erosion in deciduous teeth—An in vivo and in vitro study. J Dent 2001;29:333–340.
22. Nishino M, Arita K, Kikuchi K, et al. Hypoplasia of tooth in children with inborn errors of metabolism [in Japanese]. Shoni Shikagaku Zasshi 1990;28(2):503–509.
23. Al-Malik MI, Holt RD, Bedi R, Speight PM. Investigation of an index to measure tooth wear in primary teeth. J Dent 2001;29(2):103–107.
24. Wiegand A, Müller J, Werner C, Attin T. Prevalence of erosive tooth wear and associated risk factors in 2-7-year-old German kindergarten children. Oral Dis 2006;12(2):117–124.
25. Salas MM, Nascimento GG, Huysmans MC, Demarco FF. Estimated prevalence of erosive tooth wear in permanent teeth of children and adolescents: An epidemiological systematic review and meta-regression analysis. J Dent 2015;43(1):42–50.
26. Kreulen CM, Van 't Spijker A, Rodriguez JM, Bronkhorst EM, Creugers NH, Bartlett DW. Systematic review of the prevalence of tooth wear in children and adolescents. Caries Res 2010;44(2):151–159.
27. Lussi A, Jaeggi T, Zero D. The role of diet in the aetiology of dental erosion. Caries Res 2004;38(Suppl 1):34–44.
28. Ito E, Inoue Y. The International Classification of Sleep Disorders, third edition. American Academy of Sleep Medicine. Includes bibliographies and index [in Japanese]. Nihon Rinsho 2015;73(6):916–923.
29. The glossary of prosthodontic terms. J Prosthet Dent 2005;94(1):10–92.
30. Hublin C, Kaprio J, Partinen M, Koskenvuo M. Sleep bruxism based on self-report in a nationwide twin cohort. J Sleep Res 199; 7(1):61–67.
31. Rintakoski K, Hublin C, Lobbezoo F, Rose RJ, Kaprio J. Genetic factors account for half of the phenotypic variance in liability to sleep-related bruxism in young adults: A nationwide Finnish twin cohort study. Twin Res Hum Genet 2012;15:714–719.
32. Tachibana M, Kato T, Kato-Nishimura K, Matsuzawa S, Mohri I, Taniike M. Associations of sleep bruxism with age, sleep apnea, and daytime problematic behaviors in children. Oral Dis 2016;22:557–565.
33. John MT, Frank H, Lobbezoo F, Drangsholt M, Dette KE. No association between incisal tooth wear and temporomandibular disorders. J Prosthet Dent 2002;87:197–203.
34. Bell EJ, Kaidonis J, Townsend GC. Tooth wear in children with Down syndrome. Aust Dent J 2002;47(1):30–35.
35. Saeves R, Espelid I, Storhaug K, Sandvik L, Nordgarden H. Severe tooth wear in Prader-Willi syndrome. A case-control study. BMC Oral Health 2012;12:12.
36. Olczak-Kowalczyk D, Korporowicz E, Gozdowski D, Lecka-Ambroziak A, Szalecki M. Oral findings in children and adolescents with Prader-Willi syndrome. Clin Oral Investig 2019;23:1331–1339.
37. Hidas A, Noy AF, Birman N, et al. Oral health status, salivary flow rate and salivary quality in children, adolescents and young adults with ADHD. Arch Oral Biol 2011;56:1137–1141.
38. Hidas A, Birman N, Noy AF, et al. Salivary bacteria and oral health status in medicated and non-medicated children and adolescents with attention deficit hyperactivity disorder (ADHD). Clin Oral Investig 2013;17:1863–1867.
39. Ertugrul CC, Kirzioglu Z, Aktepe E, Savas HB. The effects of psychostimulants on oral health and saliva in children with attention deficit hyperactivity disorder: A case-control study. Niger J Clin Pract 2018;21:1213–1220.
40. Coughlin CG, Cohen SC, Mulqueen JM, Ferracioli-Oda E, Stuckelman ZD, Bloch MH. Meta-analysis: Reduced risk of anxiety with psychostimulant treatment in children with attention-deficit/hyperactivity disorder. J Child Adolesc Psychopharmacol, 2015;25:611–617.
41. Erenberg G. The relationship between Tourette syndrome, attention deficit hyperactivity disorder, and stimulant medication: A critical review. Semin Pediatr Neurol 2005;12(4):217–221.
42. Chau YC, Lai KY, McGrath CP, Yiu CK. Oral health of children with attention deficit hyperactivity disorder. Eur J Oral Sci 2017;125(1):49–54.
43. Bimstein E, Wilson J, Guelmann M, Primosch R. Oral characteristics of children with attention-deficit hyperactivity disorder. Spec Care Dentist 2008;28(3):107–110.
44. Dobry Y, Braquehais MD, Sher L. Bullying, psychiatric pathology and suicidal behavior. Int J Adolesc Med Health 2013;25:295–299.
45. Folayan MO, Oginni O, Arowolo O, El Tantawi M. Association between adverse childhood experiences, bullying, self-esteem, resilience, social support, caries and oral hygiene in children and adolescents in sub-urban Nigeria. BMC Oral Health, 2020;20(1):202.
46. Dorian B, Garfinkel PE. Stress, immunity and illness—A review. Psychol Med 1987;17:393–407.
47. Donoghue C, Meltzer LJ Sleep it off: Bullying and sleep disturbances in adolescents. J Adolesc 2018;68:87–93.
48. Lavigne GJ, Goulet JP, Zuconni M, Morrison F, Lobbezoo F. Sleep disorders and the dental patient: An overview. Oral Surg Oral Med Oral Pathol Oral Radiol Endod 1999;88:257–272.
49. Lee B, Jeong S, Roh M. Association between body mass index and health outcomes among adolescents: the mediating role of traditional and cyber bullying victimization. BMC Public Health 2018;18(1):1–12.
50. Jackson DB. Diet quality and bullying among a cross-national sample of youth. Prev Med 2017;105:359–365.
51. Gini G, Pozzoli T. Bullied children and psychosomatic problems: A meta-analysis. Pediatrics 2013;132:720–729.
52. Heyman MB, Committee on Nutrition. Lactose intolerance in infants, children, and adolescents. Pediatrics 2006:118:1279–1286.
53. Roy-Byrne PP, Davidson KW, Kessler RC, et al. Anxiety disorders and comorbid medical illness. Gen Hosp Psychiatry 2008;30(3):208–225.
54. Langeluddecke PM. Psychological aspects of irritable bowel syndrome. Aust N Z J Psychiatry 1985;19(3):218–226.
55. Goswami U, O'Toole S, Bernabé E. Asthma, long-term asthma control medication and tooth wear in American adolescents and young adults. J Asthma 2021;58:939–945.
56. Dugmore CR, Rock WP. Asthma and tooth erosion. Is there an association? Int J Paediatr Dent 2003;13:417–424.
57. Sreebny LM, Yu A, Green A, Valdini A. Xerostomia in diabetes mellitus. Diabetes Care 1992;15:900–904.
58. Moore PA, Guggenheimer J, Etzel KR, Weyant RJ, Orchard T. Type 1 diabetes mellitus, xerostomia, and salivary flow rates. Oral Surg Oral Med Oral Pathol Oral Radiol Endod 2001;92:281–291.

59. Levine M. Communication challenges within eating disorders: What people say and what individuals hear. In: Jáuregui-Lobera I (ed). Eating Disorders: A Paradigm of the Biopsychosocial Model of Illness. London: IntechOpen, 2017:239–272.
60. Robb ND, Smith BG, Geidrys-Leeper E. The distribution of erosion in the dentitions of patients with eating disorders. Br Dent J 1995;178(5):171–175.
61. Järvinen VK, Rytömaa II, Heinonen OP. Risk factors in dental erosion. J Dent Res 1991;70:942–947.
62. Milosevic A, Slade PD. The orodental status of anorexics and bulimics. Br Dent J 1989;167(2):66–70.
63. Levin PA, Falko JM, Dixon K, Gallup EM, Saunders W. Benign parotid enlargement in bulimia. Ann Intern Med 1980;93:827–829.
64. Hasler JF. Parotid enlargement: A presenting sign in anorexia nervosa. Oral Surg Oral Med Oral Pathol 1982;53:567–573.
65. Philipp E, Willershausen-Zönnchen B, Hamm G, Pirke K-M. Oral and dental characteristics in bulimic and anorectic patients. Int J Eat Disord 1991;10:423–431.
66. Milosevic A, Dawson LJ. Salivary factors in vomiting bulimics with and without pathological tooth wear. Caries Res 1996;30:361–366.
67. Cinar AB, Oktay I, Schou L. Toothbrushing: A link between noncommunicable and communicable diseases? Oral Health Prev Dent 2015;13:515–522.
68. Roa I, Del Sol M. Obesity, salivary glands and oral pathology. Colomb Med (Cali) 2018;49:280287.
69. Orr WC. Sleep issues in gastroesophageal reflux disease: beyond simple heartburn control. Rev Gastroenterol Disord 2003;3(Suppl 4):S22–S29.
70. Meyer GW, Austin RM, Brady CE 3rd, Castell DO. Muscle anatomy of the human esophagus. J Clin Gastroenterol 1986;8(2):131–134.
71. Peters FT, Kleibeuker JH. Barrett's oesophagus and carcinoma. Recent insights into its development and possible prevention. Scand J Gastroenterol Suppl 1993;200:59–64.
72. Dodds WJ, Dent J, Hogan WJ, et al. Mechanisms of gastroesophageal reflux in patients with reflux esophagitis. N Engl J Med 1982;307:1547–1552.
73. Ing AJ, Ngu MC, Breslin AB. Obstructive sleep apnea and gastroesophageal reflux. Am J Med 2000;108(4):120–125.
74. Orr WC, Heading R, Johnson LF, Kryger M. Review article: Sleep and its relationship to gastro-oesophageal reflux. Aliment Pharmacol Ther 2004;20(Suppl 9):39–46.
75. Myers-Wright N, Cheng B, Tafreshi SN, Lamster IB. A simple self-report health assessment questionnaire to identify oral diseases. Int Dent J 2018;68:428–432.
76. Farup C, Kleinman L, Sloan S, et al. The impact of nocturnal symptoms associated with gastroesophageal reflux disease on health-related quality of life. Arch Intern Med 2001;161(1):45–52.
77. Dickman R, Parthasarathy S, Malagon IB, et al. Comparisons of the distribution of oesophageal acid exposure throughout the sleep period among the different gastro-oesophageal reflux disease groups. Aliment Pharmacol Ther 2007;26(1): 41–48.
78. Chandra A, Moazzez R, Bartlett D, Anggiansah A, Owen WJ. A review of the atypical manifestations of gastroesophageal reflux disease. Int J Clin Pract 2004;58(1):41–48.
79. Bennett JR. Heartburn and gastro-oesophageal reflux. Br J Clin Pract 1991;45:273–277.
80. Irwin RS, Richter JE. Gastroesophageal reflux and chronic cough. Am J Gastroenterol 2000;95(8 Suppl): S9–S14.
81. Smit CF, van Leeuwen JA, Mathus-Vliegen LM, et al. Gastropharyngeal and gastroesophageal reflux in globus and hoarseness. Arch Otolaryngol Head Neck Surg 2000;126:827–830.
82. Bartlett D. Intrinsic causes of erosion. Monogr Oral Sci, 2006;20:119–139.
83. Dean BB, Aguilar D Johnson LF, et al. Night-time and daytime atypical manifestations of gastro-oesophageal reflux disease: Frequency, severity and impact on health-related quality of life. Aliment Pharmacol Ther 2008;27:327–337.
84. Watanabe M, Nakatani E, Yoshikawa H, et al. Oral soft tissue disorders are associated with gastroesophageal reflux disease: Retrospective study. BMC Gastroenterol 2017;17(1):92.
85. Ganss C, Lussi A, Schlueter N. Dental erosion as oral disease. Insights in etiological factors and pathomechanisms, and current strategies for prevention and therapy. Am J Dent 2012;25:351–364.
86. Magalhães AC, Wiegand A, Rios D, Honório HM, Buzalaf MA. Insights into preventive measures for dental erosion. J Appl Oral Sci 2009;17(2):75–86.
87. Bartlett DW, Coward PY. Comparison of the erosive potential of gastric juice and a carbonated drink in vitro. J Oral Rehabil 2001;28:1045–1047.
88. Ericsson Y. Enamel-apatite solubility. Investigations into the calcium phosphate equilibrium between enamel and saliva and its relation to dental caries. Acta Odontol Scand 1949;8(3):1–139.
89. Yip K, Smales R, Kaidonis J. Tooth erosion: Prevention and treatment. New Delhi: Jaypee Brothers Medical Publishers, 2006.
90. Marouf N, Cai W, Said KN, et al. Association between periodontitis and severity of COVID-19 infection: A case-control study. J Clin Periodontol 2021;48:483–491.
91. Iwabuchi H, Fujibayashi T, Yamane GY, Imai H, Nakao H. Relationship between hyposalivation and acute respiratory infection in dental outpatients. Gerontology 2012;58(3):205–211.
92. Drugmakers report Zoloft shortage amid COVID-19. FDA News 3 June 2020. https://www.fdanews.com/articles/197425-drugmakers-report-zoloft-shortage-amid-covid-19. Accessed 15 Jan 2022.
93. Collins LM. Pandemic drinking shows alcohol misuse can be problem at any age. Deseret News 12 July 2020. https://www.deseret.com/indepth/2020/7/12/21317903/covid-19-pandemic-alcohol-drinking-addiction-alcohol-use-disorder-niaaa-george-koob-odyssey-house. Accessed 15 Jan 2022.
94. Kudo E, Song E, Yockey LJ, et al. Low ambient humidity impairs barrier function and innate resistance against influenza infection. Proc Natl Acad Sci U S A 2019;116(22):10905–10910.
95. Lowen AC, Mubareka S, Steel J, Palese P. Influenza virus transmission is dependent on relative humidity and temperature. PLoS Pathog 2007;3:1470–1476.
96. Chen L, Zhao J, Peng J, et al. Detection of SARS-CoV-2 in saliva and characterization of oral symptoms in COVID-19 patients. Cell Prolif 2020;53(12):e12923.
97. Matsuyama Y, Aida J, Takeuchi K, Koyama S, Tabuchi T. Dental Pain and Worsened Socioeconomic Conditions Due to the COVID-19 Pandemic. J Dent Res 2021;100:591–598.
98. Bardow A, Nyvad B, Nauntofte B. Relationships between medication intake, complaints of dry mouth, salivary flow rate and composition, and the rate of tooth demineralization in situ. Arch Oral Biol 2001;46:413–423.
99. Sreebny LM, Schwartz SS. A reference guide to drugs and dry mouth—2nd edition. Gerodontology 1997;14(1):33–47.
100. Ship JA, McCutcheon JA, Spivakovsky S, Kerr AR. Safety and effectiveness of topical dry mouth products containing olive oil, betaine, and xylitol in reducing xerostomia for polypharmacy-induced dry mouth. J Oral Rehabil 2007;34:724–732.
101. Wolff A, Joshi RK, Ekström J, et al. A guide to medications inducing salivary gland dysfunction, xerostomia, and subjective sialorrhea: A systematic review sponsored by the World Workshop on Oral Medicine VI. Drugs R D 2017;17(1):1–28.
102. Lobbezoo F, Aarab G, Wetselaar P, Hoekema A, de Lange J, de Vries N. A new definition of dental sleep medicine. J Oral Rehabil 2016;43:786–790.
103. Lavigne GJ, Cistulli PA, Smith MT. Sleep Medicine for Dentists: A Practical Overview. Chicago: Quintessence, 2009:210.
104. Senaratna CV, Perret JL, Lodge CJ, et al. Prevalence of obstructive sleep apnea in the general population: A systematic review. Sleep Med Rev 2017;34:70–81.
105. Durán-Cantolla J, Alkhraisat MH, Martínez-Null C, Aguirre JJ, Guinea ER, Anitua E. Frequency of obstructive sleep apnea syndrome in dental patients with tooth wear. J Clin Sleep Med 2015;11:445–450.
106. Thie NM, Kato T, Bader G, Montplaisir JY, Lavigne GJ. The significance of saliva during sleep and the relevance of oromotor movements. Sleep Med Rev 2002;6(3):213–27.
107. Janson G, Oltramari-Navarro PV, de Oliveira RB, Quaglio CL, Sales-Peres SH, Tompson B. Tooth-wear patterns in subjects with Class II Division 1 malocclusion and normal occlusion. Am J Orthod Dentofacial Orthop 2010;137(1):14.e1–14.e7.
108. Oltramari-Navarro PV, Janson G, de Oliveira RB, et al. Tooth-wear patterns in adolescents with normal occlusion and Class II Division 2 malocclusion. Am J Orthod Dentofacial Orthop 2010;137(6):730.e1–730.e5.
109. Vig KW. Nasal obstruction and facial growth: The strength of evidence for clinical assumptions. Am J Orthod Dentofacial Orthop 1998;113:603–611.
110. The World Health Report 2002: Reducing Risks, Promoting Healthy Life. Geneva: World Health Organization, 2002.
111. Beaglehole R, Irwin A, Prentice T, World Health Organization. The World Health Report 2003: Shaping the Future. Geneva: World Health Organization, 2003.
112. Eccles JD. Dental erosion of nonindustrial origin. A clinical survey and classification. J Prosthet Den, 1979;42:649–653.
113. Smith BG, Knight JK. An index for measuring the wear of teeth. Br Dent J 1984;156:435–438.
114. Bartlett D, Ganss C, Lussi A. Basic Erosive Wear Examination (BEWE): A new scoring system for scientific and clinical needs. Clin Oral Investig 2008;12(Suppl 1):S65–S68.
115. Bartlett DW. Retrospective long term monitoring of tooth wear using study models. Br Dent J 2003;194:211–213.
116. Fox PC, van der Ven PF, Sonies BC, Weiffenbach JM, Baum BJ. Xerostomia: Evaluation of a symptom with increasing significance. J Am Dent Assoc 1985;110:519–525.
117. Thomson WM. Issues in the epidemiological investigation of dry mouth. Gerodontology 2005;22(2):65–76.

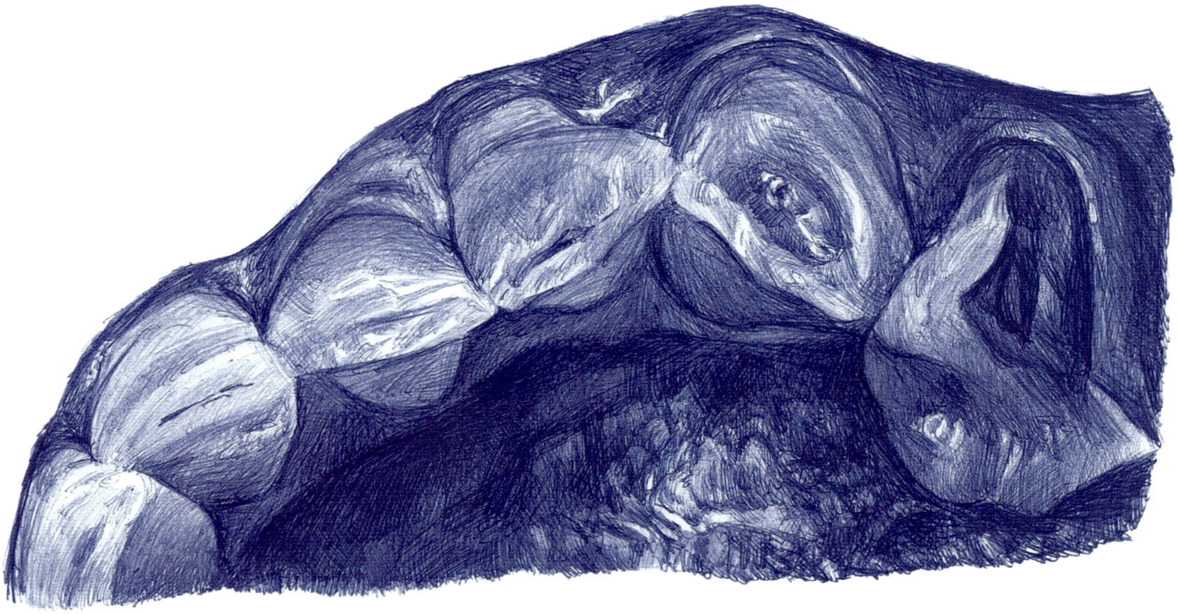

*I believe that if you show people the problems, and you show them the solutions, they will be moved to act.*

—Bill Gates, founder of Microsoft

# SECTION II ASSESSING AND TREATING TOOTH WEAR

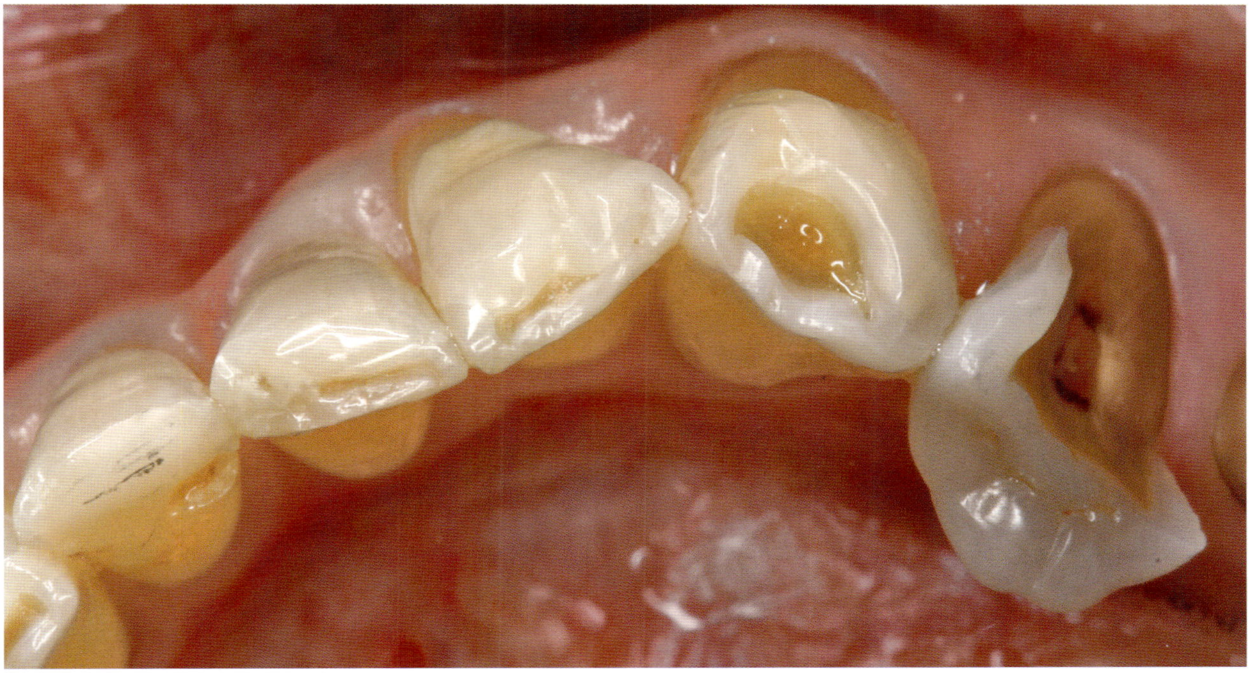

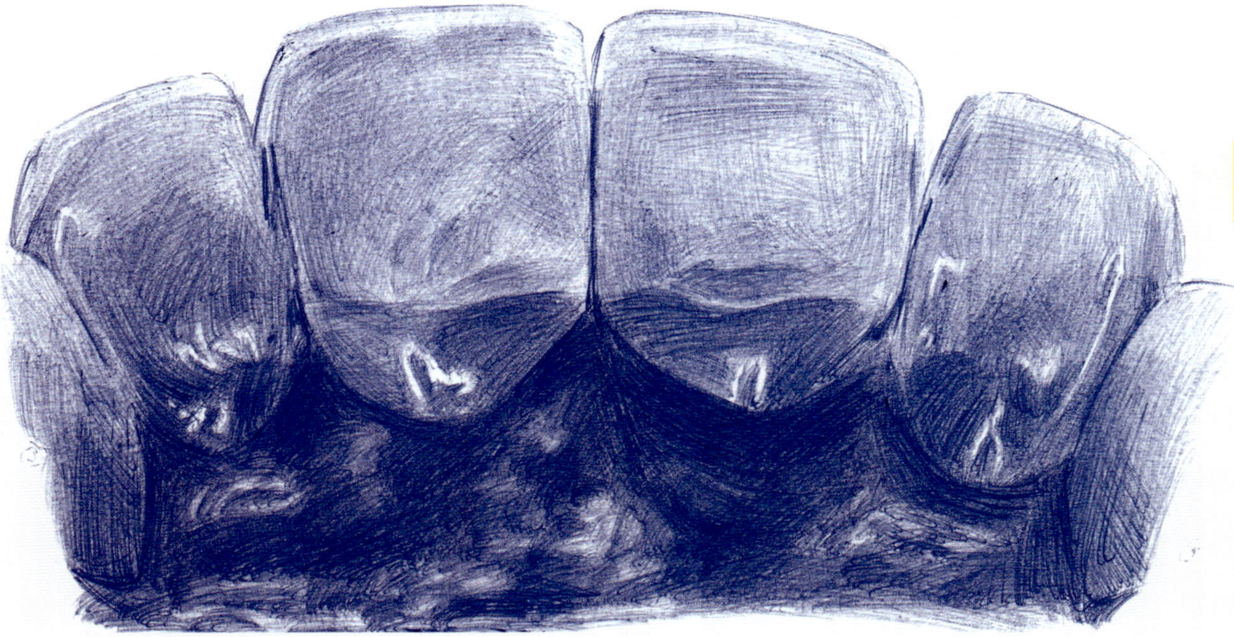

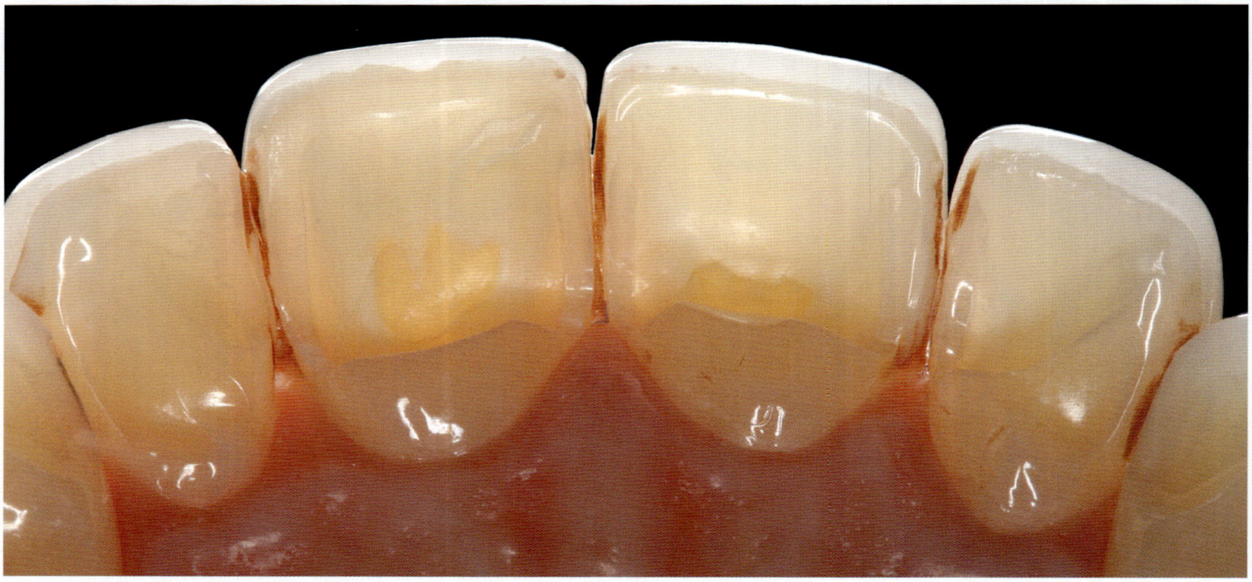

*Instead of thinking out of the box, get rid of the box.*

—Deepak Chopra, Indian physician, writer, and coach

CHAPTER 4

# DIAGNOSIS AND TREATMENT PLANNING IN TOOTH WEAR

The first contact with the tooth wear (TW) patient is, in principle, like any other. The patient's claims most probably will include, "I have a broken tooth," "My restoration has fallen out," or "I have sharp edges in my mouth." Very seldom will it be "I am wearing down my teeth."

TW patients rarely complain from pain, except for perhaps sensitivity in some areas, and they are usually unaware of the underlying condition behind their problem: the wearing of their dentition.

A good anamnesis will help in the protection and restoration of the damaged dentition. Failing to diagnose the type and severity of tooth structure loss will leave the patient ignorant of the origin and will misguide the dentist to a tooth-oriented treatment. Furthermore, a purely restorative approach may prove unable to reduce risk factors. Asking oneself, for example, why the patient has lost the protection of the saliva will help establish a preventive and maintenance program.

The psychologic aspect of the TW patient can play an important role in this last aspect as oftentimes lifestyle choices are behaviors that are difficult to share with a stranger. Contrary to patients with attrition, who usually report bruxism or clenching habits, clinical experience shows that patients with erosion may be very reserved. Unwillingness to disclose any behavioral risk patterns hinders the etiologic diagnosis of this erosive TSL and therefore the preventive and/or early treatment.

It takes a team effort to arrive at an effective and accessible treatment plan with an evidenced-based approach. Considering the patient's future needs for further treatment along with the next probable treatment will reduce invasiveness and increase acceptance.

Last but not least, choosing a workflow, focusing on the timeline, providing occlusal support quickly and predictably, and using appropriate materials should not be a phenomenal task but rather the natural consequence of a patient-centered path.

## 1. Initial Visit of the Patient with TW

As stated before, the TW patient is usually asymptomatic in the initial stages, with the exception of sensitivity or subtle anatomical changes. On the other side of the scale, in severe and advanced stages with partial or total breakdown, pain can be present due to eventual failure of a certain tooth or group of teeth. It is still infrequent to receive patients that claim TW as the reason for their visit. On top of that, it has to be acknowledged that, despite the fact that TW is increasing, evidence-based guidelines for TW screening and TW treatment options are still missing, driving the dentist to manage a sometimes complex interview.

In any case, during the intraoral exam the dentist should be prepared to detect abnormalities in the anatomy and look for signs of TW. Identification of the extension of

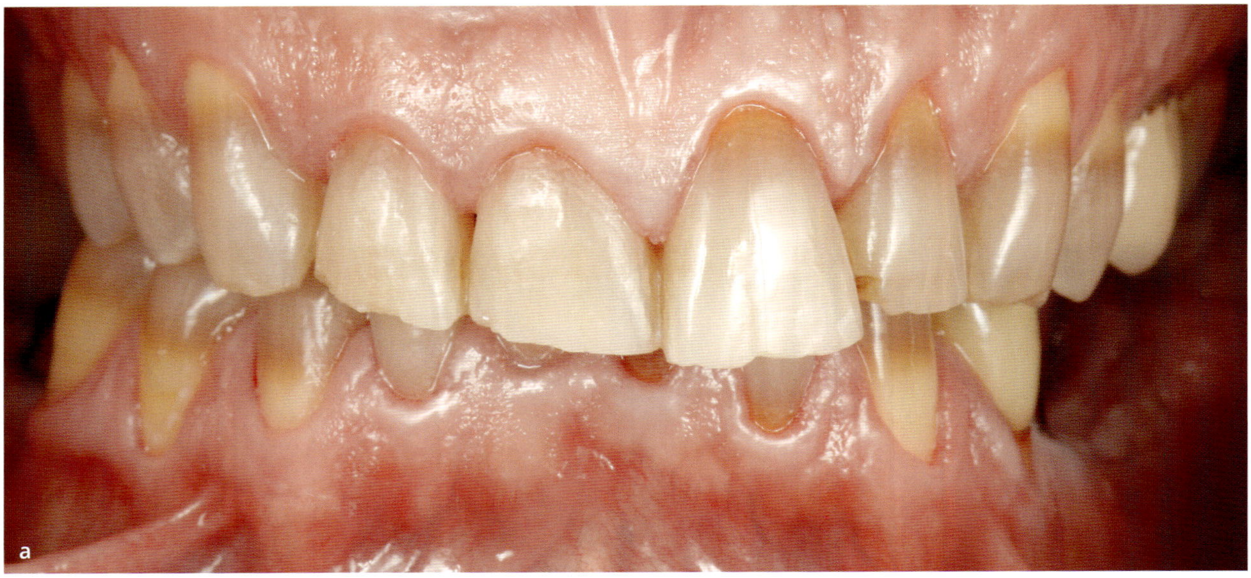

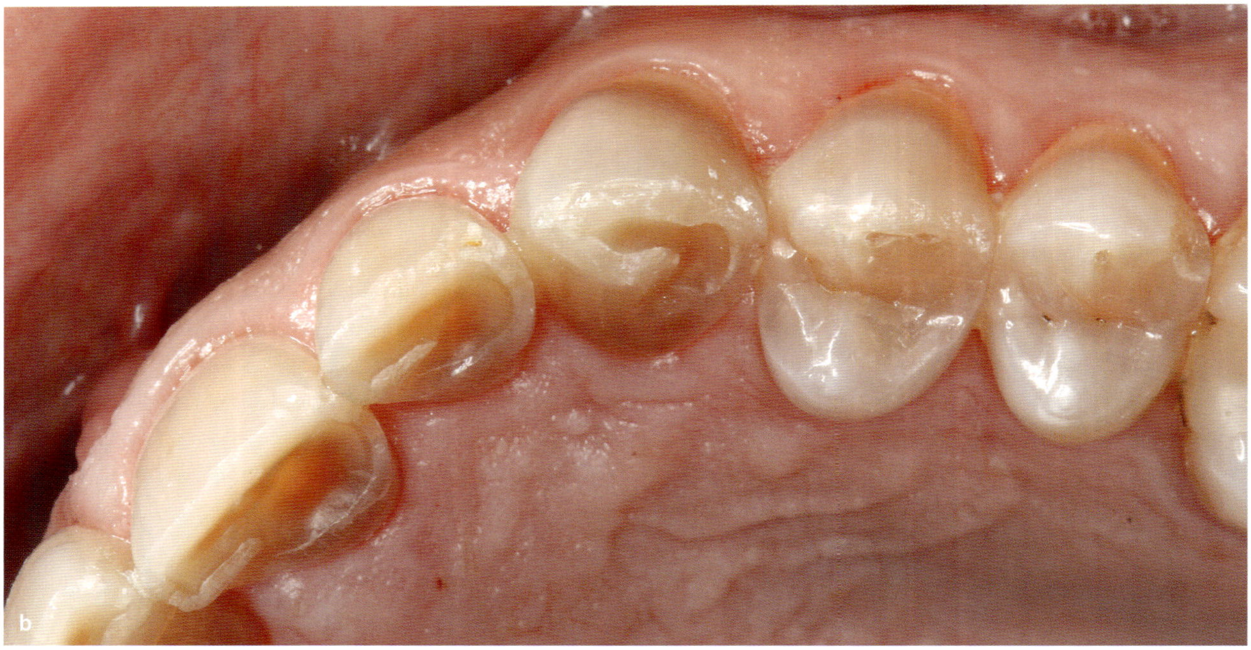

the TW damage to enamel or dentin, to the anterior or posterior regions or both, and to one or both arches should be followed by a thorough examination. Incisal edges, cusps of canines in particular as well as of posterior teeth, occlusal surfaces, and buccal and palatal aspects are not common sites for caries and receive poor attention in a general checkup. The recording of the damage, together with a general screening for caries, periodontal disease, excessive plaque accumulation, or failing restorations will lead to an overall clinical picture in which TW should frame the rest of the conditions present (Fig 4-1).

## Wear Easy Clinical Classification (WECC)

Many TW indices and TW classifications have been published; some of these are listed in chapter 3. Most of them are useful for research and for the academic world, while only a few are meant to be used at a clinical level. In order to facilitate a clinical diagnosis of TW, a simple clinical classification according to the grade or severity should be used by all members of the team. This clinical classification should be intuitive and easy to understand by all members of the TW team, including the patient. Daily applicability of a TW index should be easy and simple.

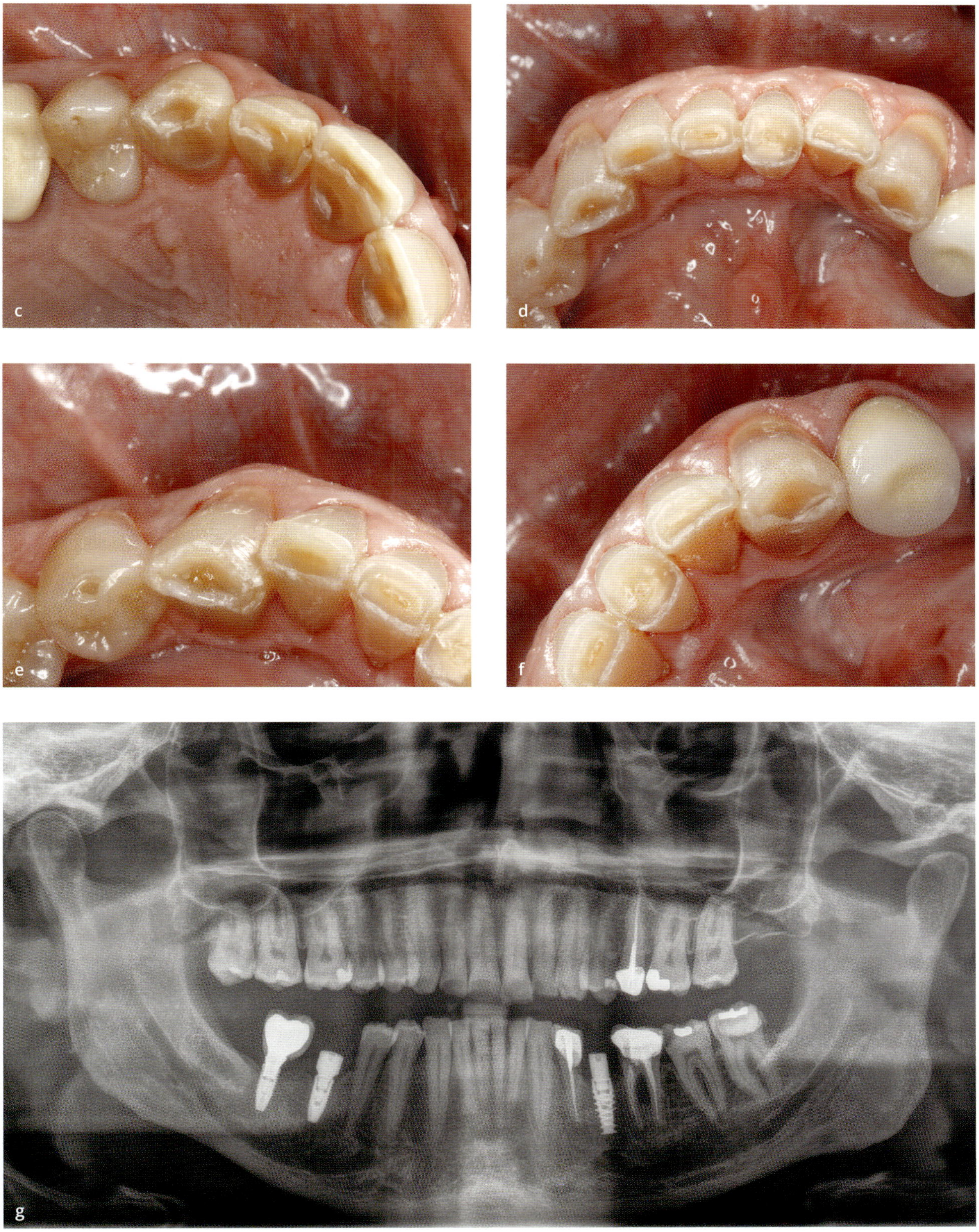


**Fig 4-1** Upon completion of this patient's first visit, the diagnosis was severe multifactorial TW affecting the anterior and posterior sectors of both arches (a to f). Insufficient occlusal support as well as a demanding lifestyle were outlined as risk factors both for the progression of TW and for the longevity of the restorations. Sustained stress due to long working hours were certainly influencing the patient's oral health and may have impeded an otherwise appropriate and sufficient previous treatment plan (g).

**Table 4-1** Wear Easy Clinical Classification (WECC) of types of TW based on severity. Incipient TW represents the lowest clinical impact, while severe TW has the highest clinical impact.

| | |
|---|---|
| **Incipient** | Incipient loss of enamel only, usually either anterior or posterior (not both). Esthetic changes are not perceptible by laypeople. Hypersensitivity or hypertranslucency may be the only sign. |
| **Moderate** | Moderate loss of enamel and dentin, anterior and/or posterior. Esthetic changes are already noticed by the patient. |
| **Severe** | Severe tooth structure loss, both anterior and posterior, that prevents normal function (chewing, speaking, or smiling) and that may challenge oral and general health with a poor quality of life, infections, fractures, and pain. Esthetic damage is evident. |

**Table 4-2** Wear Aggravation Severity Scale (WASS). If any aggravating factors are known at the time of diagnosis, the classification of TW that has been determined using the WECC is advanced to the next level of severity.

<table>
<tr><th></th><th colspan="3">TW Grade</th></tr>
<tr><th>Aggravating Factors</th><th>Incipient</th><th>Moderate</th><th>Severe</th></tr>
<tr><td>Young patient</td><td rowspan="13">↓<br>Moderate</td><td rowspan="13">↓<br>Severe</td><td rowspan="13">↓<br>Severe</td></tr>
<tr><td>Erosion process is active at the time of evaluation</td></tr>
<tr><td>Presence of etiologic factor at the time of evaluation</td></tr>
<tr><td>Erosive dietary pattern</td></tr>
<tr><td>Malocclusion</td></tr>
<tr><td>Mouth breathing, sleep apnea</td></tr>
<tr><td>Etiology of TW is not clear</td></tr>
<tr><td>Generalized TW affecting more than one group of teeth</td></tr>
<tr><td>Rate of progression is rapid</td></tr>
<tr><td>General health conditions present</td></tr>
<tr><td>Polymedication</td></tr>
<tr><td>Salivary dysfunction, hyposalivation, xerostomia</td></tr>
<tr><td>Parafunctional habits (eg, lip, nail, cheek biting)</td></tr>
</table>

A qualitative clinical classification into incipient, moderate, or severe TW would help organize the preventive and treatment approach.

A proposed Wear Easy Clinical Classification (WECC), presented in Table 4-1, is an intuitive and simple tool that can be used easily by all members of the TW treatment team.

Per the WECC, the damage can be present in anterior, posterior, or both sectors of the mouth. In the first case, the eccentric function, namely the anterior and cuspid guidance, has to be analyzed, while if the posterior dentition and/or the lingual aspects are also damaged the evaluation of the posterior occlusal plane and the posterior occlusal support are indispensable (Fig 4-2).

## Wear Aggravation Severity Scale (WASS)

The clinical application of the WECC will enable the dental team to schematically categorize damage and help in the communication between the TW team members. However, the use of a clinical classification presents only a fixed picture of the condition, while TW is a progressive condition in which risk factors may combine and accelerate the damage. In order to identify these comorbidities and better assess the TW prognosis, as well as help in the diagnosis and treatment plan, a good anamnesis is essential, putting the focus on the medical conditions, medications, and patient's lifestyle choices. These are among the aggravating conditions that have a summative effect in the TW course and prognosis. If present, they should be taken into consideration, modifying the clinical classification proposed above. Table 4-2 shows the Wear Aggravation Severity Scale (WASS) with the most commonly encountered aggravating factors and the related impact on the severity classification of TW (Table 4-2).

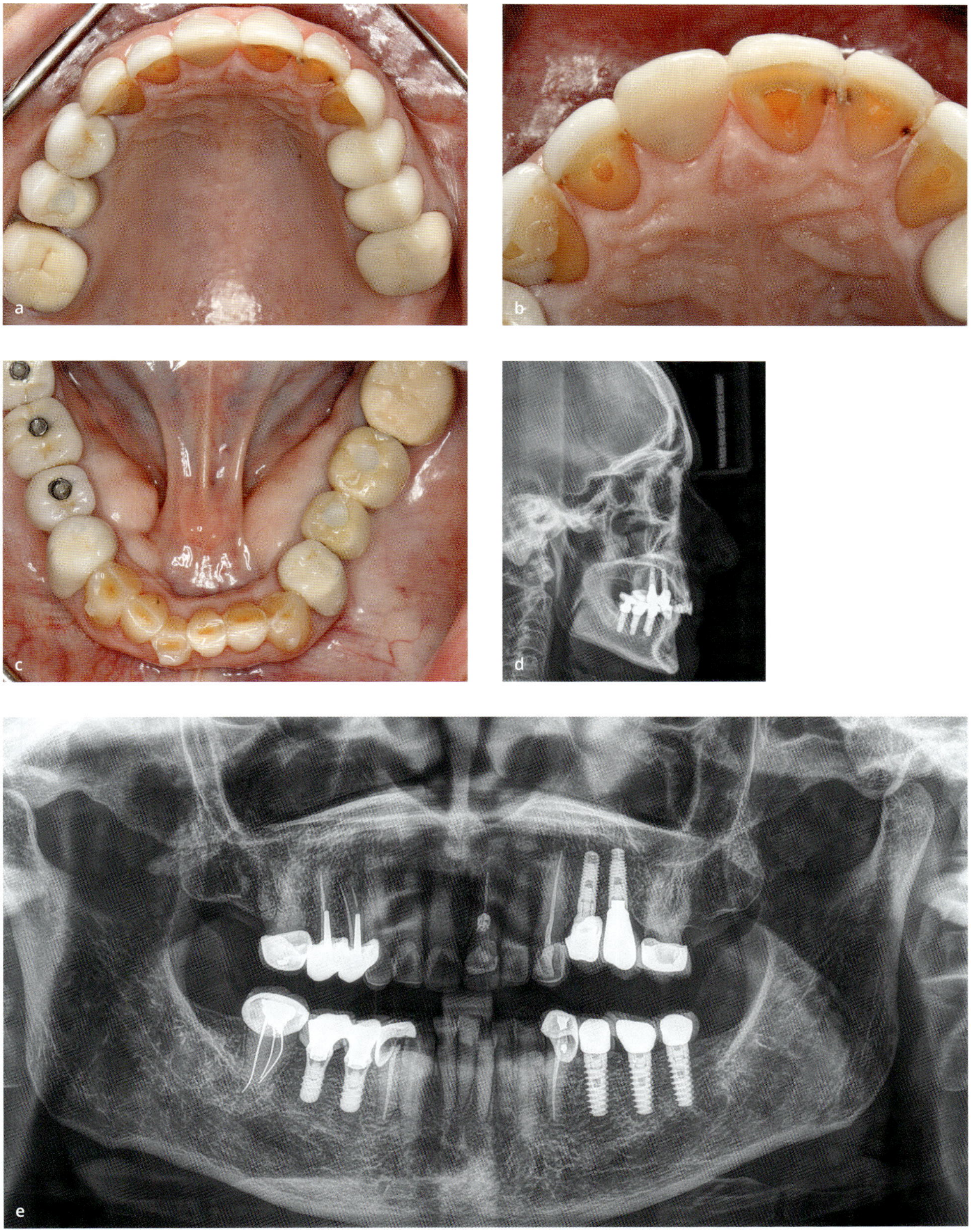


**Fig 4-2** The extensive damage to the palatal aspect of the anterior maxillary teeth indicates the needs for an extensive restoration. The patient falls in the category of severe TW. A bric-a-brac of successive partial dental treatments has failed to provide the correct occlusal support and overall protection from an active erosive attack in the presence of medication induced hyposalivation combined with GERD and tooth grinding. A compressed maxillomandibular relationship and a mandibular torus are signs of bone adaptation to parafunctional habits and premature tooth loss related to the misdiagnosed and poorly managed early TW (a to c). The study of the maxillomandibular relationship shows space for improvement both sagittally and horizontally (d). Failing previous restorations and prosthodontic interventions will have to be analyzed and included in the assessment (e).

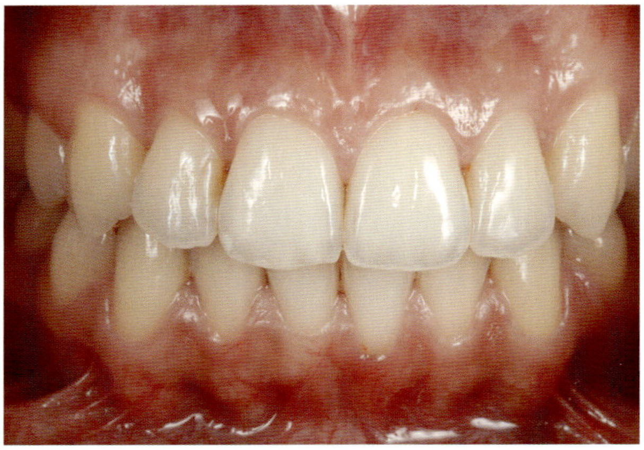

**Fig 4-3** Early detection and WECC classification of incipient TW enables the clinician to intercept future damage. Meeting the patient's expectations and wishes is critical for a good treatment outcome. (See more on this case in chapter 5.)

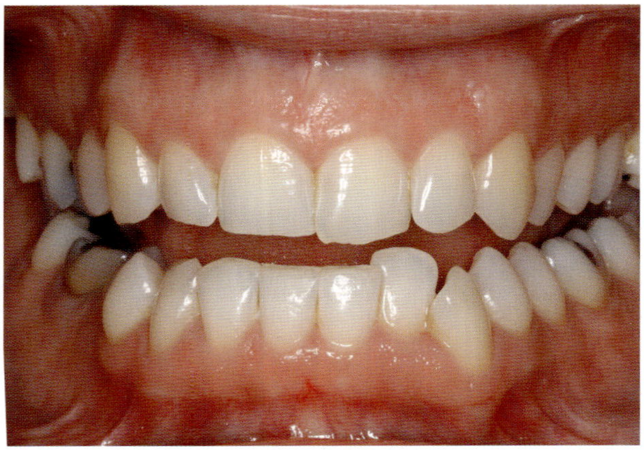

**Fig 4-4** Orthodontic evaluation and multidisciplinary treatment plan for incipient TW facilitates preservation of tooth structure and low-profile restorations. (See more on this case in chapter 8.)

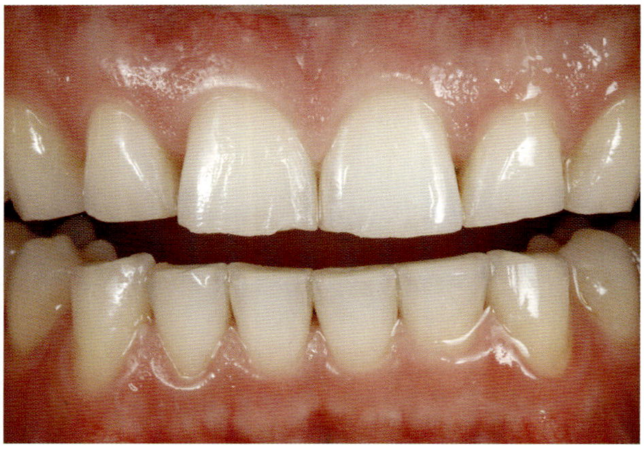

**Fig 4-5** Apparently incipient damage according to the WECC is upscaled to moderate TW as the demanding professional lifestyle and frequent international commuting is impacting the patient's sleep routine and rest time. (See more on this case in chapter 6.)

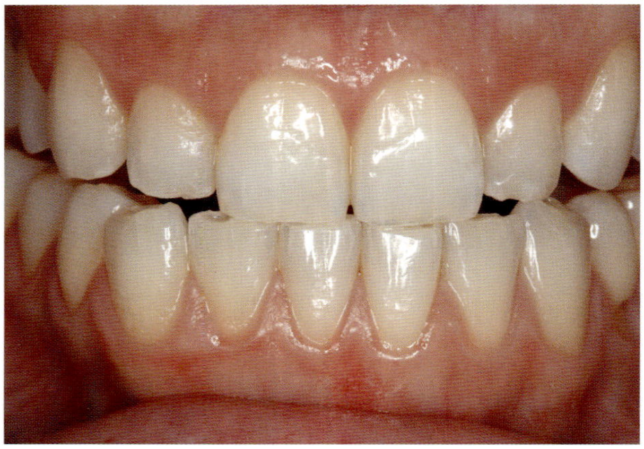

**Fig 4-6** The moderate damage to the overall dentition imposed by constant professional pressure and intercontinental time zone changes is upscaled to severe when the young age of the patient is taken into consideration.

The application of the WASS is intuitive and can be updated in the future if more risk factors and variables are determined to be implicated in the complex condition of TW. For instance, it is foreseeable that recent changes to lifestyle such us remote telework and hyperconnectivity will have an impact on oral health and TW condition in the coming years.

The WECC is therefore not a numeric anatomical/damage classification but rather an instinctive clinical classification that is easy to use and does not have a learning curve. Moreover, when additional information is gathered after the anamnesis, if an aggravating condition is detected or suspected, the WASS can move the TW grade to the next level of the severity scale or conversely bring it down to the previous level once the exacerbating condition has been eliminated or controlled. In this sense a patient who has been classified by the WECC at a certain clinical severity may return to a healthy classification or to a lesser severity grade after they have fulfilled the treatment and an appropriate personalized preventive program (PPP) is established (see chapter 10). Not all risk factors are equally easy to change, and often the TW team will be satisfied with effective control measures, ie, management (Figs 4-3 to 4-10).

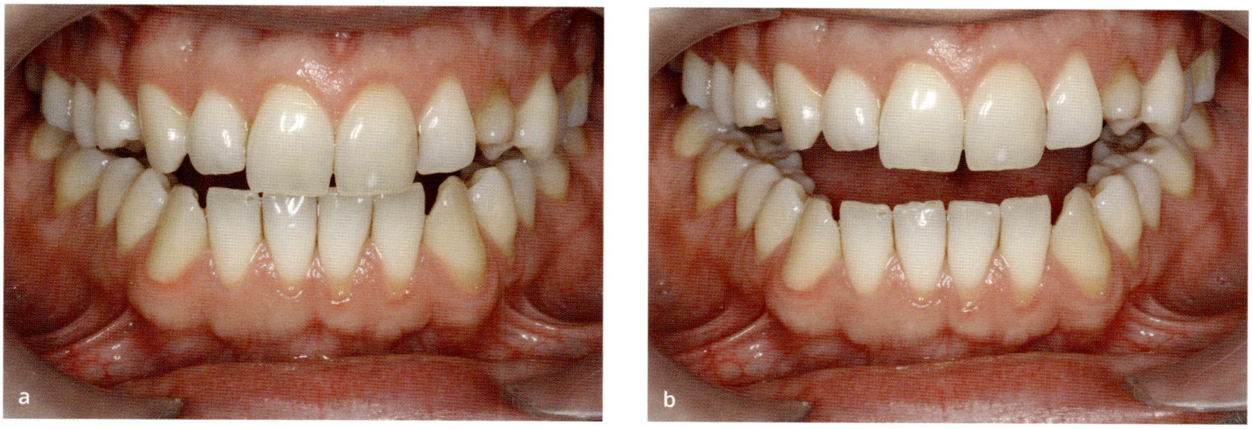

Fig 4-7 A patient classified as moderate TW by the WECC is categorized as severe as congenital agenesia and a Class III malocclusion limit the protection of efficient anterior and canine guidance. (See more on this case in chapter 8.)

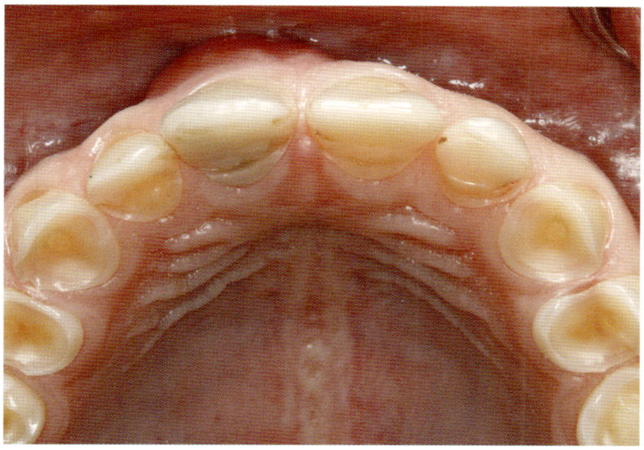

**Fig 4-8** The extensive severe damage has silently and relentlessly erased all occlusal landmarks, depriving the dentition from the opportunity to last into the fourth decade of life free of infection, even in the absence of a cariogenic risk. The clinical classification of severe TW is made easily upon examination independently of any aggravating factors. (See more on this case in chapter 9.)

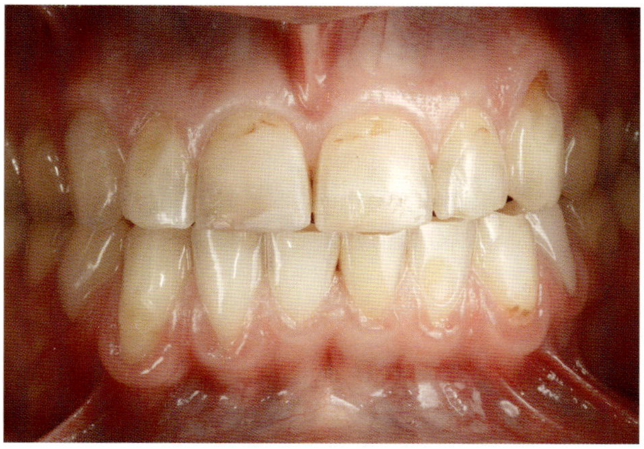

**Fig 4-9** A WECC clinical classification of severe TW is followed by the identification of a dietary erosive pattern in an otherwise health-conscious lifestyle. A comprehensive additive approach with an improvement in the occlusal support is met by the commitment of the patient, who is willing to remain risk-free. (See more on this case in chapter 7.)

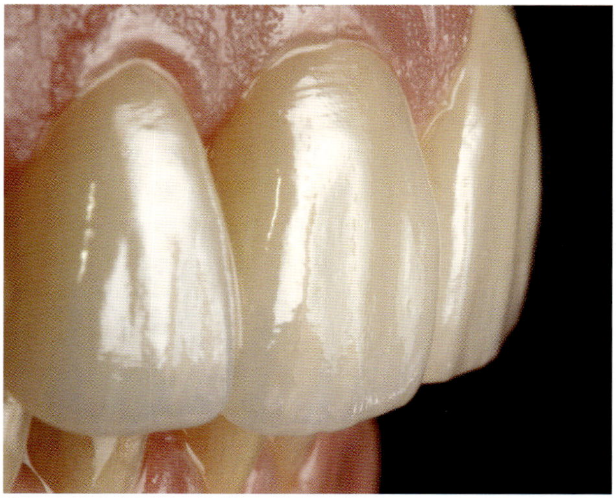

**Fig 4-10** The WASS also can have a reverse path, and a patient who was previously graded as severe can be downscaled to moderate upon completion of the treatment and establishment of a PPP. After restoration of the anterior and canine guidance, this patient with parafunctional moderate TW is monitored, with no negative events or new attrition damage detected by digital tools. (See more on this case in chapter 6.)

## 2. Anamnesis of the Patient with Tooth Wear

The medical and personal history of the patient with TW is of paramount relevance in the diagnosis and treatment plan. The concept that the medical interview is a negotiation between the clinician and the patient was introduced by physicians realizing that a negotiating strategy favored the patient-doctor relationship and helped to solve the potential future conflicts that this relationship might encounter.[1]

Within the three phases of a negotiation, it is in the exchange of information where the TW interview will be deficient because its multifactorial origin escapes the patient's usual cause-effect rationale. In addition, this interview is critical when treating individuals with eating disorders (EDs) and eating disorders not otherwise specified (EDNOS). Many authors have described a "tripartite model of influence" that includes parents, peers, and media. Nevertheless, the influence of the medical team treating these patients is not to be underestimated. Patients with EDs generally have low self-esteem and are extremely sensitive both to positive and negative remarks that can drive the patient to success, to rebounds, or to refraining from coming back to the dental office. Communication implies a bidirectional process: what is said and what is heard do not necessarily coincide sometimes. "You look great," will be interpreted by a patient with an ED as "you've put on weight," while others would generally accept it as a compliment.[2] As explained previously, commenting on patients' physical appearance should be avoided in any case. The complex emotional issues behind ED make it highly inadvisable to start directly questioning a patient who has not openly disclosed the condition. Pathologic perfectionism and lack of self-esteem may cause the patient to perceive the messages themselves as criticism. Therefore, the health care team should be aware of the possible detrimental effect that their comments may have. Not to mention that many times this type of patient is not voluntarily attending the dental office seeking help but rather is being brought by someone else (usually parents). Pushing the patient again into such a conversation with the aim of getting them to declare risky habits may create the opposite effect.

Moreover, dental fear or even dental phobia in patients with ED combined with a misguided conversation may impact negatively on whether they pursue the proposed treatment. Because of all the above-mentioned characteristics of patients with ED, it is advisable not to directly ask the patient but rather provide the opportunity for further disclosure in future visits.

**Table 4-3** Xerostomia Questionnaire. If a patient answers positively to these four questions, the match for xerostomia/hyposalivation is 95%.

| |
|---|
| 1. Does the amount of saliva in your mouth seem to be too little, too much, or you do not notice it? |
| 2. Do you have any difficulty swallowing? |
| 3. Does your mouth feel dry when eating a meal? |
| 4. Do you sip liquids to aid in swallowing dry food? |
| A positive answer to all four questions is associated with salivary gland malfunction. |

Generally speaking, using a Lifestyle and Health TW Questionnaire in the form of a standardized checklist will help in guiding the anamnesis. The questionnaire will serve in the identification of risk habits to be discussed with the patient in order to further implement a PPP. These questions should be adapted or updated depending on the location and lifestyle at a given time and modified according to clinical and academic settings (see appendix 1).

Asking the patient about the intake of medication is of high relevance as many drugs will generate hyposalivation, which has been closely linked to TW.[3]

Furthermore, the self-assessment Xerostomia Questionnaire (Table 4-3) will enable the professional to determine whether or not the patient suffers from hyposalivation, without the need to perform a salivary flow test. This questionnaire, first published by Fox et al, has proven to detect true hyposalivation (95% accuracy) when the patient answers positively to the four questions.[4] If hyposalivation is present, the WASS increases the WECC grade of severity by one level.

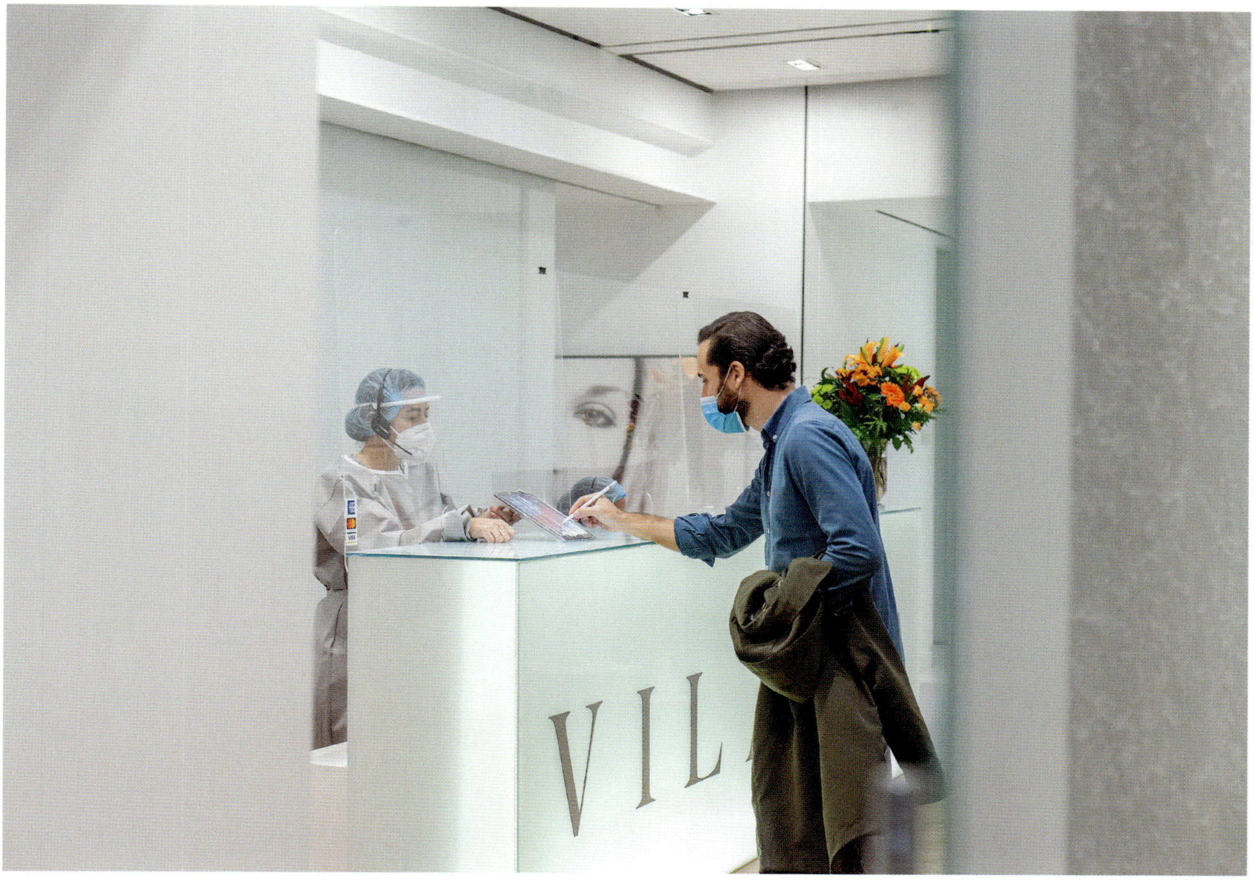


**Fig 4-11** The advent of cloud computing and "the internet of things" brings a futuristic concept to the health care field. Dentistry highly benefits from the storage of data collection. Future artificial intelligence such as face recognition technology will simplify the process to a level unthinkable today. Precision personalized dentistry is becoming a reality apace with these technologies.

## 3. Informed Consent for the Patient with Tooth Wear

Informed consent is recognized today as mandatory when practicing good dentistry. Mutual confidence is required in order to enjoy a good patient-dentist relationship; however the legal scaffold of informed consent is not only inevitable but also desirable. The capacity of the patient to understand the pathology and the benefits of the proposed treatment will aid in their decision making.

A systematic review on informed consent comprehension reveals that although patients generally seem to understand what has been explained to them, their final comprehension is limited.[5]

This is critical in TW, as restorations may only have a limited lifetime, especially in those cases where TW damage is severe at the time of diagnosis.

Repairing or replacing the proposed restorations, even further treatments, cannot be ruled out over the course of the coming years given that the TW process and its causes may well continue to remain active. Therefore, it should be anticipated and made clear to the patient that further restorations or at least partial repetitions or repairs may be necessary.

The informed consent should also include clear information about the recommendation to undergo lifestyle and nutritional modifications since otherwise TW causes will remain active, endangering the prognosis not only of the restorations but of the overall health of the patient.

A proposed informed consent for the TW patient is included in appendix 2. Legal and cultural considerations of different regions are not included and should be considered.

In the current cloud-based era it is possible to fill, store, and update the patient's documentation, self-assessment questionnaires, and files as well as personalized informed consent forms on a secure cloud-based server, avoiding mislocating files and enabling fluid update of the data (Fig 4-11).

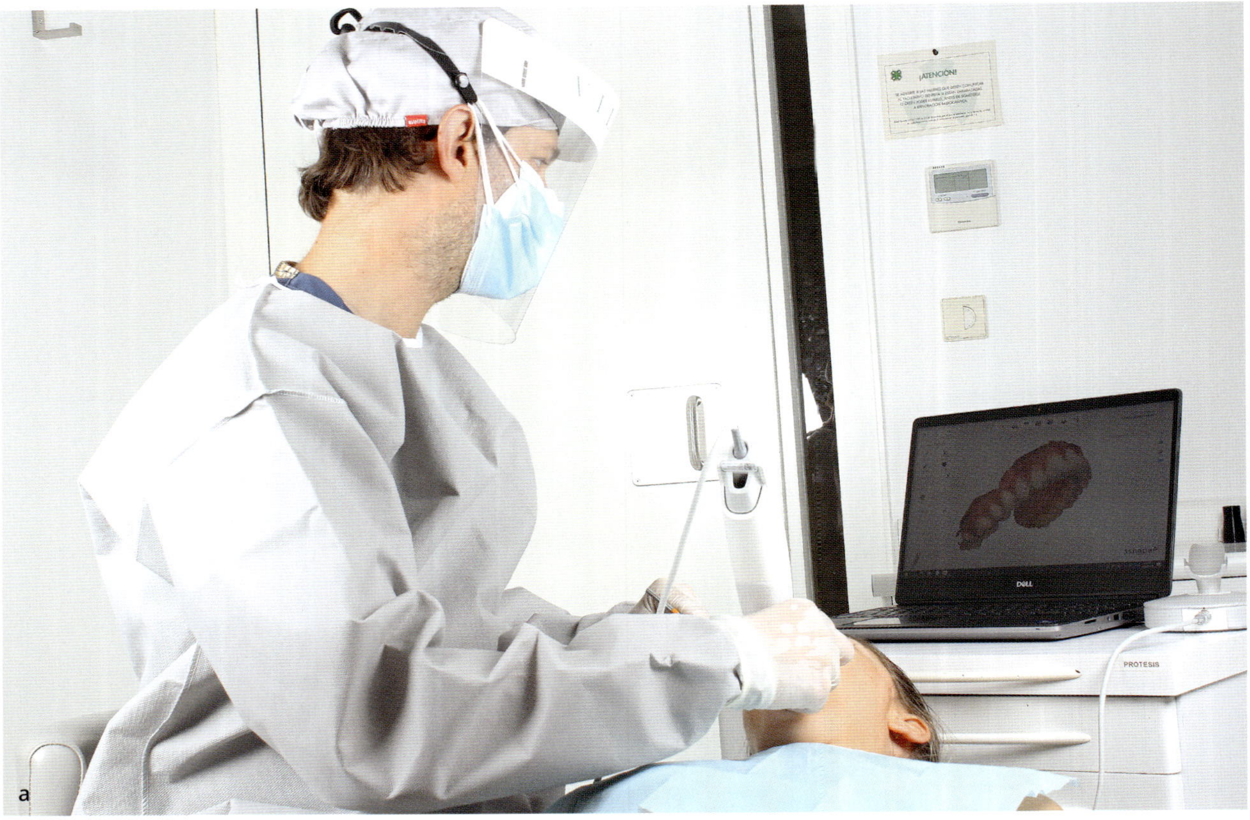


## 4. Patient-Centered Path in Tooth Wear Treatment

Back in 1999, Kokich and co-workers already stated the diverse and distinct perception of altered dental esthetics by dentists versus laypeople.[6]

Furthermore, evaluation of quality of life was proposed for the first time in medicine by Priestman and Baum in an article published in Lancet in 1976.[7] In the same line, patient-reported outcome measures (PROMs) and patient-reported experience measures (PREMs) are becoming more and more important in patient-centered care.[8] In summary, it is what the patient perceives and experiences during and after treatment that makes the difference between a poor and a good result, independent of the evaluation of the professional.

Both the US FDA (Food and Drug Administration) and EMA (European Medicines Agency) have reinforced the value of such parameters by accepting that both efficacy and improvement of quality of life could be co-primary endpoints in the evaluation of a medicament.[9,10]

If improving quality of life can be considered a co-primary endpoint in a drug evaluation process, should it likewise be regarded as fundamental when addressing a treatment strategy for a patient?

While it is true that the patient's expectations should be molded into reality by the dental team, the dentist's expectations should also be based on the needs, health, and quality of life of the TW patient, especially taking into consideration the young age at which many patients will be needing their initial treatments and the further ones to be required in the future. In this sense the dental team treating the TW patient should never lose the focus from the goal of preserving as much tooth structure as possible. Using new technologies such as STL integration and superimposition within the patient's face and cranium leads to a personalized treatment plan. The paradigmatic change to a true multidisciplinary diagnosis, together with the clinician's treatment plan presentation, which educates and advises in the decision-making process, helps not only the patient but also the dentist (Fig 4-12).[11]

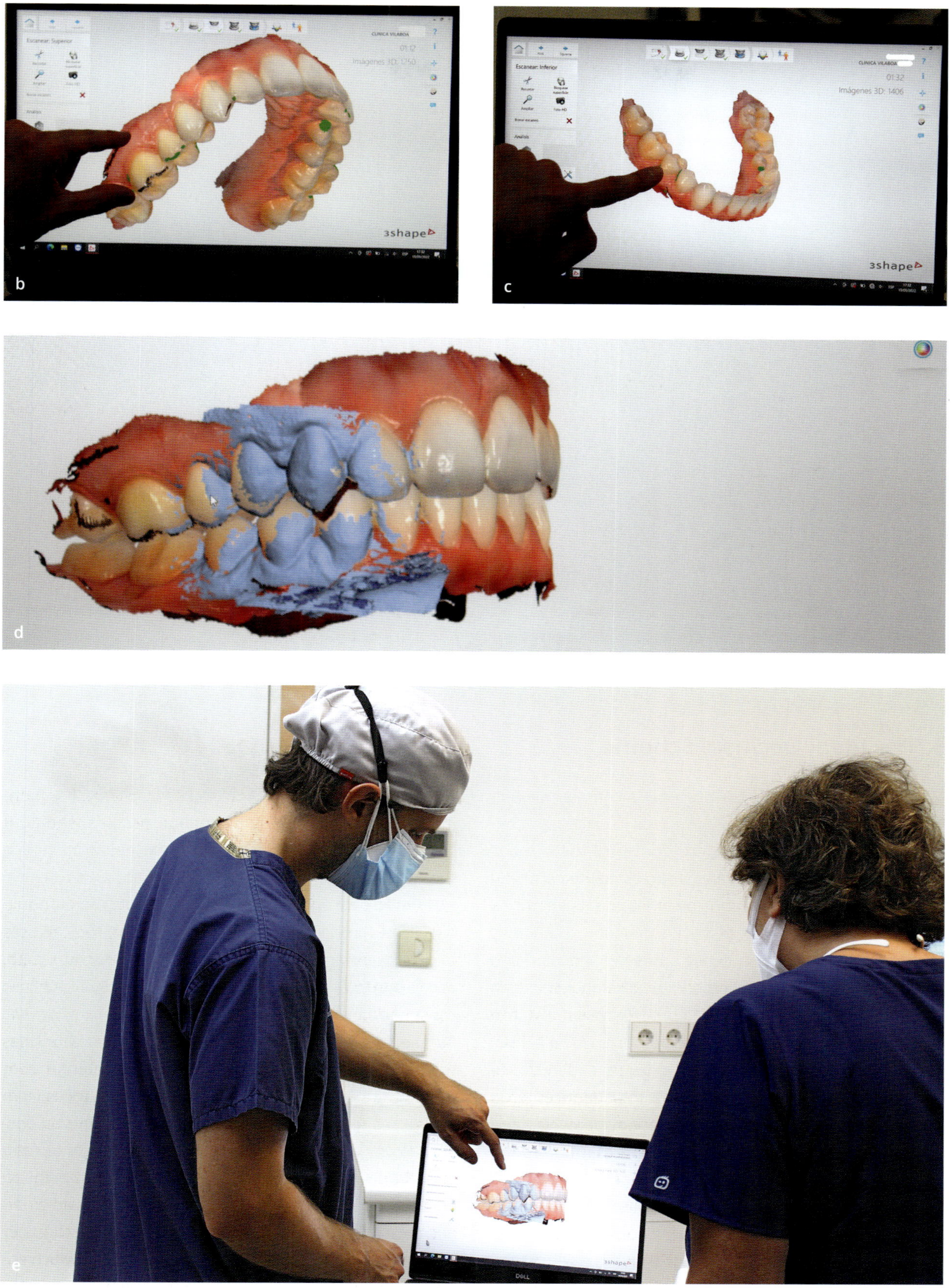


**Fig 4-12** Intraoral scans are especially useful in TW patients. EDs and EDNOS have been associated with dental phobia. A positive experience helps in the planning and treatment sessions. Noteworthy is the outstanding quality of the acquired image. The system shown in this figure is Trios 3 by 3Shape (a to e).

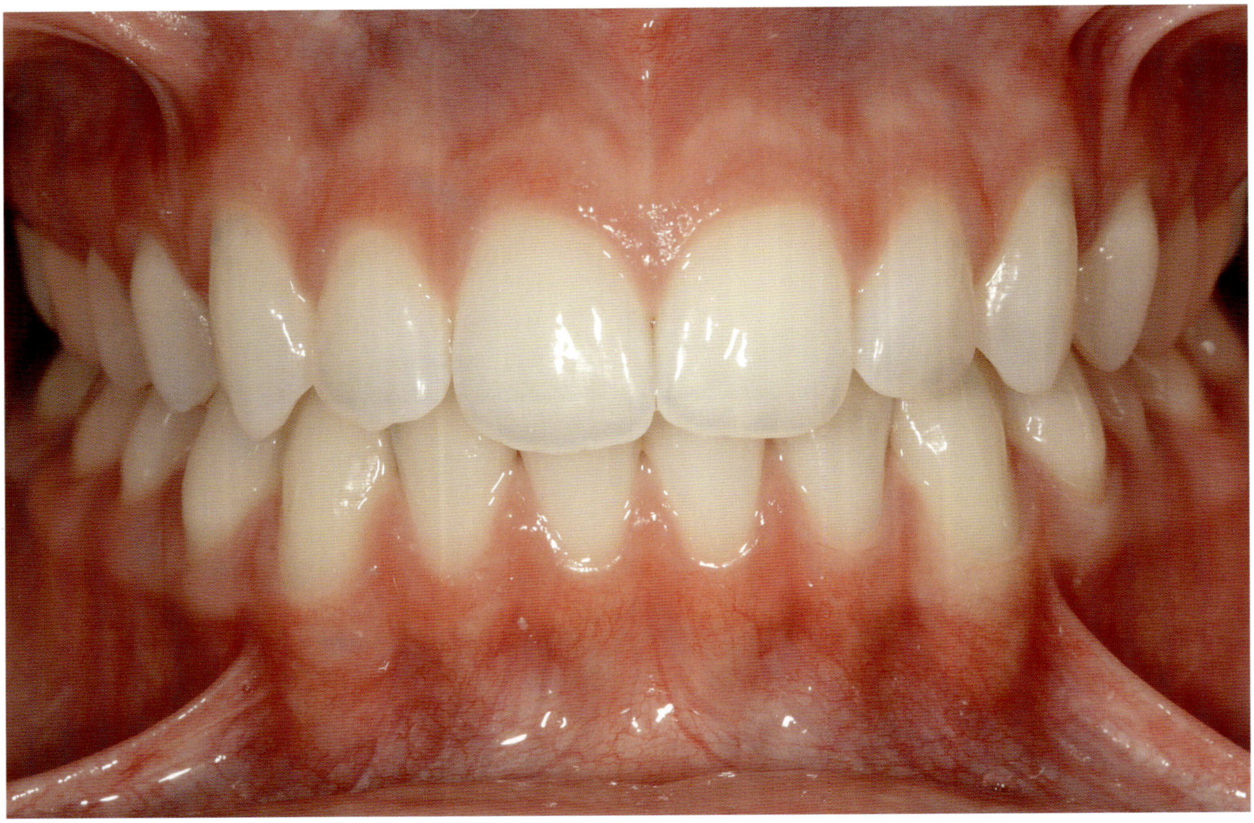

**Fig 4-13** The ideal occlusion is a safeguard for longevity and endurance of everyday challenges.

## 5. The Ideal Occlusal Scheme

The patient with severe TW presents a complex case in which the occlusion must be addressed in order to reconstruct the patient's anatomy and function. The same is true for moderate TW; however, addressing the occlusion is usually not necessary for incipient TW management.

The occlusal scenario of the TW patient is oftentimes far from ideal, that is, a mutually protected occlusion and a harmonious Class I maxillomandibular relationship with sufficient overjet and overbite to provide essential anterior guidance and canine-posterior disocclusion (Fig 4-13).[12]

A desirable freedom in centric, that is the posibility of keeping posterior contacts without interferences while having shallow anterior stops, is present only in a small percentage of the population. This is defined as a naturally occurring transition from a maximum posterior to a more anterior mandibular position while a slight anterior shift takes place.

Whatever the occlusal concept by which the restorative team is guided, it should be remembered that patients with TW benefit more from noninvasive therapy. In general, additive approaches should be prioritized versus reductive protocols. Today, the strength of evidence and clinical experience shows that recreating the full ideal anatomy of the healthy dentition not only helps in patients recovering from TW, but it also proves that all biomimetic, scientifically proven approaches to mimicking the natural anatomy of the intact tooth as part of an ideal arch is the best option to attain a successful restoration.[13]

Posterior anatomy in the patient with TW is usually damaged in moderate to severe stages, with some areas more damaged than others. TSL usually hits the most prominent parts of the occlusal anatomy by the combined action of attrition and erosion. The latter may happen by itself, independent of physical grinding, but as previously explained, often both challenges appear simultaneously. As a result of the individual's critical pH being surpassed, the mineral equilibrium on the surface of the teeth shifts toward mineral loss, resulting in rapidly occurring saucer-like lesions that will further retain acidic solutions coming either from dietary habits or from bodily fluids such as (but not exclusively) stomach acid, eventually erasing most, if not all, of the anatomical landmarks of one or both arches and altering the occlusal scheme (Fig 4-14).

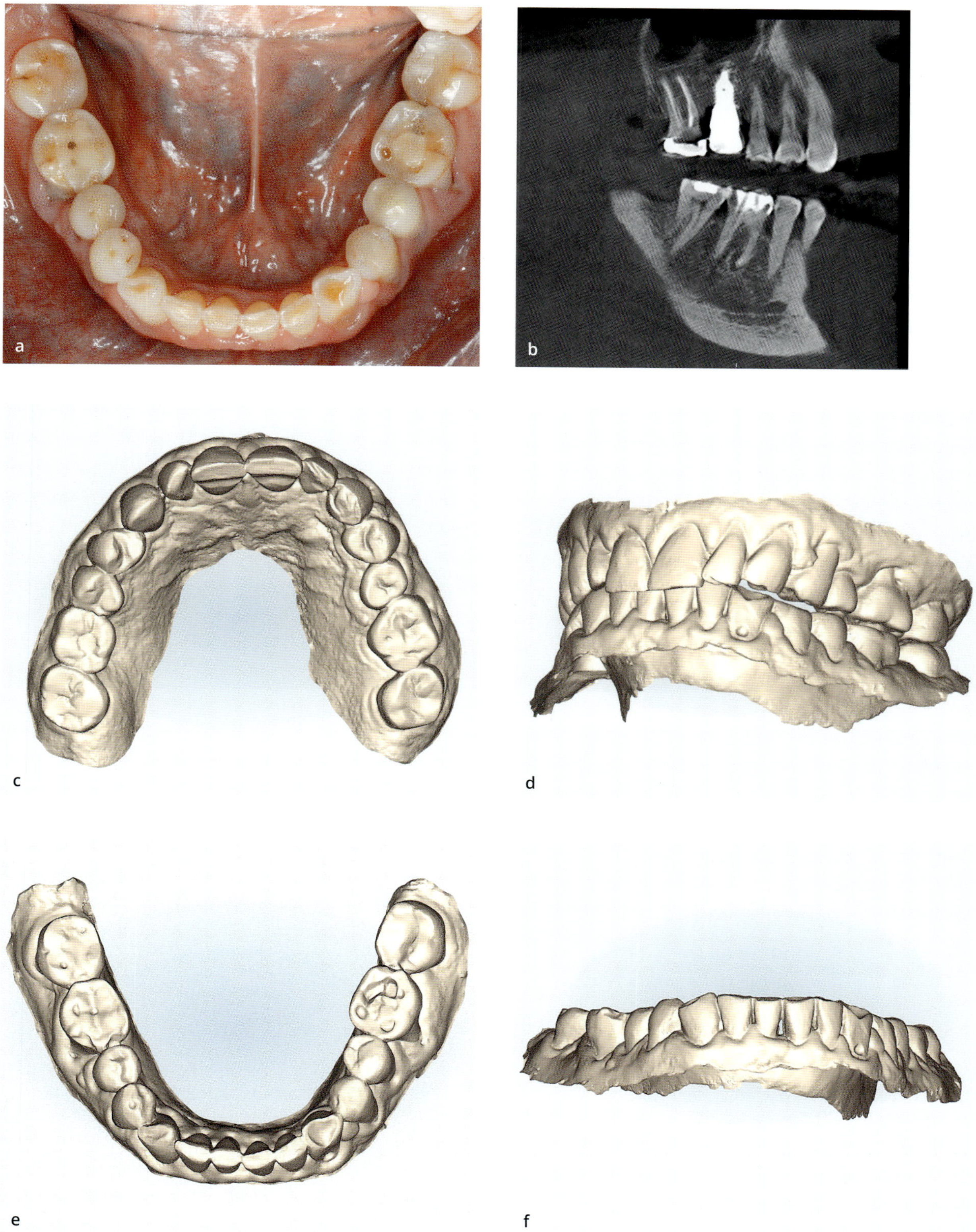

**Fig 4-14** In this patient, the previous tooth-oriented treatments had not prevented major tooth failures in a severe TW scenario. Clinical practice shows that patients with long-standing TW in severe stages often times have periapical lesions related to root fractures. It is therefore advisable to do a routine CBCT as part of the records and digital treatment planning (a and b). In doing so, if extractions and implants are indicated, the surgical planning can be built into the treatment plan, wax-up, and scheduling, with optimization of the treatment sequence. The digital-analog combination workflow boosts the possibilities of enamel preservation. The patient's intraoral situation is digitalized (c to f). *(continued next page)*

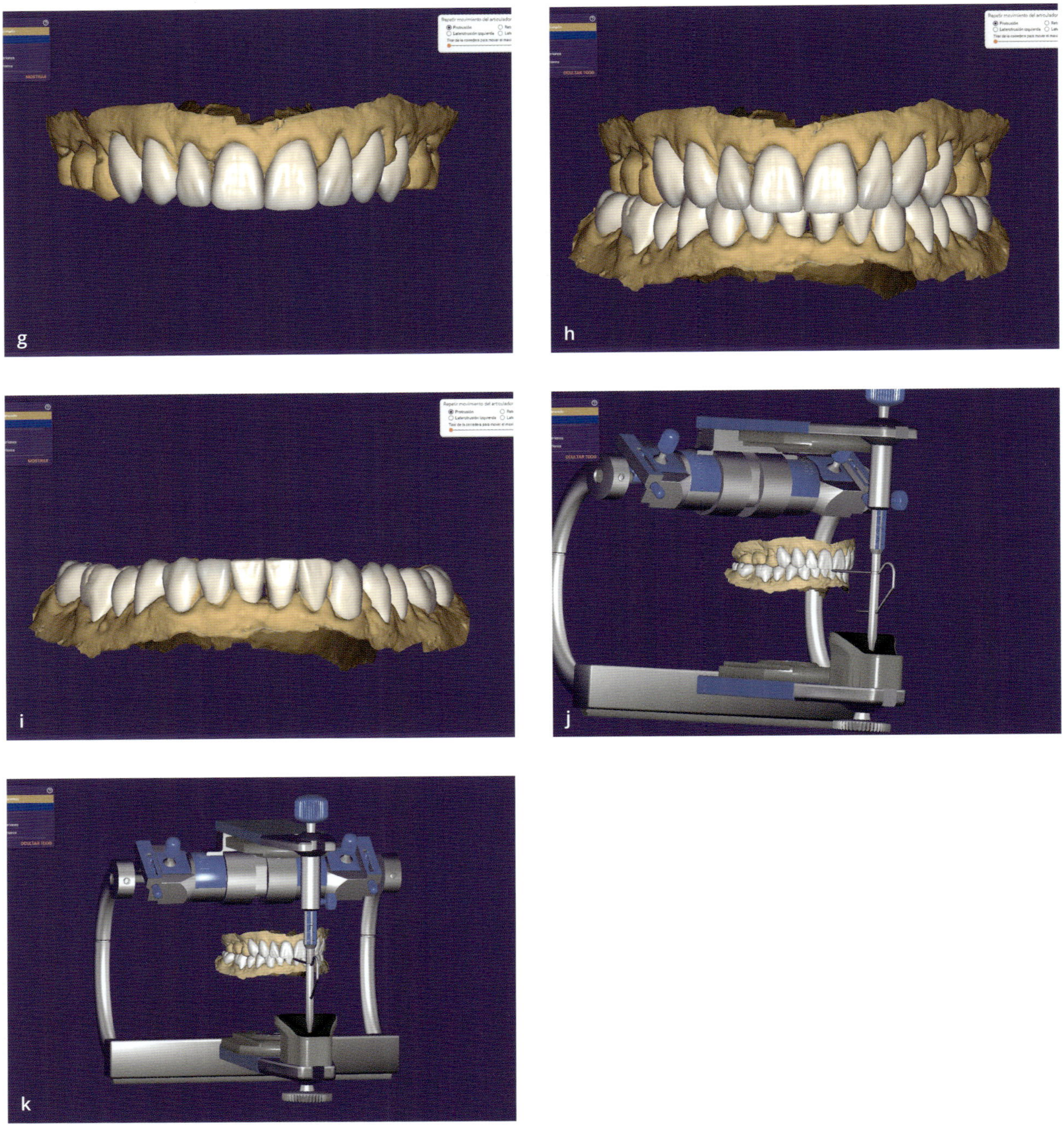

**Fig 4-14** *(continued)* A virtual full-mouth wax-up is done (g to i). In some moderate and most severe TW cases, an increase of the VDO is needed and therefore it should be contemplated from the first wax-up, otherwise extensive tooth reduction would have to be negotiated into the treatment plan. The virtual articulator allocates the vi-tual model with the virtual wax-up and the new anatomy is tested functionally (j and k).

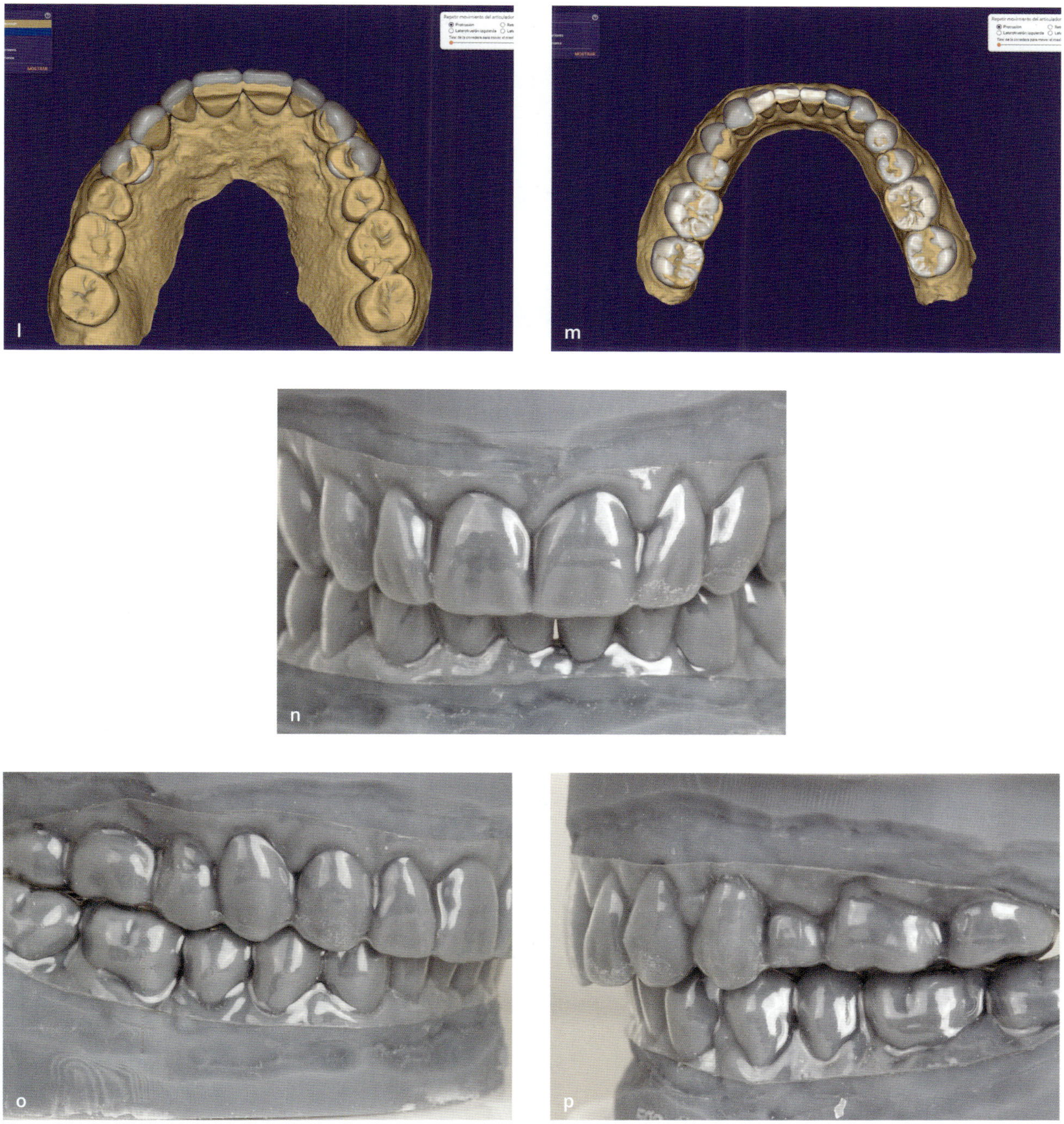


**Fig 4-14** *(continued)* The digital buildup of the buccal anatomy as well as the anterior and canine guidance is shown in the virtual wax-up along with the required restorations in the rest of the dentition (l and m). The approval of the wax-up is followed by the printing of two models, maxillary and mandibular, and the manufacturing of a set of two extra-thin, transparent, splint-like vacuum trays (n to p).

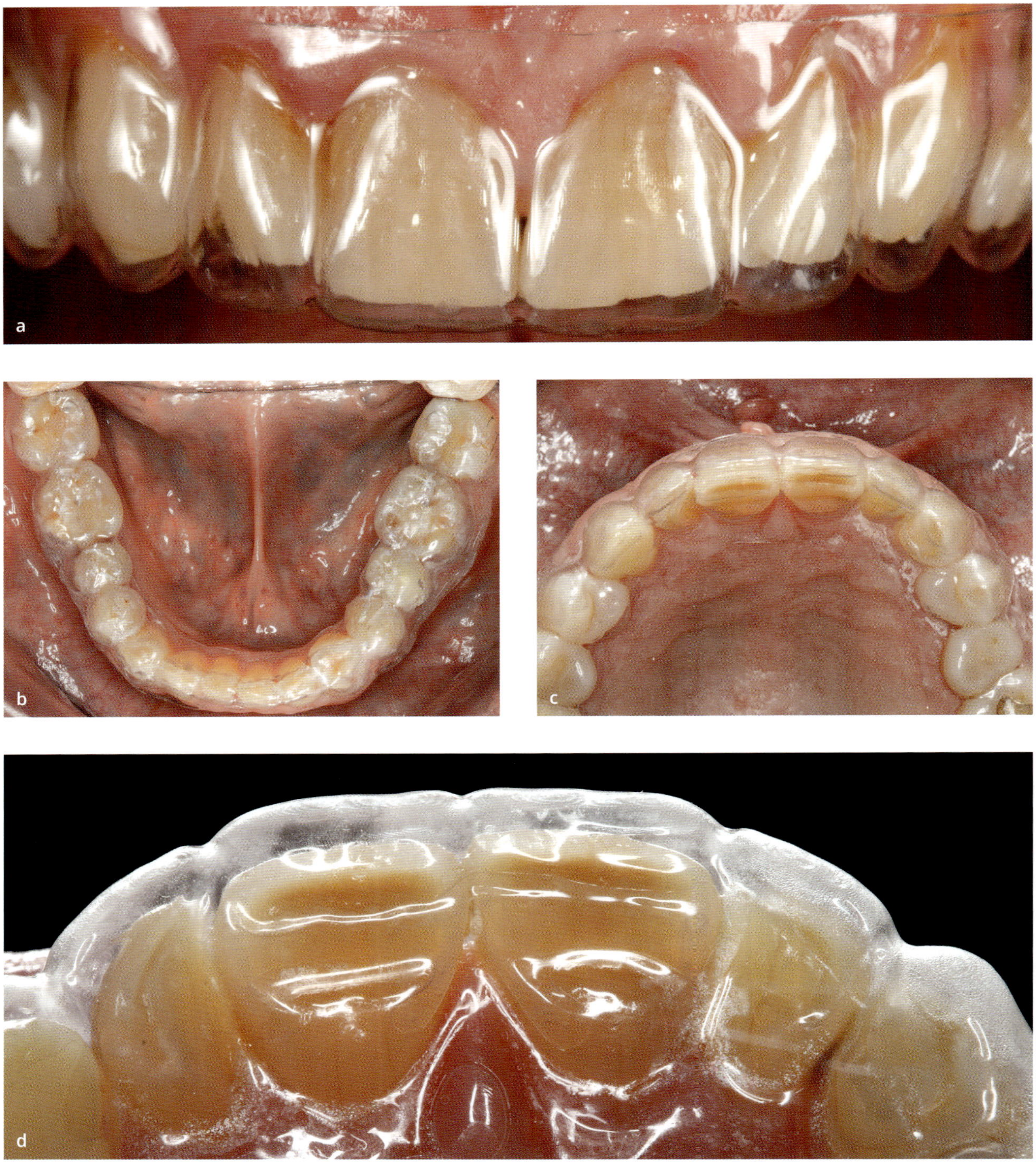


The plan behind the restoration of the worn dentition, especially in moderate to severe TW, can be hard to communicate to the patient. Anterior maxillary restorations are preferably done with indirect restorations such as porcelain laminate veneers, especially in highly esthetically demanding areas. Conceptually for many years dentists have treated merely the anterior sectors of the worn dentition since the predictable and highly appreciated esthetic improvement was easy to communicate. However, we know today that consequences of leaving sectors of the mouth untreated can be devastating. The full-arch mock-up and try-in phase can help communicate

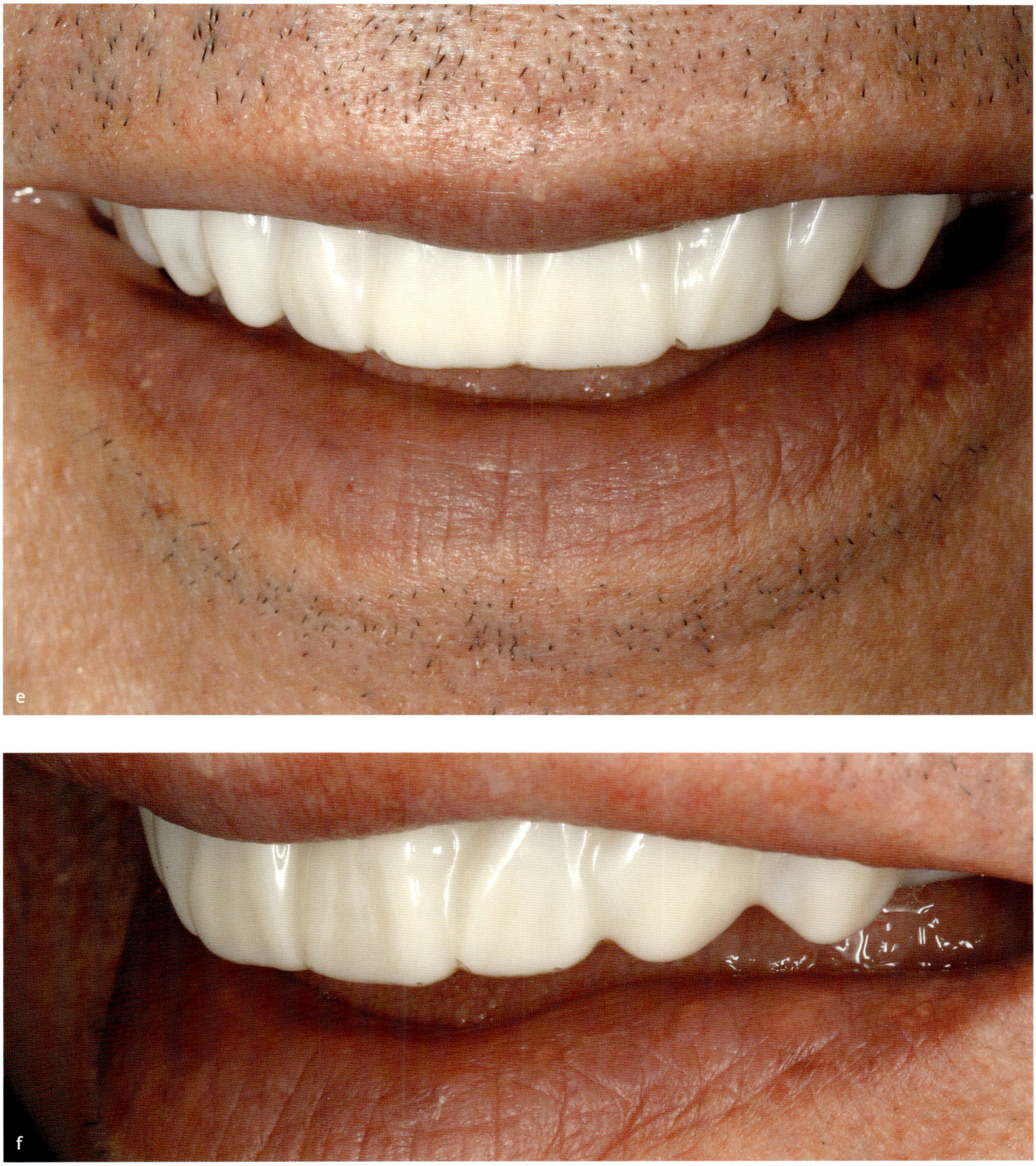

**Fig 4-15** At this point in treatment planning, the user-friendly, transparent, feather-edged, thin splints are useful for the patient to visualize the added volume and length as they show the worn anatomy and the preview of the newly restored one (a to d). If necessary, they can be also filled with try-in non-setting fluid composite for a more realistic appearance (e and f).

this information and improve the patient's understanding, resulting in a more engaging experience for all involved (Fig 4-15).

The transparent mock-up versus the traditional silicone tray and acrylic try-in can be a limitation if the dentist wants to do a mock-up for guided preparation for indirect restorations such as porcelain laminate veneers or onlays. Yet in cases of erosive severe TW, the acid might have already reduced the tooth so much that no depth preparation is needed except for rounding sharp edges or irregularities (Fig 4-16; see chapter 6 for more information).

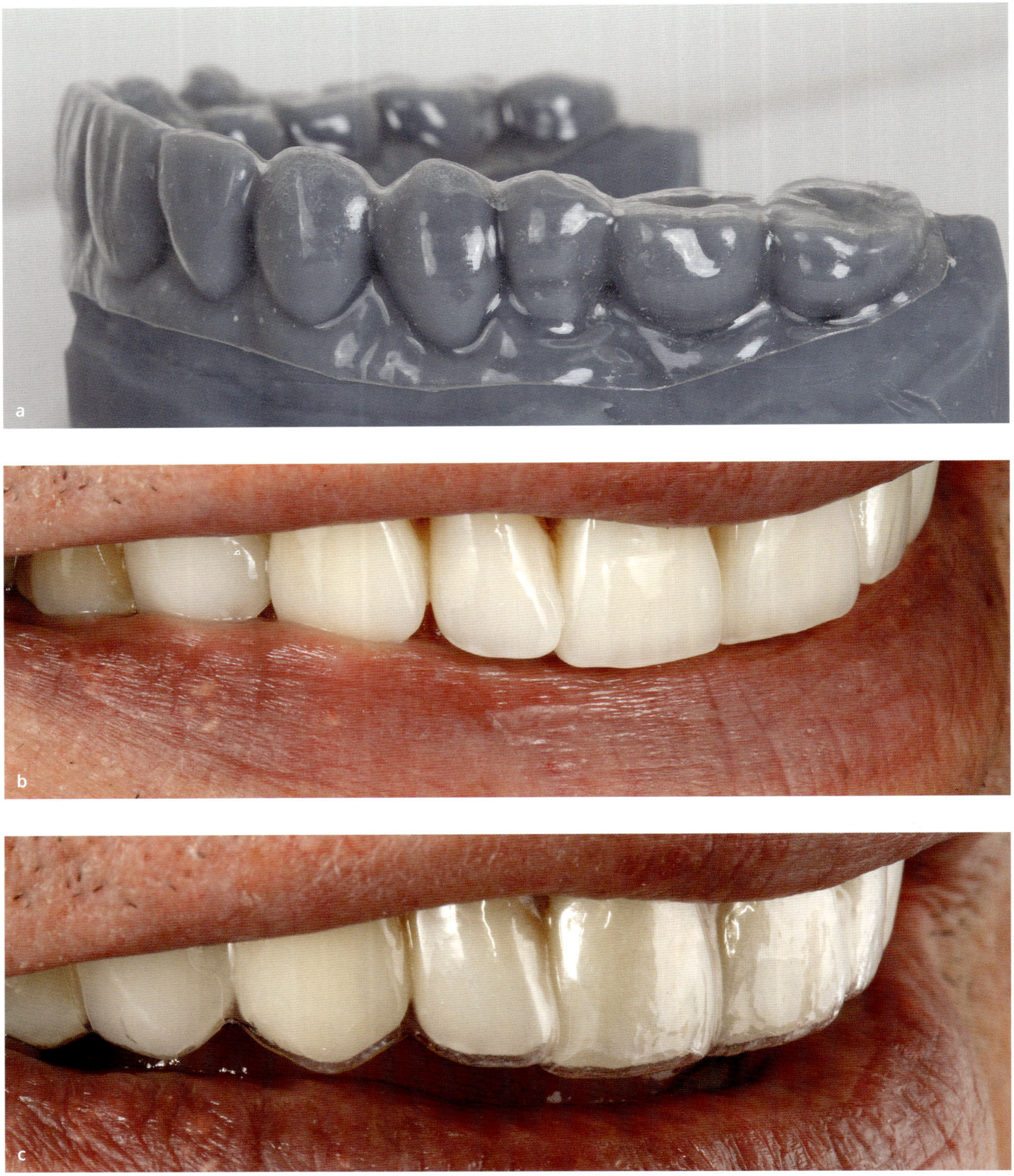

**Fig 4-16** All manual protocols such as direct freehand composite and feldspathic traditional PLVs imply slight modifications throughout the process. However, the deviation from the originally planned wax-up in the final restorative outcome should not be significant (a and b). A check of the parallelism between these two phases can be done upon completion with try-in of the transparent mock-up splints onto the finished arch (c).

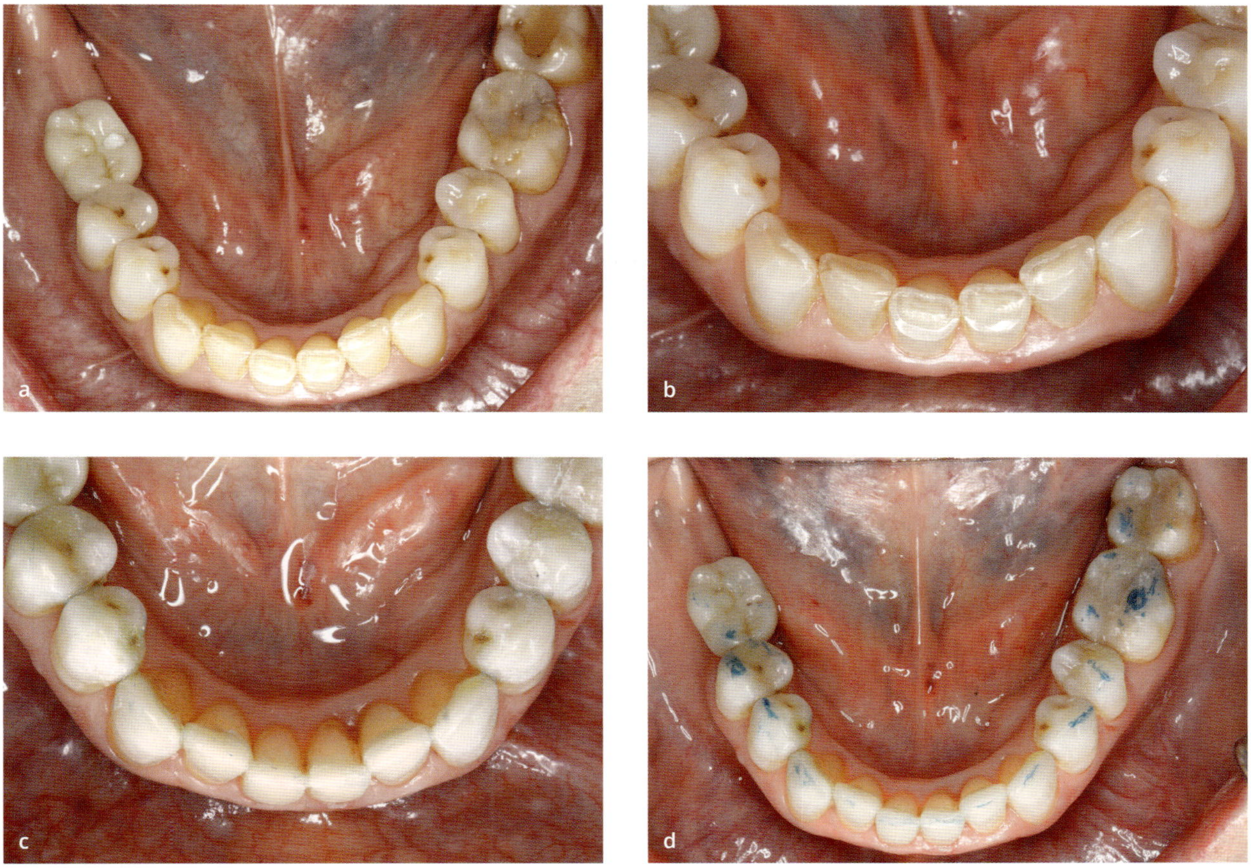


**Fig 4-17** In this case the severe TW had already caused a fracture of the first mandibular molar, which was extracted and replaced by an implant. In this scenario, the single-tooth-oriented approach should be discarded as it would irrevocably lead to the re-creation of the surrounding flattened anatomy, flat cusp inclination, shallow anterior guidance, and flat occlusal anatomy with inherent high occlusal risk (a and b). Instead, all damaged teeth should be treated accordingly to restore the occlusal support and curve of Spee. The future crown is included in the wax-up of the restored full arch from the beginning, along with the rest of the worn teeth. The material selection in this case is composite to be applied freehand chairside immediately after the single implant-retained crown is delivered. The finishing protocols and occlusal adjustment of the restorations as well as the antagonist teeth also should be scrutinized under the principle of tooth structure preservation. Occlusal evaluation after adjustment and polishing shows the final restorations contributing to a new occlusal plane (c and d).

## 6. Material Selection: When to Subtract and When to Add

In today's dentistry, material selection depends on many factors, especially in the treatment of TW cases, where the number of materials to choose from is greater.

The driving force behind material selection in treating TW should always be choosing the technology that best complies with the principle of maximum tooth structure preservation. This includes not only the material itself but also the type of treatment modality, direct or indirect, and the type workflow, classical analog or CAD/CAM digital. The dental TW team should use whatever technology and combinations thereof that best serve the preservation principle[14] (Fig 4-17).

### Repair, Repeat, and Modify

The need to repair, repeat, and modify should be anticipated in the pretreatment phase and materials chosen accordingly, ie, preferably ones that can be repaired, modified, or repeated easily.

By observing these principles, the TW team will find themselves aligned not only in the distinctive mission of restoring in a rational manner but in surviving the TW trial.

Composite reconstruction in the posterior and mandibular anterior sectors, both direct and indirect as needed, provides an easy-to-repair approach in a patient in need of protection of an eroded dentition due to acid exposure in the oral cavity. Prognosis of

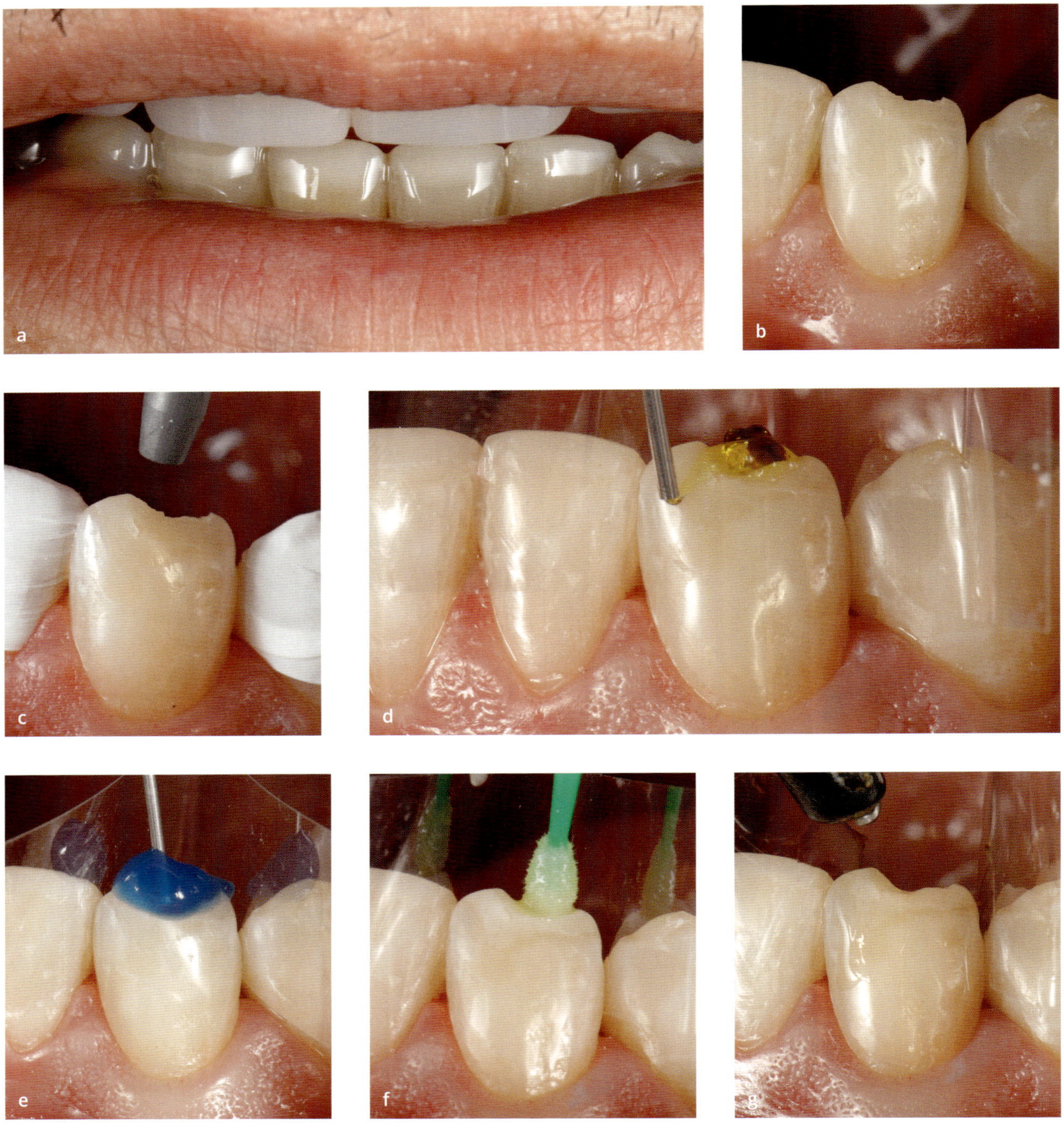


the restorations will depend on the origin of TW, the amount of remaining tooth structure before treatment, the cessation or persistence of challenge, presence of comorbidity factors, and most importantly the occlusal scheme achieved at the end of the restoration and the measures for restoration protection implemented after the treatment.

Nevertheless, composite restorations are subject to chipping or fracture. Most chipping or minor fractures can be detected at regular checkups. Whenever possible, the repair should be done immediately (Fig 4-18).

If the area to be repaired is small, the composite can be applied freehand and molded with the use of an appropriate composite spatula guided by the adjacent tooth anatomy.

Alternatively, if several fractures have to be repaired, a vacuum-formed transparent splint made from the printed wax-up model using STL or, if the wax-up was

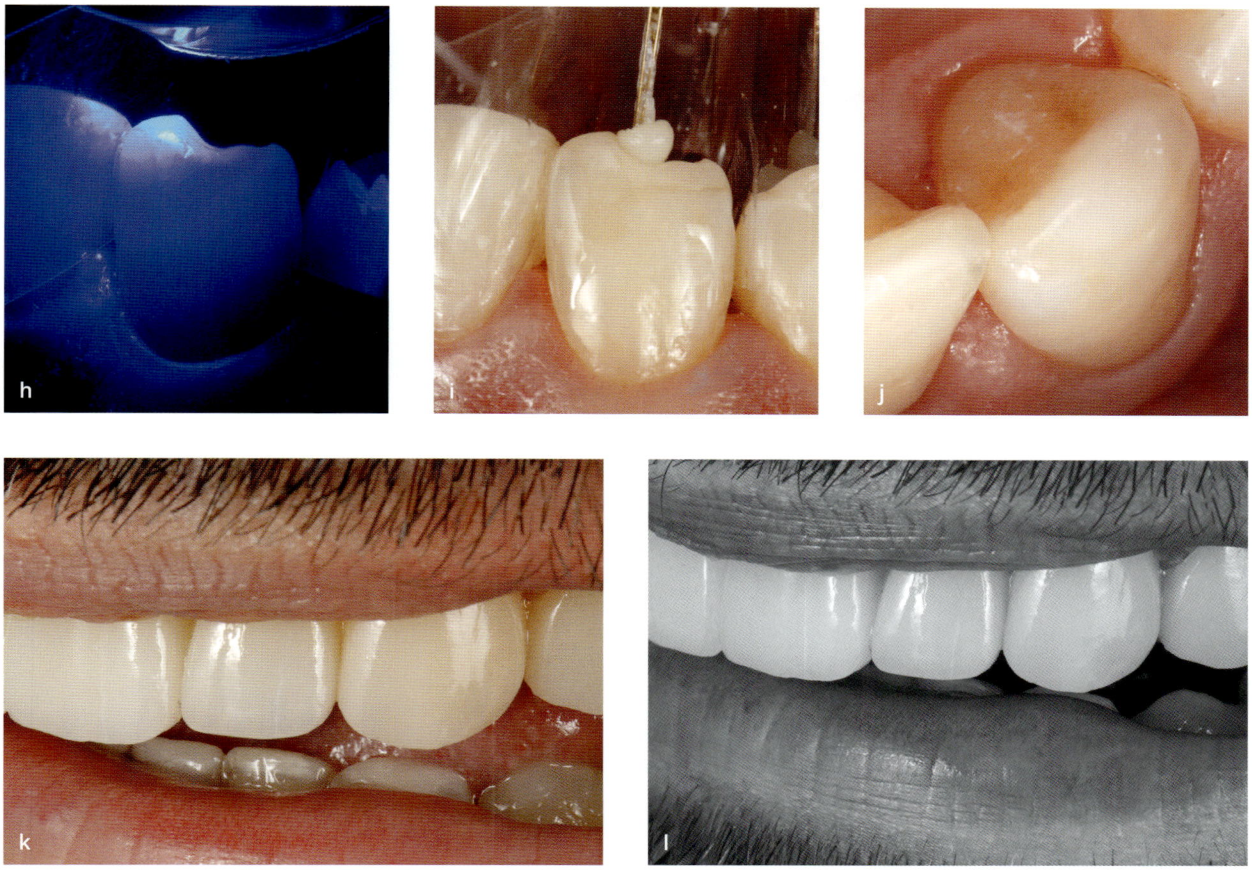


**Fig 4-18** During a regular control visit a fracture is detected within the composite mass of a mandibular canine that had been restored with direct freehand composite (a and b). The repair is done in the same appointment. The solution will be partial as the anatomically guided restoration approach also requires the visualization of the adjacent teeth during function. In order to increase the adhesion strength of the restoration, air abrasion with roughness enhancement is recommended, with polytetrafluoroethylene (PTFE) tape wrapped around the proximal teeth for protection. Use of a system such as a Microetcher (Danville Engineering) or application of 50-mm particles with a polishing system such as the EMS Air-Flow on the remaining composite adjacent to the fracture/chipping will increase the bond strength of the new composite (c). To provide a direct view of the anatomical boundaries, the white opaque tape is exchanged for a transparent matrix both distal and mesial to the tooth to be restored. An initial etching of the remaining composite mass is done for 2 minutes with hydrofluoric acid, which is then rinsed, followed by enamel etching for 30 seconds with orthophosphoric acid, which is then removed with profuse water spray, and the area is dried (Ultra-Etch System, Ultradent). After air abrasion and silanization, a light-cured adhesion system is applied, following the manufacturer's instructions, prior to adding the amount of composite suitable for repair or modification of the restoration. Restoration of the missing tooth structure is completed with strict adhesion to the manufacturer's protocol (d to i). The final anatomy is checked within the framework of the occlusion and arch (j to l).

handmade, a stone cast provides an inexpensive means of transporting the repair composite. In this case extra escape holes are advisable in order to limit the excess overflow of material as this type of mold might fit more snugly than a rigid tray (Fig 4-19).

Remaining up-to-date on adhesive protocols and advancements in these products can prove both stimulating and challenging. However, what is most important is to choose one system and strictly follow its protocol. The proceedings from the Versailles Adhesion Workshop provide a detailed explanation and interpretation of the various adhesive systems for different dental and restorative surfaces, together with their clinical application, and are an interesting read in this regard.[15]

Today, with few exceptions, the goal of maximum tooth preservation has brought unprecedented treatment modalities.[16] It comes as no surprise to the proficient reader that the general trend in TW is to follow an

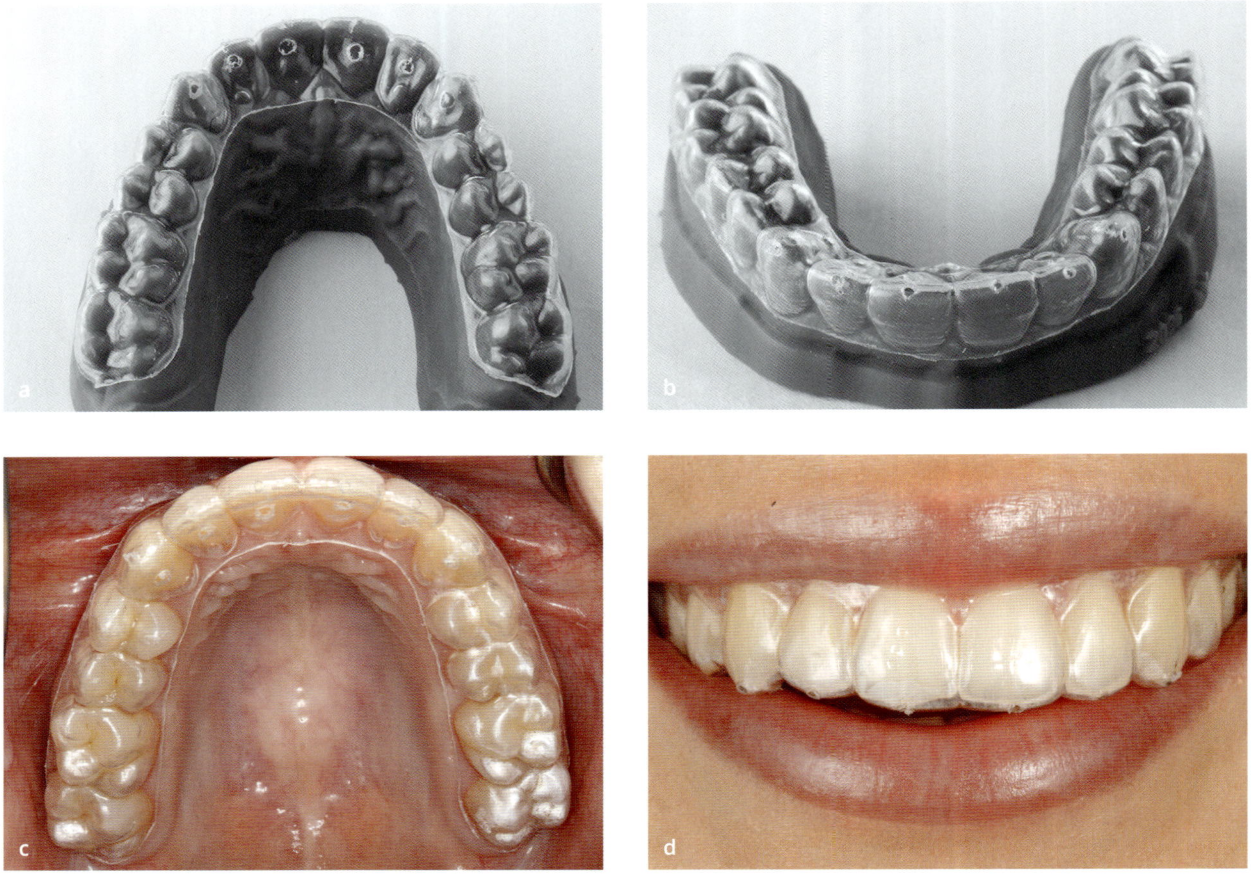


**Fig 4-19** Note the perforations at the specific sites where composite is going to be syringed (a to d). Extra holes will help control the excess material and facilitate final polishing and adjustment. Polishing of the remaining and new composite restoration is recommended with either composite polishing kits or polishing paste applied with felt brushes.

additive approach, avoiding as much as possible tooth preparation and limiting the drilling of any amount of remaining sound tooth. Generally speaking, the possibilities for no preparation or shallow preparation are greater if more teeth receive treatment. In TW, the damage affects usually several or most of the teeth in one sector, making it necessary to address even the full arch. However, this decision should derive from anatomical, functional, and conservative reasons and not from mere esthetic consideration.

Attending to the principle of enamel preservation, true additive buildups can only be achieved in direct restorative protocols with composite resin materials. Many cases of moderate TW and practically all cases of incipient TW can be treated without anesthesia as the result of not cutting tooth structure. Most of time tooth preparation is not needed or is restricted to rounding sharp edges with a medium-grain diamond bur or slight beveling in highly esthetically demanding areas (see more in chapter 5). Due to the physiopathology of TW, in principle, it is not desirable to remove remaining tooth structure to allow for the restorative procedure. Amalgams or any retentive restorations should be discarded as the type of lesion in TW does not enable any sort of mechanical retention. This applies also to temporary cements and fillings as well as glass ionomers (Fig 4-20).

The direct composite additive approach should favor building the damaged anatomical site in excess rather than below the occlusal or incisal planes, with any surplus eliminated at the adjustment and polishing phase. Occlusal equilibration or occlusal adjustment should be carefully weighed in TW patients; removing any sound

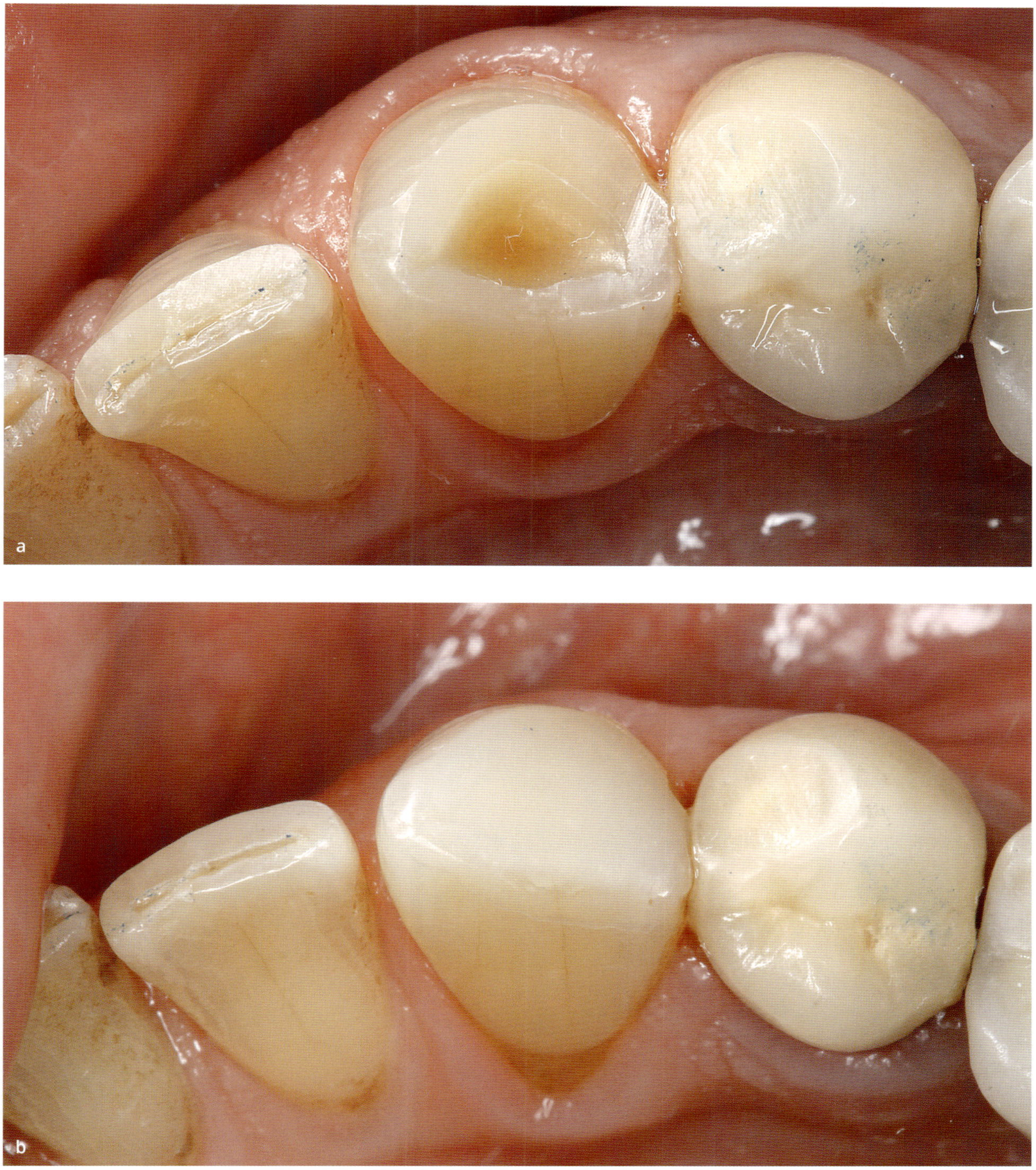


**Fig 4-20** The temporary direct composite is applied guided by the anatomical landmarks in this worn canine. The adjacent posterior sector has suffered and will need further treatment. While this treatment is carried out, protecting the exposed dentin prevents rapid wear progression or even failure of the canine (a and b).

structure may awaken tooth sensitivity. The alternative of orthodontic correction or adding to the occlusal surfaces should be considered instead.

In cases where damage has progressed to the dentin or affected several aspects of the tooth, indirect composite restorations, indirect reinforced composite blocks, or porcelain laminate veneers may be chosen depending on the site to be treated (see chapter 6). Independent of the material selection, the principle of minimal invasiveness should prevail.

## 7. Accuracy and the Preservation Principle

The accuracy of the prosthodontic and restorative therapy can be measured, for example, by the number of occlusal contacts achieved, their distribution, the time required for occlusal adjustments and polishing, the expenditure and resources invested by both the patient and dentist, and the patient's satisfaction. This is without doubt one of the most relevant aspects of everyday practice today and a major part of continuing education, with the goal of obtaining a better outcome and clear patient satisfaction. The patient with TW cannot be reduced to a damage-related category; TW management must be a patient-driven process.[17]

In other words, while some patients will react positively to a laborious prosthodontic protocol, others will veto tooth reduction unless it is clearly anticipated within the treatment plan. In this regard, the combined use of traditional and digital workflows with the purpose of preserving tooth structure is perceived as an advantage by the patient.

Within this perspective, the digitalization of the dental practice and the emerging computational technologies from artificial intelligence (AI), the internet of things (IoT), big data, cloud computing, blockchain, and the cyber security and privacy issues related to patient data sharing will inevitably transform the way TW is managed.

Some authors clearly advocate for a full digital workflow as much as possible, pointing out the unpredictable outcomes brought by analog procedures such as traditional impression making and mounting of casts on a standard articulator.[18,19] On the other hand, highly technological workflows can be perceived as senseless and expensive if the process seems an inarticulate mishmash of gadgets.

In TW, a well-integrated digital workflow combined with traditional analog processes in a hop-on, hop-off approach will bring benefits both to the diagnosis, planning, and especially treatment phases as part of a multidisciplinary approach. Superior, more accurate, more predictable, quality-controlled final outcomes will be easier to obtain even in the face of the quintessential challenge of TW. The added potential of new aspects of TW management and monitoring has only begun, as will be explained in the upcoming chapters of this book.

## 8. Traditional Acquisition of Data

Traditional prosthodontic workflows are widely used today, with a history of more than 50 years of research and development and concepts originating from an era in which many patients in their midlife required partial or full dentures.[20] Contributions to fixed prosthetic replacement are well known and have been the guidelines for generations of dentists.[21]

The prosthodontic process relies on a series of intraoral impressions either in the diagnostic phase (alginate) or later in the treatment phase (silicone or polyvinyl siloxane), that may differ in their accuracy depending on the impression material, the handling and expertise of the professional, and the quality of the stone model. In a second appointment, a facebow and a semi-adjustable articulator are used for the precise positioning of the reference planes and orientation in the three dimensions of space. Mounting of the models in the articulator should not be taken for granted as many mistakes can be made—some obvious and promptly corrected, others more difficult to detect and leading to gross misplacement of the occlusal plane in the final restorations (Fig 4-21). Therefore the mounting protocols should be reviewed and optimized with every new member of the team.[22]

During the pretreatment phase the technician is able to recreate the ideal anatomy in an additive wax-up on the stone model, based on the surrounding gingival architecture, the remaining intact teeth, and most importantly photos of the patient, taking into consideration the patient's wishes (and limitations).

Depending on the dentist's preference, the color of the wax up can vary from white to tooth color or even bright shades that may be seen better by the patient (Fig 4-22). The in vivo try-in of a mock-up is ideal for the patient to experience the planned improvements and be able to take part in the decision making[13,23–25] (Fig 4-23).

As explained before, showing the patient the new dimensions and proportions and their importance in the overall occlusal scheme is of paramount importance; therefore, anatomical restorations in the posterior sectors also should be included in the preview. This is critical in the patient with TW, who may be already accustomed to the shortening of the teeth. If any changes are done chairside, a new impression should be taken and transferred to the lab before the final restoration is started.

Advantages of this traditional flow are the design freedom and the potential for restorations that may excel both in esthetics and function (Fig 4-24).

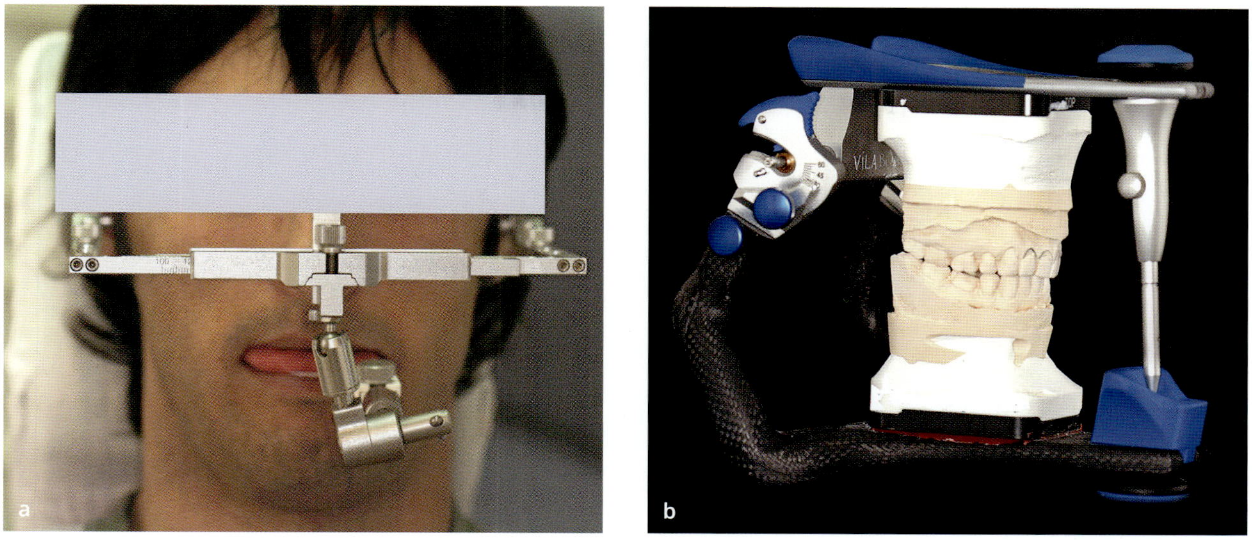


**Fig 4-21** The positioning of the occlusal plane is of paramount relevance for the final outcome. This depends on standard landmarks such as the external auditory meatus that may well be parallel to the occlusal plane, such in this case, or not. The required learning curve together with limited storage space and distance from other members of the TW team such as the lab technician all advocate for virtual scanning of the patient.

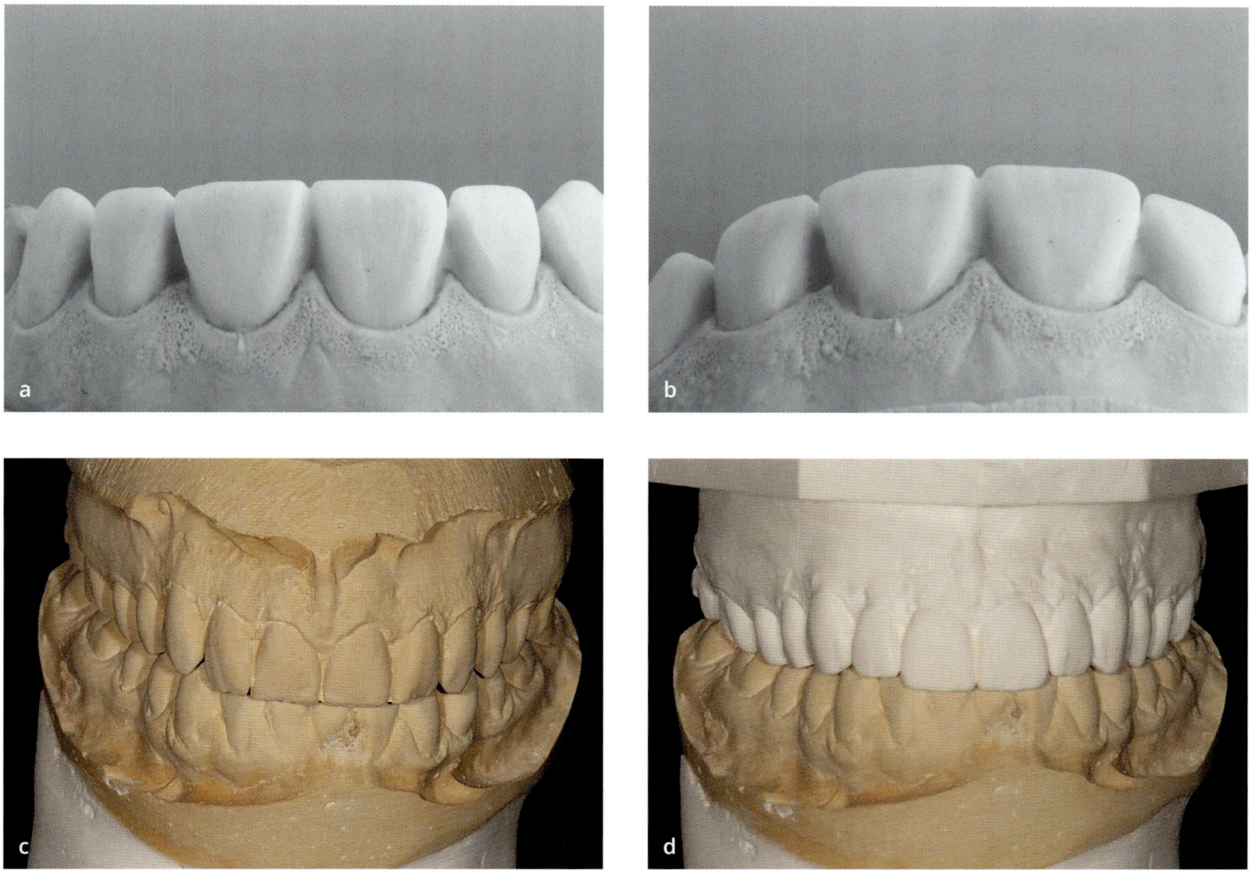


**Fig 4-22** This in vitro wax-up is a valid setup for all the professionals involved in treatment planning, but it is barely useful for the patient's understanding and even less so for the acceptance of any esthetic changes in the smile (a and b). The state of the art in this sense is delivering a try-in mock-up to the patient. The steps are well known and include the fabrication of a set of silicone transfer trays (if maxillary and mandibular dentition will be treated) and optionally silicone preparation guides from the mounted wax-up models in a semi-adjustable articulator (c to j). *(continued next page)*

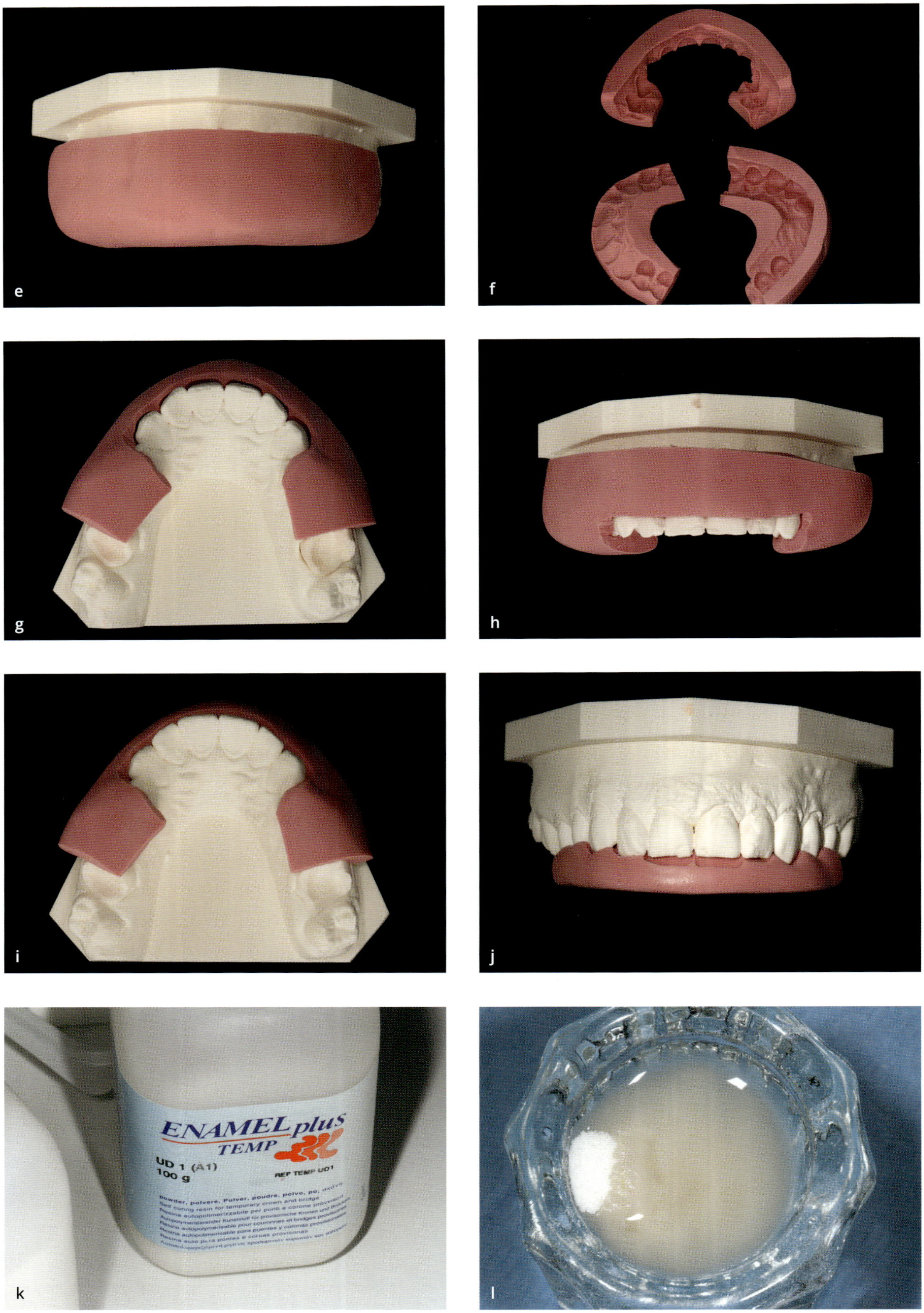
e
f
g
h
i
j
ENAMEL plus
TEMP
UD 1 (A1)
100 g
REF TEMP UD1
k
l

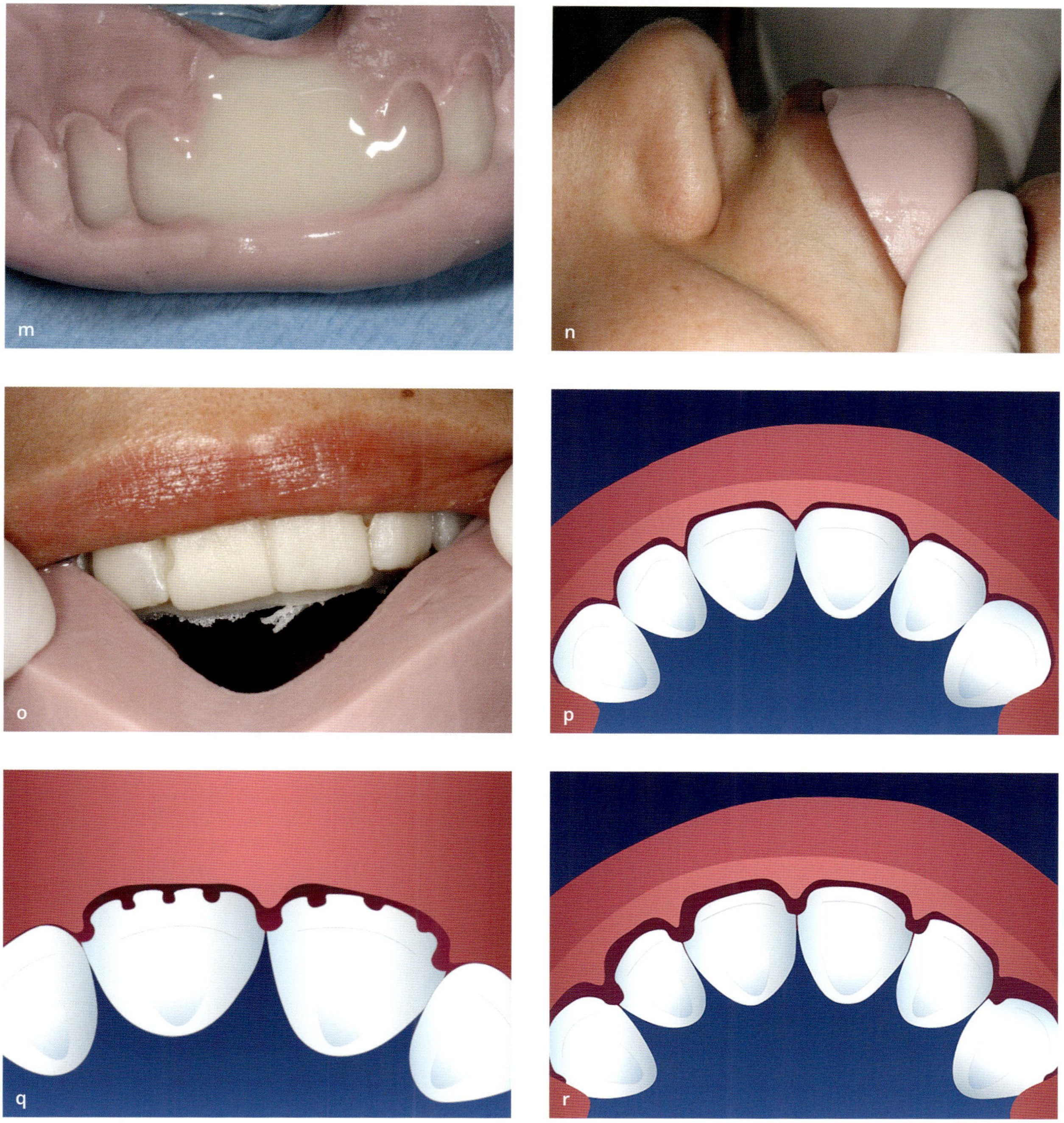


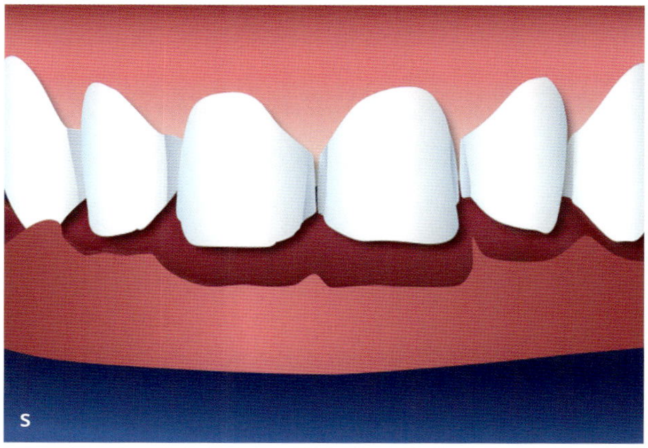


**Fig 4-22** *(continued)* Today the wax-up as well as the transport and preparation guides can be done digitally. An auto-curing resin is then mixed and delivered to the arch until it sets (k to o). This is usually done before any tooth preparation and used together with the preparation guide in order to limit the reduction of the natural tooth to what is strictly necessary (p to s). As mentioned, in patients with TW tooth reduction is minimized, but there is still use for this technique in some cases. (See chapters 6, 7, and 8.)

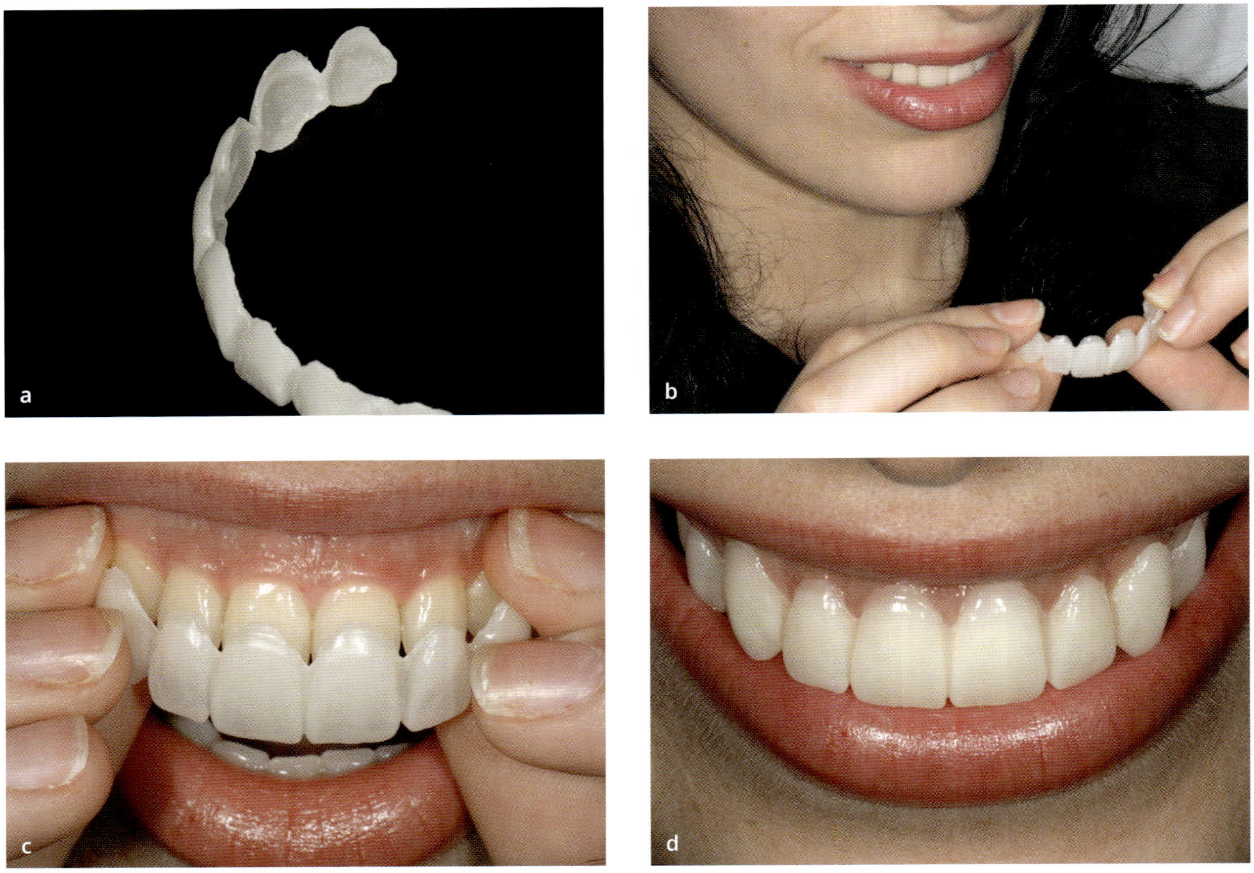

**Fig 4-23** The engaging experience of seeing smile improvements in one's face reduces the gap between what is recommended and what is wanted. In this case a young woman is trying in a cutback anterior prototype handmade from the wax-up (a to d). Pictures and video recordings should be taken with the mock-up in place in the patient's smile and rest positions as well as during excursions. If modifications are to be done, this is the correct time. This also would be the correct time to inform the patient of any tooth reduction if it is deemed necessary. The new length and volume may feel strange as the insidiousness of TW has made the patient used to an altered proportion to a large extent. Imposing abrupt changes that have not been anticipated may be a cause of unnecessary dispute as the perception of the stomatognathic system in all its complexity is not an easy task.

Drawbacks are cost and the limitations of communication of upstream and downstream data, which must be interpreted by the viewer and transferred to the lab technician and other members of the TW team in an inarticulate flow. Last but not least, the expenditure of a traditional workflow for the patient is higher as it not only includes the cost of the handmade wax-up but also the time-consuming procedure of the in vivo mock-up. Moreover, in the case that the mock-up is used as a guide for tooth preparation, a second mock-up will need to be done after the restoration of all posterior sectors is finished and before the actual tooth preparation (see the TW treatment flowchart at the end of the chapter).

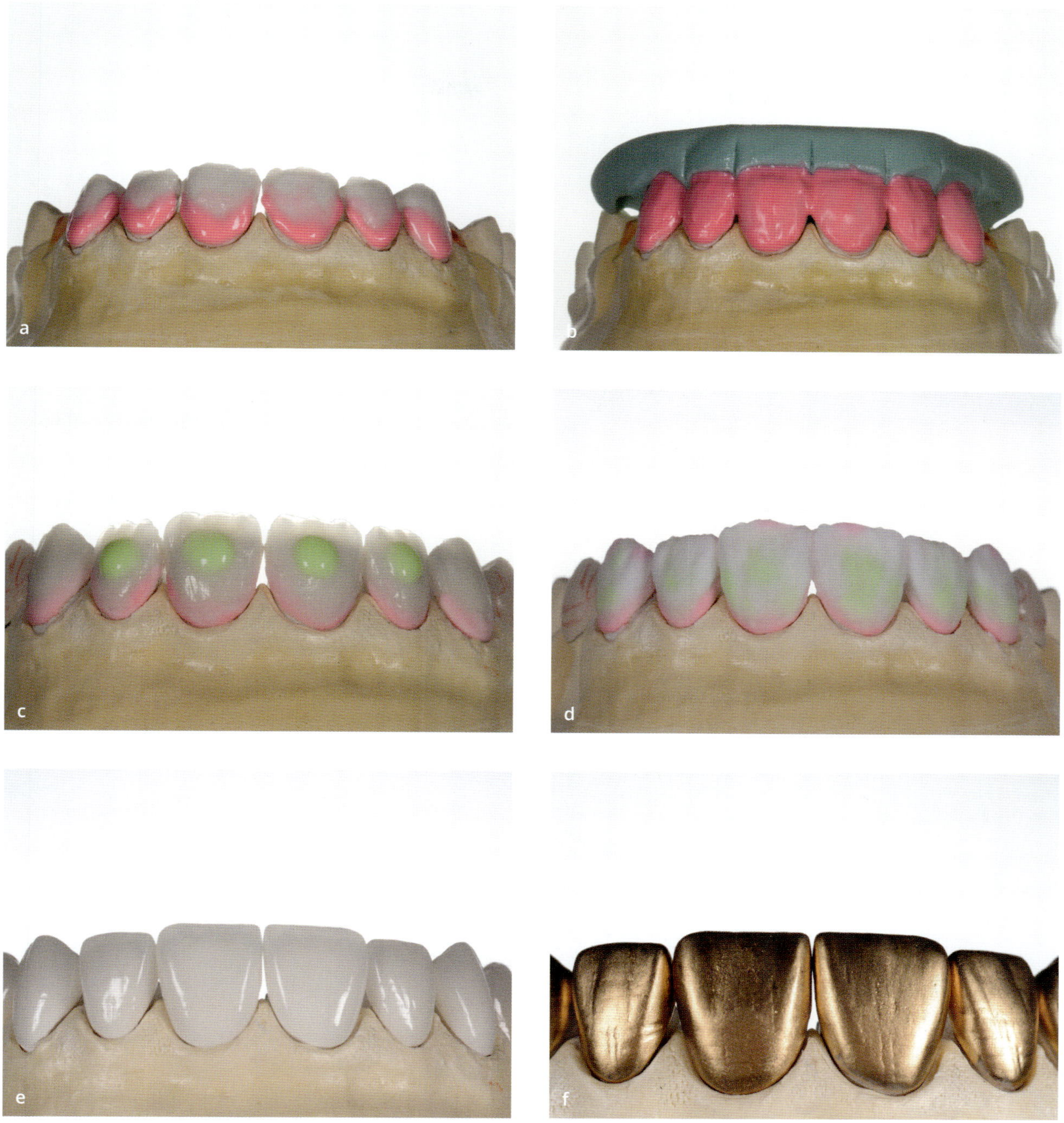


**Fig 4-24** The traditional workflow for restoration manufacturing is still a valid option in highly demanding situations (a to f). An accurate silicone impression is essential for an accurate restoration outcome. A meticulous step-by-step protocol is mandatory for a predictable flow. Any correction once this protocol has begun might mean coming back to the starting point.

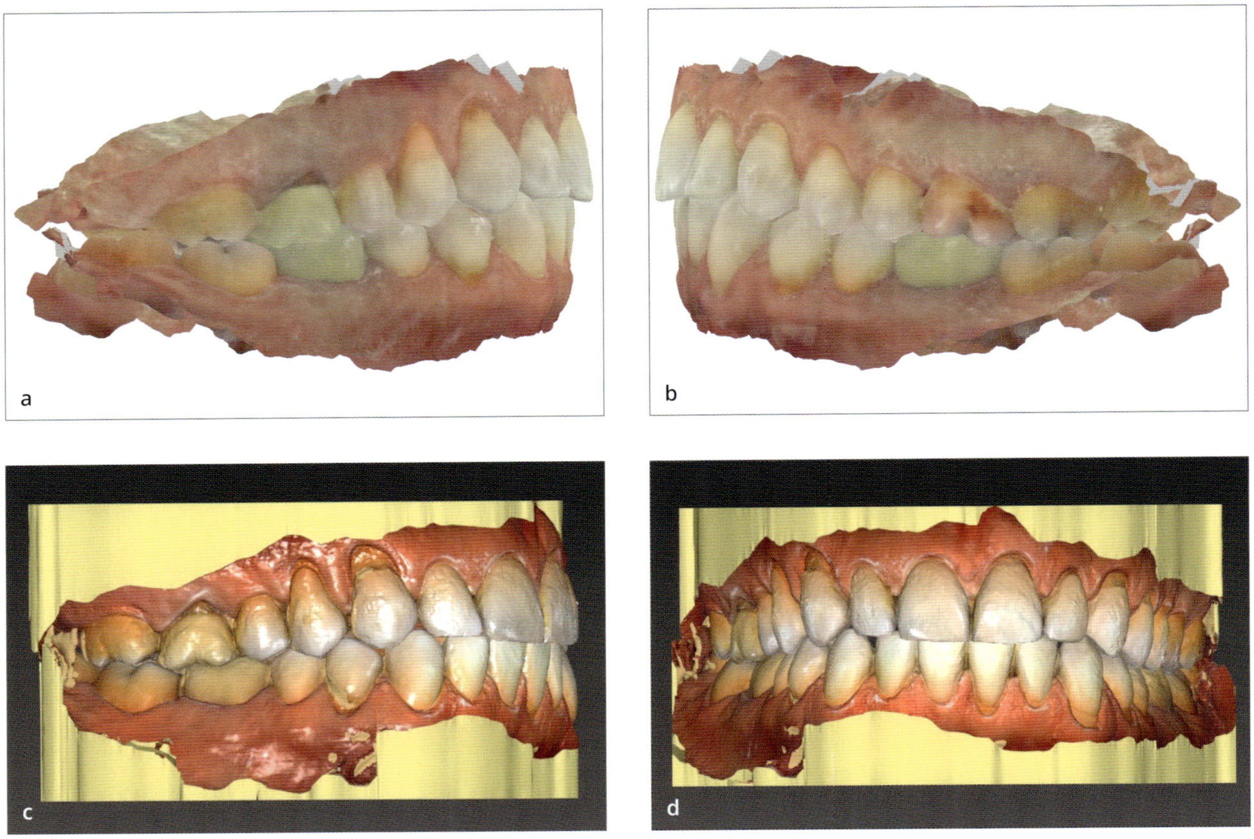

**Fig 4-25** In this patient in his fifth decade of life, the parafunctional habit has affected only several of the anterior teeth, with more damage to the tips of the canines. Once the patient's intraoral situation is digitalized, it is decided to restore the canine/anterior guidance anatomy as needed. The importance of the canine both functionally and esthetically in TW during the initial years is key for the progression and esthetic impact of TW. In this case, reconstructing the cusps of the four canines as well as the incisal edges of the four mandibular incisors with freehand composite is key to intercepting future TSL (a to h). The patient is advised to stop biting his nails and wear a set of extra-thin mouth splints during the daytime hours and to sleep with a Michigan-type mouthguard in place (i). Digitally monitoring the effect of the implemented measures will help in the management of future treatment needs. (See chapter 10.)

## 9. Digital Acquisition of Data: Cross-Mounting in the Digital Era

The visual communication with the patient was eased with the introduction of Digital Smile Design (DSD) and more recently its evolution into a truly integrated tool that can also be used along with other CAD/CAM software and 3D technology for a completely digital workflow.[19]

Whatever the type of flow, in patients with TW, the diagnosis and therefore the treatment plan should focus on the functional aspects of the damaged and eventually restored dentition rather than merely esthetics. In fact reconstructing the canine and canine guidance often is sufficient to establish protection of the rest of the anterior teeth.[26]

Frequently shallow or insufficient anterior guidance can be fixed with a minor intervention on the incisal edges of the maxillary or mandibular anterior teeth, whichever show more incisal damage. No matter the amount of damage, all TW cases should be given the same level of attention and managed similarly (Fig 4-25). In other words, applying a well-established TW protocol is an appropriate tool to efficiently treat patients with TW. In this sense a digital or a combined digital-analog workflow is of great value.

Overlapping, superimposing, and cross-mounting are all new verbs that find their way more and more into our everyday practice. Digital technologies have made a quantum leap in terms of improving the accuracy of restorative and implant dentistry (see chapter 8). Intraoral scans, STL files, and CAD/CAM 3D mounting in a virtual plane have a definitive place in our daily tasks. It is possible to acquire, diagnose, plan, design, and virtually test, both esthetically and functionally, the CAD/CAM prototype on the patient's virtual self. This can even be done within the face of the patient by means of an exciting new tool, the face scan.[27]

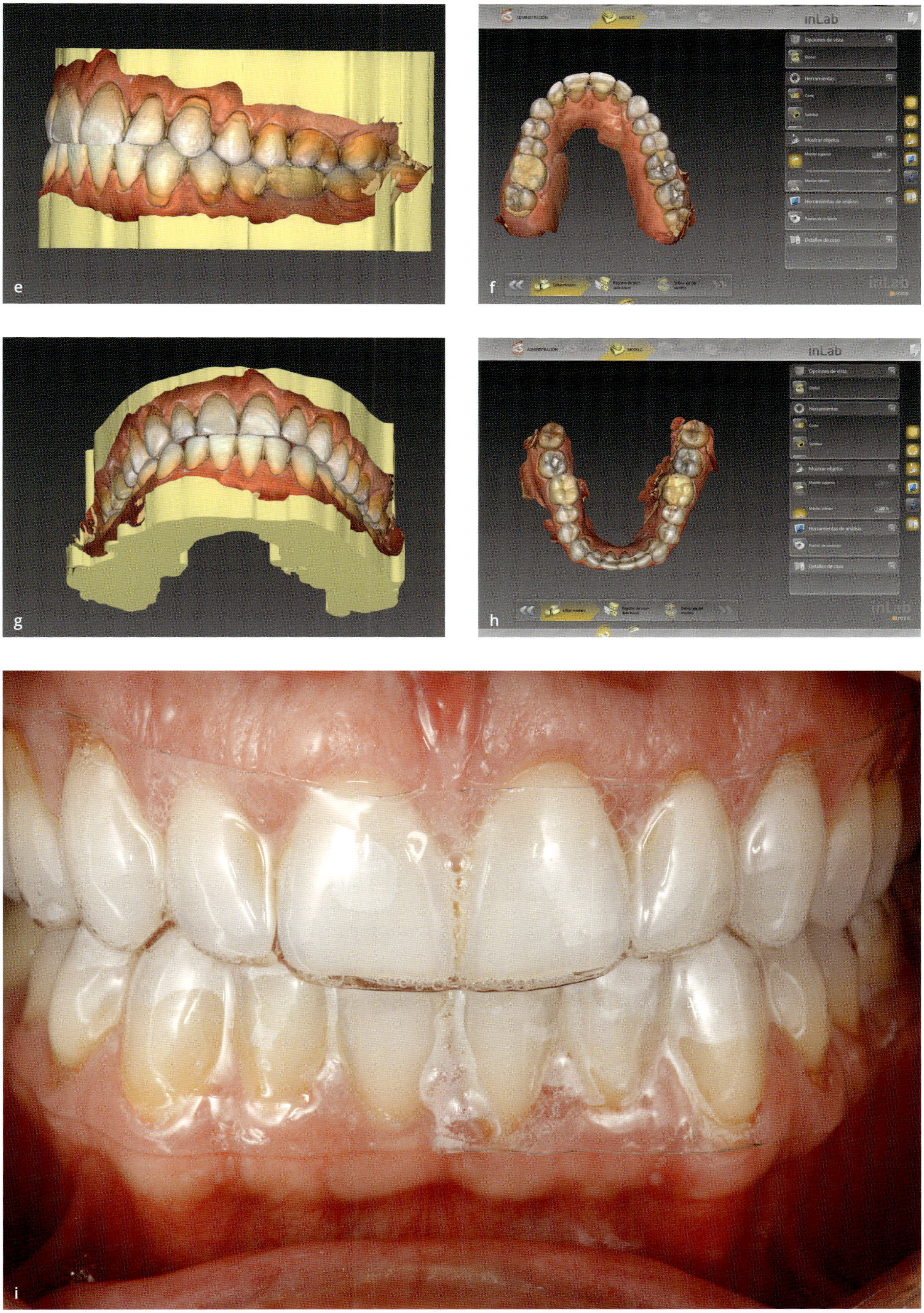
e
f
inLab
Opciones de vista
Herramientas
Mostrar objetos
Herramientas de análisis
Detalles de caso
g
h
inLab
Opciones de vista
Herramientas
Mostrar objetos
Herramientas de análisis
Detalles de caso
i

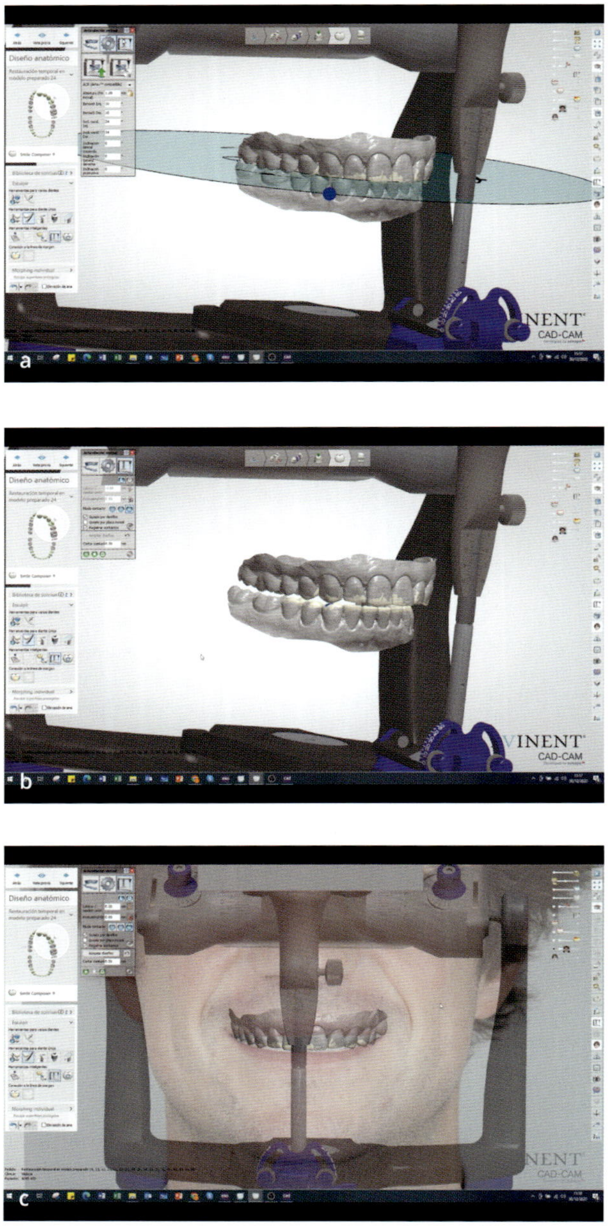

**Fig 4-26** Obtaining a face scan should be part of the digitalization at the initial phases of diagnosis. The superimposition of the digital face and intraoral scans enables a virtual wax-up that can be analyzed on the three planes of space. Any improvements necessary for esthetic or functional reasons are easily implemented with these digital tools (a to c).

There are a number of face scanning systems, some currently available and some under development. Depending on the budget and practice strategies, it may be that investing in a system proves to be pivotal in the digital journey. Even the simplest system provides a patient with a 3D image of the face that is accurate enought for 3D diagnosis and planning (Fig 4-26).

The lab technician matches the face scan and the intraoral scan. A 3D virtual articulator then can be superimposed, and a functional titration of the computer-assisted design is tested in the patient's virtual mouth. Another advantage of the virtual mock-up is the possibility of superimposing the same design onto the various intraoral scans and at the manufacturing phase (Fig 4-27).

Not having to remove the handmade mock-up and the flexibility for making instant changes digitally is a tremendous advantage to the patient in terms of time and discomfort. Notwithstanding this, an in vivo trial of the proposed restoration before manufacturing has started can and should be done in patients with high esthetic demands and in cases of comprehensive full-arch reconstructions.

This mock-up can be milled from a resin or PMMA (polymethyl methacrylate) thin transparent splint vacuum-formed from the printed wax-up model, or at this time one may choose to step out of the digital workflow and do an in vivo mock-up using a transfer tray done on a printed model to transfer tooth-colored resin material onto the teeth in an example of a hop-on, hop-off flow from a digital to a traditional workflow.

The digital steps can be outsourced to a design center or the practice's usual lab. Desk versus chairside time should spare expenses and bring benefits to the TW team, meaning not only the restorative team but also the patient. It is, however, not uncommon to see an ample display of the latest technologies to attract patients who are digital enthusiasts or to justify large fees. Conversely, this digital trend should aim to reduce time and costs both to the patient and dentist.

The advantages of the digital articulator and the virtual facebow are myriad when compared to the manual articulator. The combined use of this digital tool with CAD technology boosts the possibilities in the planning phase as well as in the treatment itself as it can prove more efficient and accurate in regard to occlusion and fit.[28]

A recent study compared the accuracy of traditional and digital articulators when measuring the quality and quantity of occlusal contacts of single zirconia crowns fabricated with a digital versus a traditional flow. A visual analog scale of occlusal comfort where 0 was intolerable and 100 was perfect found that there were no significant differences in terms of interference nor adjustment time. Moreover, the digital articulator was presumed to show a better occlusal dynamic performance of the crowns during functional movements due to the possibility of more accurate customization of the mandibular hinge axis compared to the standard semi-adjustable articulator as

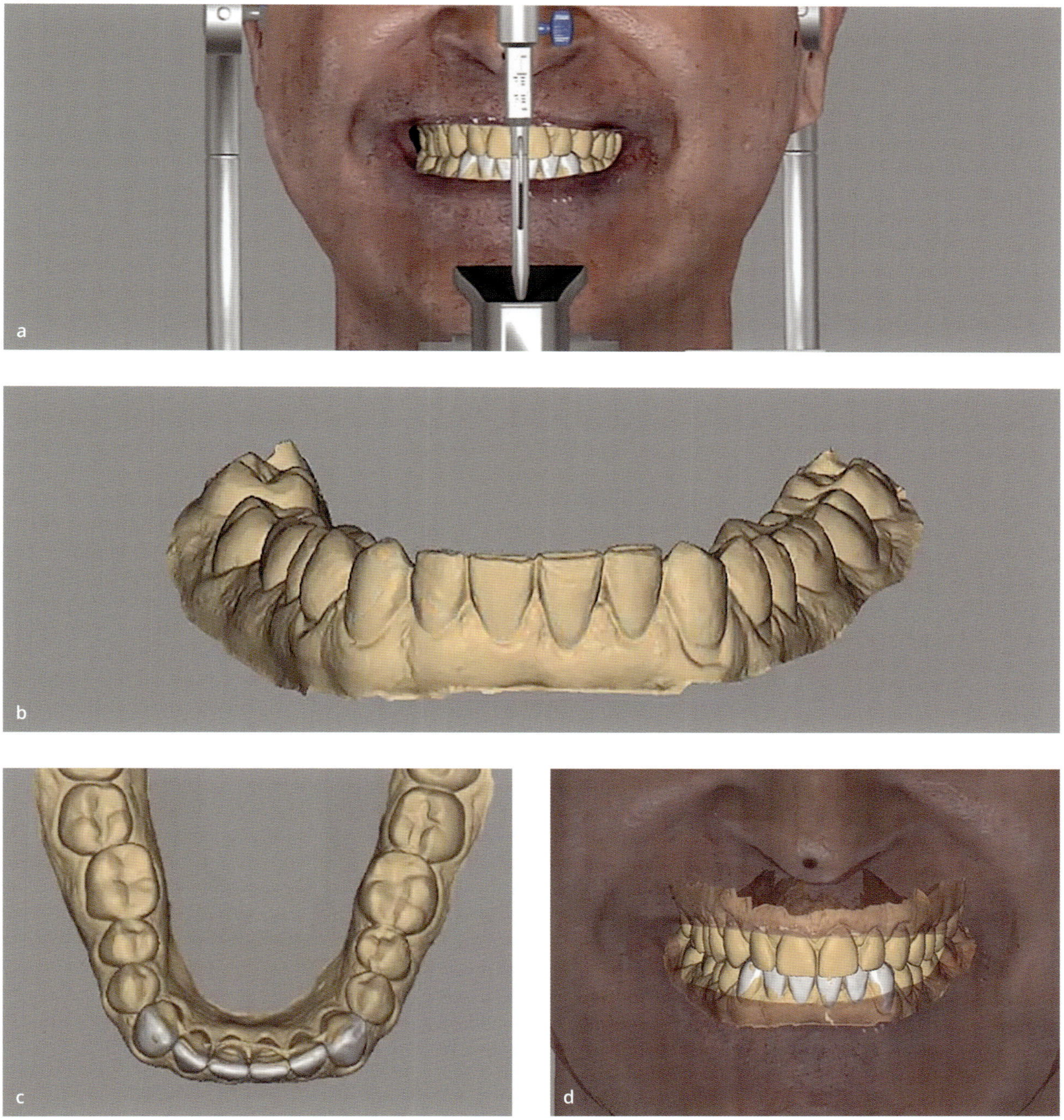

**Fig 4-27** The virtual articulator is used on the image of the patient's face obtained from the face scan. The digital wax-up is superimposed on the 3D representation of the patient during the planning and design phase. This can be shared, discussed, and modified by any member of the TW Team (a to d).

well as the simulation possibilities of the digital software. Lastly, the time spent for adjustment of the occlusal and functional aspects of the crowns showed no significance differences.[29]

Neither the previously mentioned study nor the few PROMs studies on digital dentistry included patients with TW.[30] Clinical practice also seems to indicate that, from the perspective of the patient with TW, the digital workflow, or the intentional combination of digital and analog workflows, is well appreciated. It is in the design of function, esthetics, and hygiene access that digital dentistry excels. From the dentist's perspective, accuracy as well as reduced total chairside time add to the advantage of easily making modifications. Last but not least, the timetable and treatment schedule is optimized, as most of the STLs can be superimposed. The potential for further follow-ups is a clear advantage when compared to a fully analog flow.

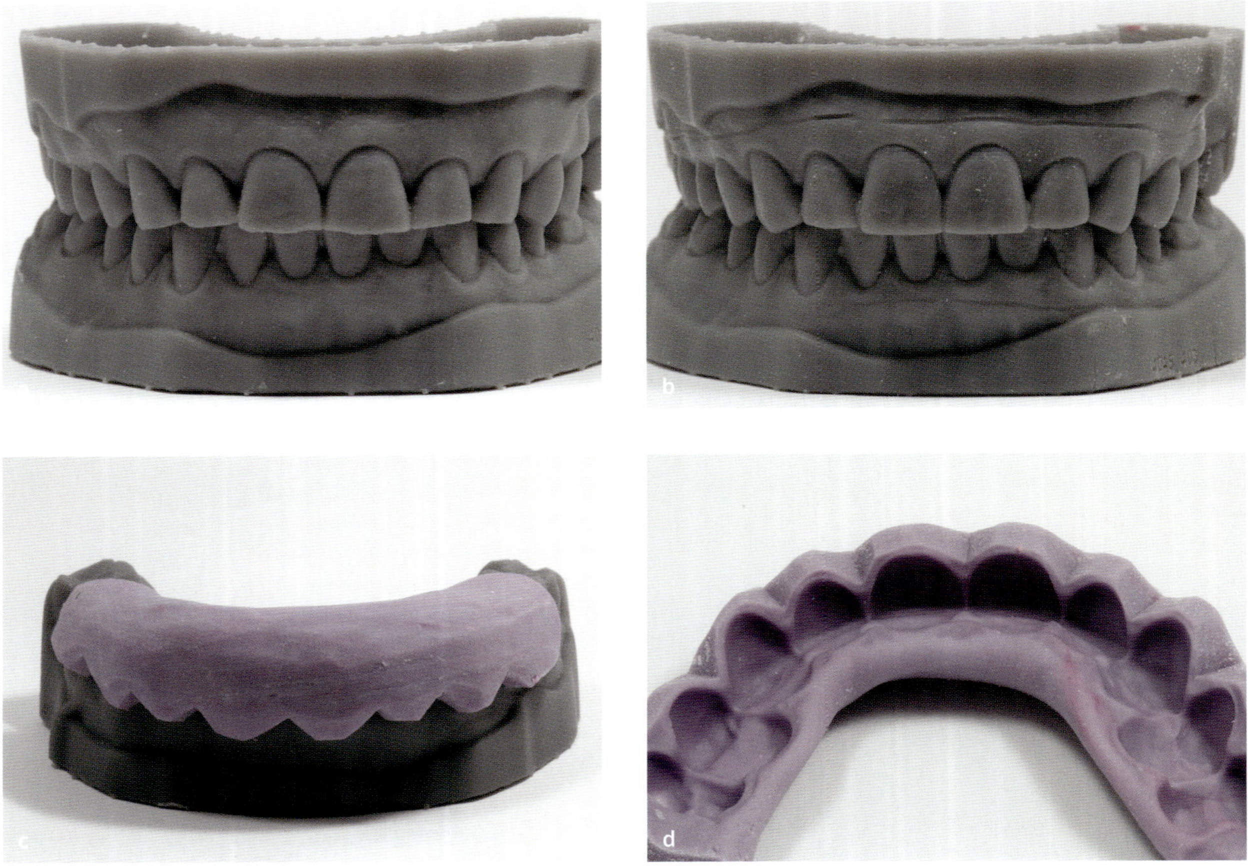


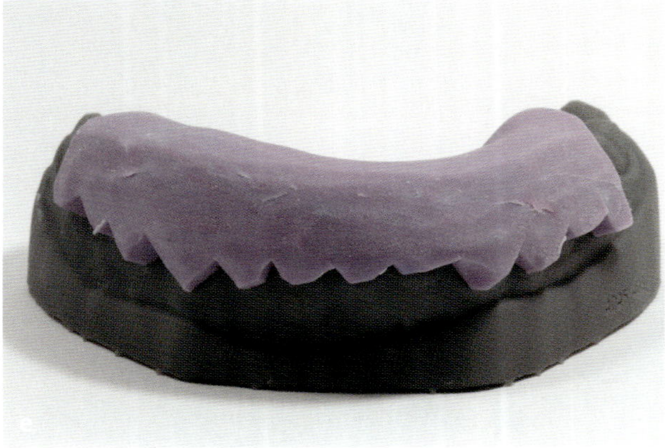

**Fig 4-28** Example of a hop-on, hop-off work flow. Printed models and a silicone transfer guide provide the dentist the opportunity to perform a direct delivery of the virtual wax-up to the mouth of the patient if a classical mock-up try-in is the desired approach. In this case an initial digital virtual workflow was changed to an analog workflow (a to m). Final monitoring is done digitally.

## 10. Traditional and Digital: Hop-On, Hop-Off Workflow

The traditional workflow data acquisition usually is followed by a handmade restoration process that counts on the excellence and experience of the lab technician for an outstanding result. In a fully digital workflow, the digital images are usually incorporated into digital planning and eventually a computer-assisted manufacturing line.

In combination workflows, traditional models and wax-ups can be scanned and then used for digital planning and vice versa. A model can be printed from the computer and from there a polyvinyl siloxane impression can be taken and a cast model poured in a traditional manner if the handmade manufacturing of the prosthetic piece is preferred. The esthetic outcome of a handmade prosthesis can excel that of CAD/CAM, given the right lab technician is available. It is feasible to jump from one workflow to the other in what can be referred to as hop-on, hop-off; no restrictions should be imposed to serve the patient with TW to the best of our abilities (Fig 4-28). (See more in chapters 6, 7, and 9.)

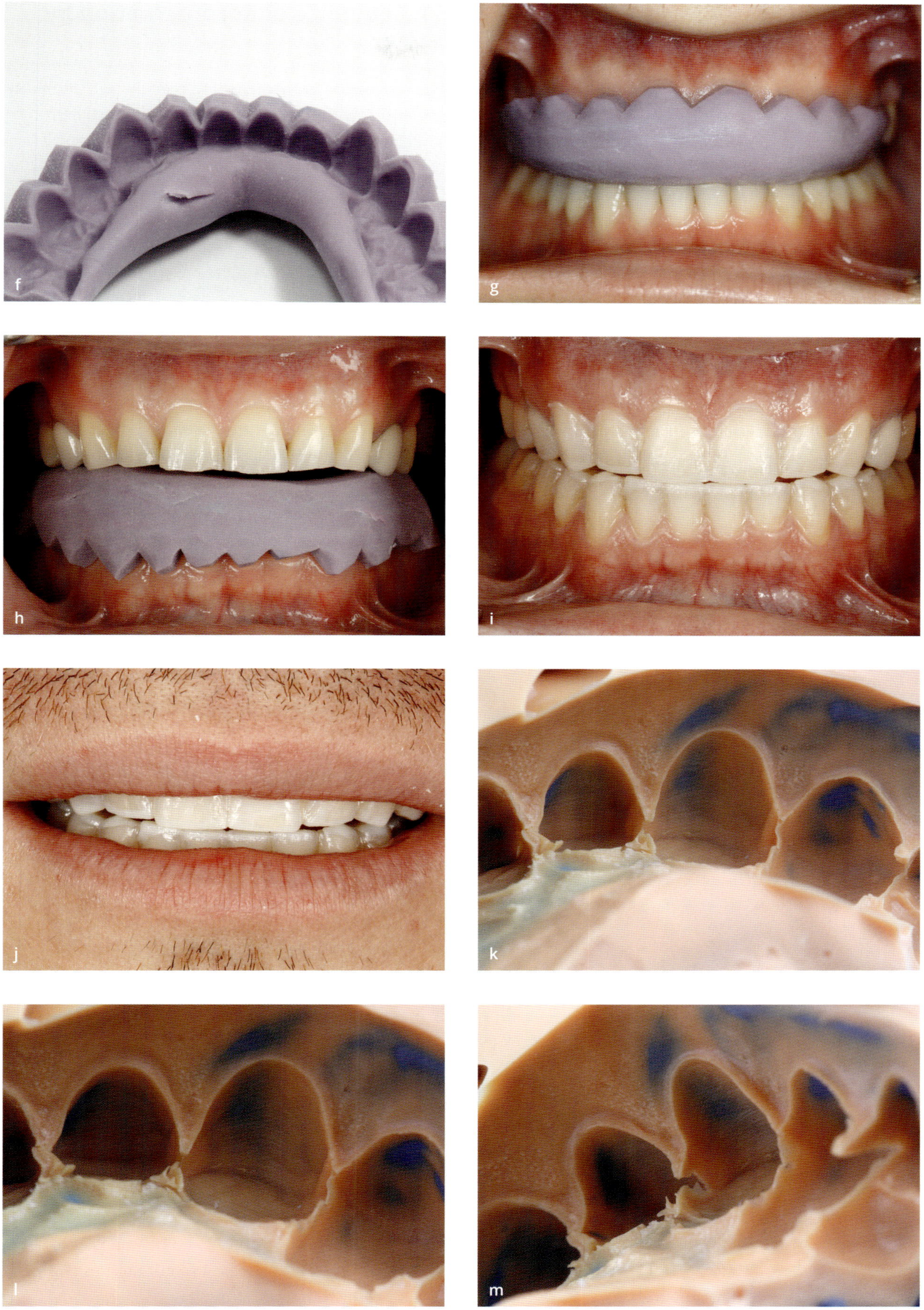

Another example of implementing a different flow is the use of intraoral scans for the monitoring of the restorations. With the advent of the superimposition software for intraoral scanners such as TimeLapse for iTero (Align Technology) or OraCheck for Primescan (Dentsply Sirona), the dentist knows where and when to modify the restorations that have become worn or defective. A quantitative comparison between two time periods is a valuable guide for the TW team. If the TW team does not have a scanning device in office, the models of the final restored dentition can be digitalized at the lab and compared to a new set of models after a certain time. A 3D computerized comparison will provide a quantitative value of how much loss has occurred. A transfer mold can be printed for the addition of the necessary amount of material.

The same protocol for repair as previously described should be followed (see Figs 4-18 and 4-19).

## 11. Sequence of Reconstruction by Sector

The elucidation between centric relation (CR) and maximal intercuspal position (MIP) for the desired interocclusal relationship should not influence the anterior incisal plane and anterior esthetics as this depends entirely on facial and tooth proportions in relation to the lips, smile, and a pleasant facial anatomy.

A virtual set-up from a digital library is done in a similar manner as the classical wax-up for an edentulous patient, only virtually. That being said, if posterior restorations are needed or if an increase of the VDO is the plan, the new posterior anatomy also can be virtually incorporated onto the virtual mock-up at this stage. This procedure can be done before the posterior restorations have been delivered, whether they may be direct composites, indirect milled tooth-colored restorations, or a combination of both.[14]

Generally speaking, mandibular (posterior or posterior and anterior depending on the needs of the case) restorations should be done first, followed by maxillary posterior restorations when needed. Maxillary anterior restorations should follow.

## 12. Key Points: TW Treatment Flowchart

**Table 4-4** TW treatment flowchart. *(continued next page)*

| TIMELINE | INCIPIENT TW | MODERATE TW | SEVERE TW |
|---|---|---|---|
| **1st Contact** | Routine visit during hygiene and prophylaxis. | New patient with tooth event or esthetic concern. Usually asymptomatic; may declare hypersensitivity or repeated infection. | |
| **1st Visit** | **Examination: Anamnesis**[a]<br>1. TW diagnosis<br>2. Localization and severity of TW: WECC and WASS<br>3. TW and Fox questionnaires<br>4. Identification of risk and etiologic factors<br>5. Profile and facial harmony, smile, incisal edges, occlusal anatomy<br>6. Anterior function (anterior and canine guidance), overbite, and overjet<br>7. Radiographs (panoramic and cephalometric) | **Examination: Anamnesis**[a]<br>1. TW diagnosis<br>2. Localization and severity of TW: WECC and WASS<br>3. TW and Fox questionnaires<br>4. Identification of risk and etiologic factors; identify missing teeth, restorations, and tooth failures<br>5. Profile and facial harmony, smile, incisal and occlusal anatomy and support; inspect for palatal damage<br>6. Anterior function (anterior and canine guidance), overbite, and overjet<br>7. Radiographs (panoramic and cephalometric), CBCT (diagnosis and treatment plan of severe TW) | |
| **2nd Visit** | 1. TW informed consent signed, photographs, video (optional)<br>2. Digital: intraoral scan in MIP, face scan optional; Analog: impressions of both arches and bite registration, stone models<br>3. Presence of malocclusion, maxillomandibular relationship (Angle class, crossbite, open bite), altered eruption, airway, Bolton analysis<br>4. Profile and facial harmony, smile, occlusal plane<br>5. Anterior function (anterior and canine guidance), overbite, and overjet<br><br>**In case of orthodontic indication, the restorative phase can be done before or after the orthodontic phase. If restorations are done first, a second data recording is done with new intraoral scans or impressions and photos before starting orthodontics.** | 1. Proceed as in incipient, but if analog flow use facebow and semi-adjustable articulator.<br>2. Record data.<br>**Orthodontic evaluation.**<br>Proceed as in incipient.<br>**In case of orthodontic indication, the restorative phase should be done after and only exceptionally before the orthodontic phase.**[b]<br>**Orthodontic path will include 3D virtual planning or handmade wax-up and provide space for rehabilitation of anterior or other damaged sectors.**<br><br>If orthodontics is discarded:<br>1. If palatal space is needed for restorations, evaluate impact of MIP and CR or VDO increase.<br>2. If occlusal space is needed for restorations, evaluate VDO increase. | |

[a]EDs should not be discussed with the patient on the 1st visit to prevent a negative reaction.
[b]Orthodontic indication for improvement of overjet, overbite, gingival outline, occlusal plane, expansion, and correction of mesial drifting (crowding). Infections and failing restorations should be addressed first.

**Table 4-4** *(continued)* TW treatment flowchart.

| TIMELINE | INCIPIENT TW | MODERATE TW | SEVERE TW |
|---|---|---|---|
| **3rd Visit** | **Restorative phase:**<br>No VDO increase is needed to restore: space is found in CR or MIP or after orthodontic therapy.<br>a. Direct freehand composite of worn teeth (anatomically guided), canine and anterior guidance and posterior defects.<br>b. Semi-direct wax-up-driven restoration, an index, mold, or modified technique can be used.<br>Occlusion control, adjust and polish, postoperative intraoral scan for monitoring (iTero TimeLapse or Primescan OraCheck); if traditional impressions: photos video. | **In vivo mock-up.** Depending on the workflow:<br>a. Wax-up or CAD/CAM mock-up try-in, record[c]<br>b. Wax-up or CAD/CAM resin cutback prototype try-in, record (impression not possible) and remove<br>c. Transparent full-contour prototype try-in to show new volume and length | |
| **4th Visit** | Dietary and lifestyle counseling. Michigan-type night mouthguard adjusted if origin of TW is mainly bruxism or attrition. Transparent day protection mouthguard delivered if erosion or daytime parafunctional habits such as lip biting, nail biting, etc are predominant factors. | **Restorative phase:**<br>1. Direct or semidirect protocols.<br>a. Direct composite is delivered freehand or through an index or mold, first in mandible, then in maxilla. Check occlusion. Adjust and polish.<br>b. VDO is increased to provide space in the anterior and/or posterior sector: Direct composite is used to restore the posterior occlusal plane with the help of an interocclusal jig with the estimated VDO or by means of an index or mold.<br>2. Indirect or semi-indirect onlays are performed.<br>a. Intraoral scan, CAD/CAM in-house milling of PICN or composite blocks enable cementation in same visit (semi-indirect) with chosen VDO.<br>b. If traditional PVS impression, send to lab. Indirect restoration cementation in 7–10 days.[d] | |
| **5th Visit** | | **Moderate or severe damage to anterior teeth.**<br>a. **Traditional workflow:** Anterior restorations prepared for PLV. PVS impression is sent to lab.<br>b. **Fully digital workflow:** Anterior restorations prepared for PLV. Preparation is scanned and STL sent to lab. | |
| **6th Visit** | | **PLV cementation and digital control**<br>Intraoral scan or impressions can be scanned for TW monitoring.[e]<br>Transparent protection mouthguard delivered.<br>Photos, videos.<br>Dietary and lifestyle counseling. | |

[c]Wax-up is used to evaluate overall esthetics and function but not as a preparation guide at this time as the restorative phase of the posterior sectors is done first.
[d]Final dimension of occlusion is checked before any restorative procedure for the anterior and canine guidance is done. If palatal restorations have been delivered, they should have been designed with the full estimated incisal length. At this stage anterior length with esthetic evaluation and phonetics are tested before the next step.
[e]Stone models can be scanned for digitalization of the TW progression by means of superimposing the STL images at different time intervals (iTero or OraCheck).

# References


1. Lazare A. The interview as a clinical negotiation. In: Lipkin M, Putnam SM, Lazare A (eds). The Medical Interview: Clinical Care, Education, and Research. New York: Springer, 1995:50–62.
2. Levine M. Communication challenges within eating disorders: What people say and what individuals hear. In: Jáuregui-Lobera I (ed). Eating Disorders: A Paradigm of the Biopsychosocial Model of Illness. London: IntechOpen, 2017:239–272.
3. Villa A, Wolff A, Aframian D, et al. World Workshop on Oral Medicine VI: A systematic review of medication-induced salivary gland dysfunction: Prevalence, diagnosis, and treatment. Clin Oral Investig 2015;19:1563–1580.
4. Fox PC, Busch KA, Baum BJ.Subjective reports of xerostomia and objective measures of salivary gland performance. J Am Dent Assoc 1987;115:581–584.
5. Moreira NC, Pachêco-Pereira C, Keenan L, Cummings G, Flores-Mir C. Informed consent comprehension and recollection in adult dental patients: A systematic review. J Am Dent Assoc 2016;147:605.e7–619.e7.
6. Kokich VO Jr, Kiyak HA, Shapiro PA.Comparing the perception of dentists and lay people to altered dental esthetics. J Esthet Dent 1999;11:311–324.
7. Priestman TJ, Baum M. Evaluation of quality of life in patients receiving treatment for advanced breast cancer. Lancet 1976;1(7965):899–900.
8. Meyer KB, Clayton KA. Measurement and analysis of patient-reported outcomes. Methods Mol Biol 2009;473:155–169.
9. Oncology Working Party. Guideline on the Evaluation of Anticancer Medicinal Products in Man—Revision 4. London: European Medicines Agency, 2013.
10. U.S. Department of Health and Human Services FDA Center for Drug Evaluation and Research, U.S. Department of Health and Human Services FDA Center for Biologics Evaluation and Research, U.S. Department of Health and Human Services FDA Center for Devices and Radiological Health. Guidance for industry: Patient-reported outcome measures: Use in medical product development to support labeling claims: Draft guidance. Health Qual Life Outcomes 2006;4:79.
11. Devigus A. Editorial: What is your treatment plan? Int J Esthet Dent 2021;16(1):7.
12. Dawson PE. Evaluation, Diagnosis, and Treatment of Occlusal Problems, ed 2. St Louis: Mosby, 1989.
13. Magne P, Magne M. Use of additive waxup and direct intraoral mock-up for enamel preservation with porcelain laminate veneers. Eur J Esthet Dent 2006;1(1):10–19.
14. Gracis S, Marinello C. Selecting the ideal esthetic restorative material: Some clinical aspects and suggestions. Int J Esthet Dent 2016;11(2):260–263.
15. Tripodakis AP, Kaitsas V, Putignano A, Eliades G, Gracis S, Blatz M. Proceedings of the 2011 Autumn Meeting of the EAED (Active Members' Meeting) - Versailles, October 20-22nd, 2011. Eur J Esthet Dent 2012;7(2):186–241.
16. Gürel G, Paolucci B, Iliev G, Filtchev D, Schayder A. The fifth dimension in esthetic dentistry. Int J Esthet Dent 2021;16(1):10–32.
17. Bartlett D, O'Toole S. Tooth wear: Best evidence consensus statement [epub ahead of print 17 Dec 2020]. J Prosthodont doi:10.1111/jopr.13312.
18. Att W, Plaster U, Brezavscek M, Papathanasiou A. Digital workflow for the rehabilitation of the excessively worn dentition. Int J Esthet Dent 2021;16(1):50–74.
19. Coachman C, Sesma N, Blatz MB.The complete digital workflow in interdisciplinary dentistry. Int J Esthet Dent 2021;16(1):34–49.
20. Lombardi RE. The principles of visual perception and their clinical application to denture esthetics. J Prosthet Dent 1973;29:358–382.
21. Shillingburg HT. Fundamentals of Fixed Prosthodontics, ed 3. Chicago: Quintessence, 1997.
22. Gracis S. Clinical considerations and rationale for the use of simplified instrumentation in occlusal rehabilitation. Part 1: Mounting of the models on the articulator. Int J Periodontics Restorative Dent 2003;23(1):57–67.
23. Bichacho N. Porcelain laminates: Integrated concepts in treating diverse aesthetic defects. Pract Periodontics Aesthet Dent 1995;7(3):13–23.
24. Bichacho N. Direct composite resin restorations of the anterior single tooth: Clinical implications and practical applications. Compend Contin Educ Dent 1996;17:796–802.
25. Bichacho N, Magne M. Controlled restorative treatment of compromised anterior dentition. Pract Periodontics Aesthet Dent 1998;10:723–727.
26. Misch CE. Guidelines for maxillary incisal edge position-a pilot study: The key is the canine. J Prosthodont 2008;17(2):130–134.
27. Reich S, Peters F, Schenk O, Hartkamp O. The face scan as a means for the visualization of complex prosthetic reconstructions. Int J Comput Dent 2016;19:231–238.
28. Solaberrieta E, Otegi JR, Goicoechea N, Brizuela A, Pradies G.Comparison of a conventional and virtual occlusal record. J Prosthet Dent 2015;114(1):92–97.
29. Zhang R, Sun Y, Liu Y, Ding Q, Zhang L, Xie Q. Occlusal assessment of zirconia crowns designed with the digital articulator and traditional methods. Int J Prosthodont 2021;34(1):13–20.
30. Joda T, Ferrari M, Bragger U, Zitzmann NU. Patient reported outcome measures (PROMs) of posterior single-implant crowns using digital workflows: A randomized controlled trial with a three-year follow-up. Clin Oral Implants Res 2018;29:954–961.

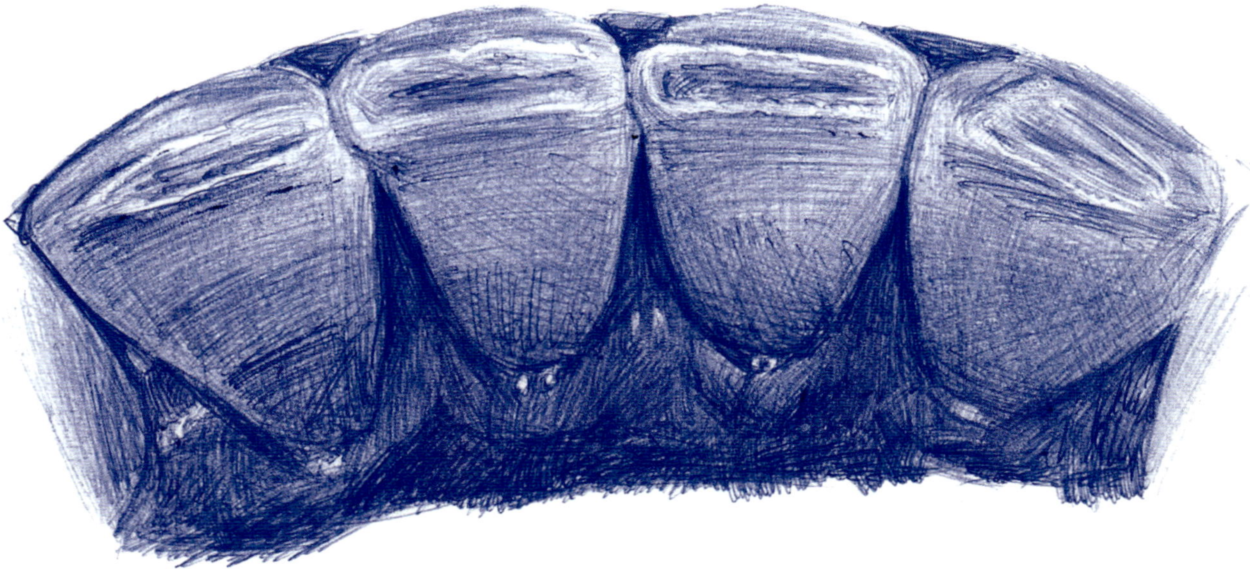

*The real voyage of discovery consists not in seeking new landscapes, but in having new eyes."*

—Marcel Proust, French novelist and essayist

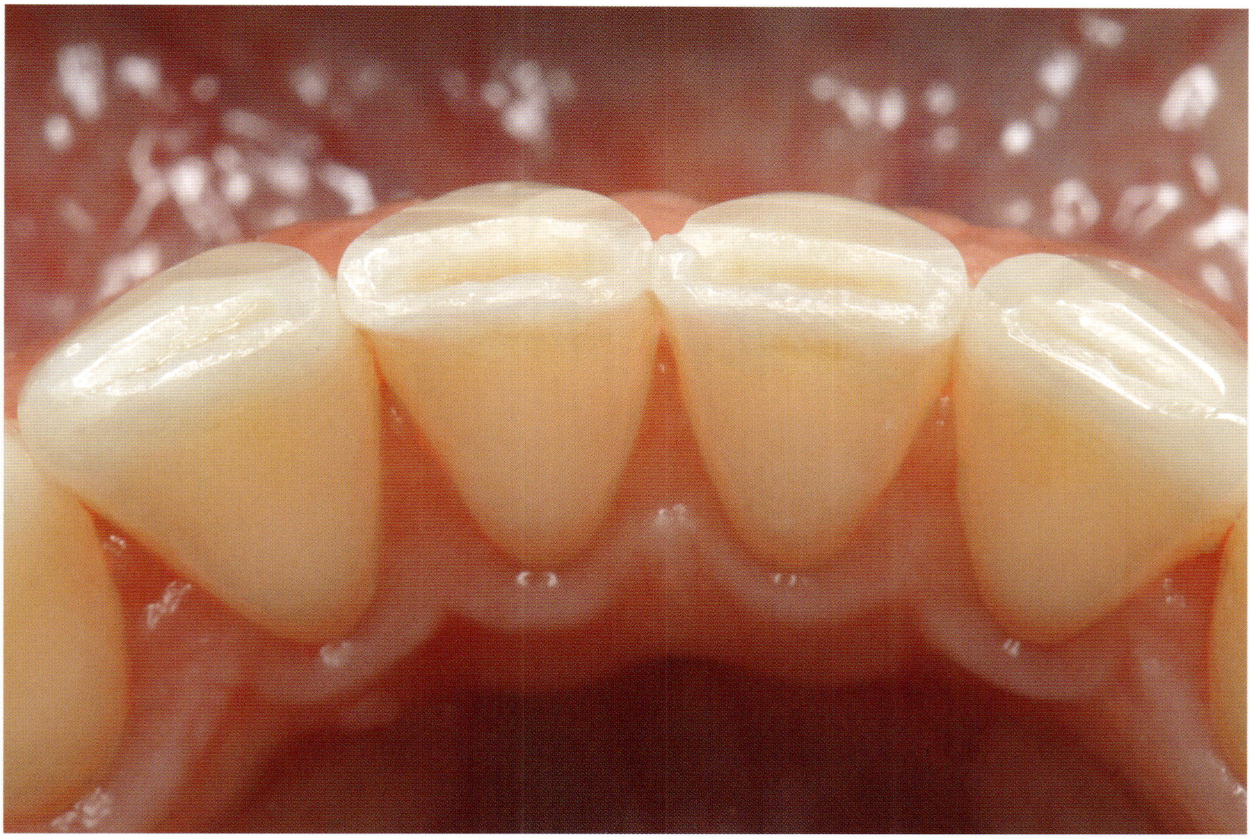

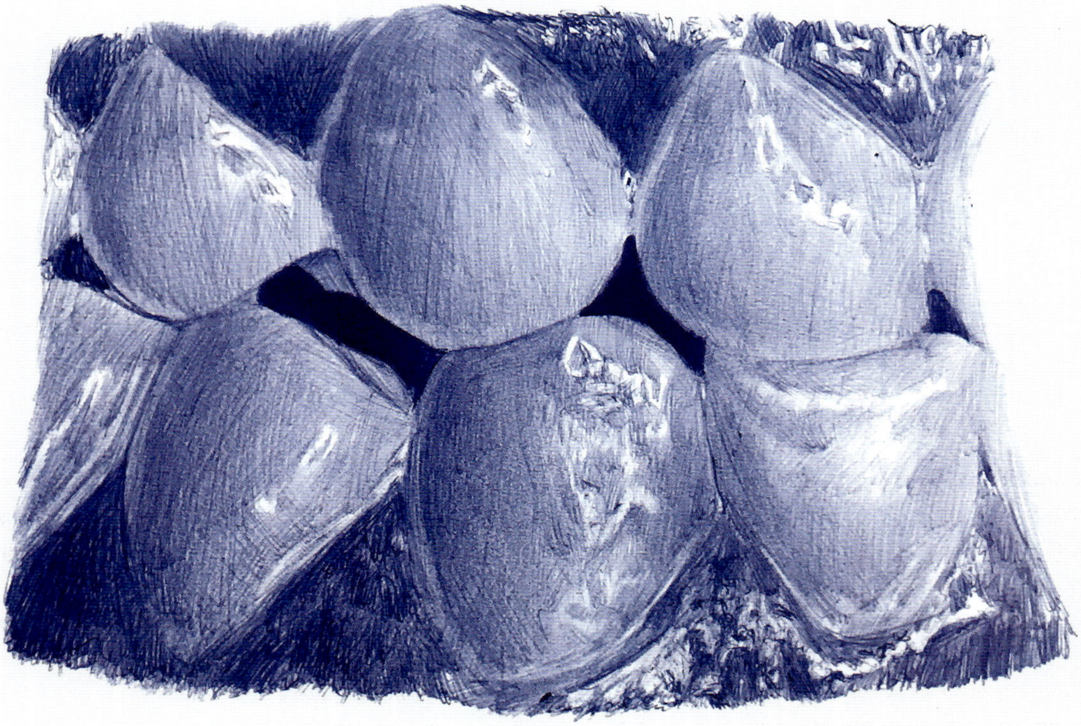

> *"Man is the meter of all things, the hand is the instrument of the instruments and the mind is the form of forms."*

—Aristotle, Greek philosopher and mathematician

CHAPTER 5

# INCIPIENT TOOTH WEAR

The early stages of oral conditions, such as incipient carious lesions and white spots, have recently been revisited in the aim of avoiding the irreversible removal of tooth structure, with some schools of thought advocating for no treatment, atraumatic restorative treatment, or sealing of the enamel lesion versus conventional cavity preparation.

Incipient tooth loss of bacterial origin (caries) has been shown to have a potential for remineralization in the early stages. In initial stages of caries, provided the surface of the lesion remains intact and the salivary flow is adequate, the remaining subsurface of the enamel acts as a matrix for more minerals to deposit.

The anatomy of the TW lesion differs from the caries lesion as the enamel is lost or thinned by a grinding force or by acidic dissolution but is not cavitated and hence provides no appropriate 3D matrix for remineralization.

The wait-and-see approach—and the reluctance of the patient to undergo treatment while asymptomatic—is behind the undesired progression to major tooth loss even in patients who regularly attend dental surgeries. Moreover, it is difficult to anticipate the rate of progression at which the damage will occur and when the patient will seek treatment again.

The decision to treat incipient TW lesions should not be judged as overtreatment (once restorative, always restorative). Instead, the benefit of a preventive and interceptive approach, with the aim of preventing further tooth structure loss and preserving as much enamel as possible, should be considered.

The advent of the additive restorative approach for incipient TW lesions, be it localized, within a sector, or even full arch, has relieved the dental professional from the dilemma of waiting until the point when restorations cannot be delayed. A good differential diagnosis, with a thorough orthodontic evaluation as well as an interdisciplinary treatment plan, is of paramount importance when working to reduce the risk of further damage and intercepting ongoing TW.

## 1. The Onset of Tooth Wear

Enamel is the hardest tissue in the human body. It has a densely mineralized structure that gives teeth their resistance to caries, abrasion, and attrition but also their brittleness. Mostly inorganic, it can only be cut by diamond. Yet it can be ground or scratched by opposing enamel, a condition known as attrition, or eroded by acids or acidic solutions, a condition known as erosion.

Enamel is mostly composed of hydroxyapatite together with other components of inferior mineral quality that vary from person to person and even within different locations in the mouth.[1] Also, the disposition of the so-called enamel rods and the thickness of enamel influences the resistance to TW.

Enamel thickness varies along the anatomy of teeth with an average thickness of 2.5 mm. It is thicker at the buccal rounded aspect of the molars and premolars, describing a sigmoid inverted curve in relation to dentin.[2] In other words, the convexity of enamel is countered by a concavity in dentin, providing areas that are stronger and designed to endure the masticatory forces. This is meaningful in the working landmarks of either arch, with unique reinforced features such as the cusps and the palatal and buccal aspects of teeth.

Enamel is a non-shedding oral tissue meant to last a lifetime. The natural balance by which teeth remain intact in the oral milieu is first broken at a micromolecular level that is invisible to the eye. By the time minor or incipient tooth surface loss (TSL) starts at a macromolecular level, important microscopic changes in the molecular morphology of the tooth have already taken place (Fig 5-1).

In incipient TW, early changes appear first predominantly in the anterior sector at the incisal edges and/or cusps of the canines. For many years, night bruxism was immediately assumed as the cause of a worn dentition. However, there is an increasing number of patients that have TW and claim not to have grinding nor clenching habits. Parafunctional habits such us nail biting, hair biting, pen biting, and lip biting cause incisal wear and may often be unreported and forgotten by the dentist (Fig 5-2).

If bruxism is the predominant cause of incipient TW, a flattening of the incisal plane will progressively affect most teeth (Fig 5-3).

In contrast, Figure 5-4 shows a patient in the second decade of life with a mandibular premolar with a dull and smoothed enamel surface, incipient saucer-like concave lesions at the tip of the canine, and cervical lesions throughout the arch. These signs are mostly seen when the major origin of TW is an erosive attack.

Moreover, both types of lesions may be present at the same time in one tooth or within the arch (Fig 5-5).

Incipient TW is usually seen in the anterior zone of the mouth first. Nevertheless, once incisal wear has started, it may eventually affect posterior teeth. Incipient damage in the posterior teeth happens initially on the tip of the cusps as a consequence of acidic and/or physical challenges but also on other sites associated with congenital or acquired enamel deficiencies (Fig 5-6).

In general terms, parafunctional habits, malocclusions, medical and psychologic conditions, and some lifestyle choices should alert the dental professional and call for a thorough screening in order to establish an early preventive or interceptive program.

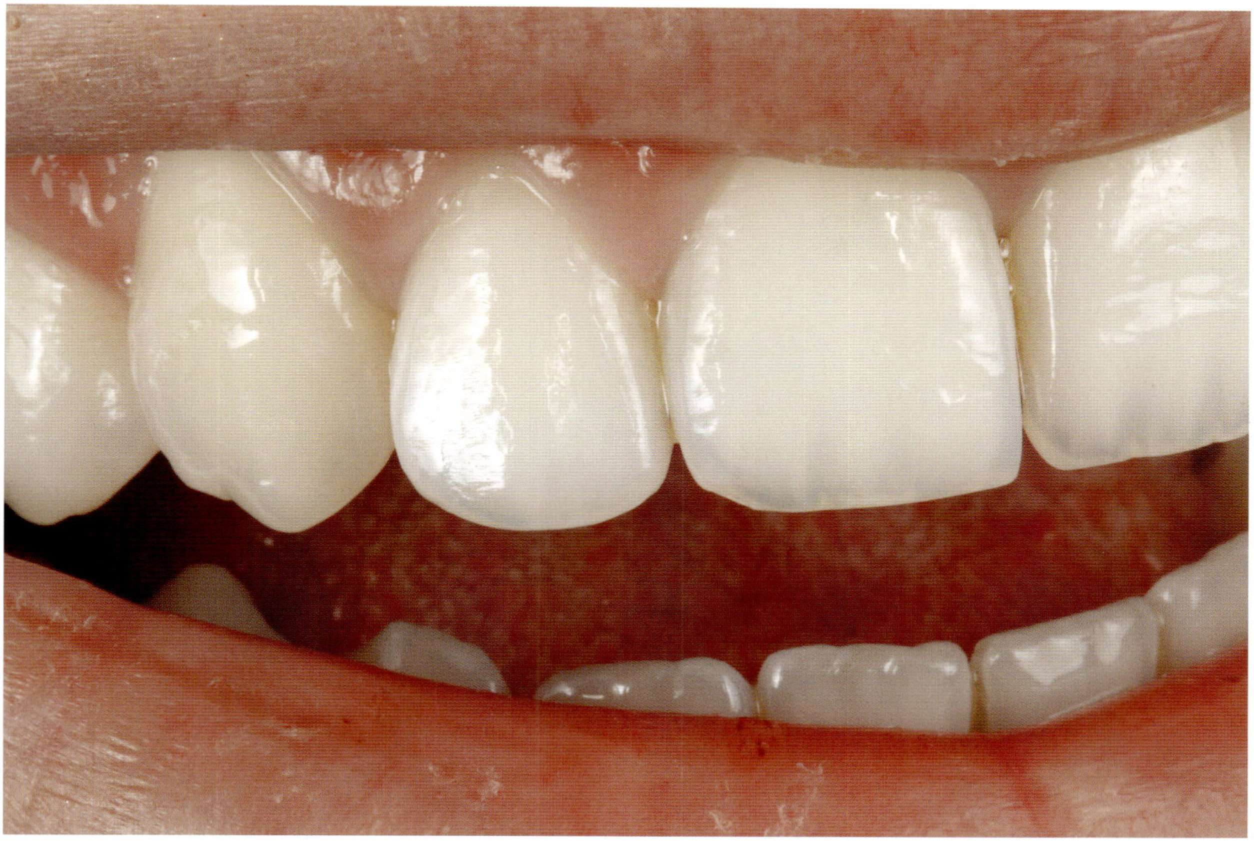

**Fig 5-1** Incipient remodeling of the incisal edge in this young girl is subtle and only visible by comparison with the adjacent teeth, which still show the elaborate incisal peculiarities. TW will be unnoticeable to the nonprofessional eye and even to the patient, who will not be able to easily detect the loss of enamel within the enamel mass, leading in this case to a narrower translucent frame at the distal angle of the right central incisor. The presence of parafunctional habits such as hair biting helps in corroborating the diagnosis.

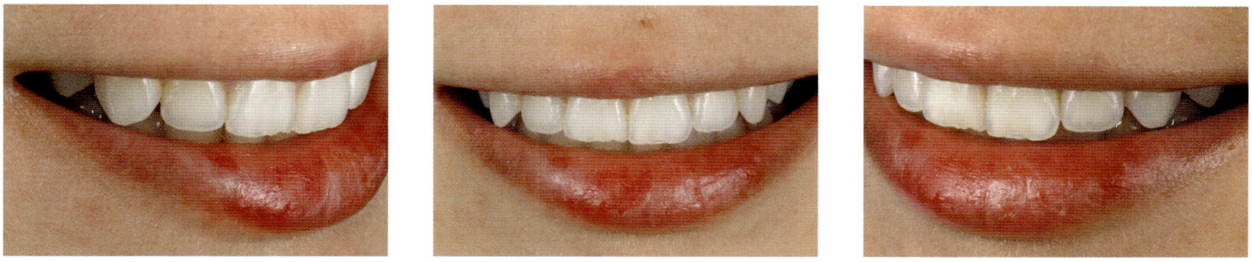

**Fig 5-2** Attention should be paid to be the anatomy of the lips. The lack of epithelial or mucosa integrity, sometimes with exposure of deep layers and bleeding, may indicate traumatic lesions from lip biting, and if so, incisal wear is frequently found. Lip biting in a shy young female has worn the incisal edges in absence of an erosive pattern (a to c). If this incipient TW occurred in later life, it could be considered physiologic or acceptable to a certain extent. The problem arises when this type of TW appears in a young dentition with a long dental life expectancy ahead.

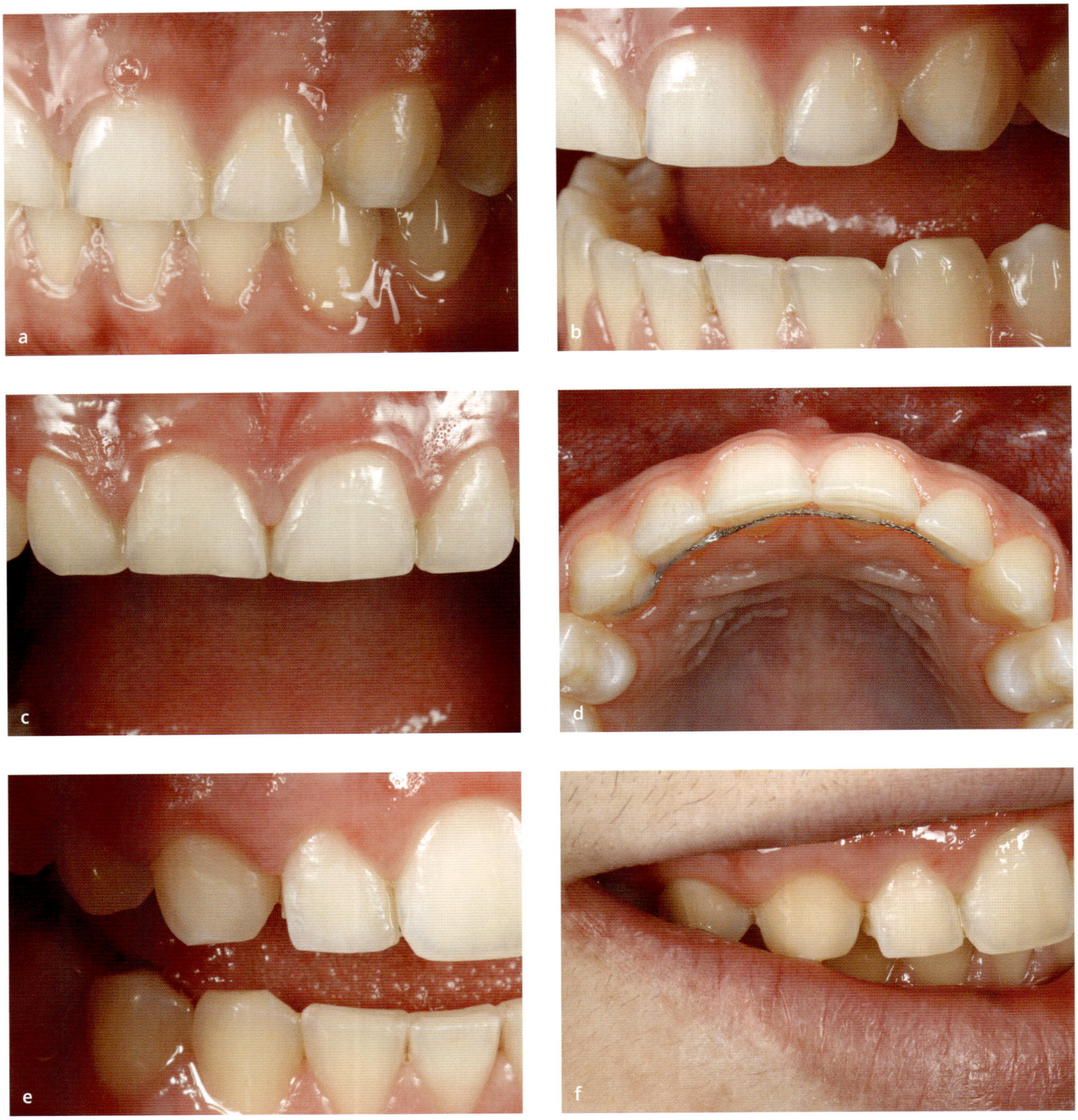

**Fig 5-3** The flattening of the incisal anatomy in this young boy (a to d) and also in his brother (e and f) is generalized but is not perceived as pathologic by the patients nor their family at this stage. At a young age, these anterior teeth show incipient TW that has affected only enamel so far but that could endanger the anterior and canine guidance and originate damage to distal teeth in a short time. In both cases, dentin is not yet exposed and no evident functional impairment has occurred at this point.

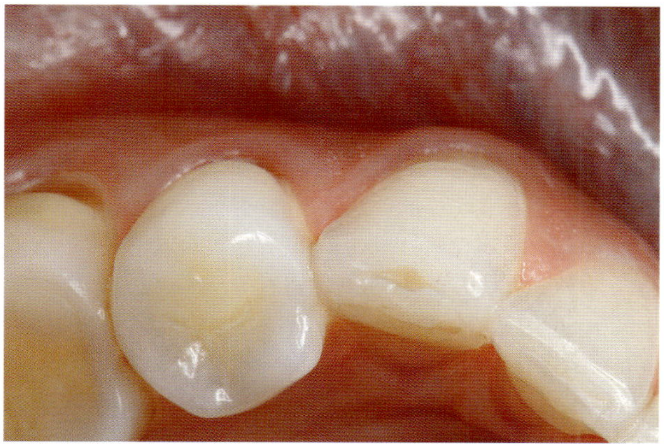

**Fig 5-4** A young woman wishing to whiten her teeth does not seem to notice the TSL, more obvious in the mandibular arch as the anatomy of the floor of the mouth acts as a container for the acidic solutions. TW in children and adolescents has been shown to hit a strikingly high percentage of the population, especially when erosion is taken into consideration. Therefore, the term incipient TW does not correspond to the age of the patient as some young dentitions can already show moderate or even severe damage. Erosive damage as seen in these mandibular teeth could easily go undiagnosed as the loss of enamel is generalized, having erased the occlusal anatomical features such as cusps and even fossae. The clean, pristine aspect of these teeth is an indication of an active erosive challenge still present. Note the adjacent canine that suffers from concomitant erosive and incipient TW due to attrition in the anterior teeth as the patient also has a lip-biting habit.

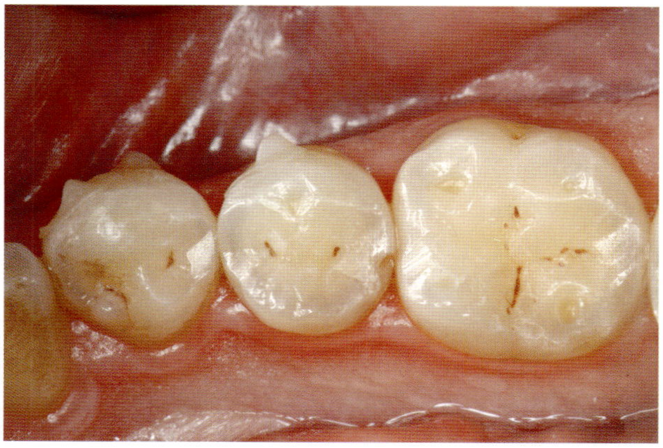

**Fig 5-5** When using magnification, it is not unusual to see the two types of major incipient TSL, attrition and erosion, in the same tooth.

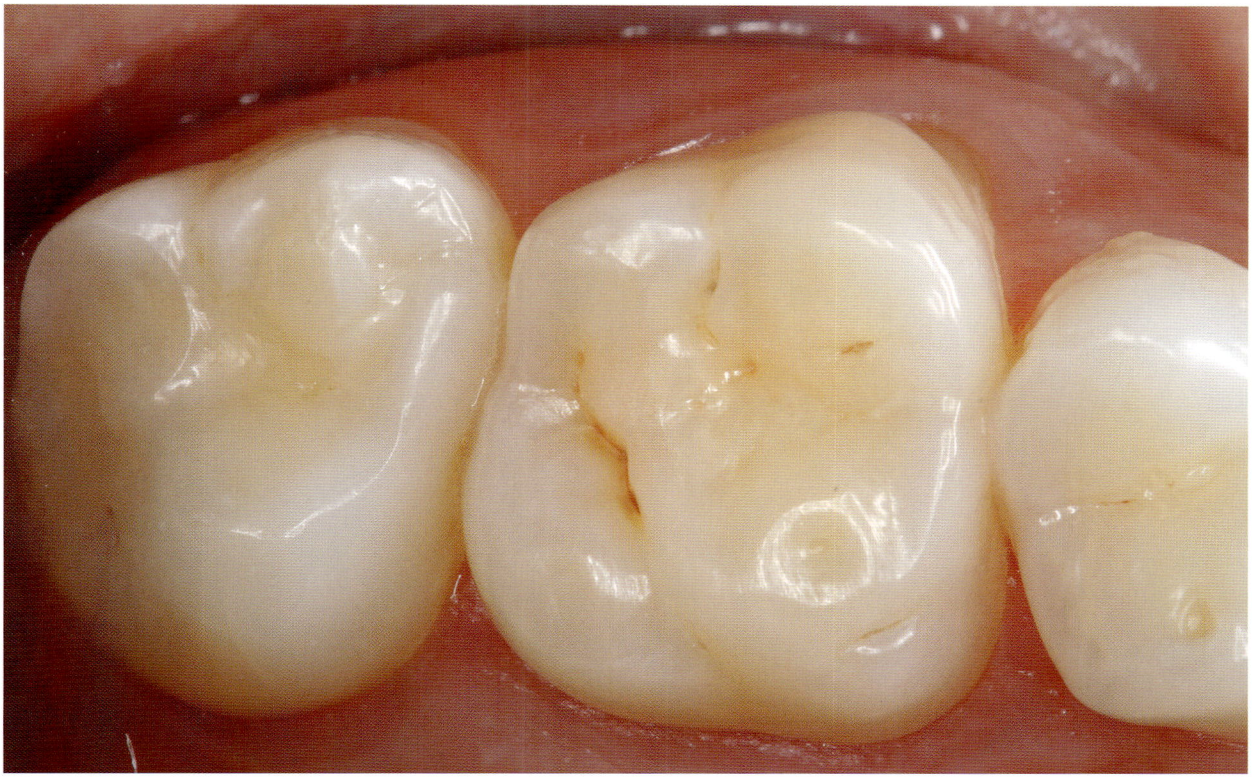

**Fig 5-6** The palatal cusps of this maxillary first molar and second premolar show incipient TW at a routine intraoral exam. Incipient TSL on the posterior areas of the mouth are often times undiagnosed as routine examination is usually oriented toward caries and infection, and therefore early detection of minor posterior TW is infrequent. Moreover, TW is not seen in radiographs unless very severe damage is already present.

## 2. Erosion and Caries: Is There a Link?

Erosion and caries have noticeable differences and share some similarities. The common feature in both conditions is a drop in pH that initiates tissue destruction, in caries from bacterial plaque metabolism, in erosion from acids of nonbacterial origin. However, this does not fully explain why research has shown a significant link between both conditions. As explained before, authors have found that children who suffer from caries are at a higher risk of developing erosion. Common nutritional risk factors, such as consumption of soft drinks, may be behind this association. Likewise, lack of an ideal amount of saliva and/or its protective factors may also explain why caries and erosion have a common etiopathogenesis.[3,4] Erosion and caries may appear in the same teeth and even tooth surfaces in certain cases, leaving for the academic realm the discussion of whether both conditions can be concomitant. In the clinical world, however, this poses further difficulty in diagnosis as the rapid tissue destruction of a caries lesion can be superimposed on a previous erosive lesion, erasing all signs of it. The opposite is also possible.

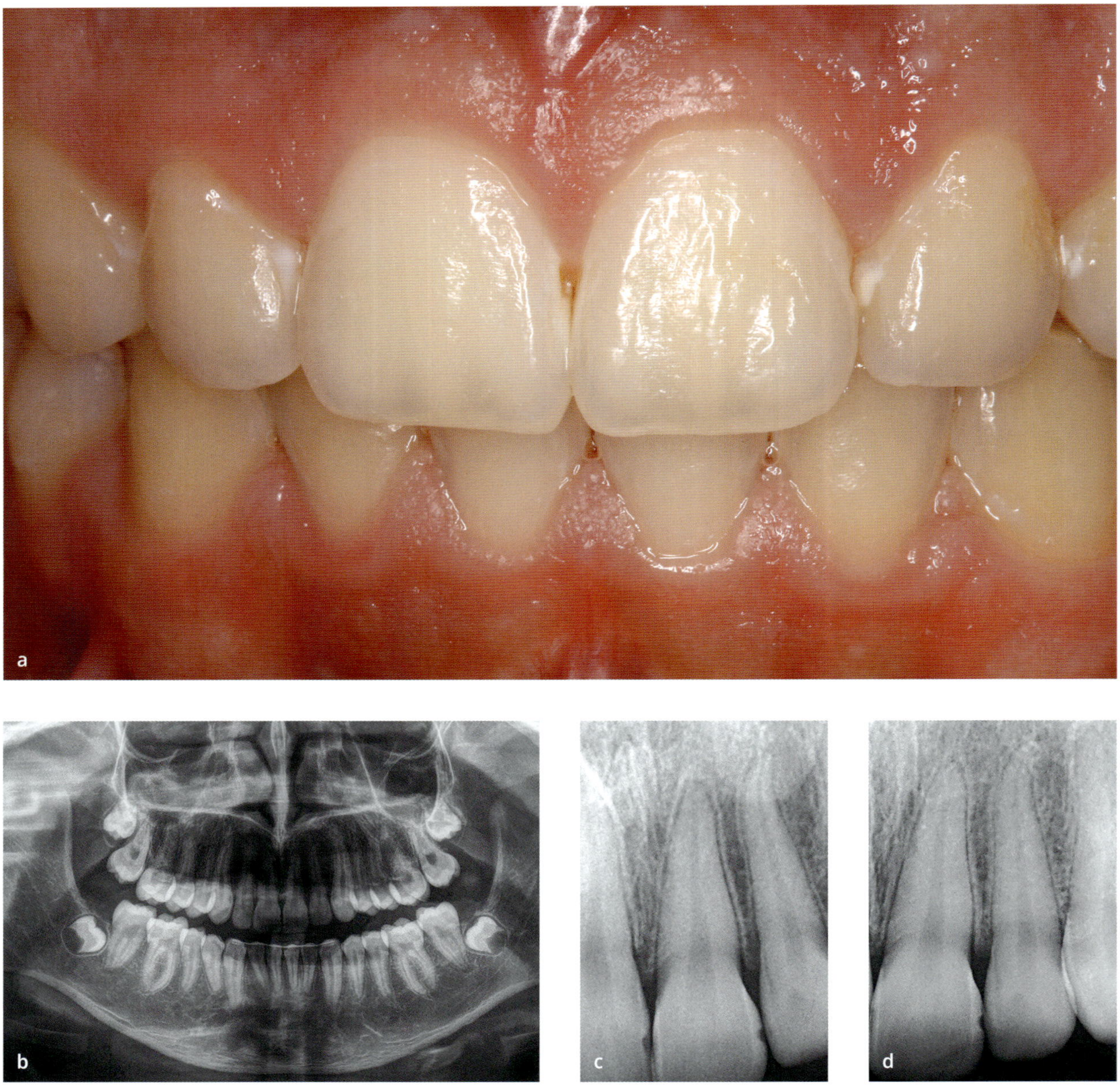

**Fig 5-7** A young male patient presents with multiple incipient caries lesions and white lesions (a to d). A history of food intolerances should alert the professional to the potential for an increased risk of erosion. Dietary counseling and hygiene maintenance are fundamental to diminishing the challenge.

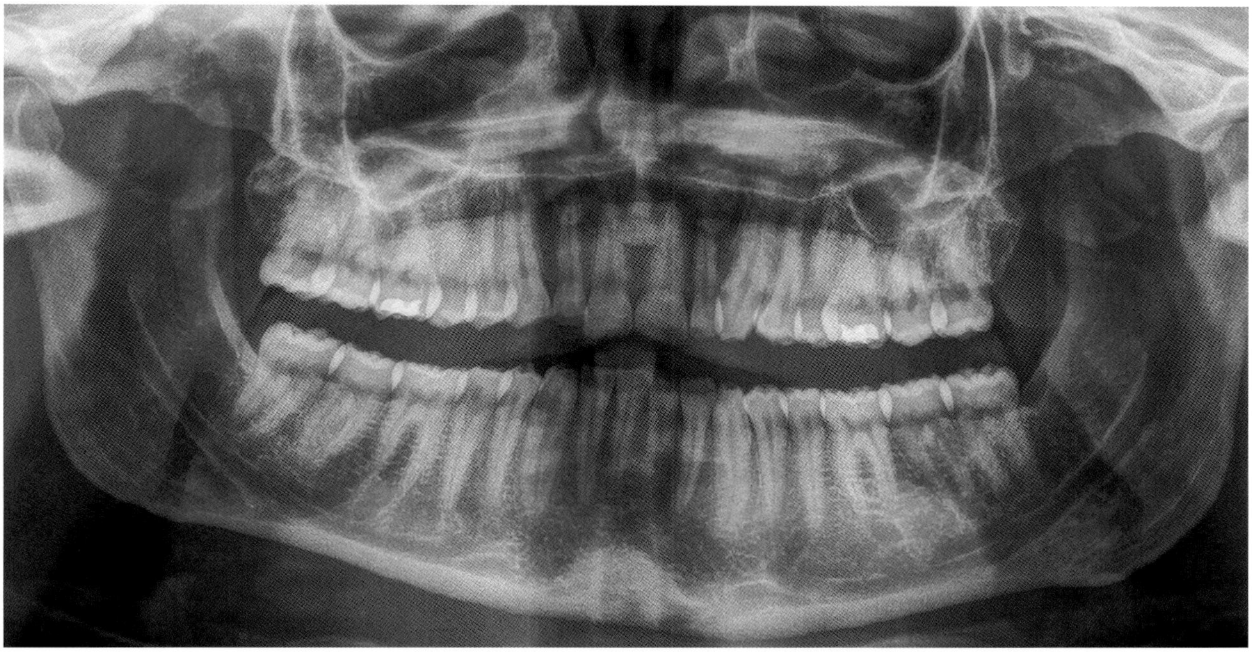

**Fig 5-8** In this radiograph of a patient with moderate TW, the wear lesions are not framed by surrounding tooth structure, and therefore there are no cavitated radiolucent images. Instead, the occlusal and incisal planes appear flat, lacking the radiodensity provided by enamel, as a long-standing erosive challenge has dissolved enamel on most of the surfaces of the teeth.

Furthermore, dietary coaching for children may revert their erosion risk, but conversely not being able to follow a noncariogenic diet will eventually lead to an erosive diet in future years.[5,6] Therefore the dental professional should know that the presence of caries may be considered a risk factor for erosion (Fig 5-7).

While erosive TW is a major factor in all age groups, genetically determined conditions render the young patient more susceptible to rapid progression and severity. It has been explained that the imperfect mineralization in hypoplastic enamel defects may lay behind a high susceptibility to acid challenge as well as caries. This is the case of molar-incisor hypomineralization, amelogenesis imperfecta, dentinogenesis imperfecta, and combinations thereof. Clinical observation of patients with amelogenesis imperfecta, with extensive tooth damage in first molars, and generalized TW in the following years is not uncommon. As explained in chapter 2, the correlation of the genes involved in enamel development with the levels of calcium and phosphorous in saliva provides a new perspective as to how scrupulous prevention measures need to be in patients with genetic enamel alterations.

Caries and erosion both start at the enamel and progress to dentin if left untreated. Nevertheless, these two distinctive conditions, caries and TW, usually pose no difficulty in the differential diagnosis and have a differentiated course and treatment modality.

The typical caries lesion appears interproximally or at the occlusal fossae, while TW damages the tips of the cusps, the buccal and palatal surfaces, and the incisal edges (Fig 5-8).

The panoramic radiograph of a patient with incipient caries shows no TW damage on the occlusal or incisal planes, which appear to have a bulky occlusal and incisal radiopaque dense enamel in the radiograph (see Fig 5-7b). Incipient caries lesions usually affect the enamel at the interproximal areas, and intraoral radiography is the standard of care for diagnosis. These tooth contact areas are predilected sites for caries lesions that show radiographically a translucent defect (see Figs 5-7c and 5-7d).

## 3. A Close-Up Look at the Incisal Edges

The incisal edge is completely formed by enamel that lacks a dentin core. Young healthy dentitions have a very pronounced mamelon-like enamel formation that will eventually disappear. The translucency of enamel at the incisal edge, with a white halo that frames it, is also typical of a young smile that has not been worn at all.

The incisal edges provide invaluable information when identifying the predominant etiology of TW and hence in stablishing a correct preventive protocol. Incisal edges can be damaged by the impact of different mechanisms.

The shortening of the incisors powered by attrition will start at the incisal edges, which will appear with a broad incisal platform. In this case, the incisal rim will look unchipped, with distinct margins, and will perfectly match the antagonist dentition upon biting (Fig 5-9).

When erosion is the principal issue, the incisors may also be short. Nevertheless, the incisal rim may then be thin and chipped with a translucency that will become more intense as enamel is chelated and starts to dissolve from the palatal aspect of the maxillary teeth (Fig 5-10).

The advent of digital technologies has been a game changer for the TW team as data recording and visualization of lesions has experienced a quantum leap with computer-aided technologies (Fig 5-11).

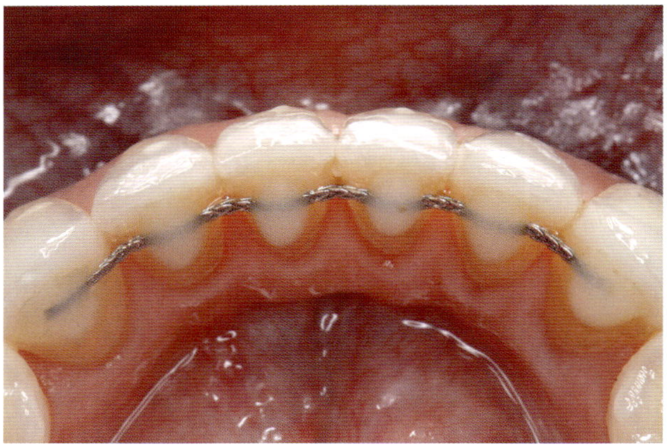

**Fig 5-9** The shortening or roughening of the incisors may go undetected at the initial stages of TW. Only a thorough intraoral occlusal evaluation will reveal the onset of the damage.

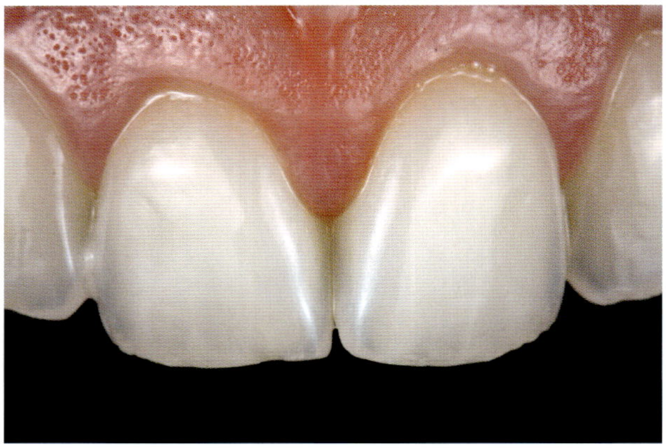

**Fig 5-10** A medical and lifestyle interview may help in determining the risk factor behind an unknown acidic challenge. The intake of anti-acne medication since this patient was a teenager has secretly removed enamel as it has altered the intraoral mineral balance with changes first at the incisal translucency of maxillary incisors.

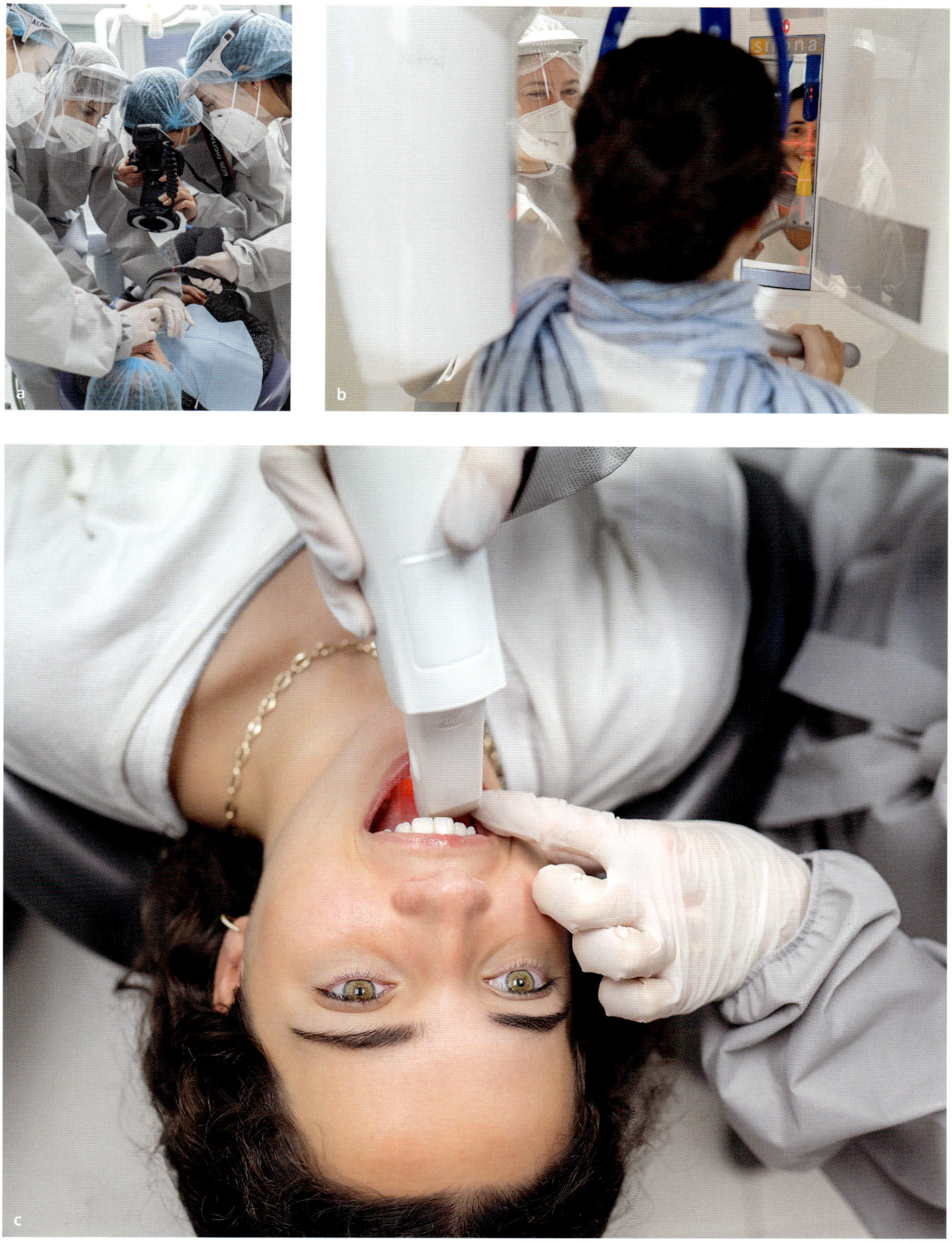

**Fig 5-11** The geography of incipient TW varies from person to person, with frequent combinations of minor anterior and posterior lesions in the same mouth from diverse origins: chemical, physical, or both. Unlike incipient caries lesions, incipient TW lesions are not diagnosed radiographically and may be missed easily. The advent of digital photography first (a) and then digital radiography (b), intraoral scanning (c), and chairside digital technology more recently (d), has empowered the TW team as incipient lesions are more evident and easier to communicate to the patient with these technologies. *(continued next page)*

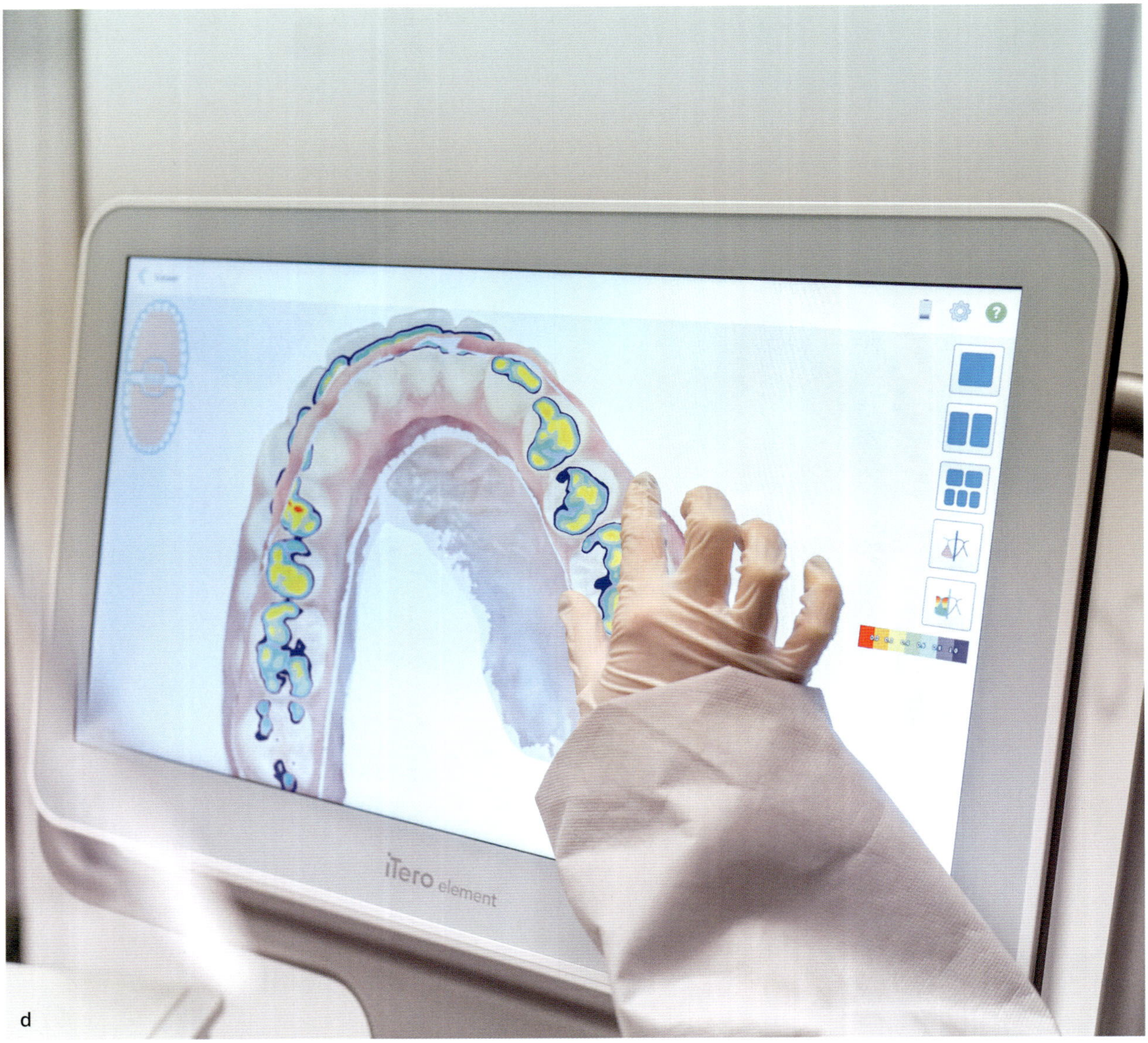


d

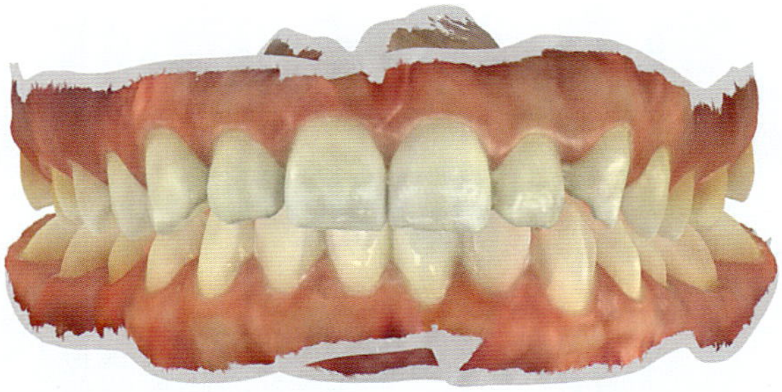

e

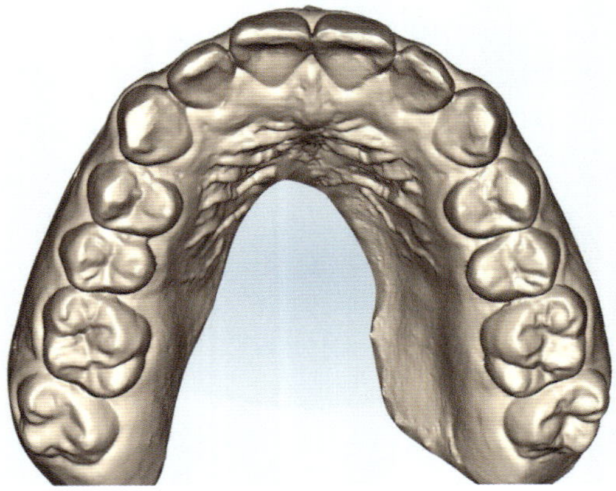

f

**Fig 5-11** *(continued)* In the intraoral digital capture image (e) and its STL rendering (f) of a young girl, the flattening of the canine and buccal premolar cusps is bright white, providing a distinctive image of the disappearance of the natural anatomy.

## 4. Anterior and Canine Guidance in Incipient Tooth Wear

Anterior guidance is a built-in natural safeguard against tooth damage arising from occlusal and masticatory forces. Canine cusps, when well aligned both in the frontal and the horizontal plane, dictate the amount of disocclusion the rest of the teeth will experience while eating or by parafunctional habits. Although described separately in the literature, anterior and canine guidance are both essential for tooth protection and work together to provide anteriorly guided disocclusion for the posterior sector of the dentition. This is an invaluable gift of nature that should be preserved and promoted (Fig 5-12).

Such protection will be present provided that the maxillomandibular relationship is stable and no external interferences or forces are present. For example, mouth breathing may disrupt anterior guidance, especially if it is accompanied by a tongue thrust habit. Not only the physical aspects resulting from an inadequate breathing pattern but also the associated buffering impairment of the saliva can ignite a combination of attrition and erosion TW on the anterior sector of the mouth, as discussed in chapter 2 (Fig 5-13).

In young patients, the threshold of TW at which anterior teeth are no longer protective against loads and forces is dependent on the overjet and overbite present when eruption is complete and whether all teeth occupy the ideal position in the arch. This unique protection is soon impaired or diminished in incipient TW, leading to further TSL. In fact, it comes as no surprise that TW will hit harder when the anterior and canine guidance are diminished or impaired (Fig 5-14).

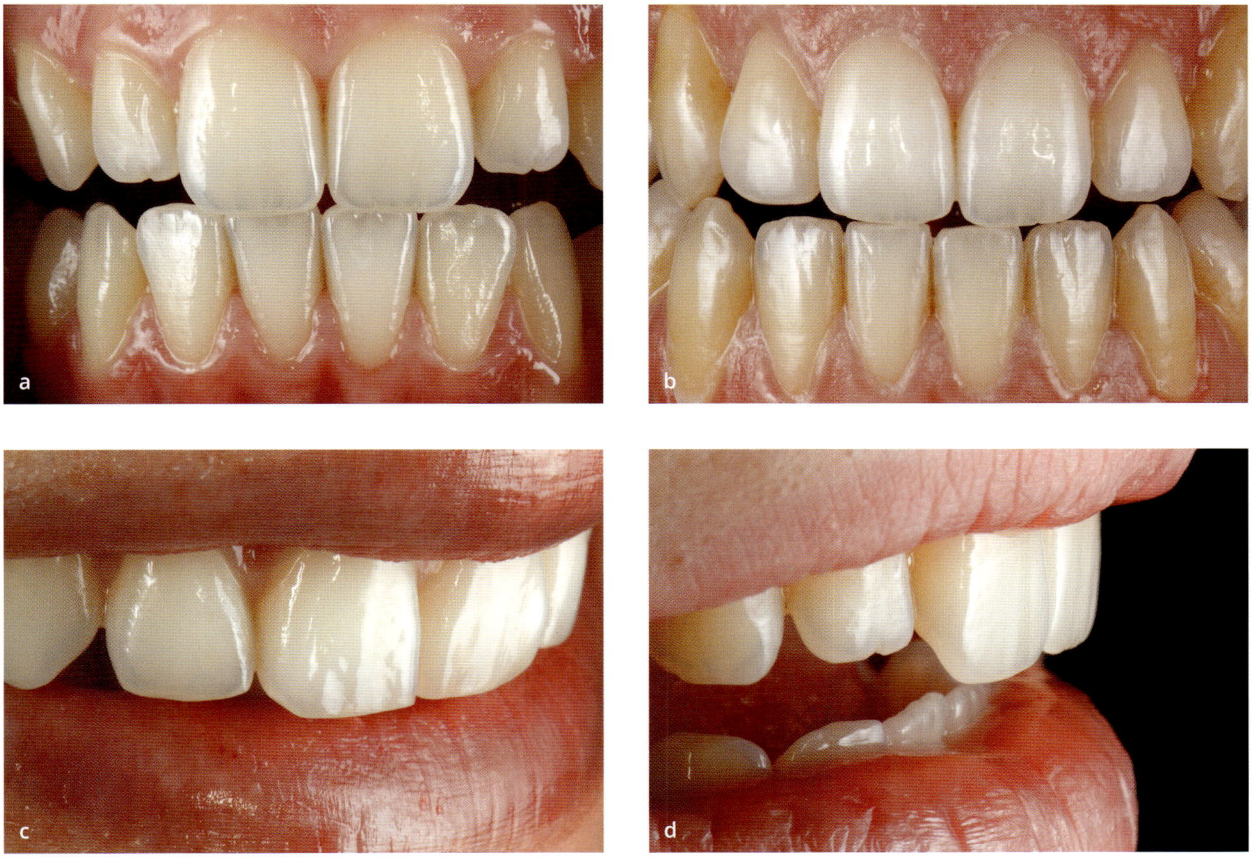

**Fig 5-12** The length of the anterior teeth is genetically determined and dictates the type and amount of posterior disocclusion during function (a to c). The incisal edges define a unique and differentiated plane in the anterior view that is an important facial reference. It not only dictates appearance and esthetics but has direct implications in phonetics and masticatory function and is considered one of the most important landmarks of a smile (d).

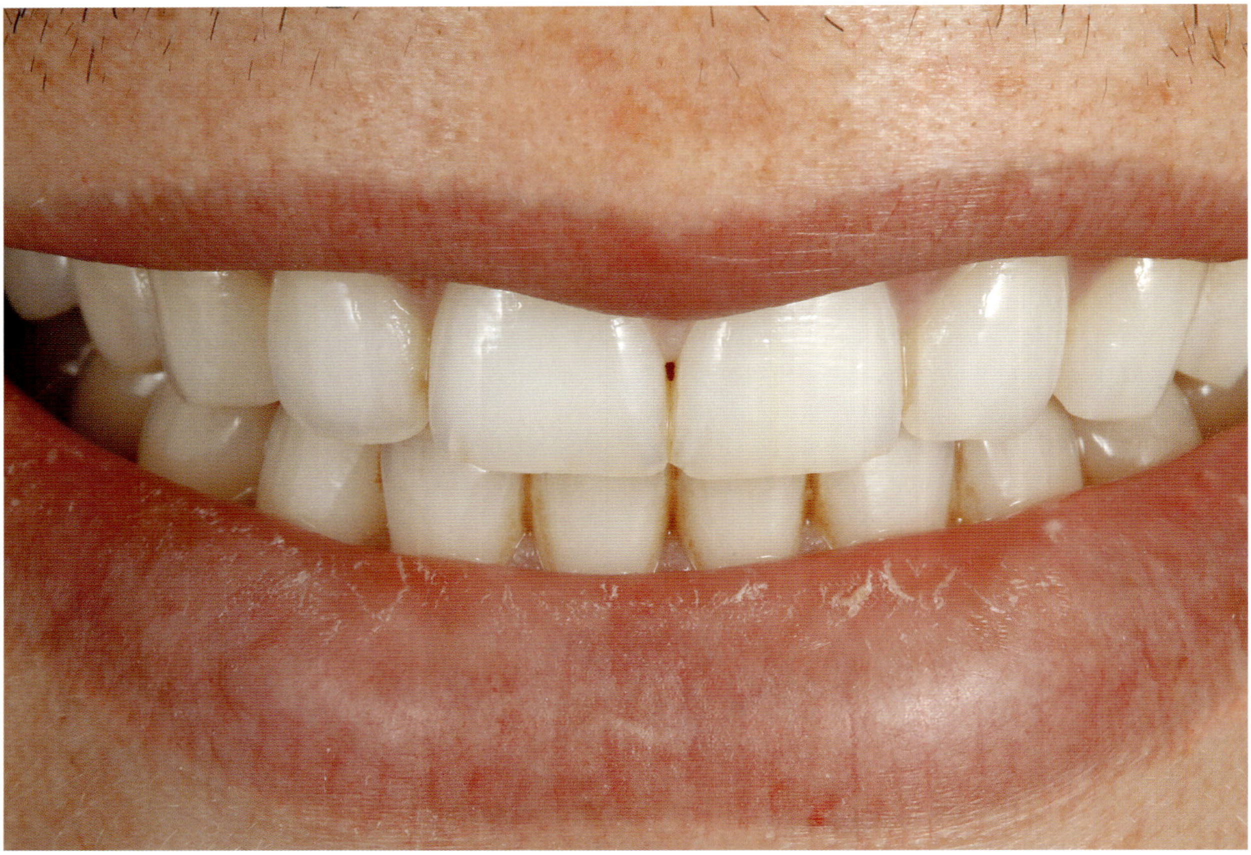

**Fig 5-13** The mouth breathing pattern in this patient contributes to dryness in the oral cavity as the excessive saliva evaporation leads to a diminished buffering and shielding capacity. Note the overall dry aspect of the teeth, which look as if they had been air dried. The incisal edges are worn, and the lower lip has a dry desquamated rough surface, typical in a mouth breathing habit.

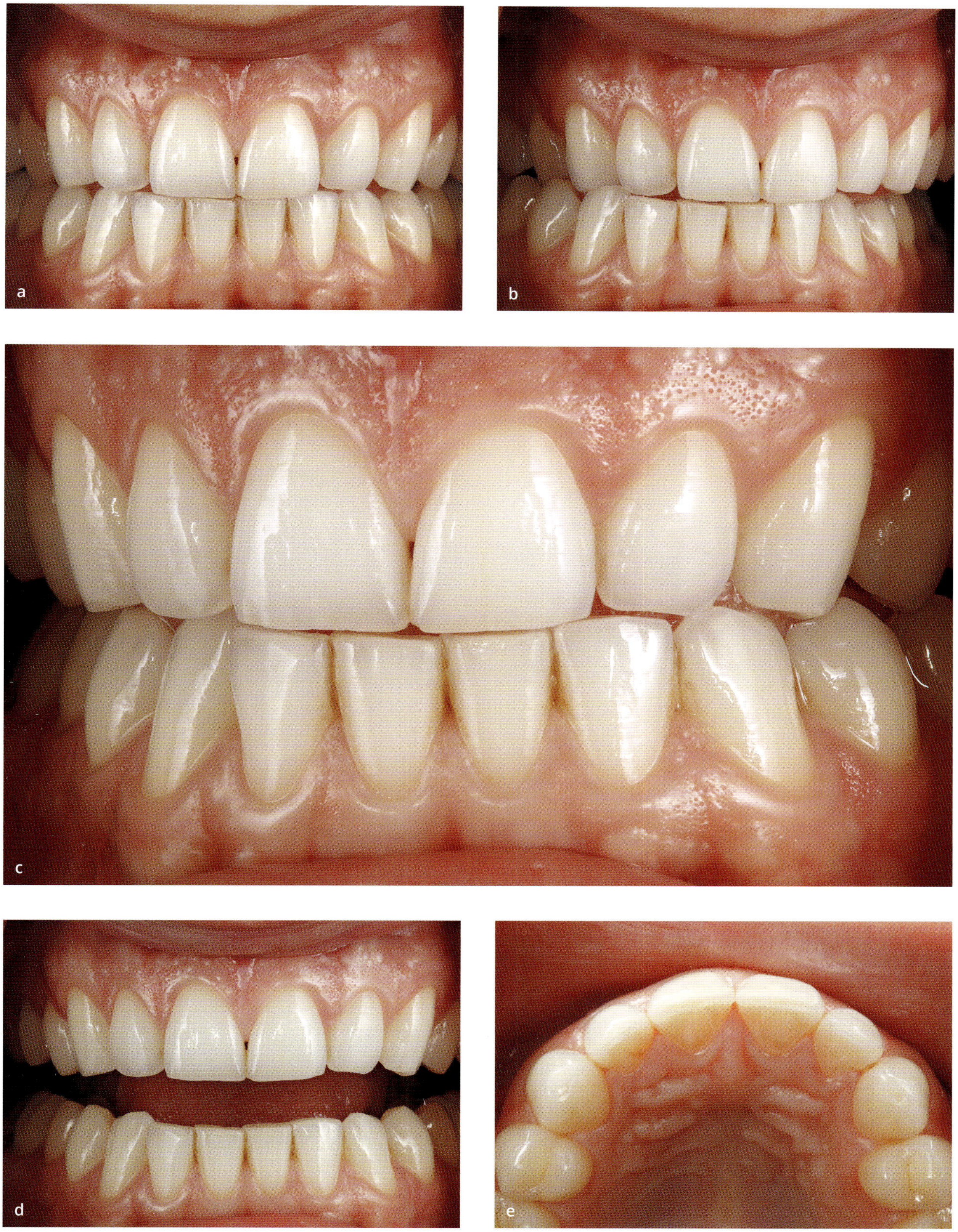

**Fig 5-14** The combined anterior and canine guidance referred to as anterior guidance is lost in most cases of TW (a to c). Detecting the onset of this impairment in incipient TW is key to the survival of the dentition. In young patients with parafunctional habits like nail, lip, or pen biting, anterior protection is soon surpassed. The advancement of anterior TW would inevitably lead to damage in the posterior areas of the mouth. Intercepting incipient anterior TW may prevent the need for extensive treatment in future years. An intraoral evaluation shows the flattening of the anterior incisal plane with initial damage to premolars but no impact as yet on the posterior occlusal plane (d and e).

## 5. Intercepting Tooth Wear with Orthodontics

There is evidence that the amount of remaining tooth structure has an indirect correlation to the survival of the tooth. Intercepting incipient TW first by means of prevention, education, and interception of risk factors and/or habits should already be part of the first line of treatment for incipient minor TW. In patients with incipient TW as well as those with moderate TW, orthodontic therapy should be evaluated as the first line of treatment and performed before or immediately after the necessary restorative phase is accomplished (see the incipient TW flowchart at the end of the chapter).

In patients with malocclusions the malposition of teeth can lead to TSL. Incipient TW in one sector can precede further adjacent loss. Once this has occurred, it will eventually lead to distant wear or fractures that are otherwise difficult to explain. The orthodontist and general dentist are not to neglect these minor but otherwise irreversible changes and should not delay combined therapy to intercept this ongoing condition, which will damage the dentition irreversibly. Whenever this is detected, it is advisable to restore it in a noninvasive manner, ideally after an orthodontic evaluation and orthodontic treatment when indicated.

In incipient TW a thorough orthodontic evaluation will provide information to the general or restorative dentist regarding the underlying 3D factors that may have caused the onset of wear. If no other aggravating conditions are present, intercepting these factors may be a wise approach to prevent further damage (Fig 5-15).

Implementing an orthodontic evaluation as a routine after a first diagnosis of TW in the incipient and moderate stages will enable the TW team to provide functional and esthetic outcomes without the need to alter natural tooth form or reduce tooth structure. Nevertheless, orthodontic therapy by itself does not restore the lost tooth anatomy that will be necessary to address, usually after orthodontic therapy (see chapter 8).

Restoration of the incipient damage is performed with direct composite without any preparation as the orthodontic therapy will not replace the lost anatomy (Fig 5-16).

Intercepting further TW even at incipient stages can save tooth structure and restorative procedures even at the expense of accepting maintenance of the interceptive treatment (Fig 5-17).

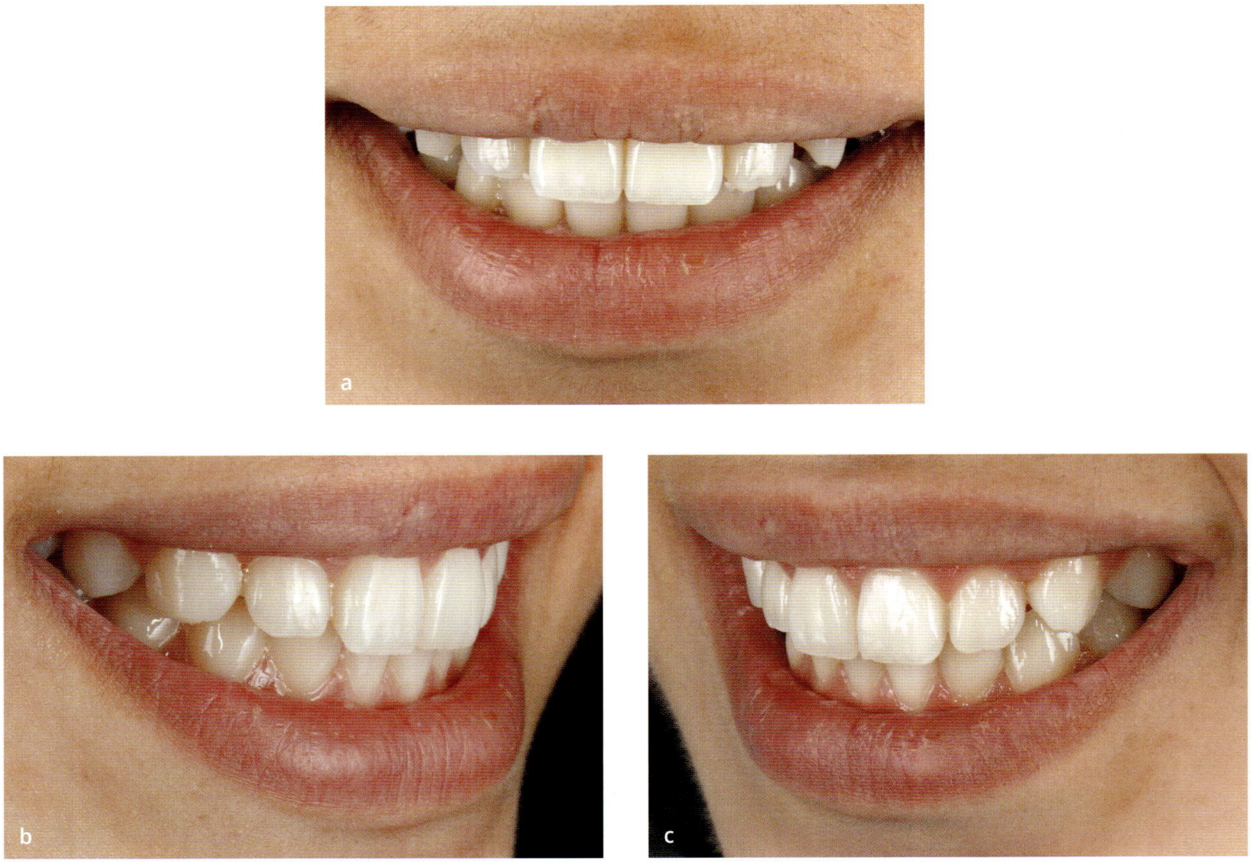

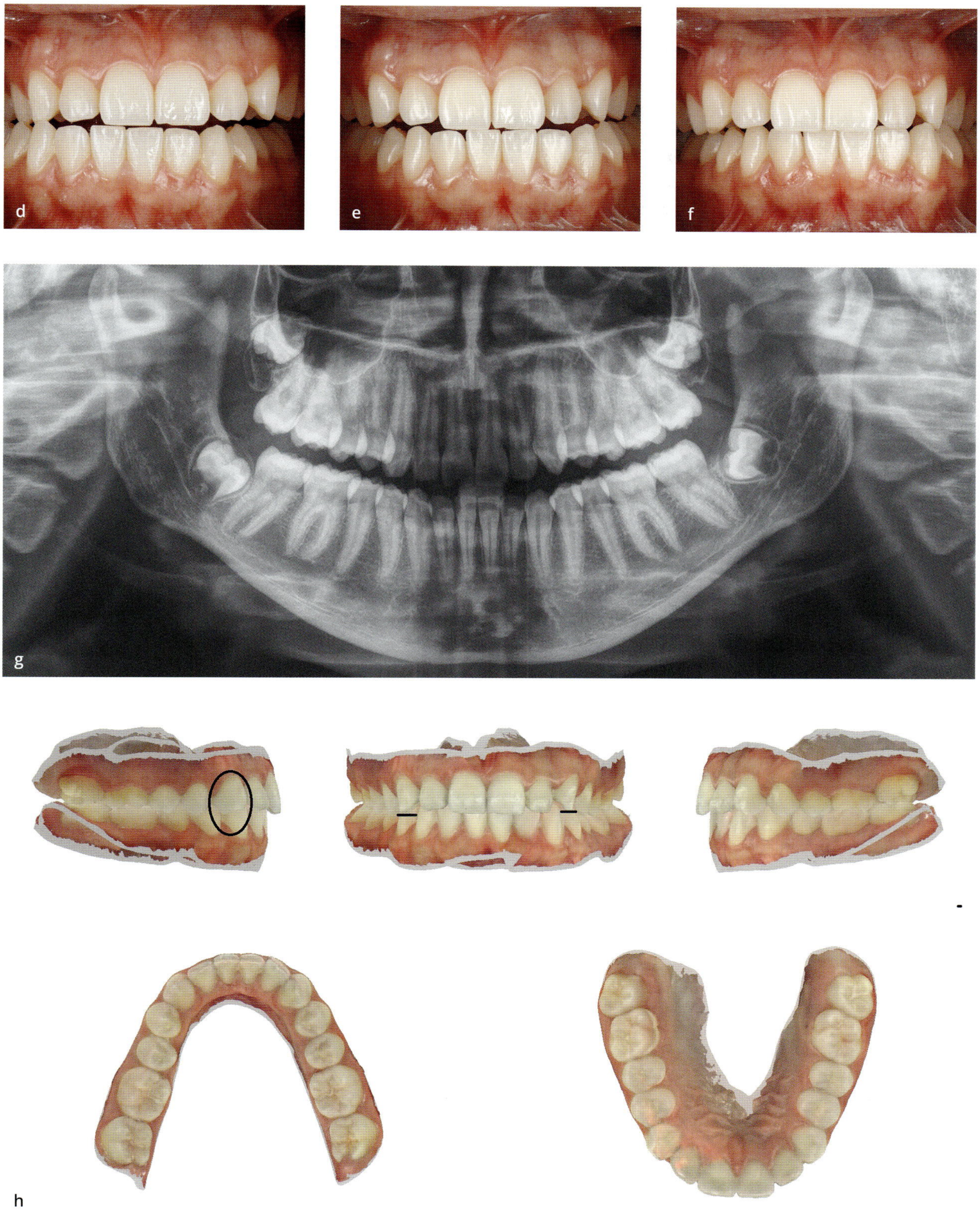


**Fig 5-15** During a regular checkup, the hygienist noticed injury to the lip explained by a lip biting habit. The occlusal anterior plane inspection shows a flattened canine cusp in the first quadrant and incomplete canine eruption in the second quadrant (a to c). Upon dynamic exploration, while anterior guidance is competent (d), canine guidance is found to be disrupted as a result of altered eruption and a parafunctional habit (e and f). TW is a dynamic, progressive, irreversible condition by which tooth structure loss leads, sooner or later, to an impairment of the protective function teeth exert on one another, as has happened to the canine of the first quadrant. The absence of wear in the contralateral canine due to incomplete eruption does not imply less TW risk. The radiograph shows an incomplete eruption of the maxillary left canine in an otherwise healthy environment (g). The intraoral image acquisition is performed as part of the orthodontic evaluation (h).

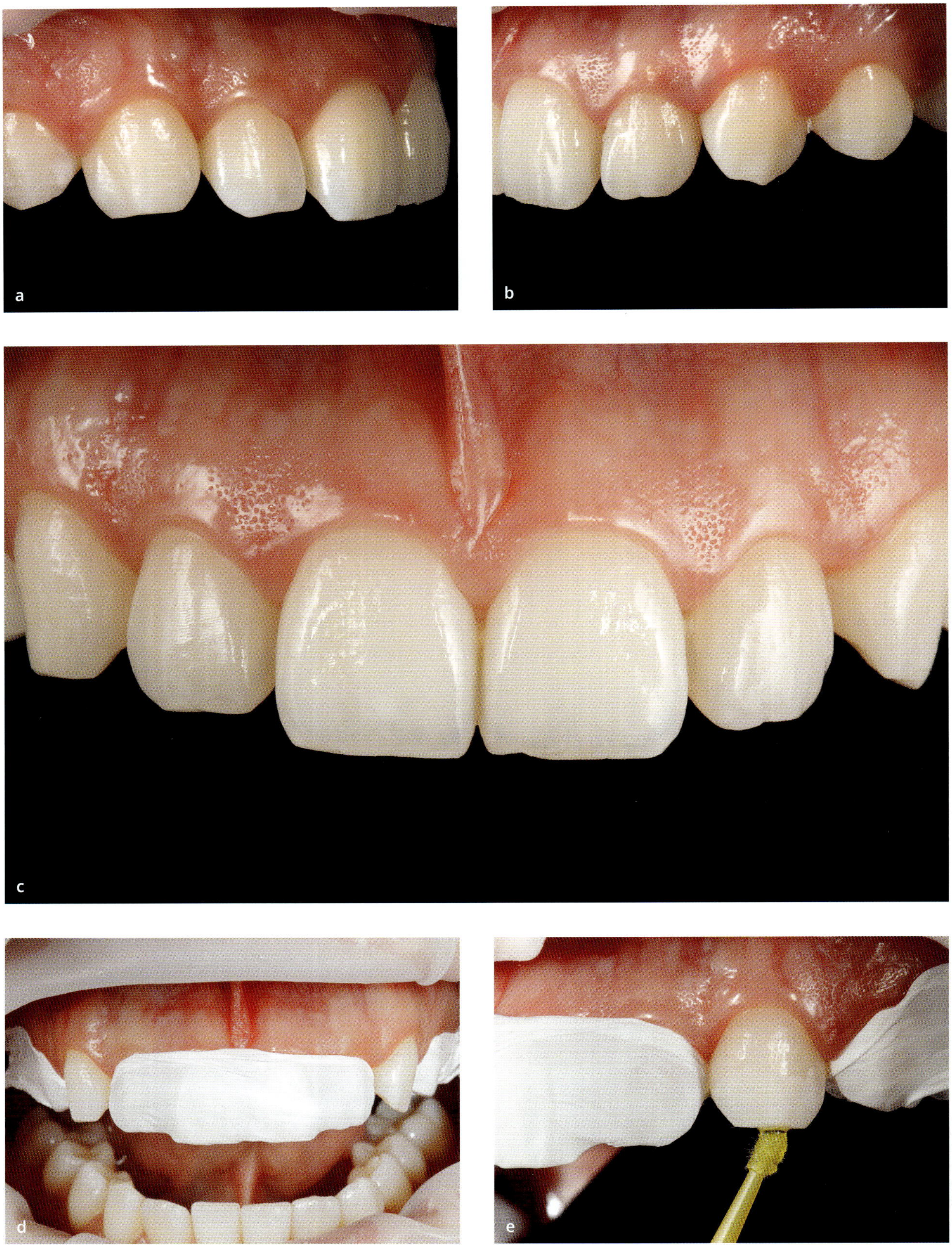


**Fig 5-16** The operator will clean the enamel surface and isolate the tooth from adjacent teeth with an easy-to-remove interproximal barrier that enables references with adjacent teeth. Calibration of the amount of material to be used is easier if adjacent neighbor teeth are visible while performing the restoration (a to d). No enamel removal nor beveling is done. The enamel etching is followed by application of adhesive and restorative material (e). Final buildup is tested facially (f to i) and intraorally, both in MIP and discursive movements (j to m). Note the injuries in the lower lip caused by the lip biting habit.

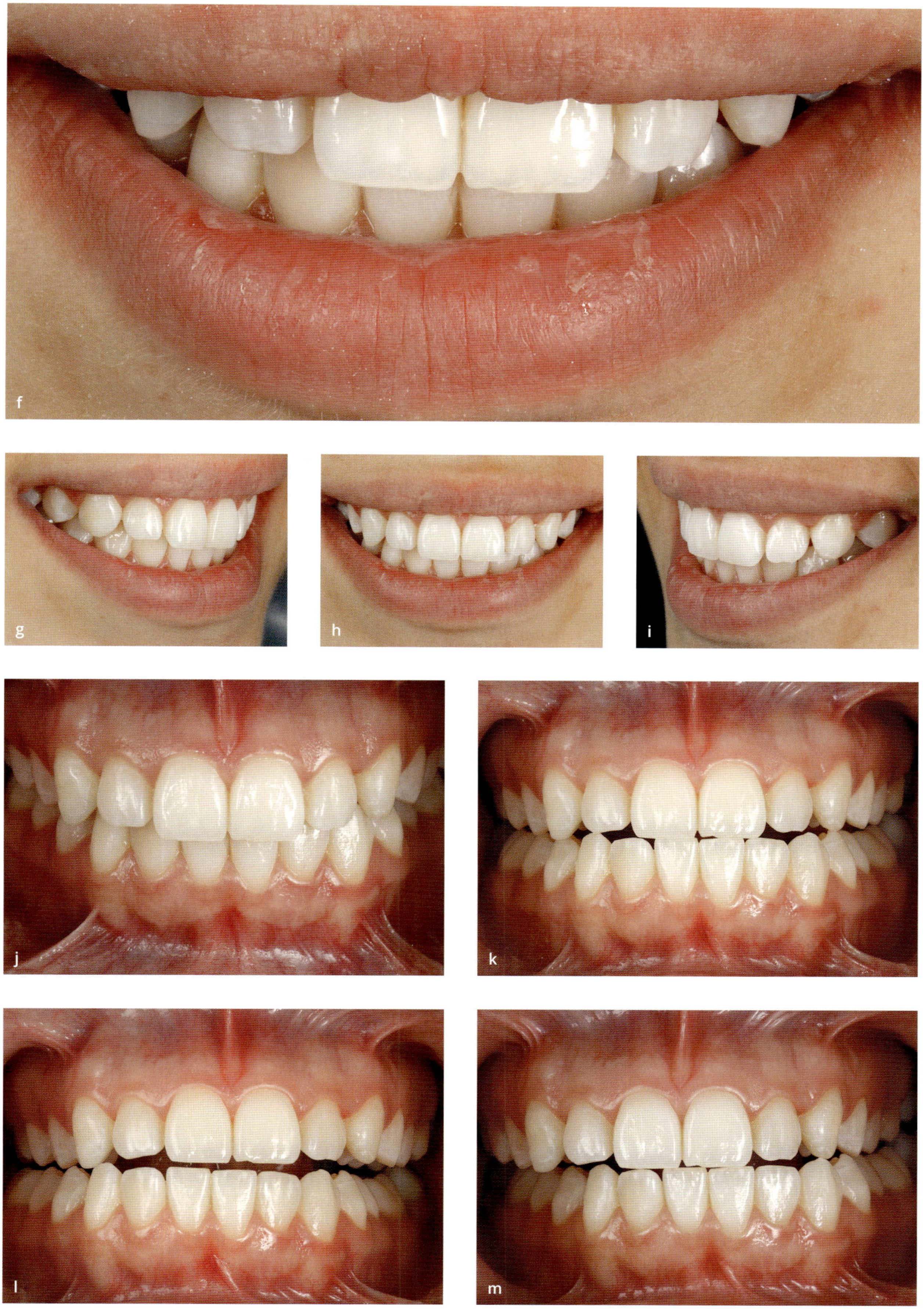
f
g
h
i
j
k
l
m

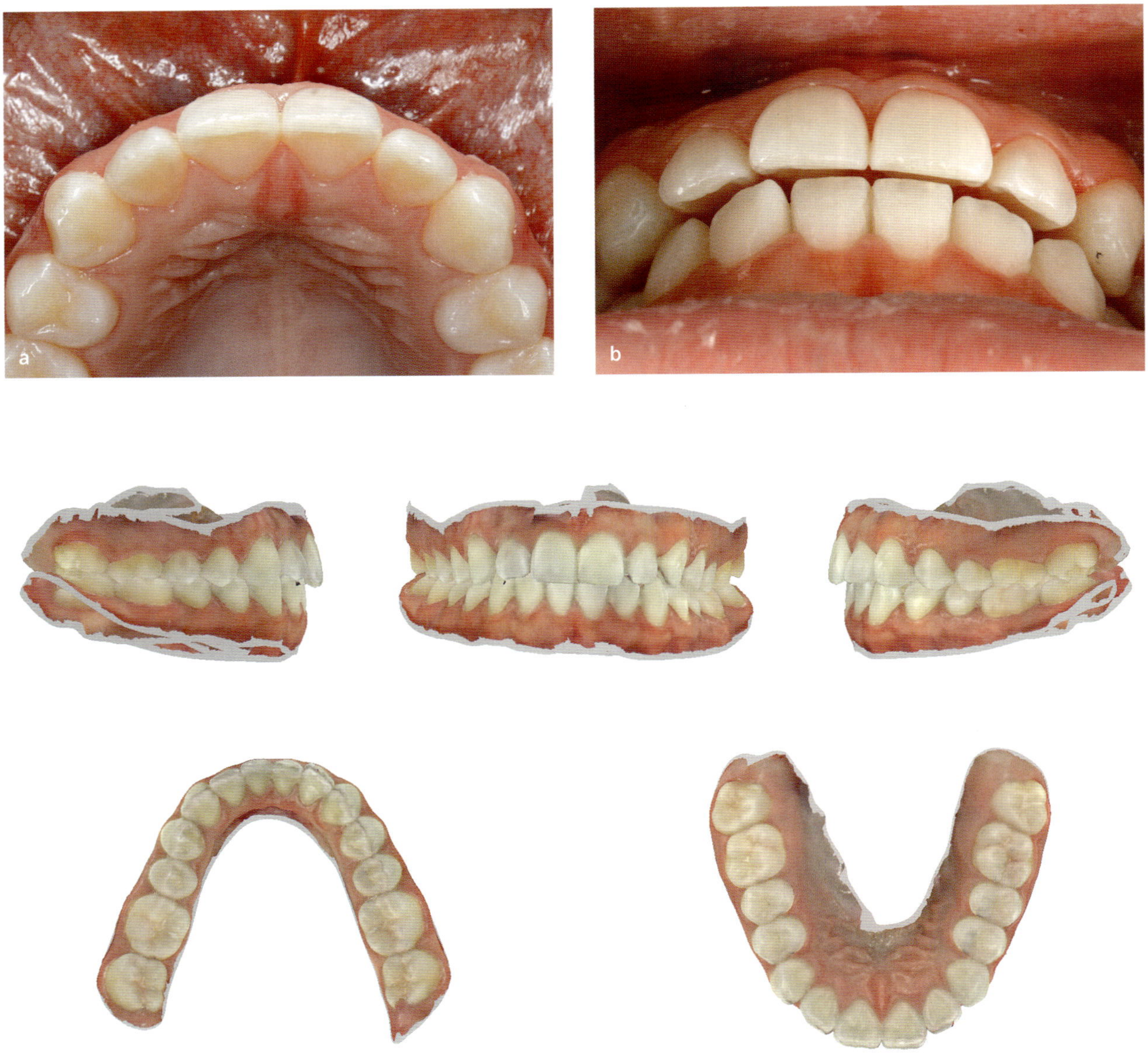

c

**Fig 5-17** In this case the tooth structure damage was repaired prior to the orthodontic treatment. The orthodontist planned to correct the interincisal relationship as well as to resolve the incomplete eruption of the canine in the second quadrant (a and b). An intraoral scan is taken after restoration of the damaged teeth, and a digital protocol is chosen for the orthodontic mechanics. Wearing the mouth splint 22 hours a day is an additional aid in stopping a lip biting habit when present (c).

## 6. Restoration of Canine and Anterior Guidance

Direct composite restorations have a long history of success in modern dentistry. They are the standard of care for partial esthetic restorations of the anterior teeth. Today, composite restorations are recognized as the least invasive and the first choice for the treatment of Incipient TW for their excellent esthetic properties and noteworthy longevity.[7] Interestingly, contrary to what could be expected, the type of composite or curing mode seems to have no impact on restoration performance, while environment and number of operators has the potential to impact the longevity or failure.

Restoring the anterior guidance with a simple direct composite restoration guided by the anatomical form is an effective procedure to regain the loss of anatomy and function. By doing this, a number of patients with no TW yet on the rest of the teeth can be saved from the wear that would otherwise follow.

Surprisingly, despite a noticeable amount of tooth structure loss, patients with TW seldom experience TMJ problems, which has led a good number of experienced clinicians to treat TW patients in their usual occlusion. While this might be arguable in advanced cases of TW cases, it can be acceptable for incipient TW, benefiting from the contemporary concept described as "comfortable occlusion" by some authors.[8] Incipient TW per se does not impact the vertical dimension of occlusion (VDO), and therefore there is no need for VDO augmentation. Not needing to choose between MIP and CR for VDO augmentation does not mean that occlusal discrepancies should be overlooked, as these can trigger a parafunctional habit.

Notwithstanding that, only when the TW has evolved to a severe level should the TW patient be considered in need of a full-mouth rehabilitation. Otherwise, the consensus on using direct composites for the worn dentition in the early stages, both anterior and posterior, offers a cost-effective line of treatment.[9,10]

Applying direct composite fundamentals for the rehabilitation of the incisal edges of the anterior teeth, sometimes maxillary only and other times also mandibular, requires expertise of the operator. If other space or anatomical issues occur in the same patient, the dentist might choose indirect restorations such as porcelain laminate veneers with a minor-preparation approach. However, the evolution of composites has made it simpler for the general dentist or prosthodontist to achieve a more than acceptable result, providing an accessible, affordable, and repairable treatment that should be the first line of intervention for incipient TW once wear has occurred. In moderate to severe TW, indirect restorations, be it composite, reinforced composite, or porcelain, require a material selection analysis that is much simpler in incipient TW. In minor TW, the damage is often so incipient, all it takes is to build up the tips of the cusps or fill a notch on the incisal edge (Fig 5-18).

Similarly, restoring the canine guidance with a simple direct composite restoration guided by the anatomical form and by the occlusal plane of the adjacent premolar and lateral and central incisors is an effective procedure. By doing this, a number of patients with no TW on the incisors can be saved from incisal wear that would otherwise follow after canine wear.

Adhesion to enamel, present in all cases of incipient TW, is by far the most predictable and least technique sensitive. Nevertheless, some dentin exposure may be seen even in early TW cases. These scenarios also benefit from direct composite restorations, provided a correct adhesive protocol for enamel and dentin bonding is issued.[11] Adhesive protocols may be cumbersome, especially if several operators in the same practice each have their preferred system.

While one-step etching protocols are usually avoided for indirect restorations, some one-step self-etch protocols after enamel etching show strong bonding to dentin and enamel. However, the three-step etch-and-rinse is considered the gold standard.[12] As mentioned previously, survival of restorations is improved when treatment is performed by a single operator.[13]

The cost of these restorations is another advantage, but what is more outstanding is the feasibility of true add-on applications. Removing sound enamel is not a prerequisite, nor is enamel beveling a mandatory protocol, to improve the life expectancy of the restoration. Direct composites can be done in combination or as adjuvant therapy with indirect restorations such as porcelain laminate veneers (PLVs), especially in more advanced cases of TW. Preserving tooth structure as much as possible should not be a limitation but a source of inspiration as nature has been generous in the exuberant anatomy of the oral tissues (Fig 5-19).

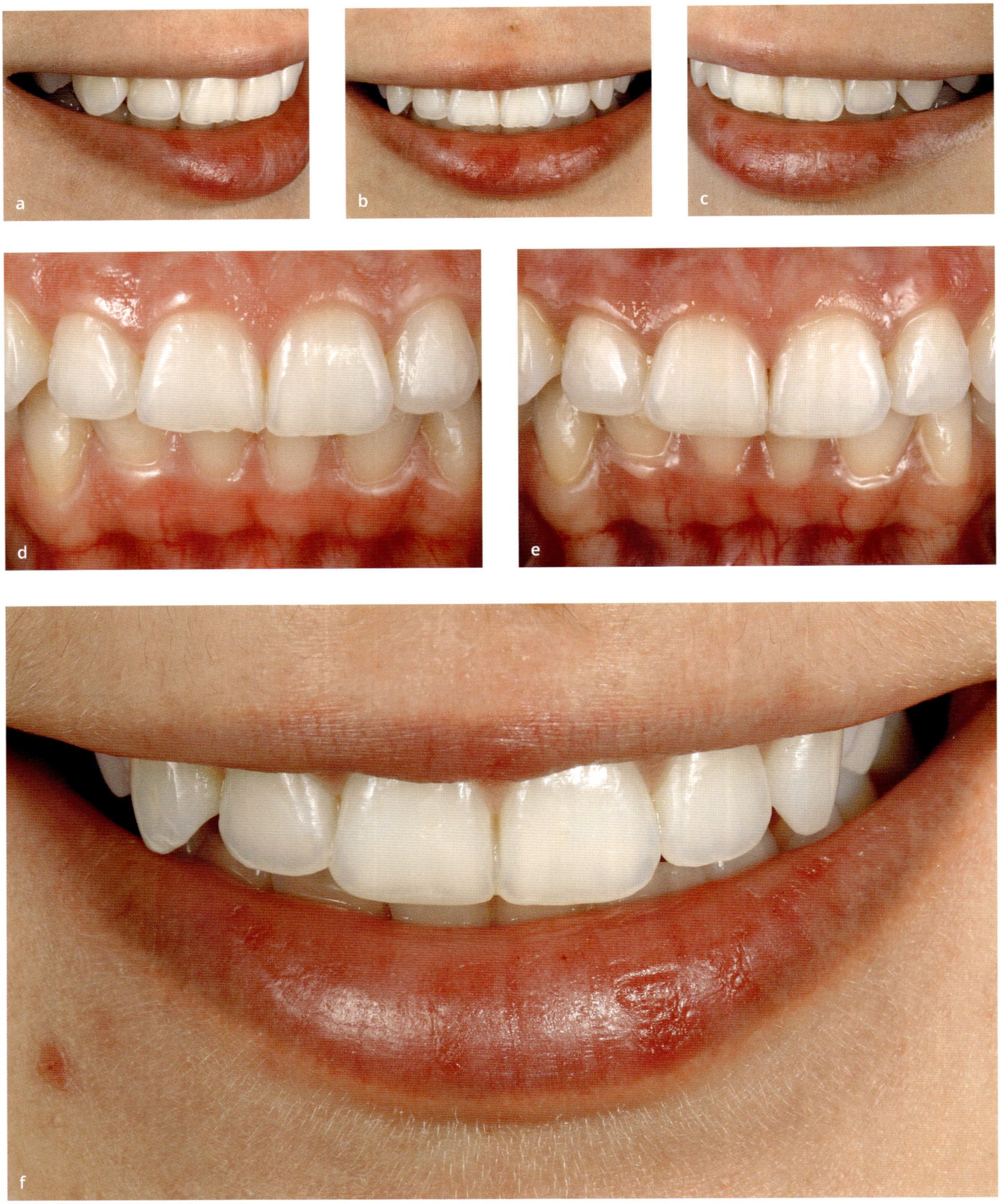

**Fig 5-18** A lip biting habit is identified during the first visit after observing the lip lesions in this young woman (a to c). Early detection of TW enables a minimal intervention at the incisal edges of the two maxillary central incisors. In minor TW, the damage is often so incipient that all it takes is to build up the tips of the worn cusps or fill the notch on the incisal edges. Incipient TW does not usually benefit from a mock-up in vivo trial as the patient can perceive the cost of the overall intervention as being too high and rule out the treatment. That being said, it is up to the dentist to choose to do a direct additive gap restoration with or without the aid of a silicone guide. Depending on the number of teeth to be restored, a silicone guide can be considered excessive, although it can be of help if the damage extends to all anterior teeth (d and e). Important as it is to restore the damage as soon as it is diagnosed, discussing habits and lifestyle choices with the patient is mandatory for long-term success. Within days after having finished the incipient TW restorations in this case, the lip biting lesions have started to heal, a sign of good prognosis associated with stopping the parafunctional habit (f).

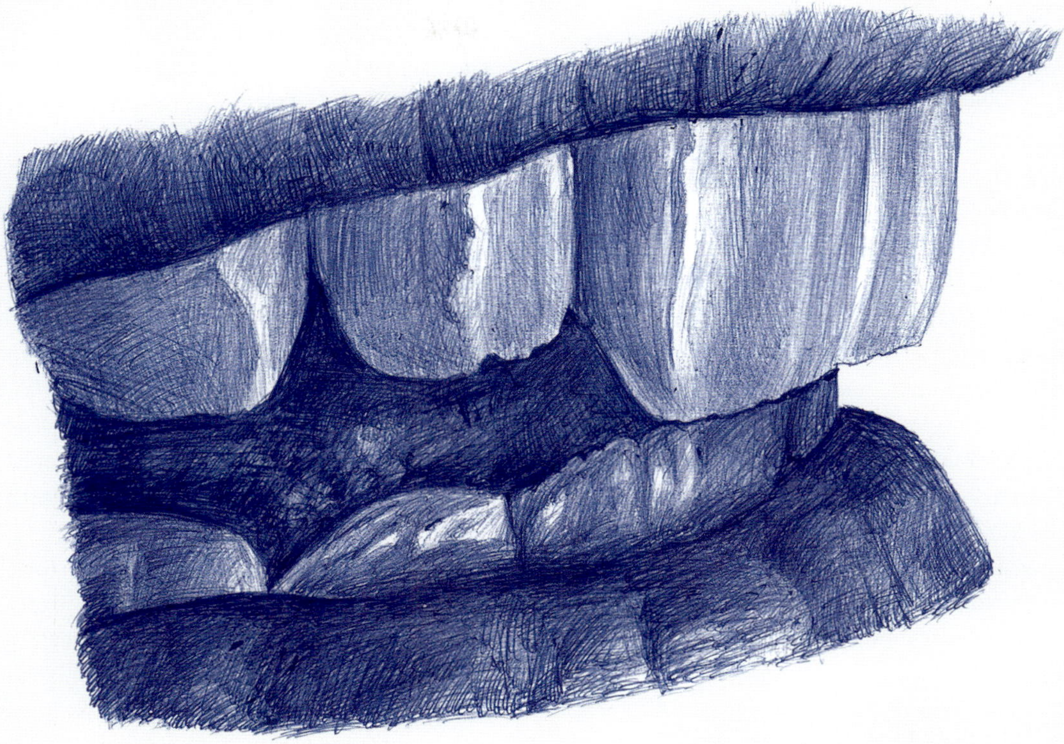

**Fig 5-19** In intercepting TW, the aim is to protect all remaining anatomy using a multidisciplinary team approach. A single restorative treatment may be insufficient to substitute the lost tissue as all the strain is put on the longevity of the restoration.

## 7. Intercepting Incipient Erosive Damage

Microscopic dissolution and chelation of minerals on the enamel surface caused by acidic challenges soften the enamel, which is then made more susceptible to mechanical wear such as chewing, toothbrushing, and even tongue and cheek rubbing, accounting for the insidious multifactorial TW origin. As detailed in chapter 2, enamel solubility is not fixed by a limited pH value of 5.5; it depends on the quality and quantity of enamel, the duration and intensity of the acid attack, and the capacity of saliva to prevent the damage, namely the amount of salivary flow. More saliva brings in more ions (calcium and phosphate), together with the micromolecular built-in defensive properties of the salivary flow.[14]

In situations in which an erosive challenge is suspected or expected, such as the environmental change in oral conditions associated with certain medications, a home prevention program should be established, as explained in chapter 10.

A group of patients especially vulnerable to erosion and demineralization is the cohort affected by polypharmacy and cancer treatments. In these patients, who have extremely acidic oral conditions, the lack of saliva has a fatal impact on tooth integrity. A few published protocols have aimed to stimulate saliva and at the same time provide a barrier, ideally to protect not only enamel but also dentin in this critically acidic oral milieu, in order to prevent further mineral loss.[15] Stimulation of salivary production by means of topical everyday hygiene measures with a compound delivered via toothpaste, mouthwash, spray, or gel has shown to effectively and safely increase salivary flow even in patients with hyposalivation from polypharmacy and severe xerostomia in patients undergoing radiation for head and neck cancer.[16,17]

Once the damage to the teeth is present, chairside strategies using adhesive systems and/or direct or semidirect composite can be helpful as a temporary measure until either the erosive condition is well identified and managed or the challenge has ceased. Using adhesive systems and/or resins to form a barrier between the acid and the tooth has proven beneficial. The drawback is the longevity of the results being linked to the duration of the coating. Some authors recommend reapplying adhesive systems every 3 months, while using filled resins or flowable composites may be more durable.[18] In incipient TW the principle to protect enamel calls for direct or semidirect protocols with composite, which will need to be reapplied periodically while the risk factors are still present.[19]

Of particular difficulty is the early management of erosive damage to the palatal aspect of teeth. The asymptomatic nature of the somewhat flat lesions as well as their hidden location hinder early diagnosis. Moreover, incipient physical tooth loss can be stimulated by acid dissolution of enamel originating either intrinsically (eg, gastric acid), environmentally (eg, soft drinks, dietary changes), or biologically (eg, congenital conditions, medications, mouth breathing, salivary dysfunction, psychologic status, or sleep disorders). Establishing the origin may be arduous as several factors can have a summative effect, leaving the TW team without an etiologic diagnosis. That being said, the clinical diagnosis of erosive TW should not be overlooked. In this situation, high translucency on the incisal third of anterior teeth may be the only sign, especially as oral changes can be subtle and mostly evident at a microscopic level (Fig 5-20).

Controlling or changing TW risk factors, especially those of erosive origin resulting from lifestyle choices, is a phenomenal task from the dentist's perspective. Nevertheless, not doing anything will lead to macroscopic changes in tooth anatomy and eventually function. Therefore, it can be agreed with the patient to restore and protect tooth structure with a chairside protocol. A digital model is useful as a baseline record for future monitoring and also for treatment planning (Fig 5-21).

Color and form are often a concern in patients with erosion, as a long-standing demineralization challenge may have changed the appearance of the teeth. In cases in which an improvement of color and/or form is expected or intended as a result of the treatment, it is advisable to do a mock-up and try-in in order to decrease the chance of unnecessary surprises from the patient's point of view (Fig 5-22).

The improvement of the patient's smile shown in Fig 5-22 could have also been achieved with buccal restorations, either direct or indirect, such as porcelain laminate veneers. However, by doing so, the incipient palatal damage would not have been protected, leading eventually to dissolution of all or most of the palatal anatomy. This formerly typical approach is falling out of favor as more and more patients show unceasing progression of palatal damage after being treated with this modality. A semidirect protocol in the case of treating multiple teeth can employ flowable composite if the area in question is not a high-friction area, as is the case with palatal areas. On the other hand, in order to facilitate application in the case of occlusal or palatal restorations, the use of molds or guides is helpful.[20] The rigidity and fitting of the mold is key for the ease of the procedure (Fig 5-23).

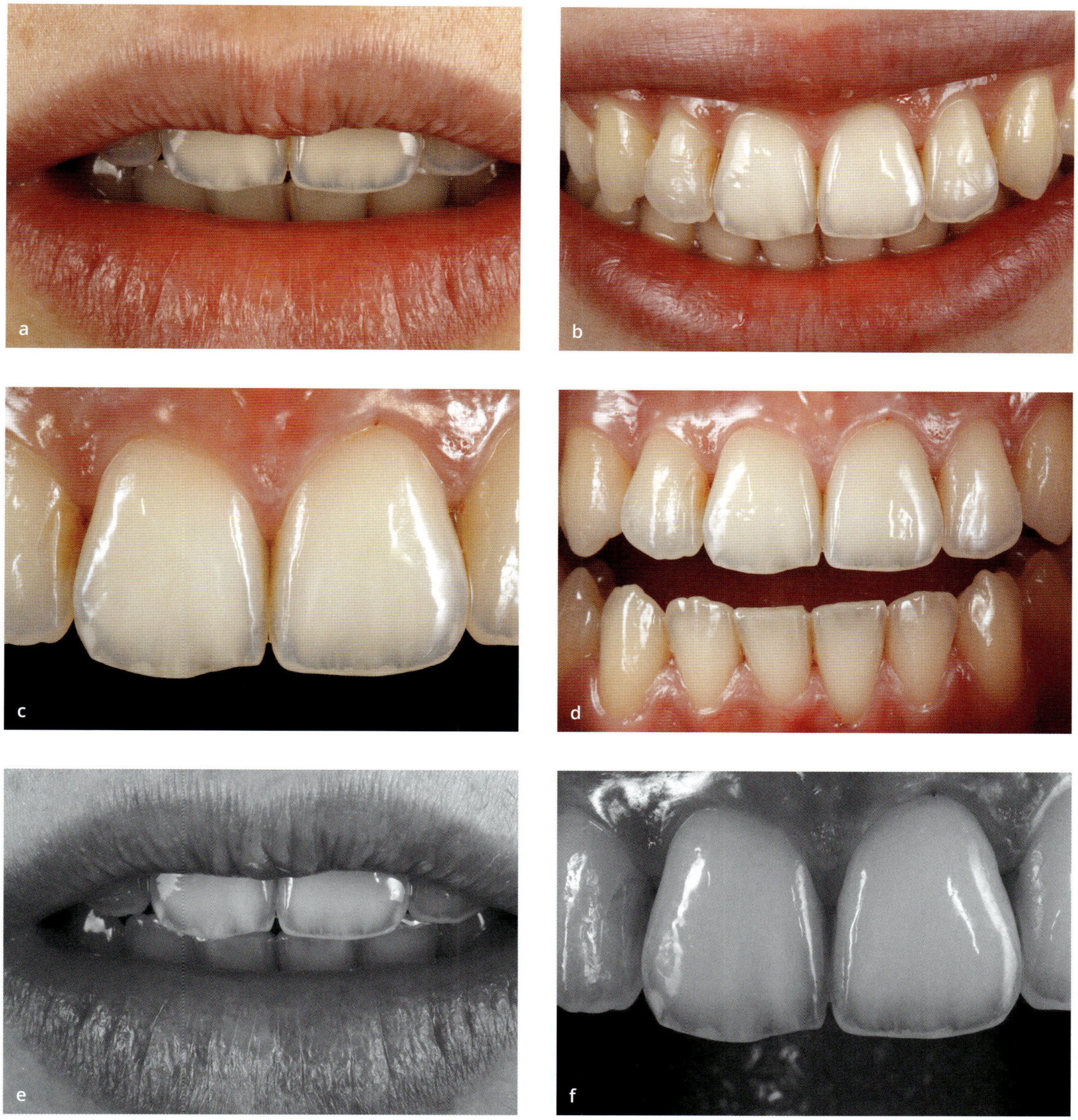


**Fig 5-20** A young female patient presented with a recent change in the appearance of her anterior teeth, which have turned gray-blueish. The examination identifies an increase of translucency affecting the maxillary anterior teeth, a sign of an erosive environment. The presence of a palatal fixed orthodontic retainer has probably protected the central and gingival third, while the incisal palatal third has subtly thinned as a consequence of the erosive challenge (a to c). Signs of neither attrition nor abrasion are found (d). A black-and-white series of images shows a jelly-like appearance related to the increased incisal translucency (e and f).

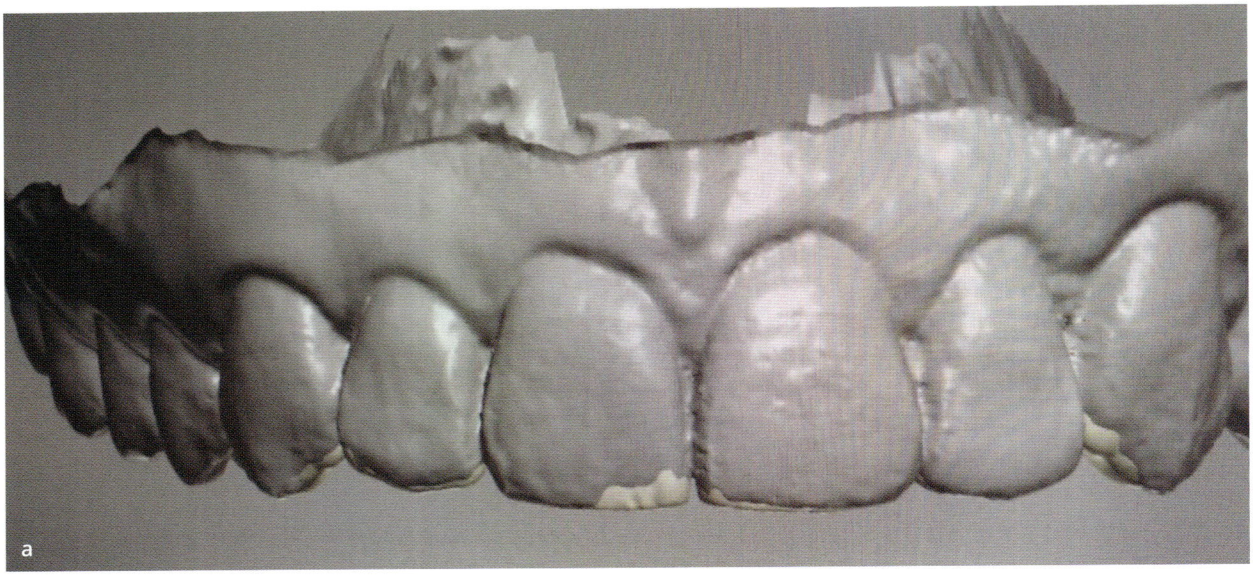
a

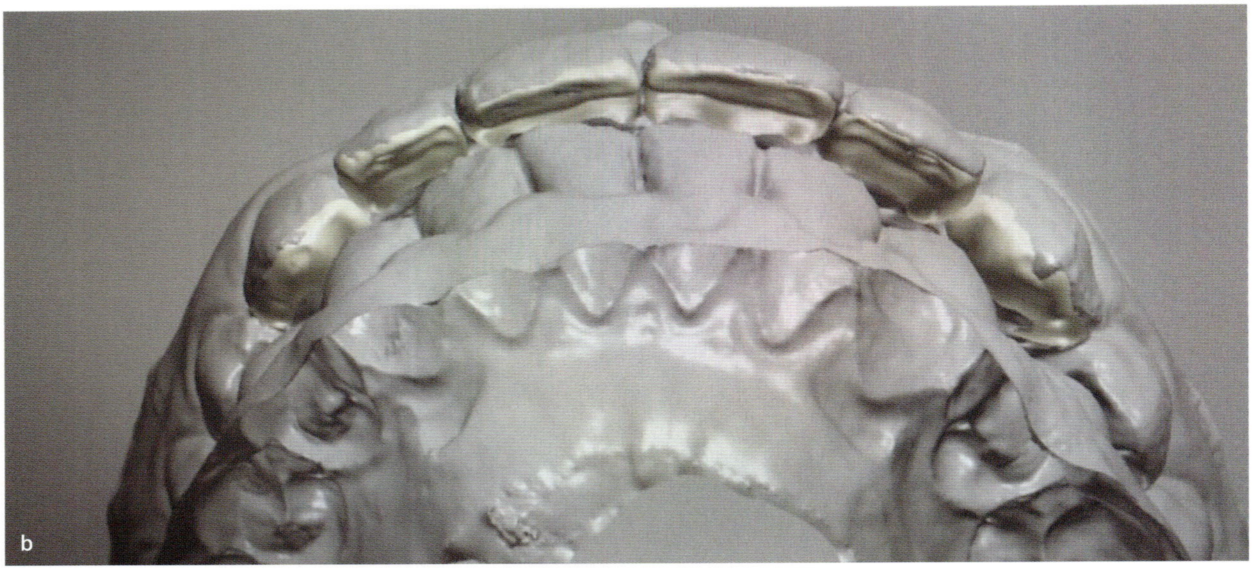
b

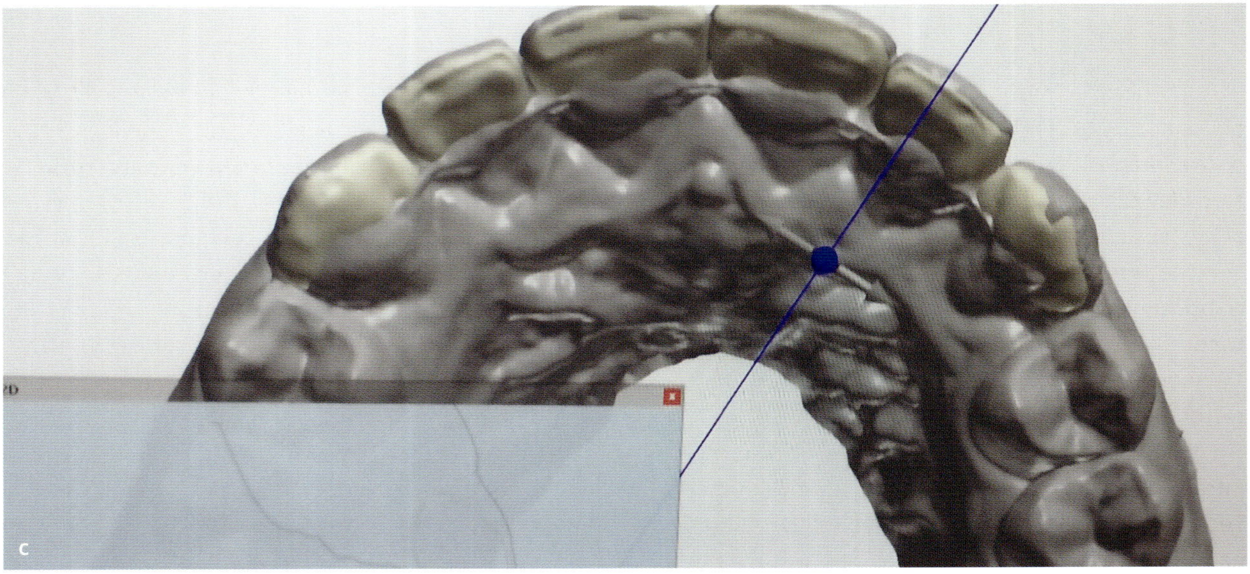
c

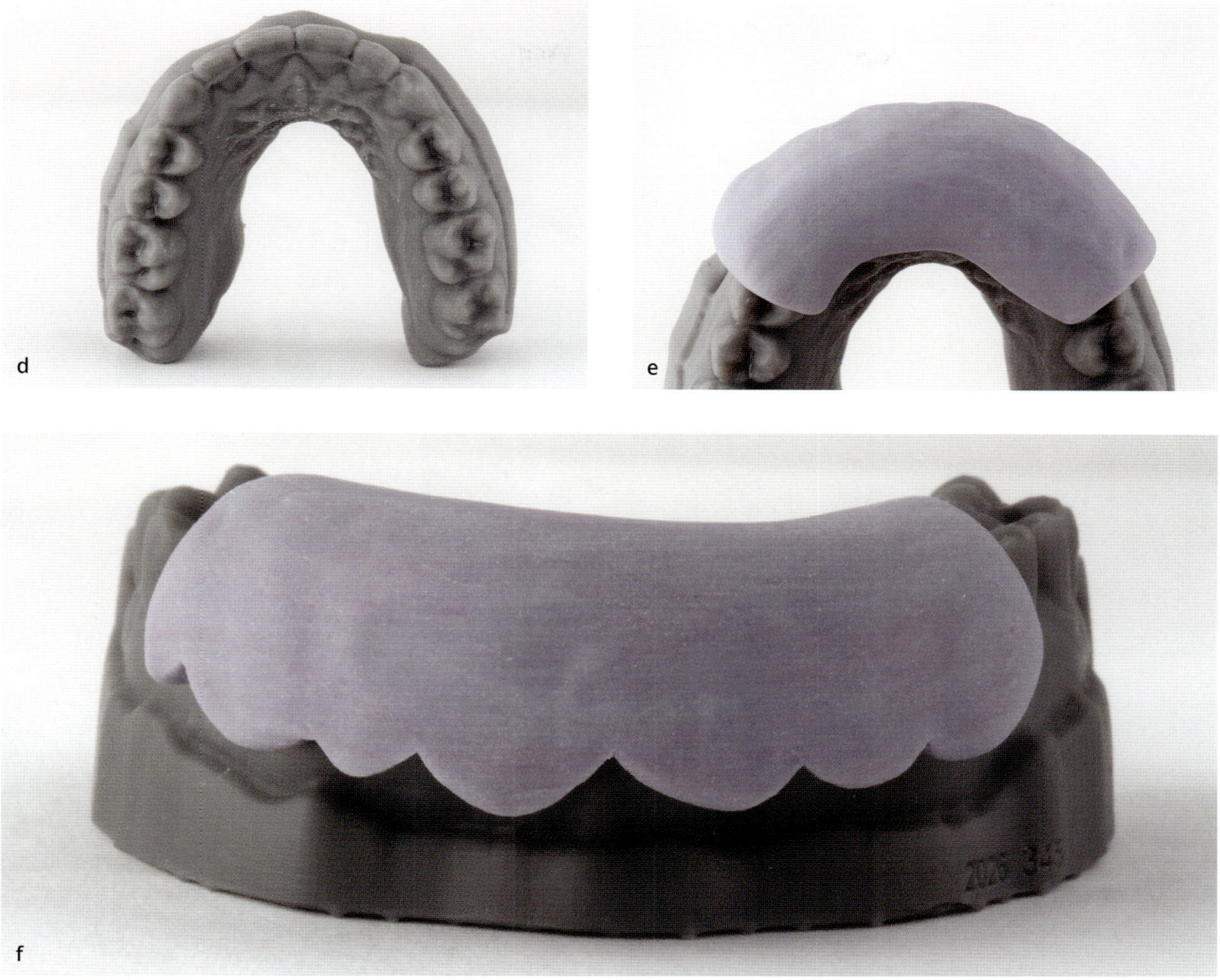

**Fig 5-21** The STL of the initial intraoral scan of the same patient is used to create a digital wax-up, namely of the palatal aspect of the teeth, without having to remove the fixed retainer. The buccal aspect of the teeth is not included in the wax-up as they are not suffering except for some minor changes in the incisal borders of two teeth (a). The digital setup is checked to make sure there will be no occlusal interferences (b). An estimated volume of 0.5-mm thickness is added digitally onto the palatal incisal half of the six maxillary anterior teeth (c). A model is printed with the additions of the wax-up (d), and a sturdy silicone index is made that covers the palatal aspect of the maxillary anterior arch. The unaltered vestibular anatomy helps in the positioning of the tray (e and f).

Whenever possible, relative isolation of the teeth to be treated will help the operator control contamination of the surfaces. Likewise, individualization might require extended time in the initial stages but will reduce efforts at the finishing phase (Fig 5-24).

The combination of adhesive protocols with direct composite applied with the aid of a 3D reservoir can be used for extended periods of time if the monitoring of TW shows insufficient protection or if deterioration of the restorations is seen.

With the advent of the superimposition software for intraoral scanning, such as TimeLapse for iTero (Align Technology) or OraCheck for Primescan (Dentsply Sirona), the dentist knows where and when to modify the restorations that have become worn or defective. A quantitative comparison between two time periods is a valuable guide for the TW team (see chapters 3 and 10).

Patients should be informed that TW is an irreversible chronic and cyclic lifetime condition and that restorations will need to be repaired or replaced in order to prevent the tooth from being exposed again to the wear factors. Restorations will also be subject to material wear and/or fractures that are to be anticipated and discussed with the patient, independently of the material selection. Therefore, choosing a repeatable protocol and a repairable material will delay the need for more invasive treatments (Figs 5-25 and 5-26).

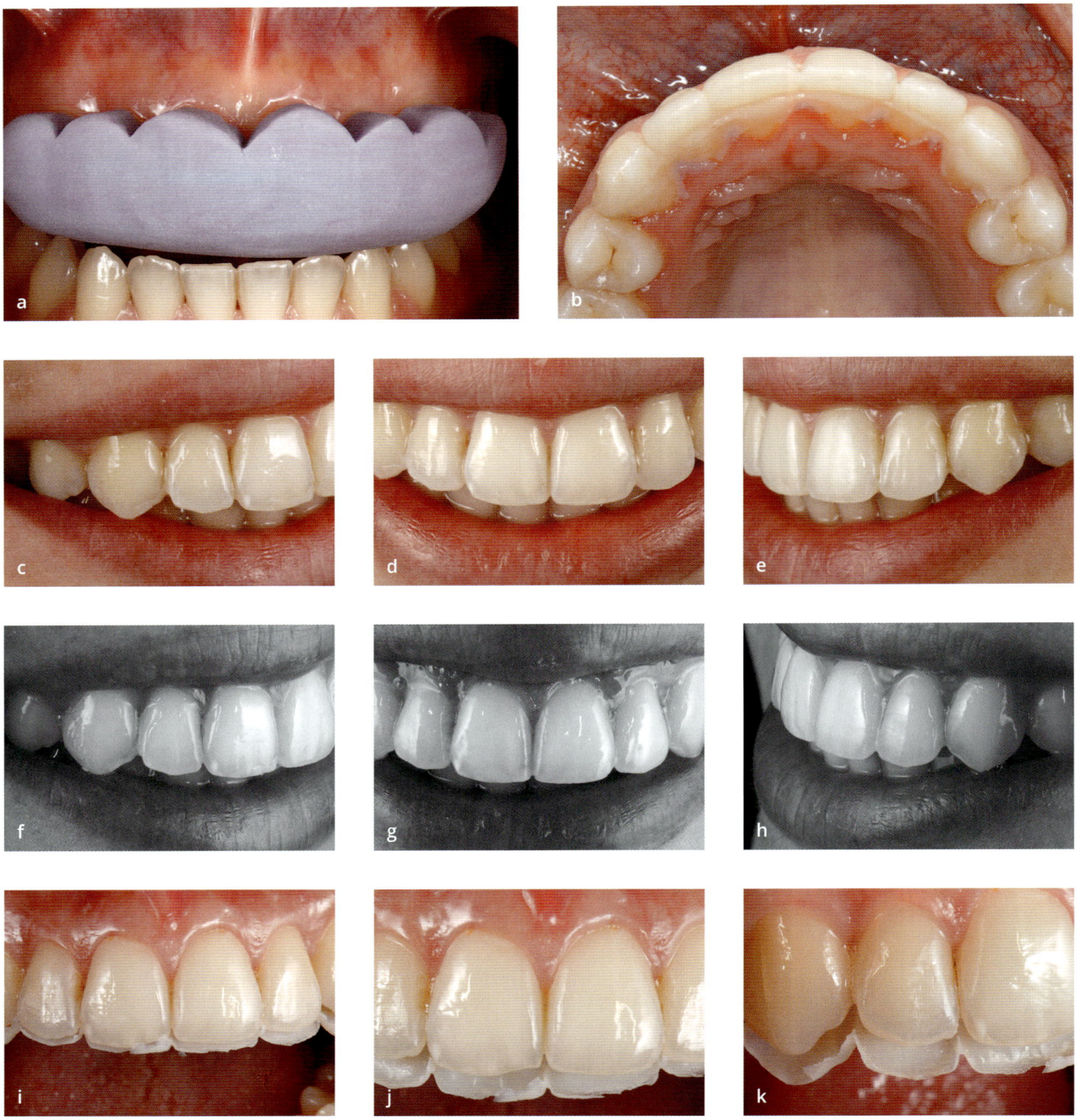


**Fig 5-22** For the mock-up stage, a simple tooth-colored acrylic resin material (in this case Enamel Plus, Micerium) is applied mostly to the palatal aspect of the silicone tray and transported onto the maxillary teeth, which have been isolated with petroleum jelly, once the maxillary fixed retainer has been removed (a and b). Excess resin is trimmed, and digital photos are taken to evaluate the improvement in value and chroma as a result of the thickening of the palatal aspect. No material has been added to the labial aspect, which is in contrast to what has long been the tendency: to address the labial and not the palatal (c to h). The resin palatal mock-up is removed easily as the maxillary teeth have been coated with an isolating gel prior to the application of the acrylic resin (i to k).

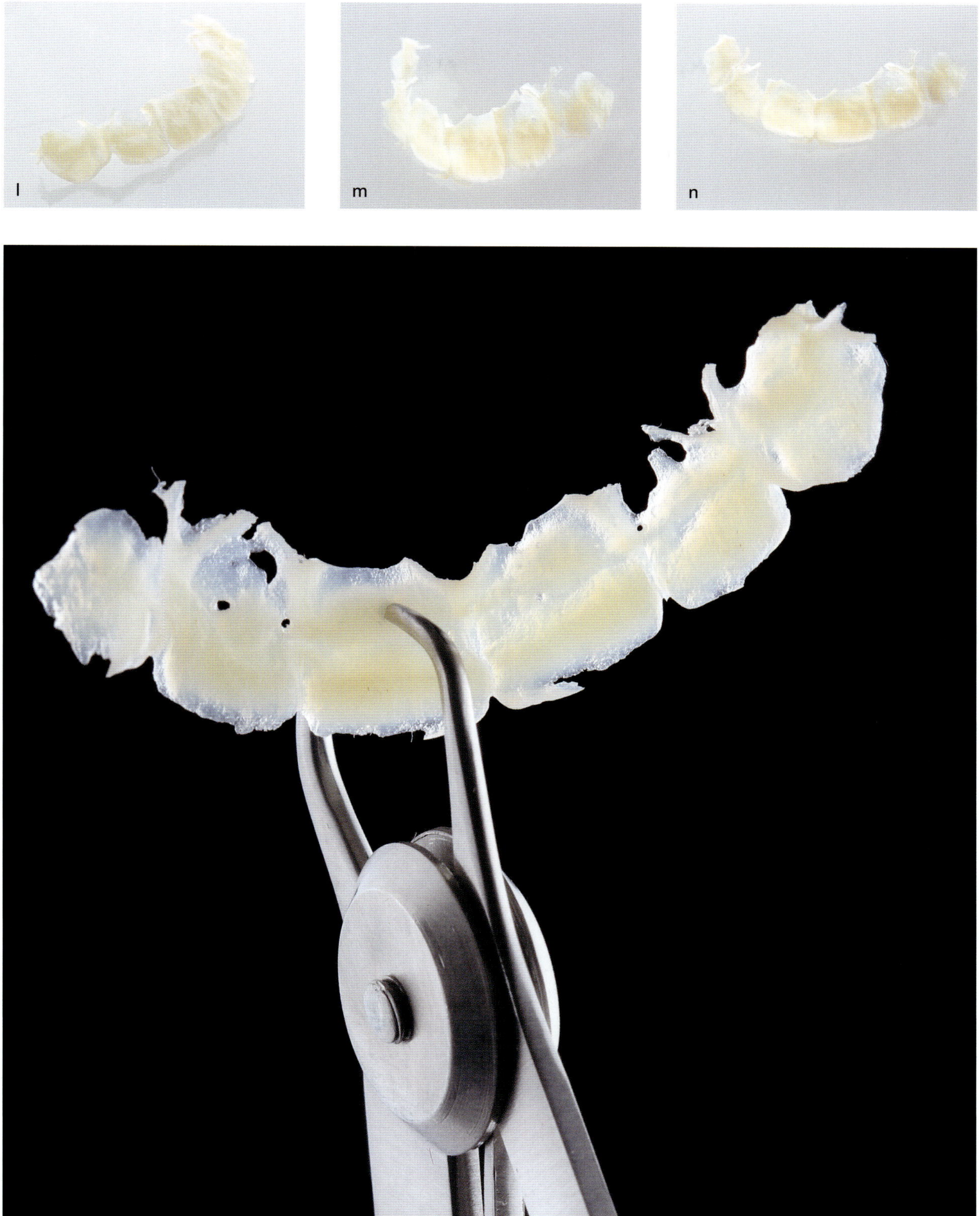


**Fig 5-22** *(continued)* No acrylic is added to the vestibular aspect. The overall thickness of the mock-up is quite thin as the lesions are incipient, and no extra restorative space has been provided, nor has any VDO alteration been contemplated (l to o).

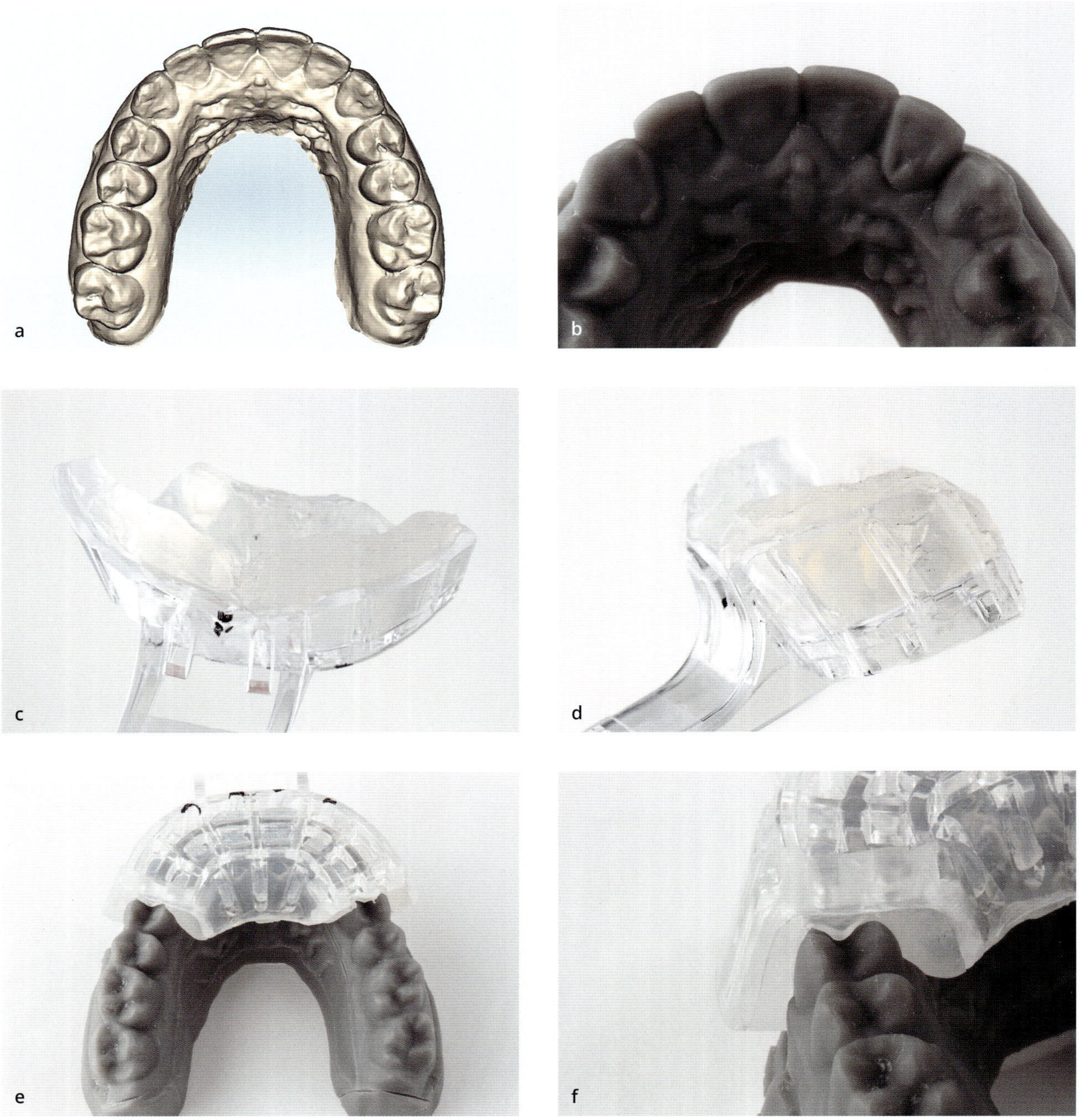


**Fig 5-23** For the treatment phase, a new digital scan of the same patient is taken after removal of the fixed orthodontic retainer, and the initial digital wax-up is superimposed and positioned on the lingual aspect of all six maxillary anterior teeth, from which a new model is printed (a and b). The mold to be used should be transparent to enable light curing of the composite. A prefabricated transparent impression tray can be used, trimmed, and relined with transparent silicone on the final wax-up to get a tight fit once it is placed intraorally on the adjacent untreated teeth (c to f).

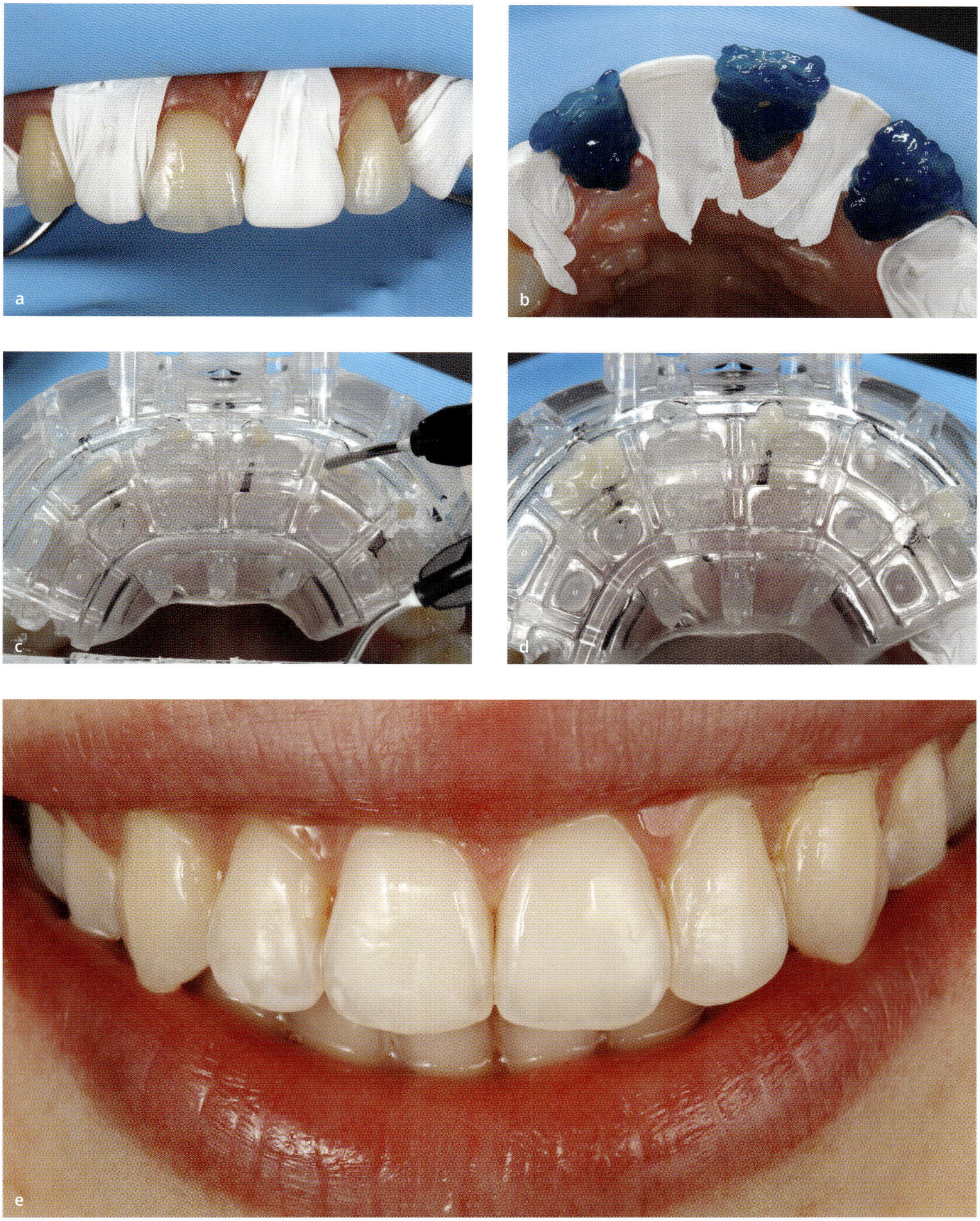

**Fig 5-24** When using a mold, a critical point will be separating teeth after treatment. Any means to prevent unwanted splinting, such as PTFE tape applied to the adjacent teeth is advisable (a and b). In this same patient, as teeth will be treated continuously one at a time, the process has to be repeated until all six teeth are finished. A flowable composite is selected as the restorative material, and six channels, one for each tooth, are drilled completely through the rigid transportation tray for the material to be injected through them with a syringe (c and d). When the procedure is finished, new digital images are taken. The subtle change that incipient erosive TW had caused in these teeth is no longer visible as the flowable composite has thickened the palatal enamel (e). The low value and the hypertranslucency of these anterior teeth have improved simultaneously when the incipient TW lesions have been addressed.

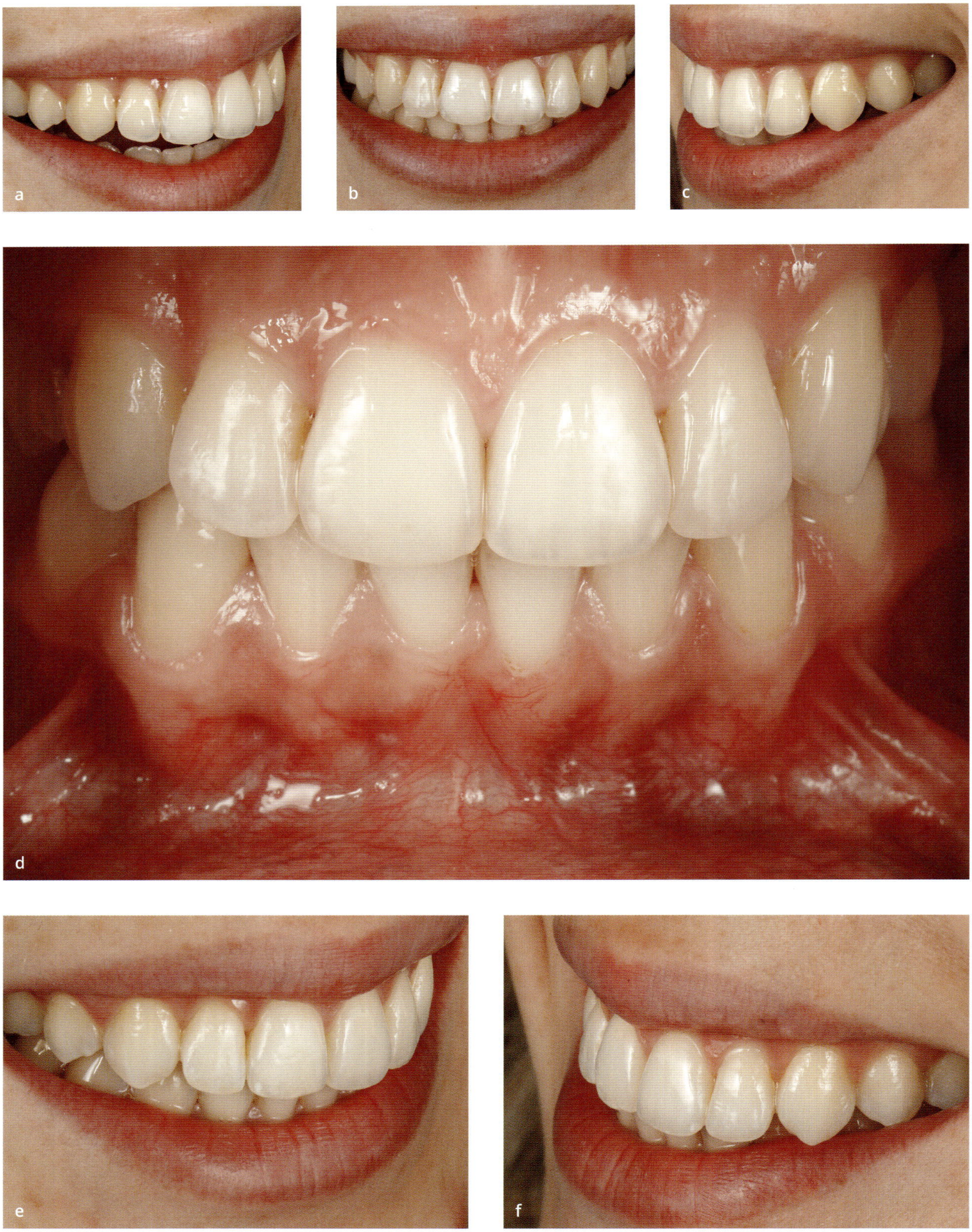


**Fig 5-25** The preservation of all tooth structure has proved an effective means of reverting the signs of incipient erosive damage in this same patient. The overall integration of the treated teeth has been achieved without masking the color change, which would have necessitated an irreversible tooth reduction (a to f). The anticipation of future interventions should be explained to the patient. A final model, either printed or cast, and a mold (e and f) can be made, along with a mouthguard that safeguards both teeth and restorations (g and h) and should be worn when teeth are more susceptible, especially but not exclusively at night. The final STL has more than a forensic value as it will be used in the future checkups to assess relapse or TW progression (i).

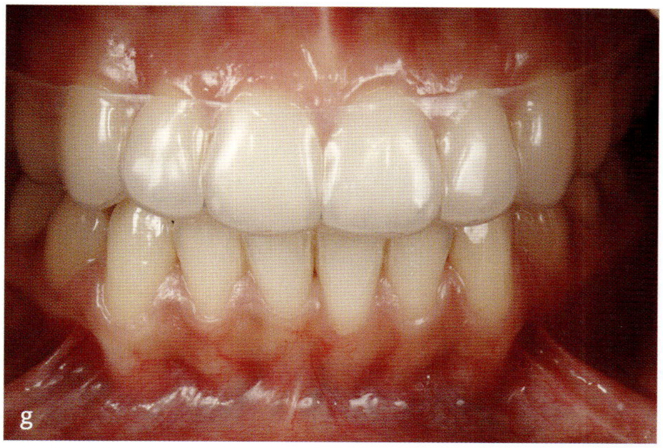
g

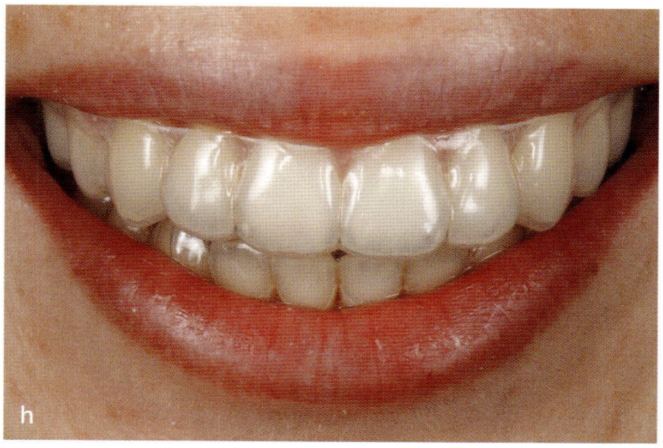
h

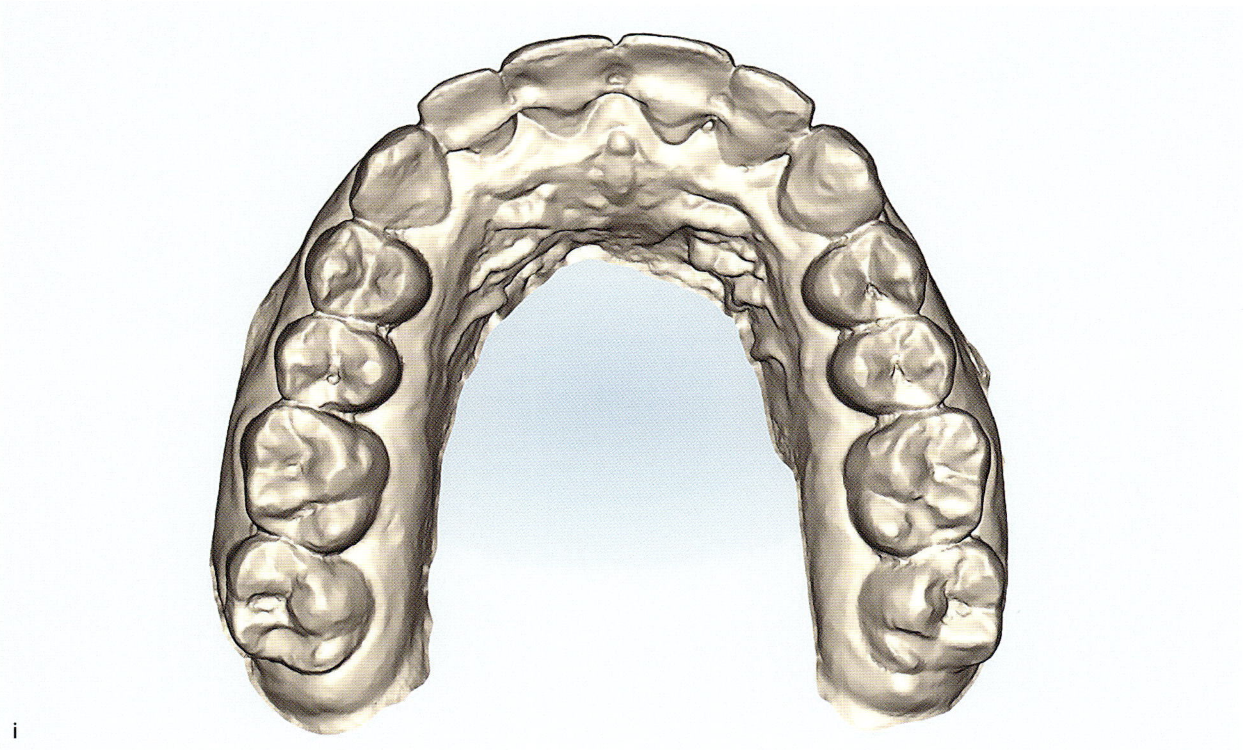
i

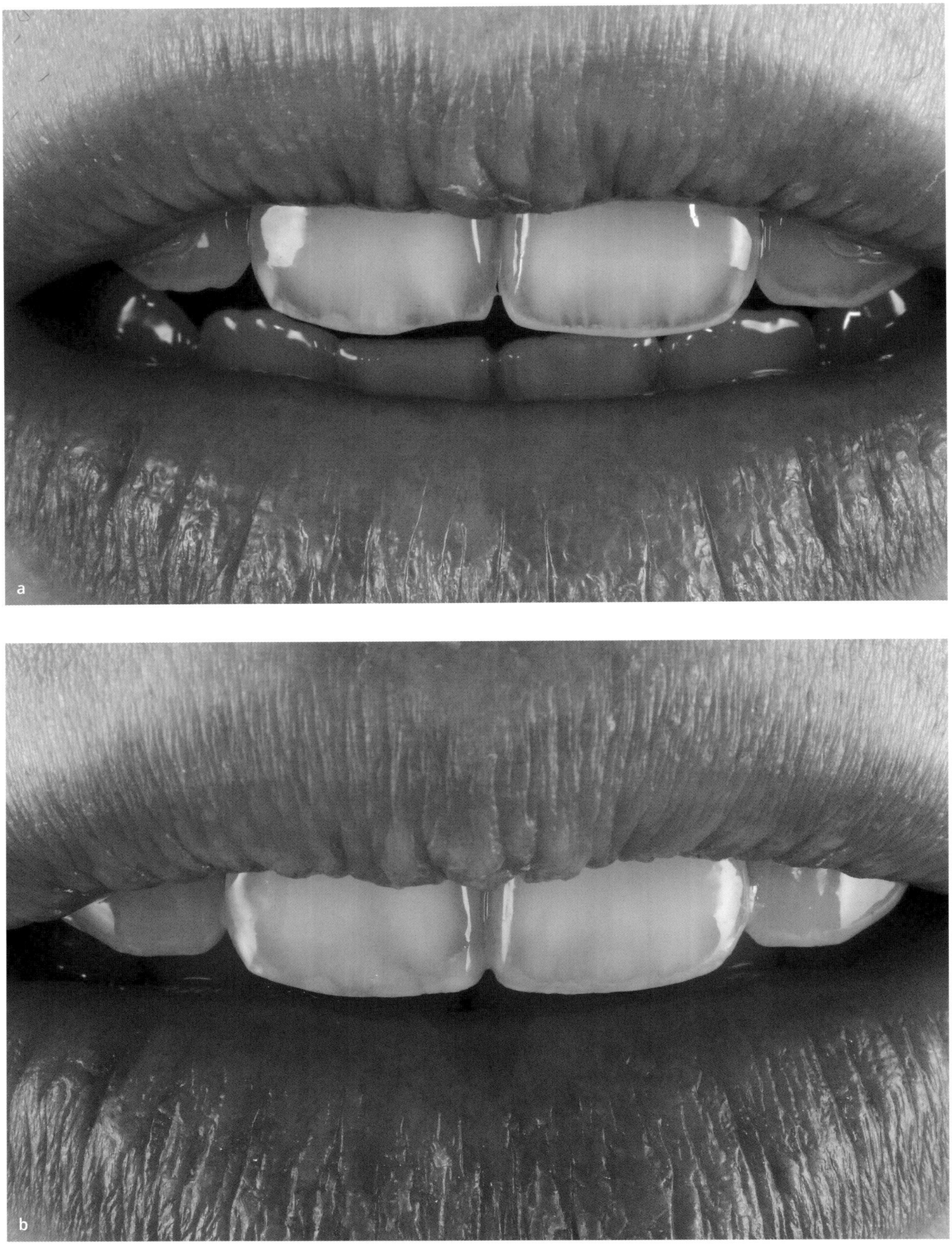

**Fig 5-26** The black-and-white images of the same patient show that the process of an additive mock-up has helped in diagnosing disease causation, in this case an erosive challenge to an otherwise young and healthy dentition. The initial smile is subtly improved when the palatal mock-up is delivered and tried in the mouth (a and b). The final detailed images of the six maxillary anterior teeth with the definitive palatal restorations show the good response to a limited intervention that has saved tooth structure and diminished the probable number of future complications (c to e).

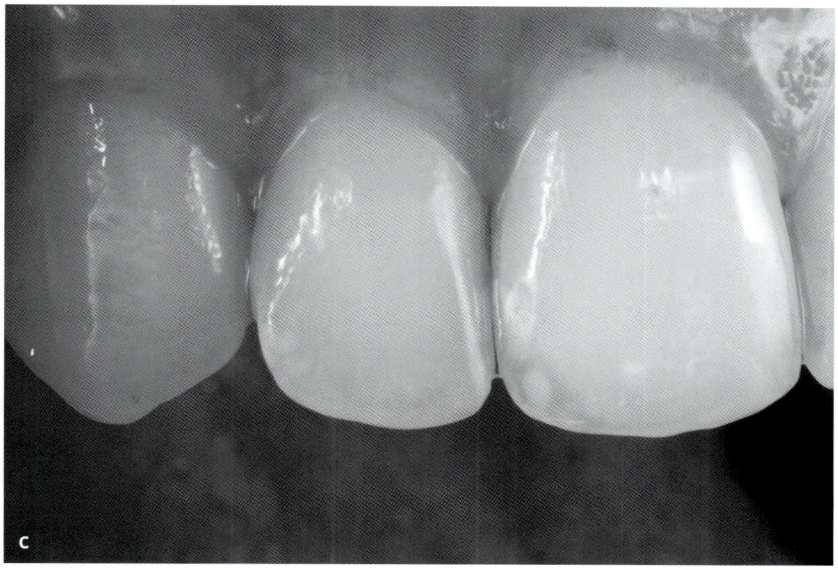
c

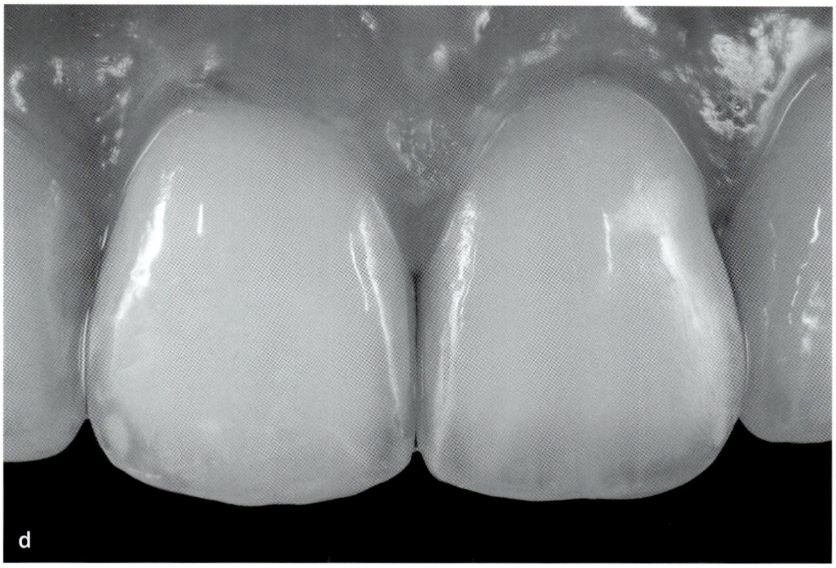
d

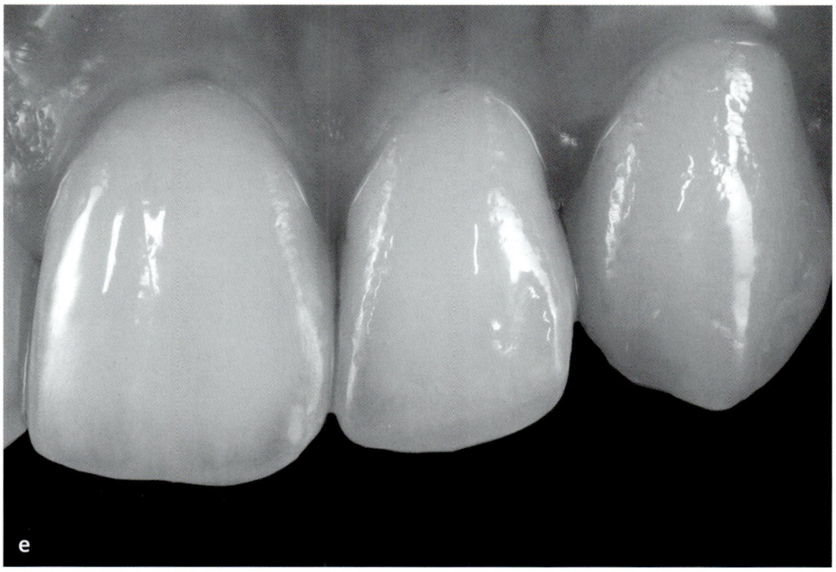
e

## 8. Key Points: Incipient TW Flowchart

**Table 5-1** Flowchart for incipient TW.

| | |
|---|---|
| **1.** | **Anamnesis and TW questionnaire**<br>■ WECC and WASS evaluation |
| **2.** | **Orthodontic evaluation**<br>**If indicated:**<br>■ Anterior wear: If incisal edges are worn out, build up with direct composite.<br>■ Posterior wear: If cusps are worn out, build up with direct composite.<br>■ Orthodontic treatment can be done before or after restorative phase.<br><br>**If not indicated:**<br>■ Restorative phase is followed by diet and lifestyle coaching.<br>■ If additional restorative/esthetic needs are contemplated, porcelain laminate veneers may be an option. |
| **3.** | **Personalized preventive program** |
| **4.** | **Mouthguard protection, individualized depending on type of TW (primary origin)** |
| **5.** | **Periodic TW monitoring and regular checkups**<br>■ Intraoral scanning with time-elapse comparison |

## References


1. Dawe C. What is the critical pH and why does a tooth dissolve in acid? J Can Dent Assoc 2003;69:722–724.
2. Bazos P, Magne P. Bio-Emulation: Biomimetically emulating nature utilizing a histoanatomic approach; visual synthesis. Int J Esthet Dent 2014;9:330–352.
3. Kazoullis S, Seow WK, Holcombe T, Newman B, Ford D. Common dental conditions associated with dental erosion in schoolchildren in Australia. Pediatr Dent 2007;29(1):33–39.
4. Young WG, Khan F. Sites of dental erosion are saliva-dependent. J Oral Rehabil 2002;29(1):35–43.
5. Al-Malik MI, Holt RD, Bedi R. Erosion, caries and rampant caries in preschool children in Jeddah, Saudi Arabia. Community Dent Oral Epidemiol 2002;30(1):16–23.
6. Dugmore CR, Rock WP. The prevalence of tooth erosion in 12-year-old children. Br Dent J 2004;196:279–282.
7. Dietschi D, Shahidi C, Krejci I. Clinical performance of direct anterior composite restorations: A systematic literature review and critical appraisal. Int J Esthet Dent 2019;14:252–270.
8. Devigus A. What is your occlusion style? Eur J Esthet Dent 2013;8:355.
9. Loomans B, Opdam N, Attin T, et al. Severe tooth wear: European consensus statement on management guidelines. J Adhes Dent 2017;19(2):111–119.
10. Poyser NJ, Briggs PF, Chana HS, Kelleher MG, Porter RW, Patel MM. The evaluation of direct composite restorations for the worn mandibular anterior dentition—Clinical performance and patient satisfaction. J Oral Rehabil 2007;34:361–376.
11. Spreafico RC. Composite resin rehabilitation of eroded dentition in a bulimic patient: A case report. Eur J Esthet Dent 2010;5(1):28–48.
12. Van Meerbeek B, Peumans M, Poitevin A, et al. Relationship between bond-strength tests and clinical outcomes. Dent Mater 2010;26(2):e100–e121.
13. Burke FJ, Lucarotti PS, Holder RL. Outcome of direct restorations placed within the general dental services in England and Wales (Part 2): Variation by patients' characteristics. J Dent 2005;33:817–826.
14. Dawes C, Dong C. The flow rate and electrolyte composition of whole saliva elicited by the use of sucrose-containing and sugar-free chewing-gums. Arch Oral Biol 1995;40:699–705.
15. Wiegand A, Gutsche M, Attin T. Effect of olive oil and an olive-oil-containing fluoridated mouthrinse on enamel and dentin erosion in vitro. Acta Odontol Scand 2007;65:357–361.
16. Martín M, Marín A, López M, et al. Products based on olive oil, betaine, and xylitol in the post-radiotherapy xerostomia. Rep Pract Oncol Radiother 2017;22(1):71–76.
17. Ship JA, McCutcheon JA, Spivakovsky S, Kerr AR. Safety and effectiveness of topical dry mouth products containing olive oil, betaine, and xylitol in reducing xerostomia for polypharmacy-induced dry mouth. J Oral Rehabil 2007;34:724–732.
18. Azzopardi A, Bartlett DW, Watson TF, Sherriff M. The surface effects of erosion and abrasion on dentine with and without a protective layer. Br Dent J 2004;196:351–354.
19. Azouzi I, Kalghoum I, Hadyaoui D, Harzallah B, Cherif M. Principles and guidelines for managing tooth wear: A review. Int Med Care 2018. doi: 10.15761/IMC.1000112.
20. Dietschi D, Saratti CM. Interceptive treatment of tooth wear: A revised protocol for the full molding technique. Int J Esthet Dent 2020;15:264–286.

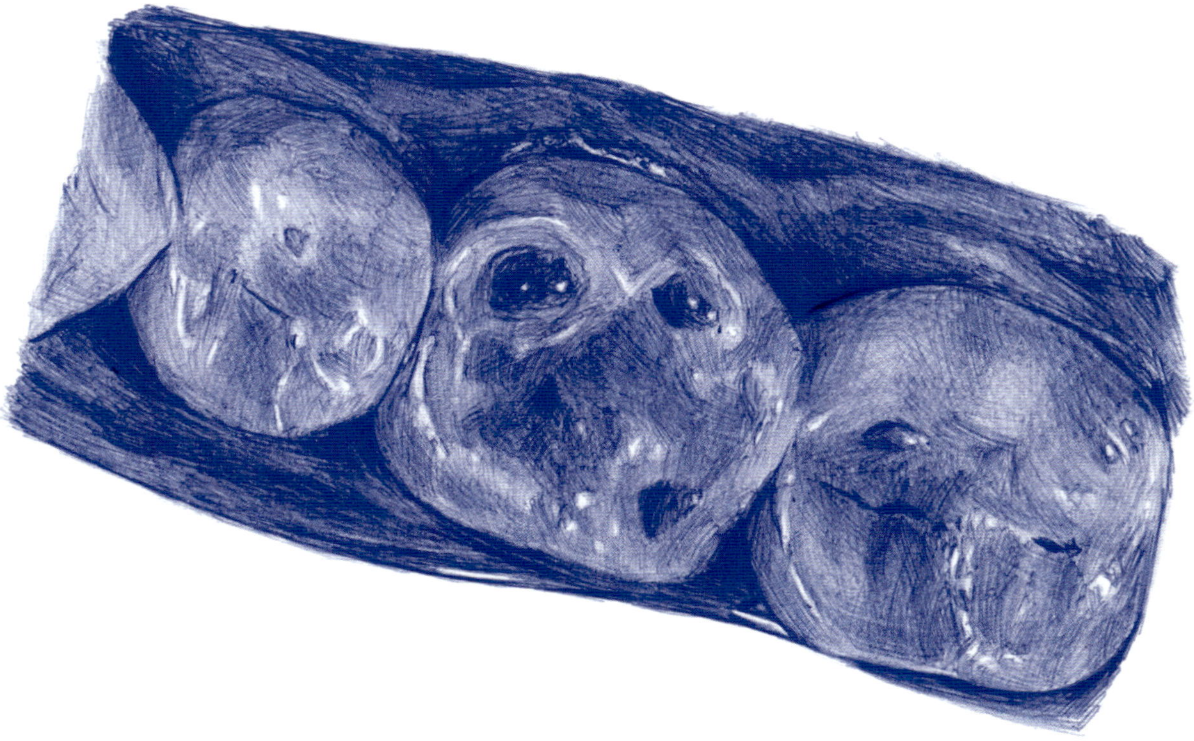

*No matter how great your dedication is, you never win anything on your own.*

—Rafa Nadal, Spanish tennis player

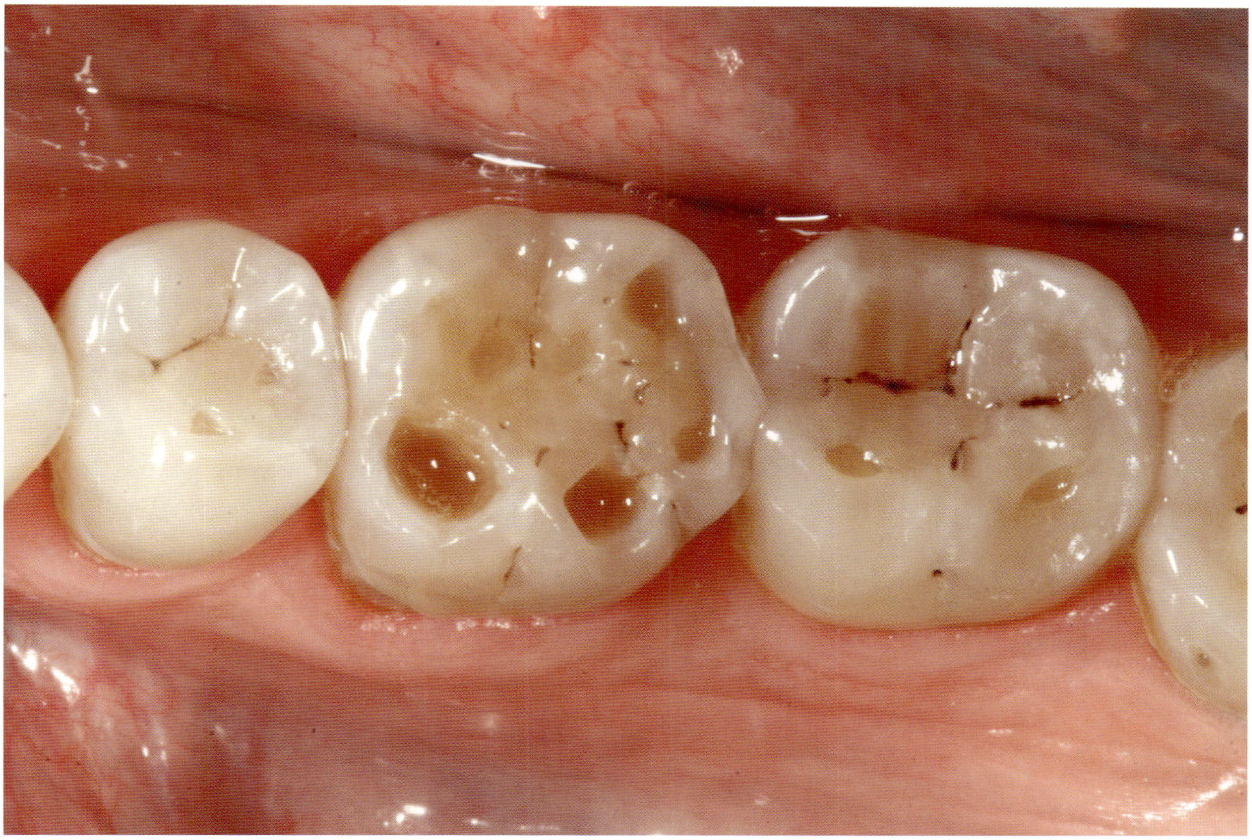

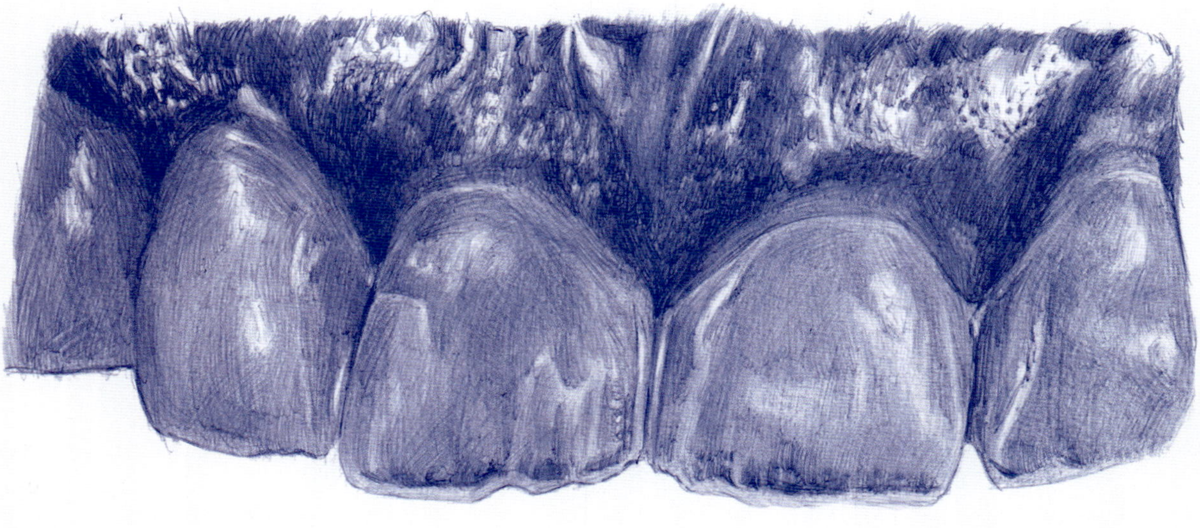

*The positive thinker sees the invisible, feels the intangible and achieves the impossible.*

—Sir Winston Churchill, Prime Minister of the United Kingdom

CHAPTER 6

# MODERATE TOOTH WEAR: TREATMENT STRATEGIES

Early incipient TW occurs usually in young, even very young patients, whose wear damage is localized in enamel, mostly in the anterior sector of the mouth. An uneventful function in the absence of pain is maintained along with so-called normal esthetics.

The majority of times, these patients either are not closely examined or encounter more times than desired a clinician reluctant to intervening. It is in the more advanced cases, usually in adults but increasingly in young patients, when the damage is quite clear, that clinicians feel more comfortable proposing a treatment.

While it is true that the damage might be small initially, the evidence shows that the remaining tooth structure is fundamental for the life expectancy of a tooth.

Regardless of the apparent simplicity of the additive adhesive procedures, TW management remains a challenge for the general dentist.

In this sense, moderate TW represents the quintessential challenge as it is sometimes difficult to fully comprehend what lies behind the physiopathology of nonbacterial TSL.

From the restorative-prosthetic point of view, the moderate TW patient should not fall under the classical full-mouth rehabilitation category. However, despite the fact that the destruction is not yet so severe, both arches should be addressed comprehensively.

In fact, in treating moderate TW there is a very thin line between under- and overtreatment. Choosing to treat only the most damaged teeth or the deepest lesions is the quickest way to treatment failure and a damaged patient-dentist relation. Instead, evaluating the damage and planning a treatment, respectful of the remaining tooth structure, is a clinically proven option to success and patient compliance.

## 1. Moderate TW: The Space Issue

The line between physiologic, age-related wearing of the dentition and abnormal pathologic TSL has been classified through a number of scales and models as described previously.

The distinction from incipient TW lies in the fact that in moderate TW both anterior and posterior teeth can be affected, posing a 3D challenge, as usually there is no apparent interocclusal space to deliver restorations without making space for them by reducing the amount of tissue.

Therefore, the intrinsic challenge is finding the space to deliver the restorations without sacrificing sound structure. Consequently, deciding to treat the case with orthodontics by finding free space in CR or otherwise to increase the VDO with restorative means and choosing the path—direct, indirect, or a combination of both—can be overwhelming to the untrained dentist (Figs 6-1 to 6-3).

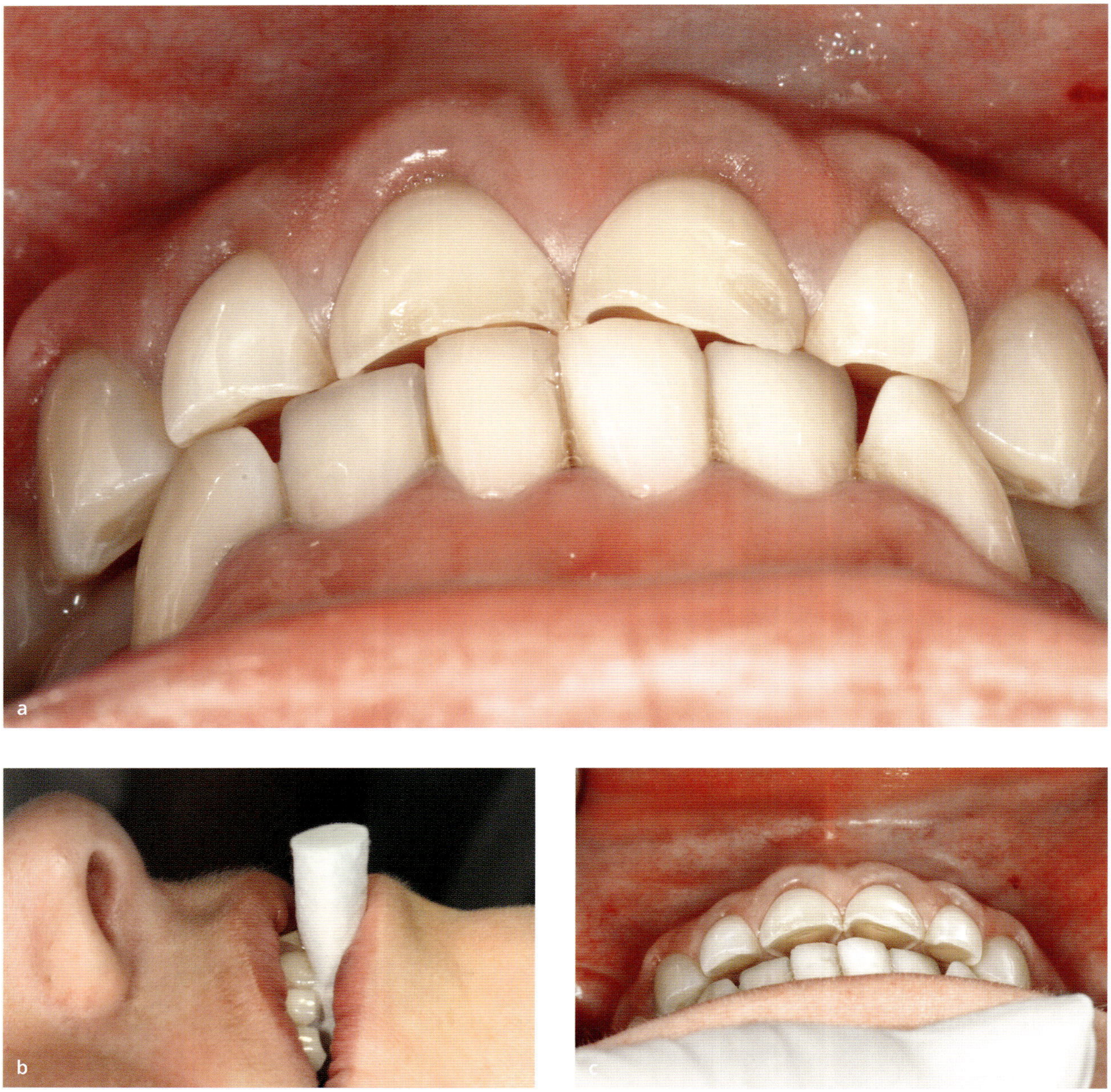

**Fig 6-1** A chairside hand manipulation revealed space in CR. A minor interference was adjusted, and a maximum of posterior contacts together with anterior PLV was able to stabilize the TW pattern over 20 years (a to c). (See chapter 7.)

For this reason, for many years it was common for exclusively the anterior teeth to be addressed with either direct composite or with indirect porcelain laminate veneers that only protected and restored the labial aspect, leaving the palatal of the maxillary teeth and occlusal of the posterior teeth untreated and unprotected from TW (Fig 6-4).

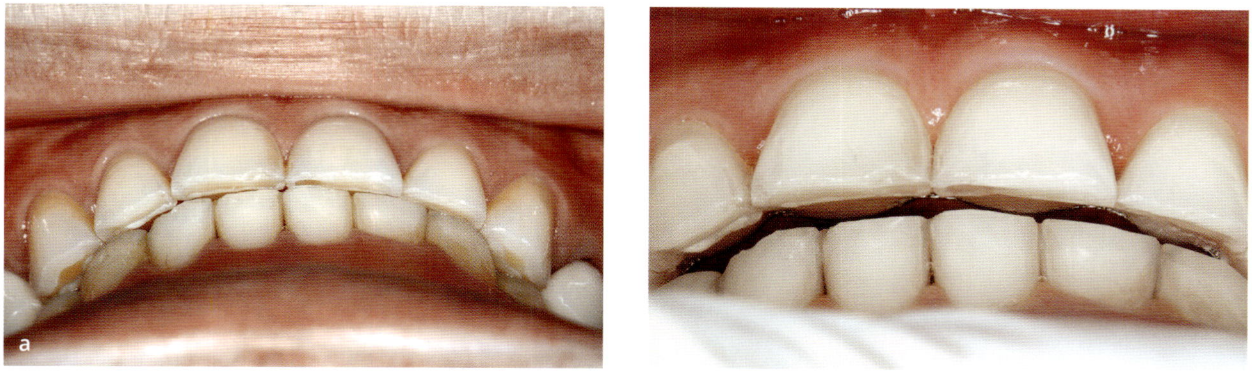

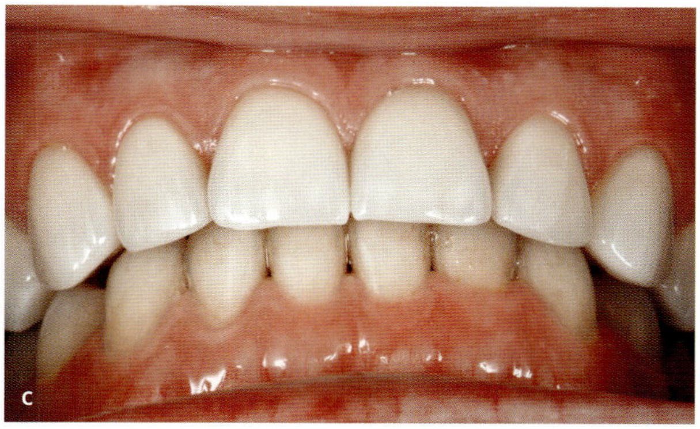

**Fig 6-2** An increase of the VDO solves the lack of interocclusal space as the manipulation in CR is not able to provide any space for the patient (a to c).

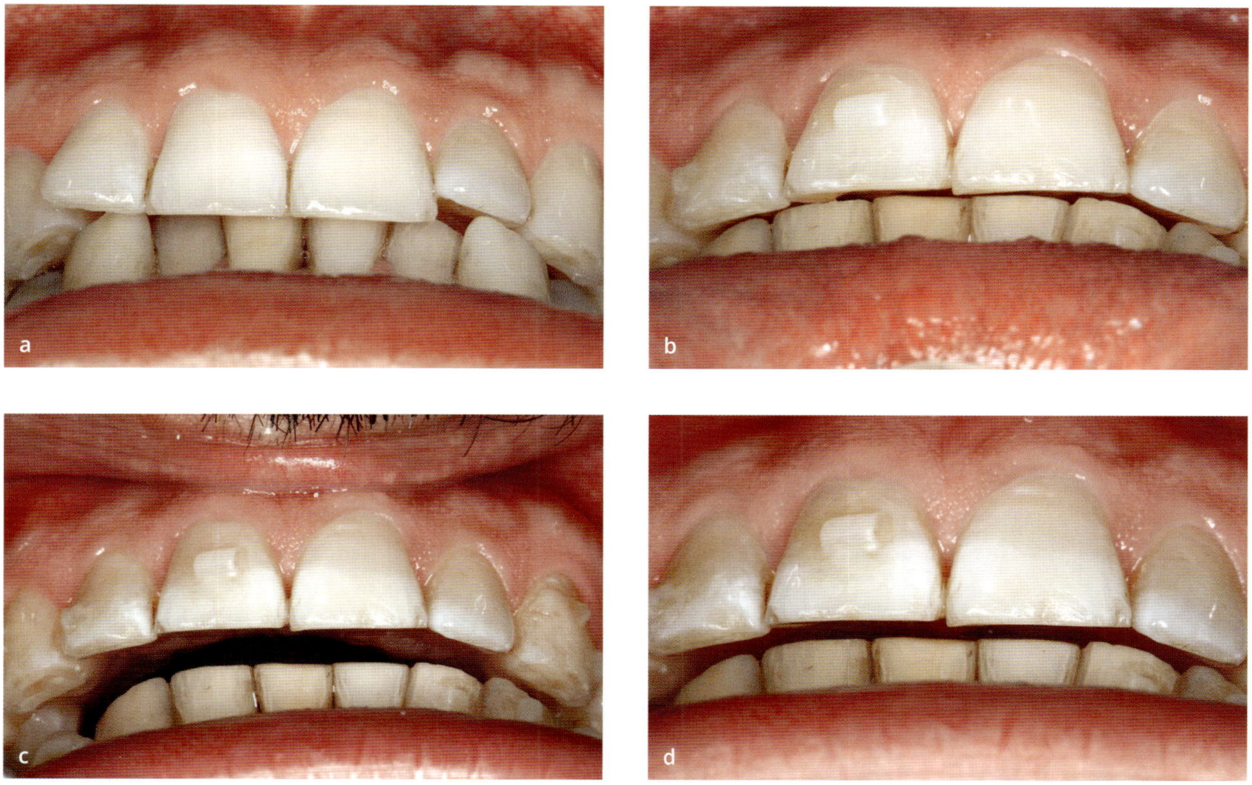

**Fig 6-3** An orthodontic path is chosen for a patient with a dentoskeletal Class II malocclusion (a). In the first months of orthodontics, the crowding has been resolved, but the interocclusal space is still insufficient (b). The CR proves the mandible to be too retrognathic and is discarded as tooth shape and form world need to be altered to enable anterior tooth function (c). At the end of the orthodontic phase, the posterior mandibular teeth are restored with an increase of 0.5 mm of the VDO. The correct tooth alignment and interocclusal space saves tooth structure (d).

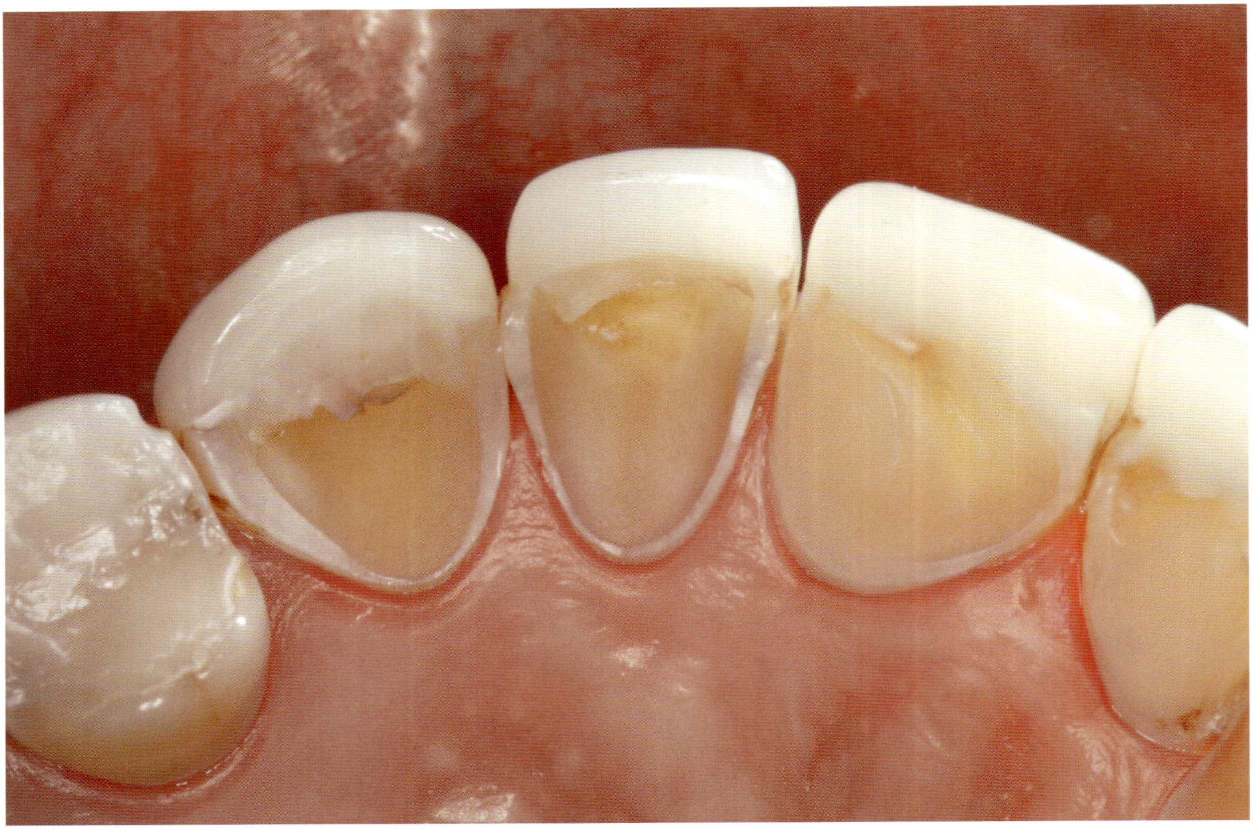

**Fig 6-4** This mode of treatment was the trend in the late 1980s and early 1990s, driven by the aging of the smile and the impact on esthetics and not based on the diagnosis of TW. Today it is not advisable to take such a partial approach, addressing only the vestibular defects, as time shows that the damage will go on irreversibly. Instead, the interocclusal space has to be found to provide the possibility of protecting all the worn surfaces with an appropriate adhesion protocol.

## 2. Adhesion to Worn Surfaces

Different types of TW produce various alterations in the tooth substrate that may negatively impact the final adhesion.

It has been reported that adhesion is greater when acid etching is performed on cross-sectional/transverse enamel prisms, while it is lower when acid etching is performed on longitudinal enamel prisms.

When restoring eroded occlusal surfaces, enamel prisms are exposed following a cross-sectional pattern, thus allowing optimal adhesion forces with conventional adhesion protocols (Fig 6-5).

In TW, especially in the moderate and severe stages, when indirect restorations are required, additional adhesion procedures may be beneficial. Such is the case with concepts such as immediate dentin sealing.[1]

When restoring eroded palatal surfaces, additional procedures have been recommended. If the restorations to be performed on the palatal aspects of maxillary incisors are "V" veneers (vestibulopalatal veneers), the challenge will be that traction forces will be added to the compressive forces. The use of "V" veneers results in more tooth reduction, another cause for worry regarding adhesion. Thus, optimization of the acid etching with prior aluminum oxide microabrasion might be beneficial (Fig 6-6).

If the selected restorations are exclusively palatal, then the standard acid-etch technique followed by a regular adhesion protocol will be enough to withstand the compressive forces[2,3] (Figs 6-7 and 6-8). Another benefit is the independent path of insertion, leading to more tooth structure preservation.

Adhesion to acid-eroded dentin is less predictable than to regular dentin; therefore, authors have recommended other steps such as rubbing with 5% sodium hypochlorite for 1 minute prior to the adhesive protocol. The rationale behind this is mainly its deep-cleaning properties and deproteinizing ability.[4]

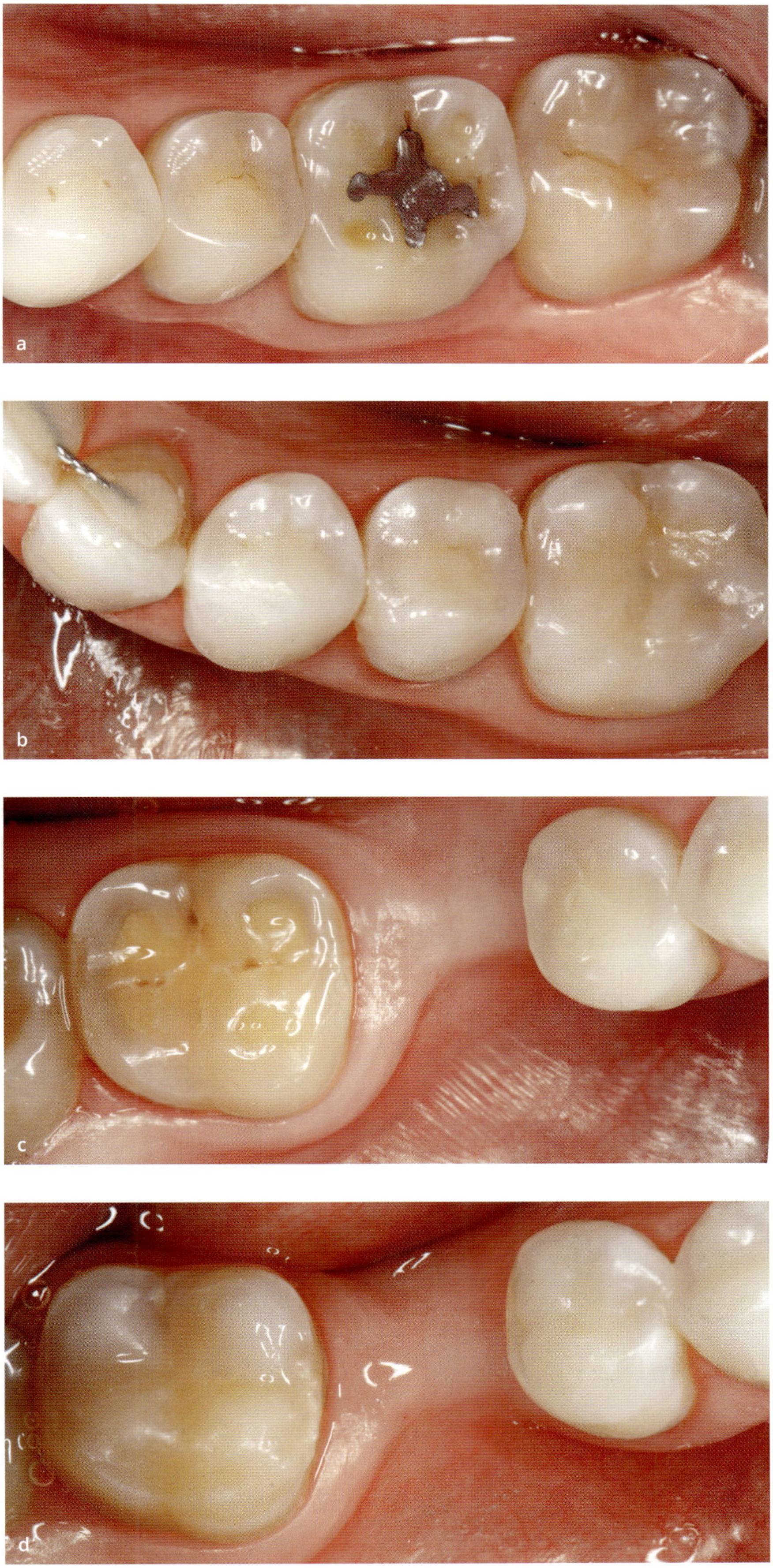


**Fig 6-5** The evolution in adhesion technology deserves to be recognized as fundamental for the noninvasive TW treatment modality. Moreover, additive concepts in the severely eroded dentition safeguard the remaining fragile "last frontier" before pulpal consequences. In this young girl, the erosive challenge will irrevocably destroy the anatomy of the teeth. A thorough anamnesis is not fruitful in revealing the erosive origin. Direct freehand composite is accepted by the patient, who was unaware of her TW (a to d).

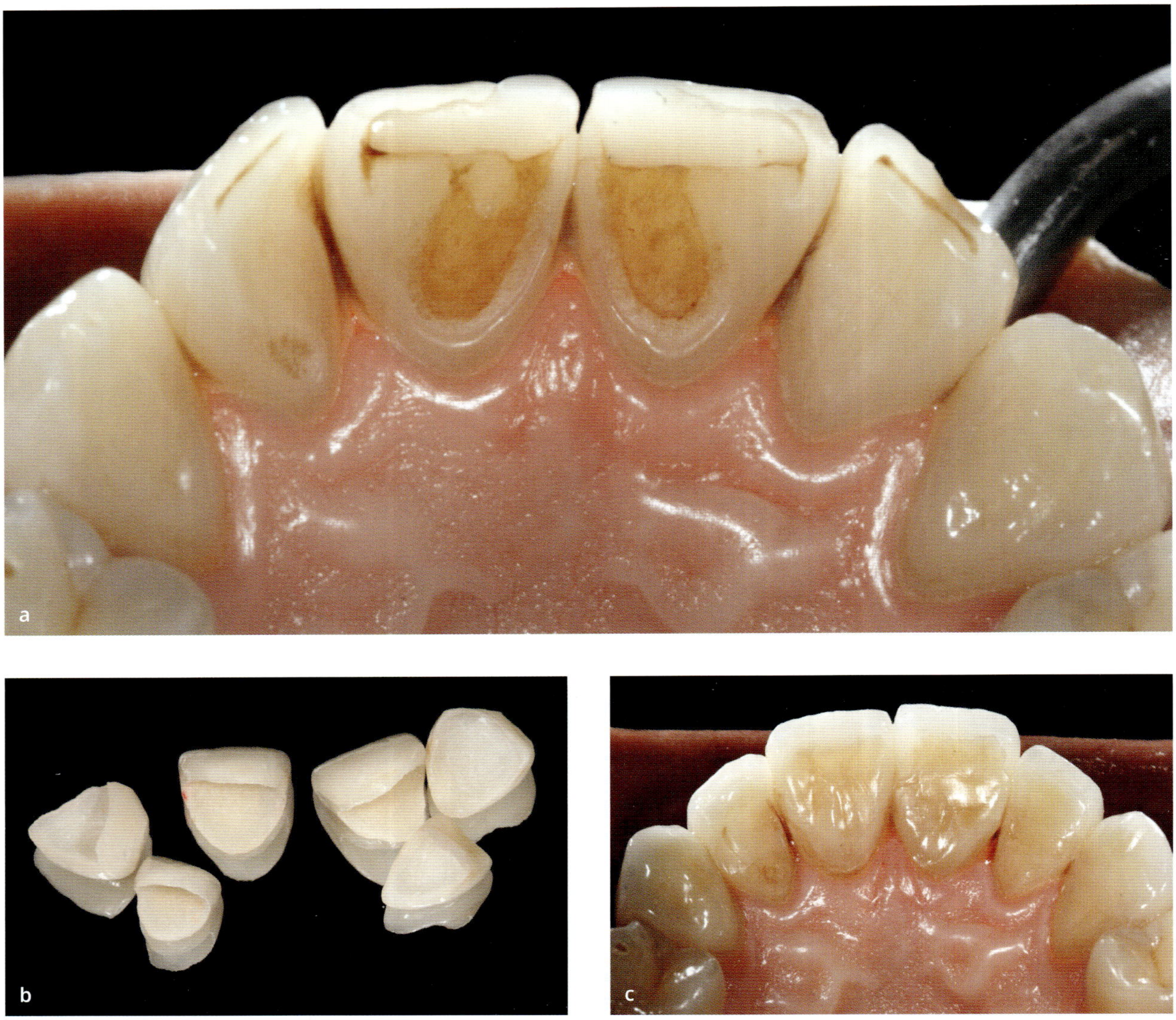


**Fig 6-6** Polymedication-induced xerostomia and intense stress in a young adult are behind the erosive signs (a) and impaired esthetics of the smile. "V" veneers were performed in feldspathic porcelain. Note the different palatal extension of the veneers depending on the extent of the palatal damage (b and c).

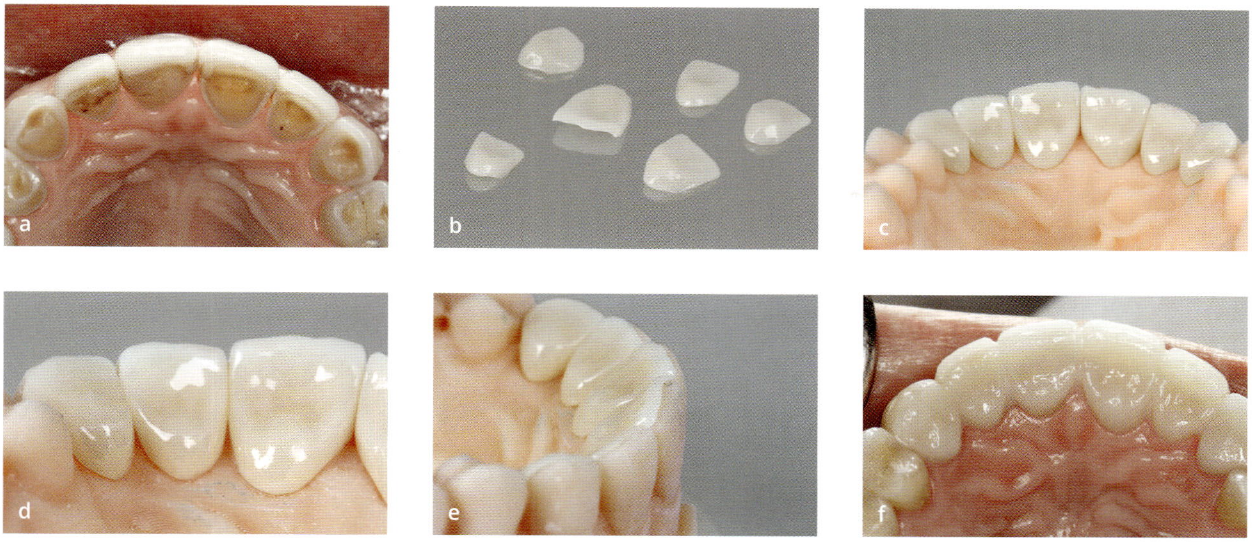

**Fig 6-7** It is increasingly common to see patients in the dental office whose previous treatment only addressed the vestibular erosive defects, leaving the palatal aspect of the teeth untreated. When vestibular PLVs are still in good service, functionally and esthetically, an option is to place palatal PICN or composite onlays. In this case the erosive damage (a) was treated with palatal CAD/CAM composite restorations (b to e) and no-prep onlays that do not overlap incisally as the existing vestibular restorations are being maintained (f).

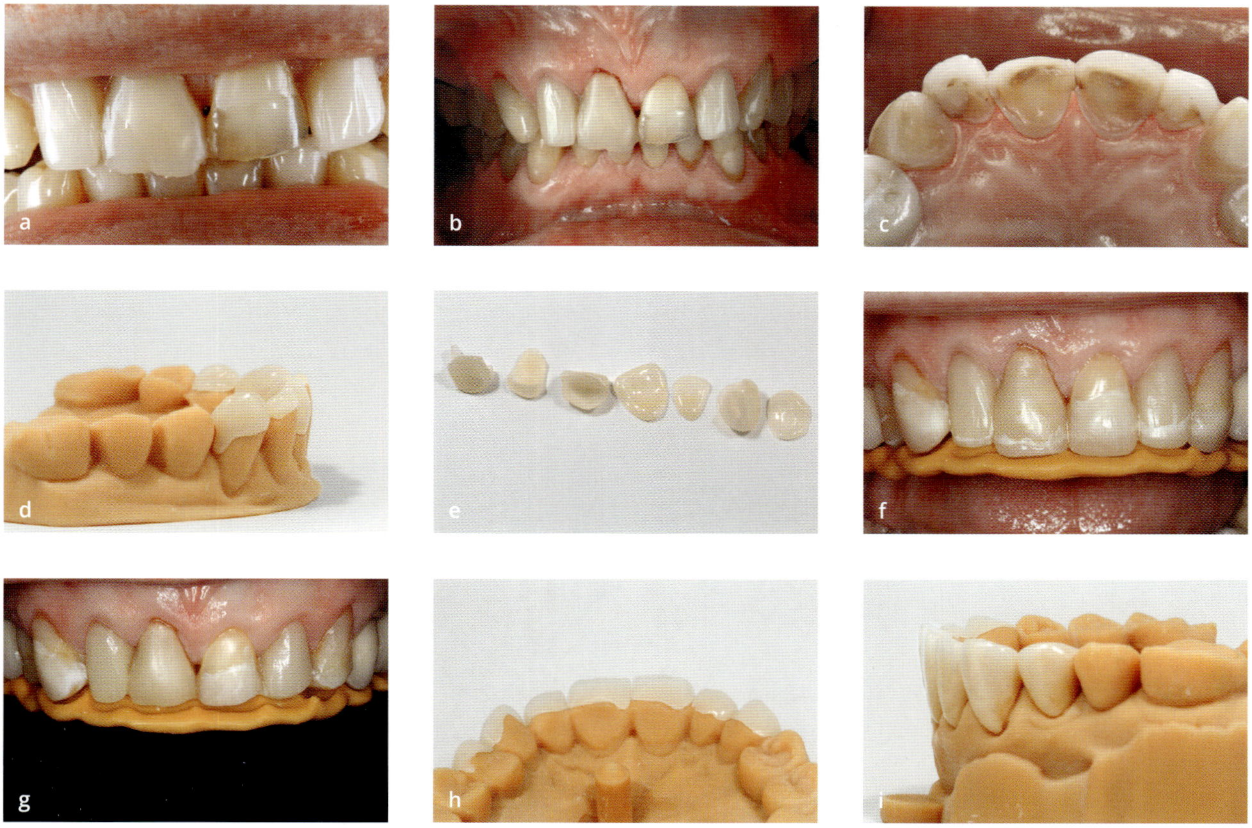

**Fig 6-8** In this case, no-prep palatal onlays are cemented first, rehabilitating both the palatal and incisal surface (a to e). Preparation for vestibular laminate veneers is performed later in the usual manner, providing space for incisal coverage (f to j). The palatal onlay will be overlapped incisally by the vestibular veneer.

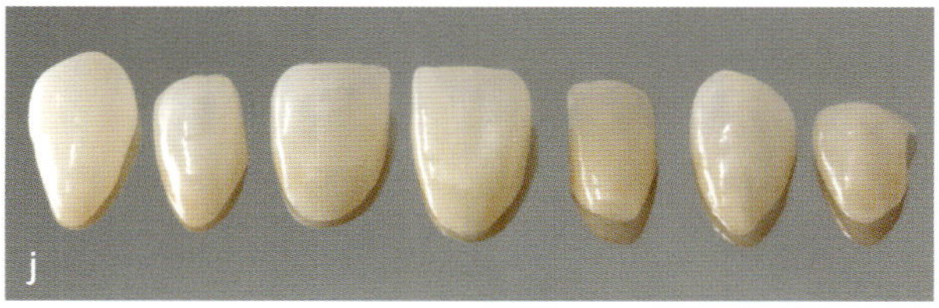

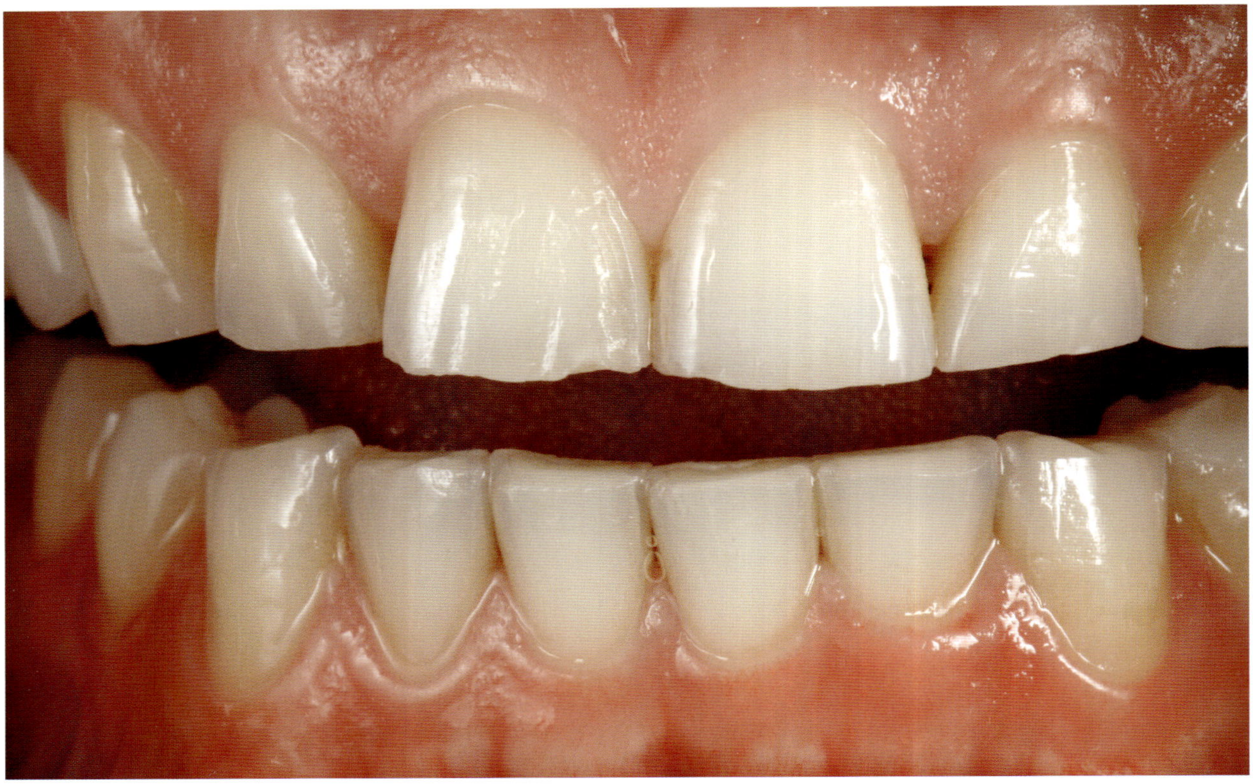

**Fig 6-9** Concomitant attrition and erosion is behind this moderate case of TW in a young patient in his early 30s.

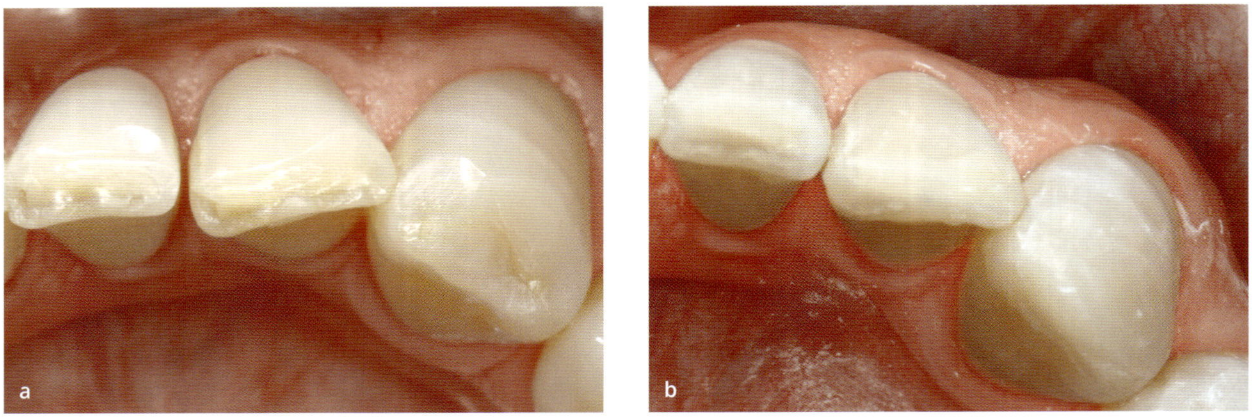


**Fig 6-10** Restoring the damaged structure with direct freehand composite in an anatomy-guided protocol is easy and affordable and can be repaired and updated when needed (a and b). The need for the same procedure in other areas of the mouth can be evaluated.

When facing abrasion or attrition cases, significant morphologic changes of the dentin have to be taken into consideration.[5,6]

Sclerotic exposed dentin creates difficulty for optimal adhesion. Several factors, such as the presence of an external mineralized bacterial layer or partially blocked dentinal tubules are behind the low final adhesion values, especially when self-etch adhesive systems are utilized.[6–9] In order to increase adhesion, some authors have recommended eliminating the sclerotic dentin layer with a fine diamond bur or aluminum oxide microabrasion prior to the application of the adhesion protocol.[2] However, the presence of hypersensitivity prior to treatment should be taken into consideration, and potential adhesion-enhancing procedures should be weighed carefully as any dentinal preparation in TW patients risks the onset of chronic pain (see chapter 7).

In those cases where erosion is combined with attrition or abrasion, the acidic dissolution will impede the formation of this sclerotic layer with the outcome of an acid-eroded surface easier to adhere to (Figs 6-9 and Fig 6-10).

## 3. Composite for Moderate Tooth Wear: Direct Versus Indirect

Composite resin materials are today the gold standard for partial anterior and posterior restorations. From the field of esthetic restorative dentistry in the anterior dentition to the restoration of TW, direct composites have demonstrated good performance.[10,11]

### Direct Freehand Composite Restorations

Interestingly, despite the demanding conditions of the worn posterior dentition, direct composite restorations have demonstrated good survival and performance for the posterior areas of the worn dentition, even in cases in which a vertical buildup is needed.[12,13] In addition, direct composite restorations offer an optimal approach to the reconstruction of worn mandibular anterior dentition as well as good performance in the rehabilitation of canine cusps (Figs 6-11 and 6-12).

Recently survival rates of direct hybrid composite resin have been rated from 50% to 99.3 % in the restoration of worn teeth in the short to medium term.[14]

However, the drawback of direct composite therapy is the artistry and creativity necessary to obtain natural results. A standard direct restoration is often not satisfying to the operator, who struggles to capture the anatomy, texture, and value of the adjacent teeth. While this may be an unattainable goal in some hands, there are very good guidelines for improving in this field.[15]

Since the development of the hybrid and microhybrid family of composites in the last decades of the 20th century until today, a quantum leap has occurred in the understanding that the enamel acts as a transparent shield, while it is in the core of the dentin that the color resides. The first is responsible for the value of the tooth, while the second will dictate the chroma of a given tooth.

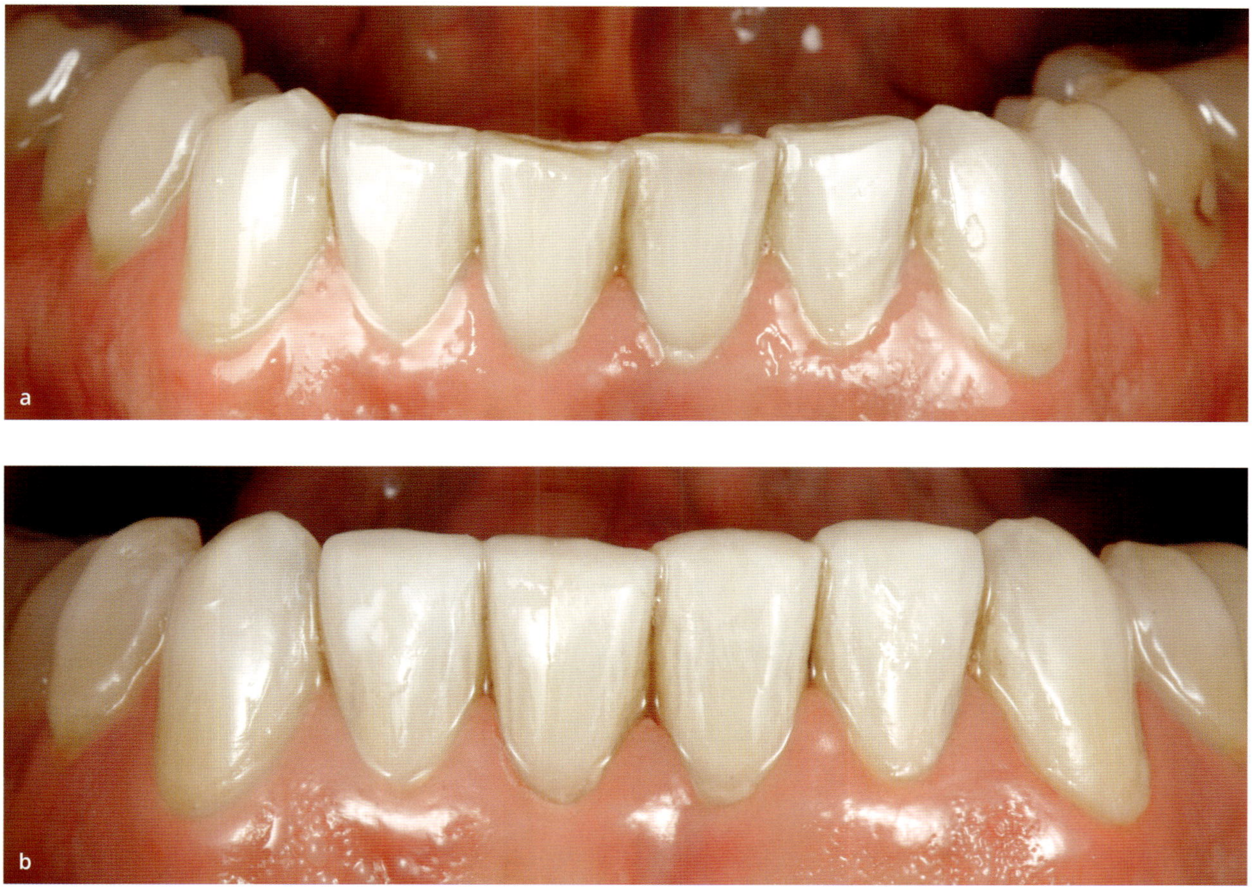


**Fig 6-11** It is common to perform restorations of the anterior mandible with direct composites in the patient with TW, provided the damage does not pass certain limits. Whether direct freehand anatomy-guided or semidirect with the aid of a wax-up-derived silicone guide, composites (eg, Filtek Universal by 3M) behave functionally and offer an overall satisfying outcome. The patient must know that repolishing, refurbishments, or repetitions should be expected (a and b).

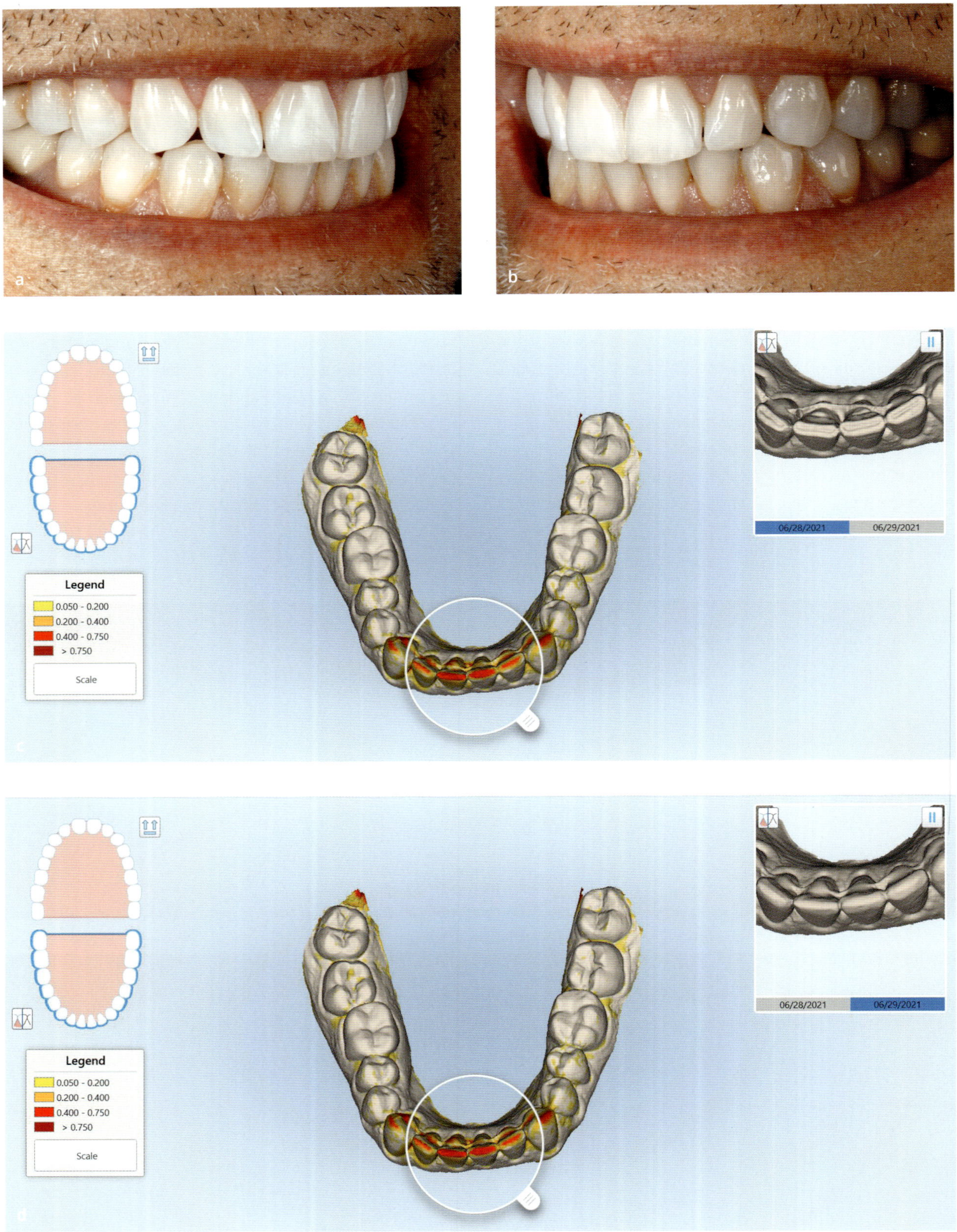


**Fig 6-12** Preserving an ideal occlusal scheme with a competent anterior and canine guidance is an adequate modus operandi to restore and prevent further wear. The use of additive composites (eg, Empress direct flow nanohybrid composite by Ivoclar) with the absence of tooth reduction is certainly indicated. Parafunctional habits have caused the damage in this case. Wearing an Essix-like soft mouthguard is highly recommended during the day in order to deprogram the damaging habits. Long-term monitoring of the survival of restorations can easily and automatically be done with the aid of a software comparative program (eg, Primescan OraCheck by Dentsply Sirona or iTero TimeLapse by Align Technology) (a to h).

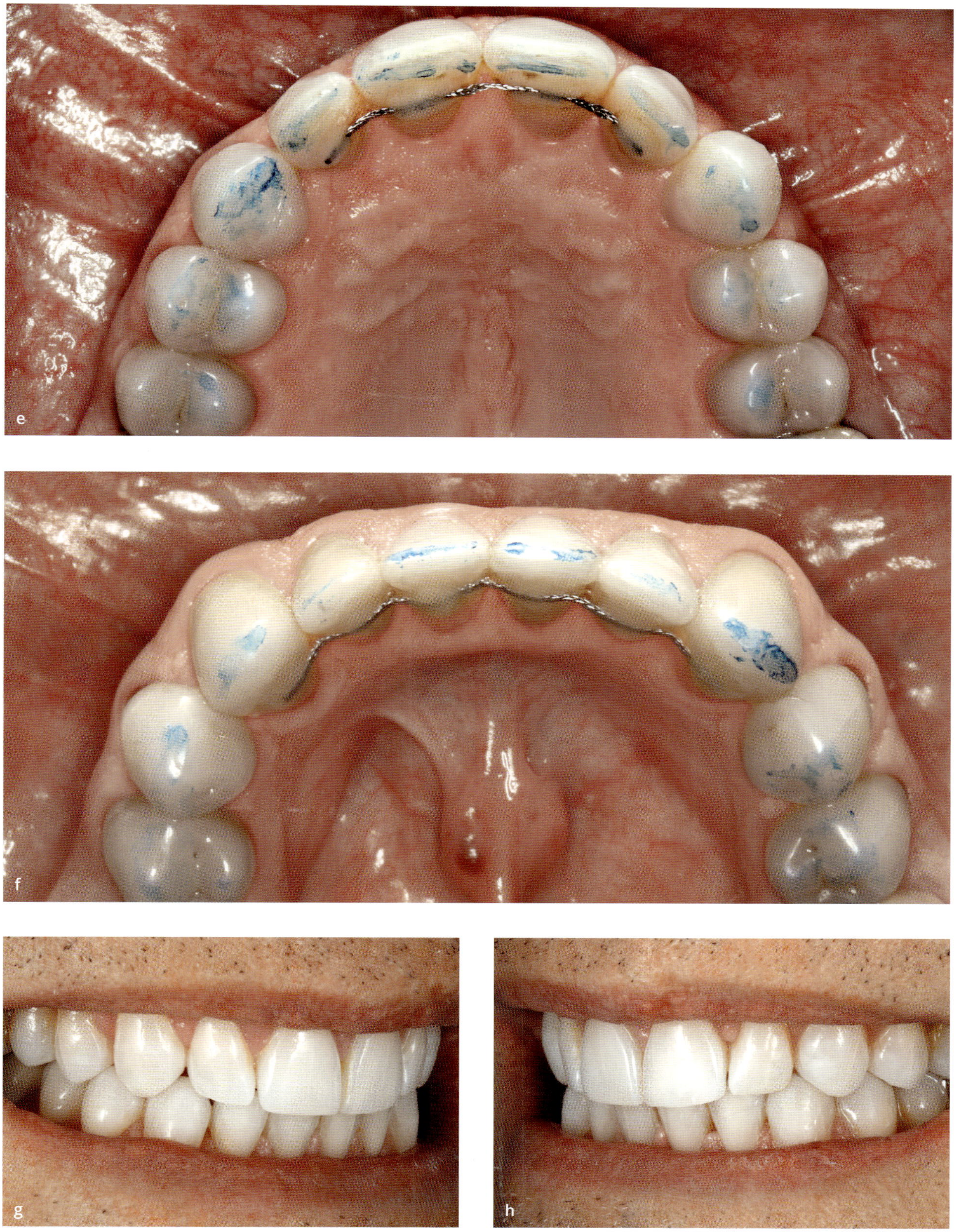


**Fig 6-12** *(continued)*

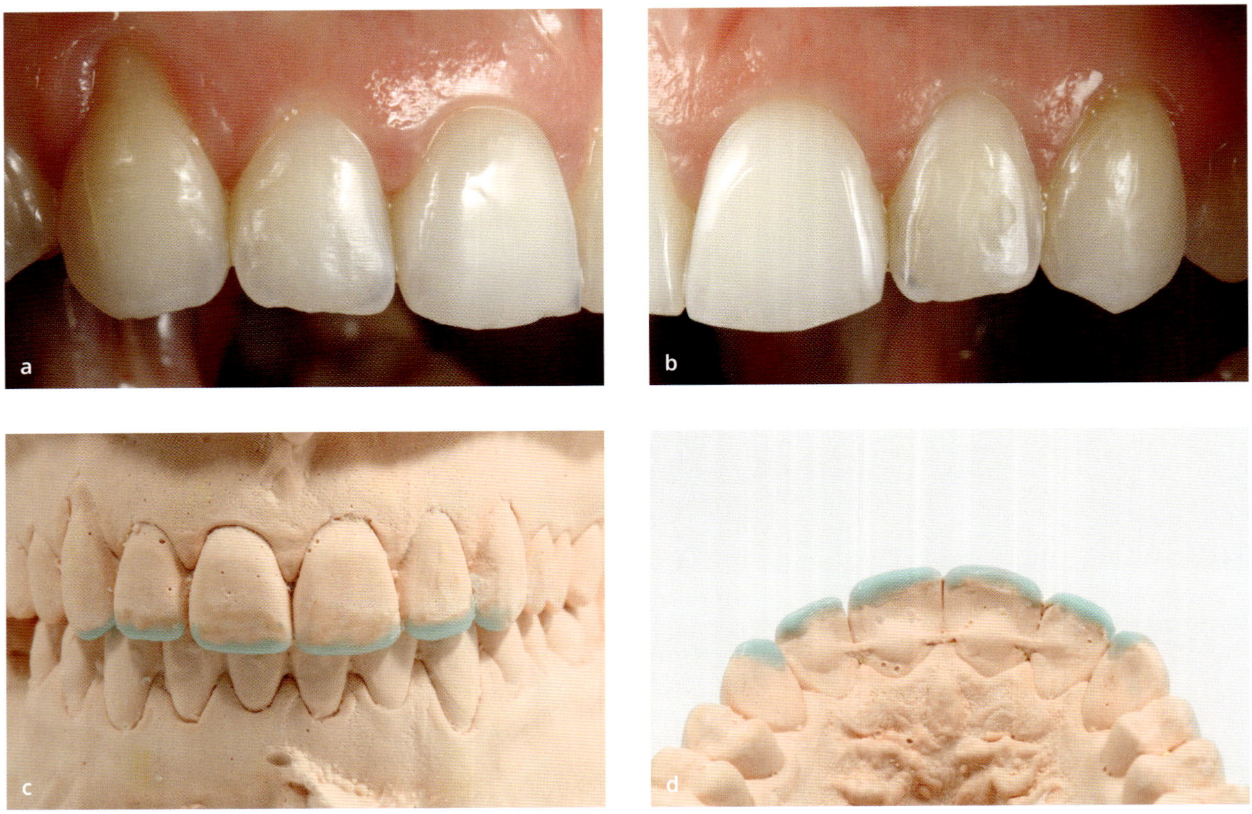


**Fig 6-13** A young girl is diagnosed with incipient TW that, in consideration of her age and the absence of a clear origin of wear, is upgraded to moderate TW (a and b). For multiple anterior restorations it is advisable to use a wax-up (c and d) of the ideal anatomy and produce a silicone index (palatal silicone index is by far the most widely used) that can assist during the reconstruction of the incisal wear. This is considered a semidirect protocol as a lab step is necessary as is a second appointment.

The trend today is to choose from several values of enamel composite (low, medium, and high) and several chromas of dentin composite. However, these techniques are not foolproof, and the finishing-polishing phase is critical for a natural final outcome.

In this sense, there are a number of schools of composite technology, which aim to bring the restorative dentist closer to the goal of imitating nature. Some have given rise to layering techniques and stratification protocols that aim to eliminate a complex armamentarium.[11,16]

Nevertheless, despite some simplified approaches, it is fair to recognize the masterpieces that some authors are able to create, with a seamless transition between natural and restorative substance.[17] A parallelism can be found in the masters of art whom are able to capture life on a flat canvas. Even though a sincere and honest effort should be made toward attaining the best esthetic result, it is in the patient's satisfaction where the dentist should be rewarded. This is even more critical if the dentist's concept of excellence would mean choosing a technique and material that would require more tooth structure sacrifice.

## Semidirect Composite Restorations

The difficulty of freehand composites can be overcome or at least reduced with the aid of an anterior wax-up and a silicone palatal guide. By doing this, a predictable outcome that avoids unnecessary stress and frustration will be accessible to every TW team (Fig 6-13).

Direct posterior composite restorations are less demanding than anterior composites from an esthetic perspective but pose a higher difficulty in cases where the anatomical destruction is extensive and the desirable anatomical or defect-oriented procedure cannot be performed.

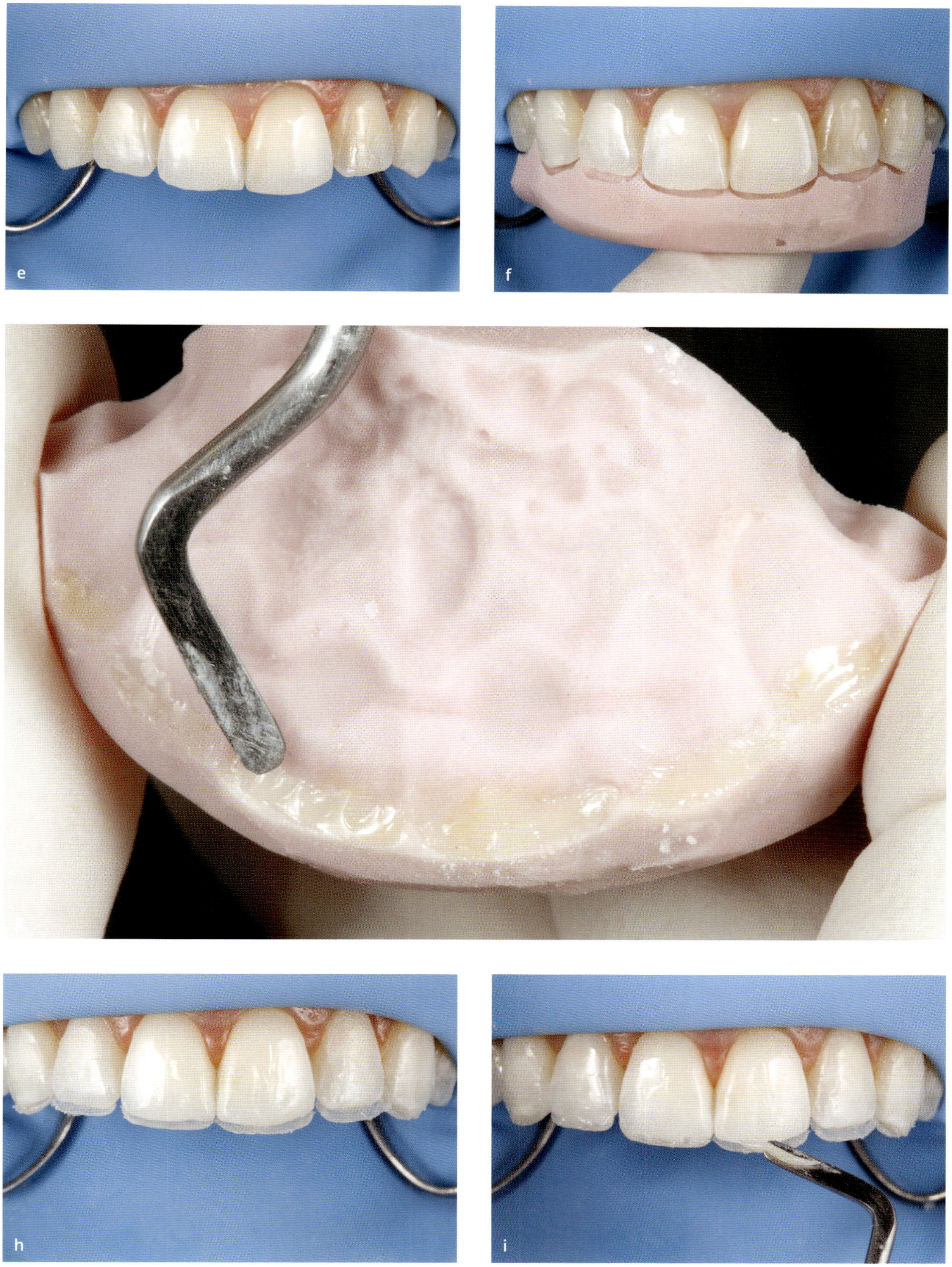


**Fig 6-13** *(continued)* Alternatively, an in-office wax-up can save one appointment. In this case it was deemed that the scope of the restoration did not justify outsourcing the wax-up. The simple procedure is an accessible treatment that provides efficient restoration with no sacrifice of the anterior tooth anatomy (e to j). Traslucent enamel composite is the sole approach for these incisal build-ups. Gingival inflammation is often times found in patients with erosive challenges (see chapter 3). *(continued next page)*

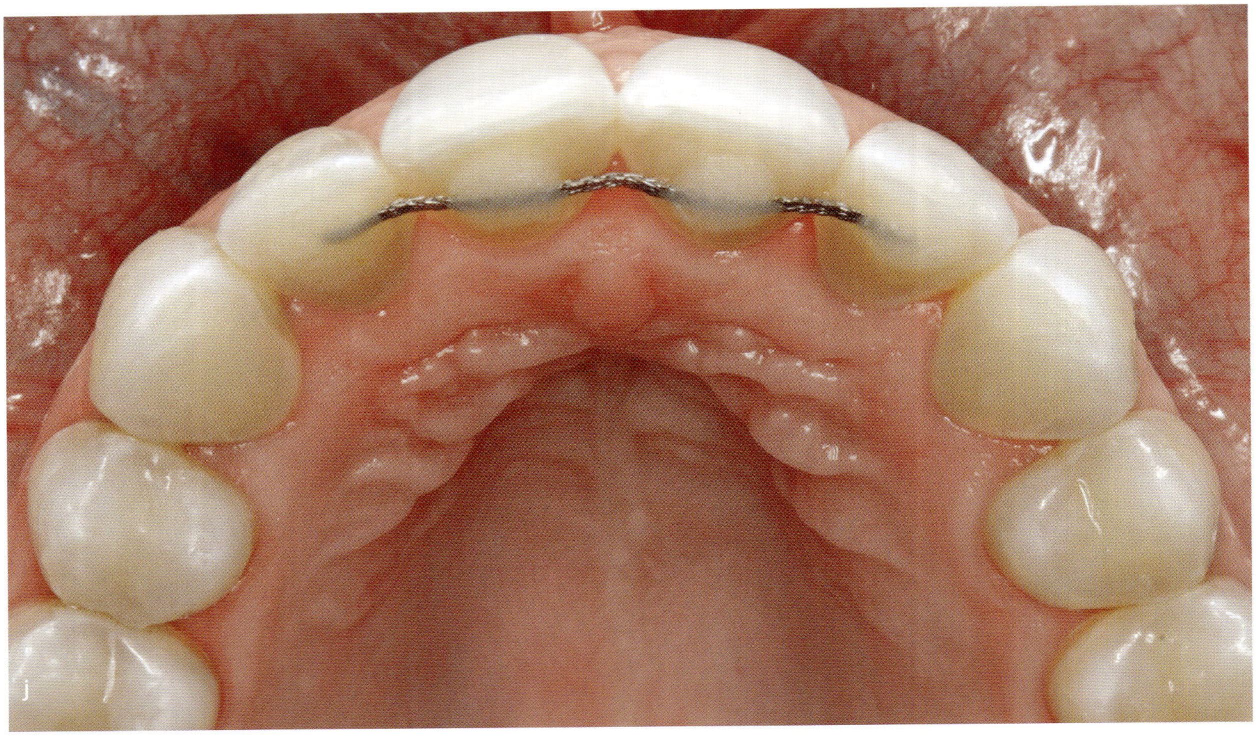

**Fig 6-13j** *(continued)*

In these cases, a number of techniques have been presented in order to transfer the wax-up, based on the estimated missing posterior anatomy, to the occlusal surfaces of the patient in a semidirect protocol. In this case, a transportation reservoir tray, be it silicone or a CAD/CAM relined resin template, is derived from the wax-up on the stone model or printed copy from the digital wax-up, loaded with the chosen composite material, and placed on the section to be restored.

Using an injectable flowable composite through a silicone or rigid tray is a fast and simple method that is indicated for lesions of limited extension or for transitional buildup of the damaged and worn dentition[18,19] (see chapters 4 and 5). Recent descriptions of the index and molding techniques explain in detail the importance of the mold or transportation tray.[20,21]

These techniques are not free of difficulties and drawbacks. A proof of this is the updates and modifications that have been published with the goal of simplifying the procedure and obtaining more precise results. Special attention needs to be paid at the occlusal embrasures if restoration of adjacent teeth is done at the same time because the composite resin may have invaded these embrasures. Interestingly, a newly published modification of the molding technique solves one of the critical issues in the restorative phase of the posterior teeth: the tedious individualization of the restored tooth once the composite is light cured.[21]

Whatever the restorative choice, the application of a standardized finishing and polishing protocol is important in achieving an acceptable result. This is particularly so in the case of nanofilled composites. Derived from nanotechnology, the amalgam of these composites is based on a cluster of nanoparticles whose intrinsic size and hardness variations might pose a challenge if a coarse bur brings them out.[22] On the other hand, the high strength, low wear, and excellent mechanical properties make them ideal for TW cases, especially in posterior lesions and in mandibular anterior teeth.[23]

## Indirect Composite Restorations. Accuracy of Diagnosis

When facing a patient with decades of TW evolution, it is mandatory to start with a solid diagnosis of the oral tissues. Good 3D diagnostic systems and new head positioning possibilities enable sharper images and less radiation (Figs 6-14 and 6-15). Assessing pulp vitality and apical health is critical and may change treatment decisions. Sometimes, long-term pulp damage cannot be totally discarded nor should preventive devitalization be completed. If an endodontic treatment is required in the future, PICN onlays can be perforated and easily repaired without endangering the durability of the restoration.

With the use of 3D imaging, it is more feasible to maintain tooth vitality for a long time.

In moderate to severe TW, indirect restorations are needed whenever the physical or esthetic performance of the direct restorations may be judged to be insufficient or inadequate. New preparation guidelines that facilitate optimal optical blending of the restoration to the tooth as well as enable adequate flow of resin during cementation should be taken into account as classical onlay/inlay preparation has given way to a more natural preparation referred to as *morphology-driven preparation*.[24]

Composite blocks can be used for posterior occlusal and anterior palatal onlays or overlays. One of the advantages is the possibility of milling thin margins with composite and composite-based materials such as polymer-infiltrated ceramic network (PICN; eg, Enamic by VITA) as they can be milled even down to 0.2 to 0.3 mm if needed (Fig 6-16). The advantage of such thin structures is to allow for a shallow tooth preparation or avoiding it altogether. The negative effect of such a thin restoration is that the thin, fragile margin might not endure the full milling process or might break during cementation; however, these thin margins will be embedded in the luting composite and polished after polymerization without any detectable gap.

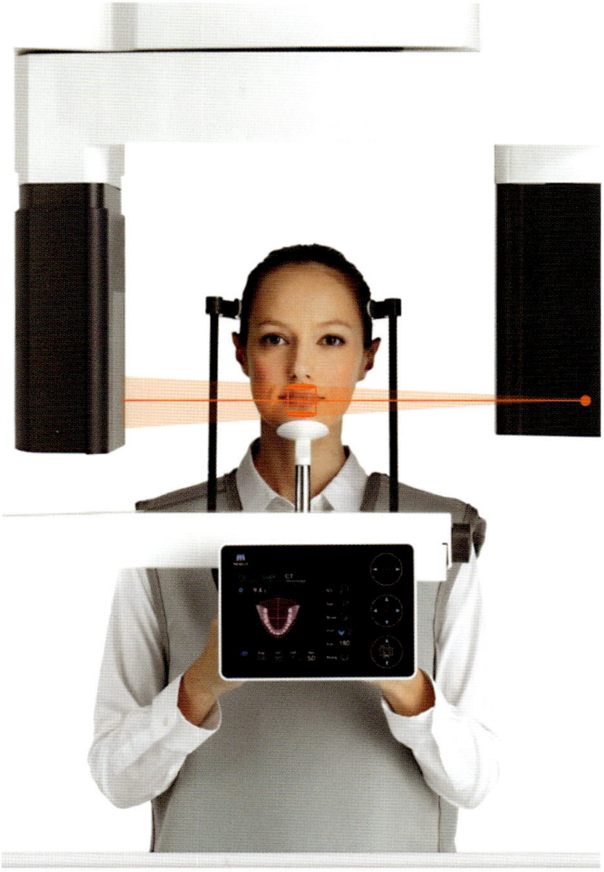

**Fig 6-14** Veraview X800 system by Morita shows a relaxed individually fitted head positioning that enhances image quality and facilitates accurate diagnosis. The operator faces the patient, ensuring there are fewer positioning errors. (Courtesy of Morita.)

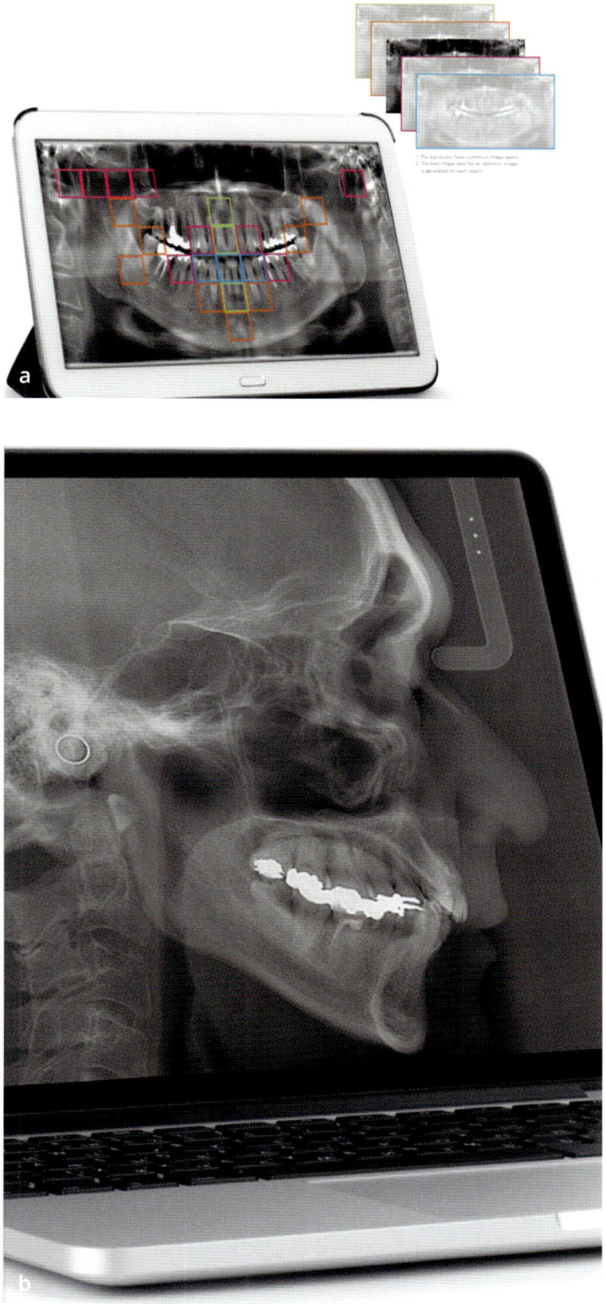

**Fig 6-15** Network connection facilitates communication among the TW team, which includes the patient, and results in a higher compliance and acceptance (a). Cephalometric images for treatment planning and control are possible because of improvements in the X-ray exposure and dosage, enabling facially oriented TW treatment planning (b).

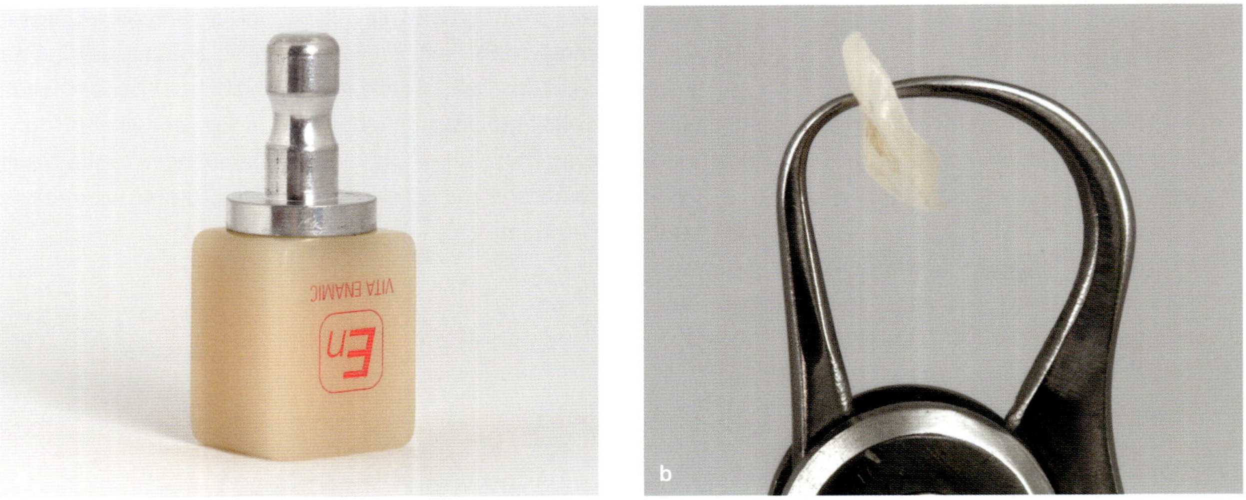


**Fig 6-16** In posterior moderate TSL the choice between indirect restorations varies from PICN (eg, Enamic by VITA) (a) to composite, both with good performance in thin depths of 0.5 mm or even less (b). PICNs have occlusal load–absorbing properties that may be more suitable for cases where high occlusal load is expected, especially as they fulfill the prerequisite of being easily repaired, adjusted, or modified. Nevertheless, in cases for even shallower lesions, there is still an indication for direct composite restorations with the virtue of not removing sound tooth structure at all.

## Dental Restoration Repair: The Case of Japan

Repairing defective restorations is an effective means of increasing restoration survival. Even more, following the Minimata Convention, it was recommended that all new graduates from 2020 onwards should have the knowledge, skills, competence, and confidence to effectively restore the damaged and diseased posterior teeth with state-of-the-art resin composite systems.[25]

Less invasive and clinically simpler procedures are finding their way into clinical practice. A recent university-based retrospective study in a susceptible group of patients with high caries risk has proved that the reparation of old existing restorations increases the survival of failed primary tooth restorations.[26]

Repairing dental restorations, namely defective resin composite restorations, has received the attention of educators in more Japanese dental schools in comparison to other schools abroad.[27] In a recent survey, the most used approach for composite repair was a flowable resin composite.[28,29] The trend has been followed in other countries, such as the US, Canada, Scandinavia, the UK, and more.[27,30–32]

Japan has become the country with the longest life expectancy in the world, with an increasing group of aging individuals affected by moderate and severe TW. Longevity, nutrition and dietary habits, hyperconnectivity, commuting, and stress in the middle age decades of life all add up. Concomitantly, people in Japan are wanting to keep their natural teeth for longer.[33]

Manual skills and digital technology together with composite science have reached outstanding levels in Japan.[11,28] Taking into consideration all that is mentioned above, it is only logical that undergraduate programs in Japanese universities have introduced the study of the reparability of dental restorations. Deep knowledge of the types of restorations and their specific repair procedures is mandatory. In this sense, being able to trace details regarding the type of composite used in an existing restoration is an important factor in the success of its reparation[34] (see more on the value of keeping the same doctor in chapter 10).

Japanese gastronomy has a well-deserved reputation and has seen unprecedented worldwide expansion. Nonetheless, inclusion of vegetable oils such as soybean oil may be advisable in order to protect teeth against TW, especially with erosive dietary patterns. Soybean oil has proven benefits to general and cardiovascular health as a source of polyunsaturated fatty acids. Essential and vegetable oils have been studied in regard to their effect on the acquired enamel pellicle in initial erosion[35–37] and as plaque-removing agents. The availability of soybean oil in Japan makes it a good candidate for further studies.

## 4. Palatal Restorations for Tooth Wear

The well-explained and well-structured three-step technique developed by the Geneva group, a sandwich technique in which the anterior teeth of the maxilla are restored palatally with indirect composite laminates and immediately after with labial porcelain laminate veneers, is a good option[38–40] (Fig 6-17).

The palatal reinforced composite indirect veneers protect the damaged area where TSL has taken place, be it through partial or a total coverage of the palatal aspect of the anterior teeth. In cases where the VDO has been increased in order to be able to deliver the posterior and/or anterior restorations to the rest of the teeth, it is also possible to close the gap created between the maxillary and mandibular anterior teeth with palatal veneers on the maxillary anterior teeth. This approach prevents the team from delivering artificially long mandibular incisors in order to achieve interincisal function. Palatal no-prep onlays also rehabilitate the worn incisal third. The palatal veneers are cemented with a composite cement.

The palatal onlays will reproduce the final length as they cover the worn incisal edge of all anterior teeth (see Fig 6-7f). Once this has been implemented on the incisal edge of the palatal veneers, they will be reduced to enable the wrapping of the labial porcelain veneers, which will be restoring the anterior guidance and the esthetic needs of the case. Therefore, this extra length of the palatal veneers will reproduce the length of the in vivo mock-up, which was approved by the patient and phonetically and functionally tested.

Some clinicians will still prefer to restore the damage directly with direct composite freehand restorations.[41] In localized lesions, this might be a practical approach as the manipulation and placement of the milled palatal pieces is more difficult the smaller they are.

In some cases, the situation might be more complex. One can encounter extensive and deep palatal erosion, and still the posterior sectors might be unharmed, for example, in cases of erosion caused by gastric acid, such as repeated vomiting or reflux. In the case of vomiting, the downwards position of the head explains why the front teeth get harmed most. In such situations it is sometimes difficult to find an indication to increase the VDO, and alternatives such as orthodontics or exploring the existence of a naturally occurring freedom in centric will help in solving the dilemma.

As explained before, some patients naturally benefit from what has been traditionally recognized as *freedom in centric*. This means that the patient keeps a maximum number of posterior contacts within the movement from MIP to CR, with a comfortable occlusion in both positions dictating a slight space between the maxillary and mandibular anterior teeth.[42] Also described as *freeway space*, this should only happen naturally and should not be the result of a dental procedure or be in conflict with natural tooth form. In other words, some patients cannot benefit from CR because their dentoskeletal condition would require alteration of tooth form to enable anterior contact[43] (Fig 6-18).

This approach might be a good option in cases with a strong component of erosive wear. On the contrary, in cases with damage caused by attrition or clenching, this approach might have the opposite effect as patients might not tolerate the loss of free space and start behaving as in a restricted envelope of function.

In addition, not all patients have this convenient space between CR and MIP. In patients treated in the past with orthodontics, it is not unusual to find a Class I occlusion with CR and MIP coinciding. If space is needed for reconstructions, another round of orthodontic therapy or a restorative increase of the VDO if posterior teeth are in need of restorations are good alternatives to subtractive methods.

In patients in whom a skeletal discrepancy is limiting the reconstruction in occlusal schemes different from MIP, an augmentation of the VDO should be considered (Fig 6-19).

Generally speaking, if such free space is not present, ie, in cases where interocclusal restorative space is missing between the maxillary and mandibular anterior teeth, especially with a mechanical component, a strong recommendation for orthodontic therapy should be discussed with the patient (see chapter 9).

### Indirect Composite Onlays and PLVs

While the use of composite veneers on the palatal aspect of the anterior teeth seems to be the standard protocol, there are some authors who also advocate for their indication on the labial aspect of anterior teeth.[44]

An easier lab technique and a lower cost for composite veneers need to be taken into consideration in certain circumstances, both for palatal and labial indications.[45] Another main reason to consider composite veneers is better absorption of occlusal forces by composite versus porcelain, together with enamel-forgiving wearing properties. Therefore, some authors see these as being indicated for patients in whom attrition is a major cause of TW.

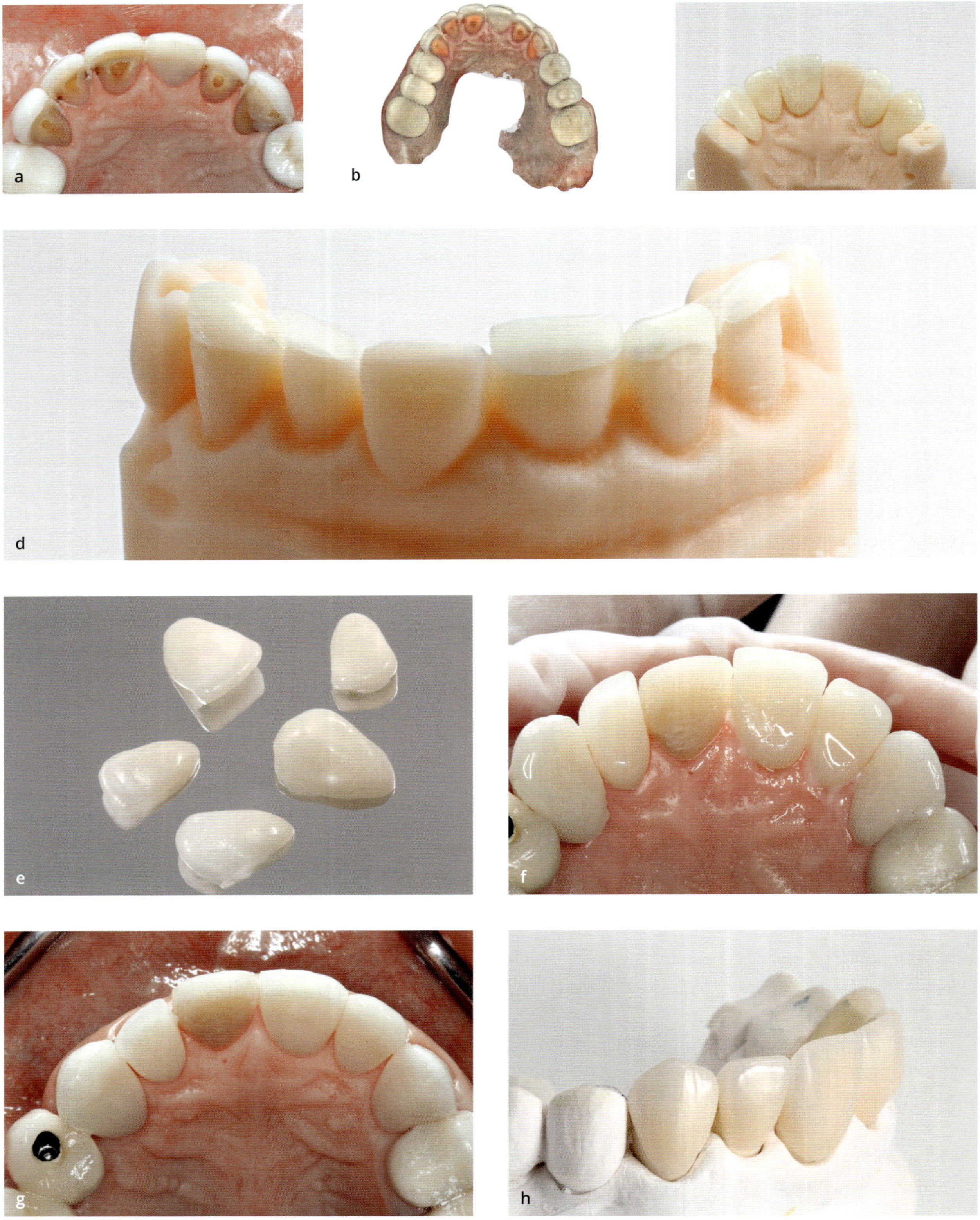

**Fig 6-17** Chronic asthma medication intake and GERD are the most probable causative factors in this patient. In addition, a restricted envelope of function has contributed to severe palatal wear and destroyed the anterior protection of the mouth in function (a and b). After orthodontic treatment (Invisalign, Align Technology) the new overjet provides interocclusal space for the palatal onlays that will restore the damaged palatal surfaces. In this case the apparently aged dentition does not correspond to the patient's age and even less to her long life expectancy. Splitting the needed anterior reconstructions into two distinctive indirect restorations done one at a time, first palatal (c to f) and then labial (h), not only may be more advantageous retention-wise but also certainly helps preserve tooth structure. The smile improvement is the consequence of the comprehensive rehabilitation of the TW collapse and restoration of the worn dentition (i to k).

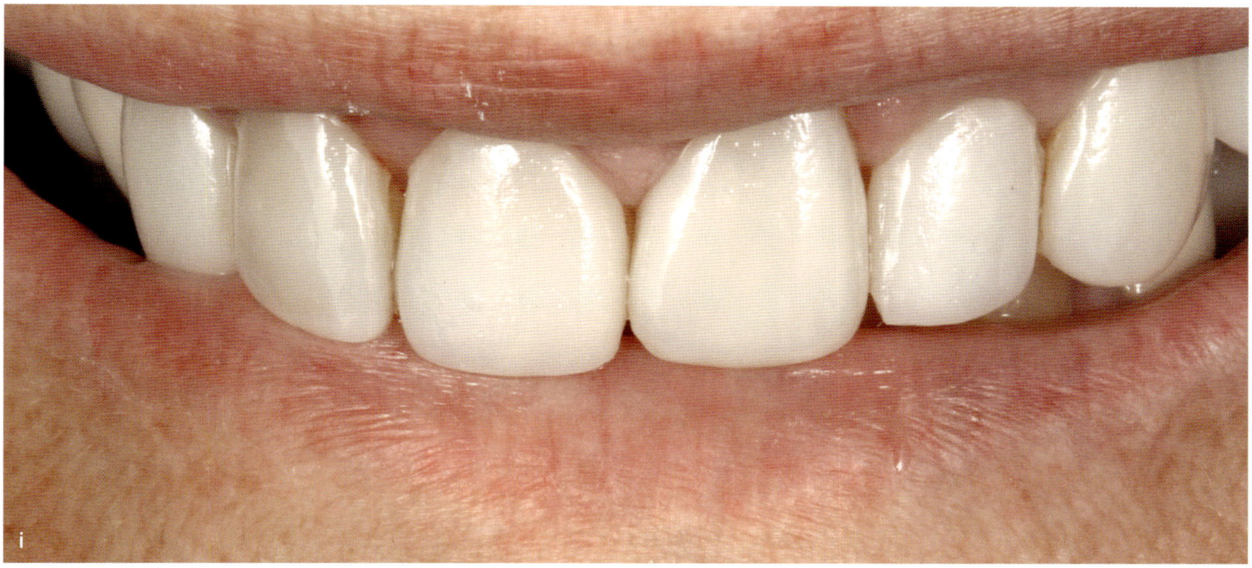
i

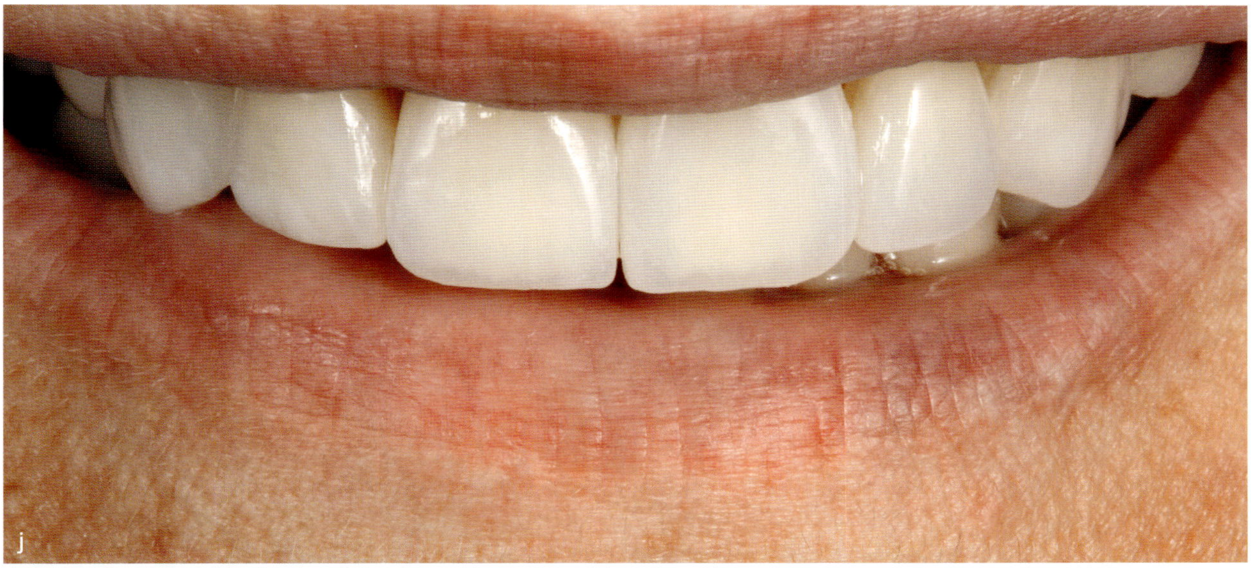
j

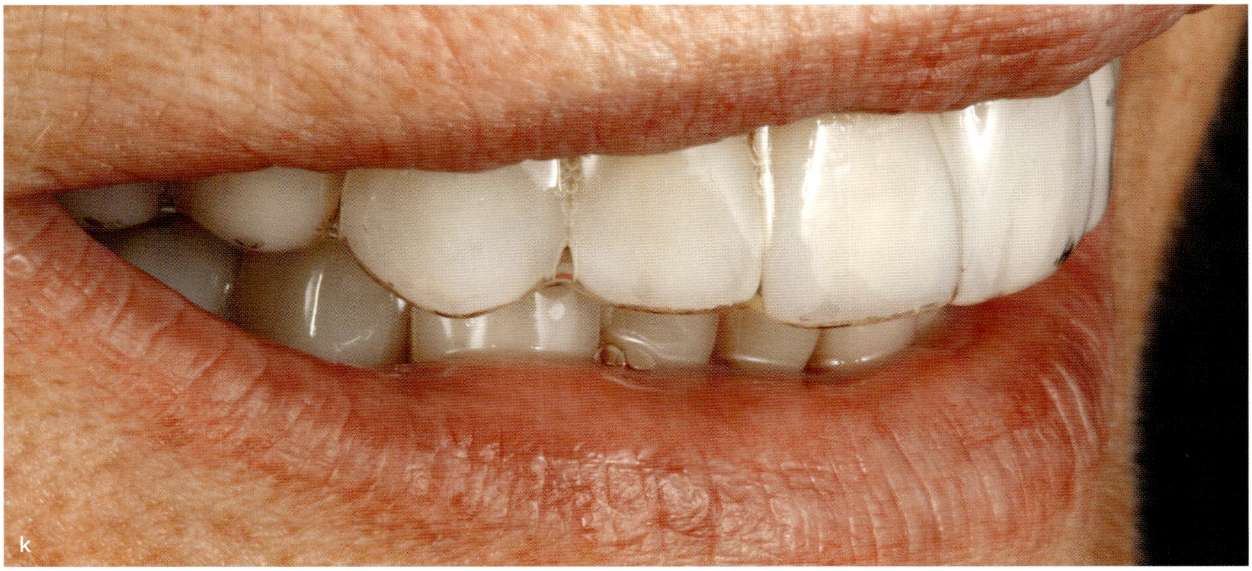
k

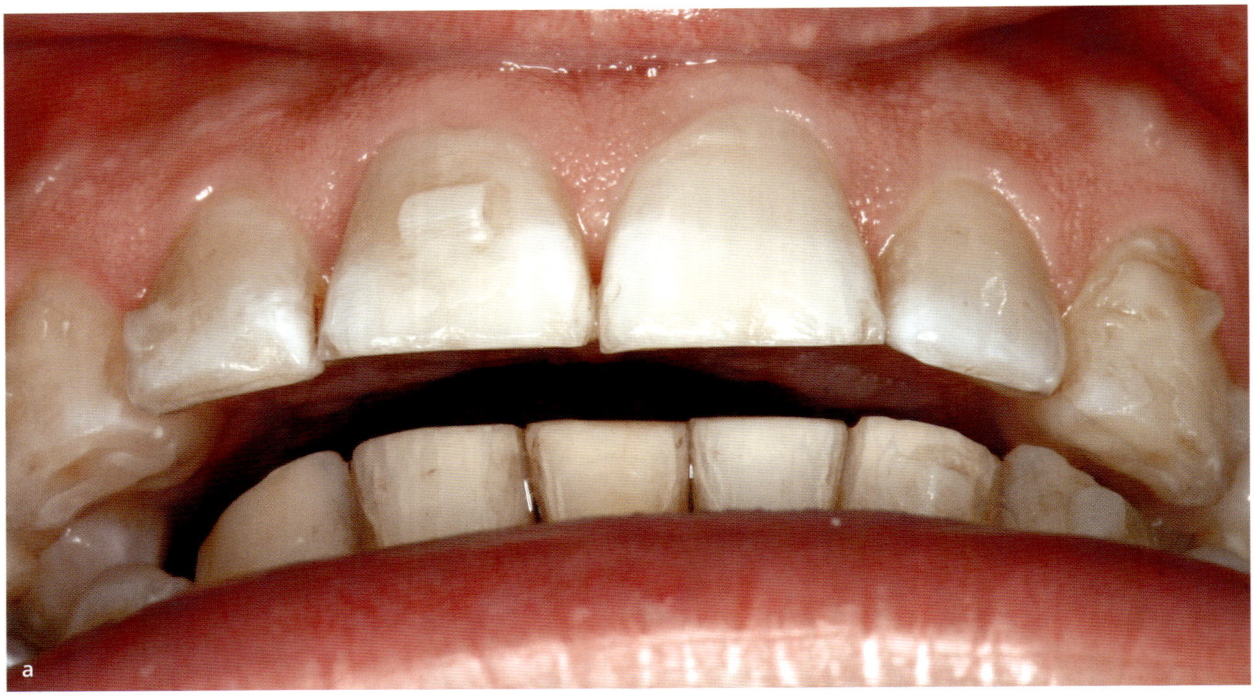


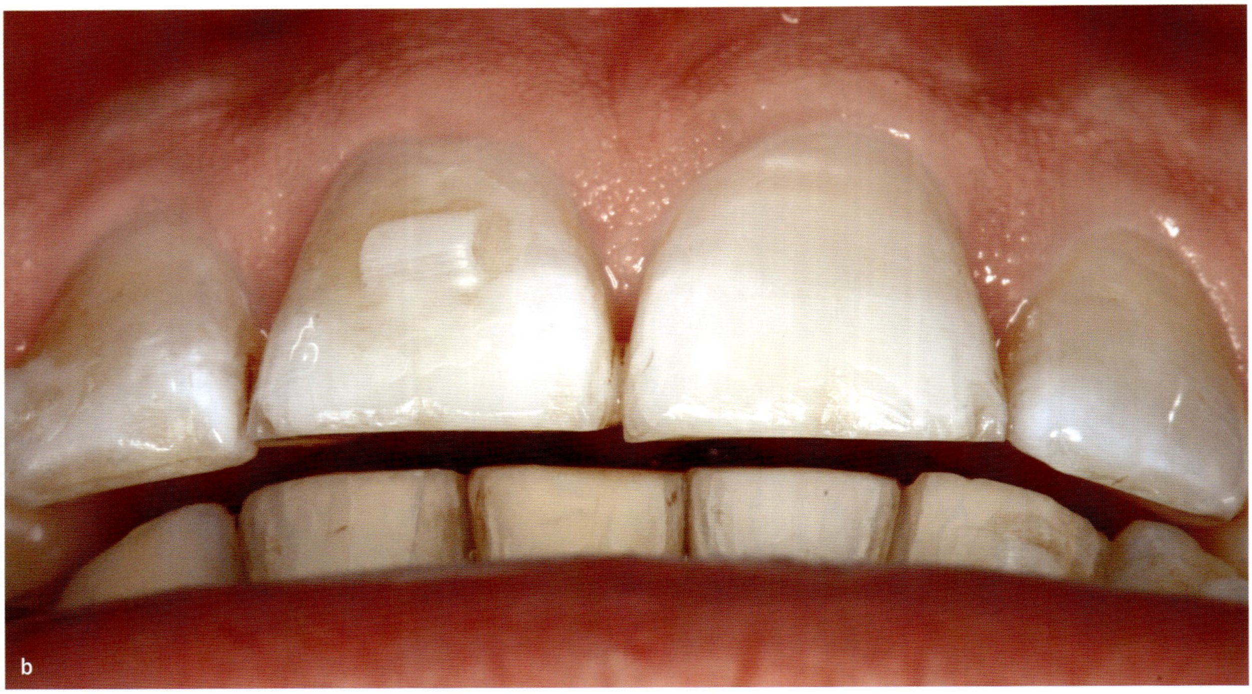


**Fig 6-18** In this case, a Class II dentoskeletal condition prevents the restorative team from using CR as the occlusal reference (a). Instead, orthodontics and restorative increase of the VDO permits restoration of anterior guidance (b).

However, the long-term stability of porcelains, together with outstanding esthetics, make these the first choice in cases where the treatment involves the labial aspects of the anterior maxillary teeth.

In a recent meta-analysis, the risk of failure of indirect composite veneers was higher than that of porcelain veneers, with the latter showing the highest survival rate and the former having the highest fracture rate.[46] The evidence shows that porcelain laminates have a better prognosis compared to indirect composite veneers. Noteworthy is the possibility of using ultra-thin porcelain, ranging from 0.3 to 0.5 mm, which exhibits higher mechanical strength in this extreme thinness.

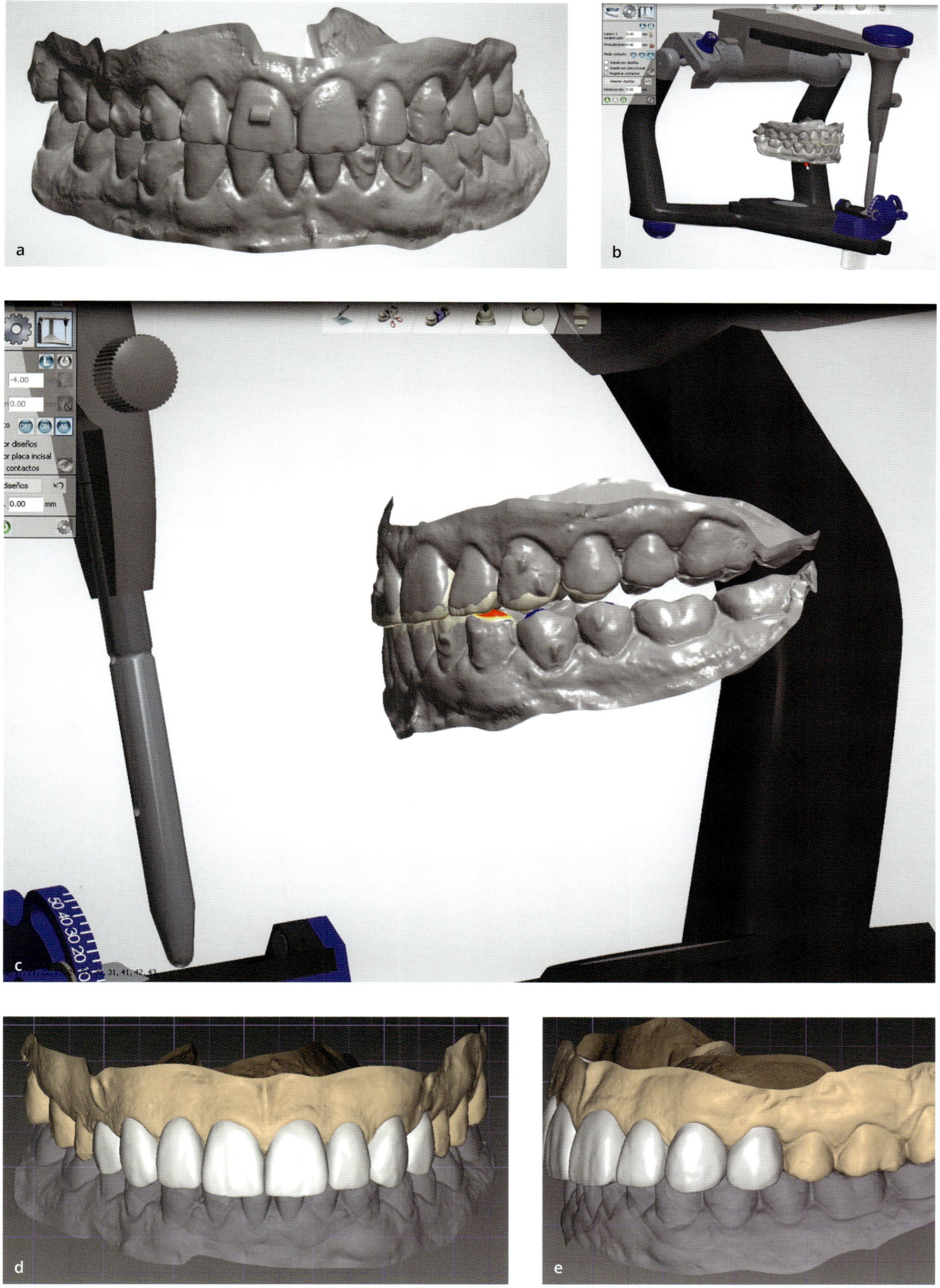


**Fig 6-19** A virtual articulator and wax-up is analyzed with the STL of the final orthodontic result once the VDO has been increased by restoring the damaged mandibular dentition (a to e). The VDO has been augmented by approximately 0.5 mm.

## 5. Porcelain Laminate Veneers for Tooth Wear

The advancement of the powerful engineering of CAD/CAM technologies in dental science and materials has created a paradigm shift in addressing TW, widening the spectrum of patients even at early stages (minimum to moderate tooth loss) that may benefit from a patient-oriented safe and effective treatment plan that ideally should be established and performed using an uncomplicated workflow to achieve final reintegration as soon as possible (see chapter 1). Prevalence of TW varies from one population group to another, but overall, one-fourth of the general population is affected by TW, and 30% of children and adolescents exhibit TW. This is even more relevant in the adult group, where severe TW reaches high levels.

As has been said before, from a restorative perspective, the TW patient, at least in the moderate stages, should not fall under the classical full-mouth rehabilitation category. However, both arches should be addressed comprehensively.

It is important to take into consideration that the worn tooth is already in a compromised flexural and overall situation, and further debilitation might endanger the strength of the final outcome. It is otherwise advisable to accept a volume increase of some microns, as this is well tolerated in clinical practice by the lips and the gingiva if the margins are juxta- or supragingival.[47] When preparing the teeth for PLVs in a patient with TW it should be kept in mind that the TSL has "prepared" the tooth already. Ideally, the gingival margin of the PLV should be left in enamel, avoiding as much as possible a composite-dentin or composite-cementum interface, as these have shown to have rougher surfaces after polishing regardless of the polishing protocol.[48]

One of the reasons for placing a subgingival margin for PLVs is to obtain margin stability over time. Interestingly, the location of the interface has been shown to be a major factor in staining and secondary caries subsequent to bacterial adhesion and composite microleakage derived from composite roughness.[49]

In fact, surface roughness is responsible for staining proclivity.[50] Therefore, in patients with TW, whenever possible the PLV margin should be left in enamel, where roughness after finishing is less than in other substrates. Also, preparing into dentin or cementum demands more sacrifice of tooth structure.

On the other hand, in thin biotypes and in the presence of gingival dehiscences, the association between the emergence profile and future gingival retraction has been widely explained. In order to avoid a bulky restoration, a chamfer preparation at the gingival margin is needed if the tooth color substrate is dark at the gingival interface or if it is not possible to provide extra-thin restorations at this critical area.

However, overpreparing for PLVs severely weakens the tooth.[51] Therefore, whenever possible, extra-thin feather-edge margins will enhance tooth preservation and enable supragingival termination of the PLV.

Final polishing is done with interproximal polishing strips, finishing with the finer grain. A thin knife-edge fine tungsten carbide bur can be used without pressure, following the gingival architecture of the porcelain laminates to engage any excess resin. The incisal envelope is addressed from the palatal aspect using the same light pressure either with a fine tungsten round bur or an extra-fine bullet diamond bur. In case an adjustment needs to be done to improve incisal contact stability in anterior guidance, the same type of burs are used followed by silicone points (Figs 6-20 and 6-21).

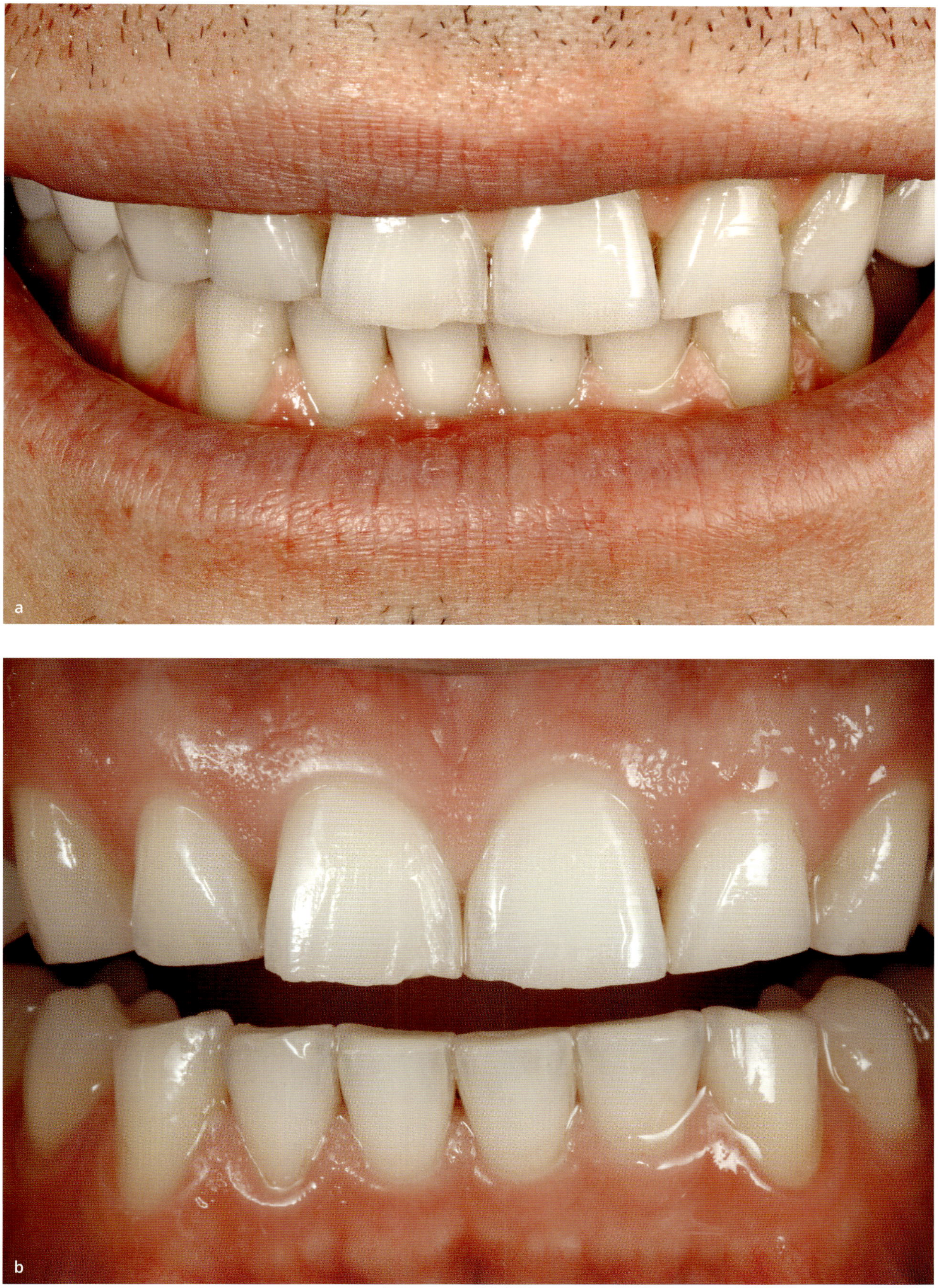

**Fig 6-20** A young male in his early 30s presented with the complaint of asymmetry is his anterior teeth. The patient has incipient TW that, due to his young age and parafunctional habits, is upgraded to moderate TW (a and b). *(continued next page)*

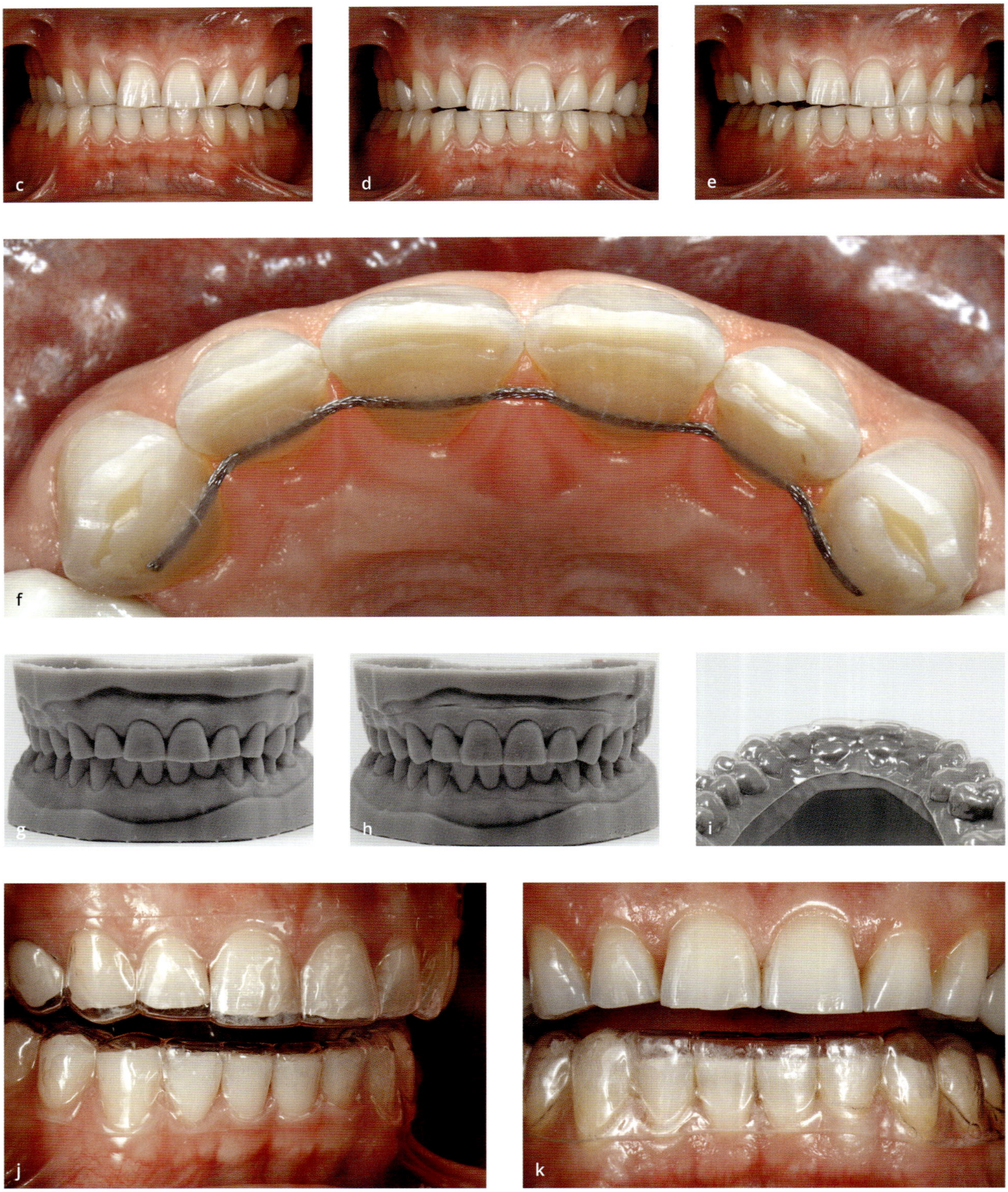


**Fig 6-20** *(continued)* The functional analysis shows that TW has deprived the dentition of anterolateral protection (c to e). The patient has restorative needs in the posterior sectors that present an opportunity for a moderate VDO increase due to the loss of anterior and canine guidance and flattening of the incisal smile line. Anterior teeth have been deprived of their enamel covering at the incisal edge and already show dentin that may also suffer from concomitant or successive erosive damage as well as saucer-like flattening of the original enamel anatomy. This might be overlooked, as the lesion, described as cupping, might still be surrounded by a shell of enamel and is better seen when inspected from an occlusal view (f). Two printed models show the flattening of the worn dentition (g). A digital wax-up and a set of printed models are done at the lab (h). A mock-up extracted from the wax-up will serve as the blueprint for the rest of the treatment. This mock-up includes all anterior and posterior mandibular teeth with restorative needs and the six maxillary anterior teeth that need rehabilitation of anterior and canine guidance. A transparent Essix-like vacuum-formed mouthguard is tried on by the patient, enabling a preview of the length and volume that is intended to be added (i to k).

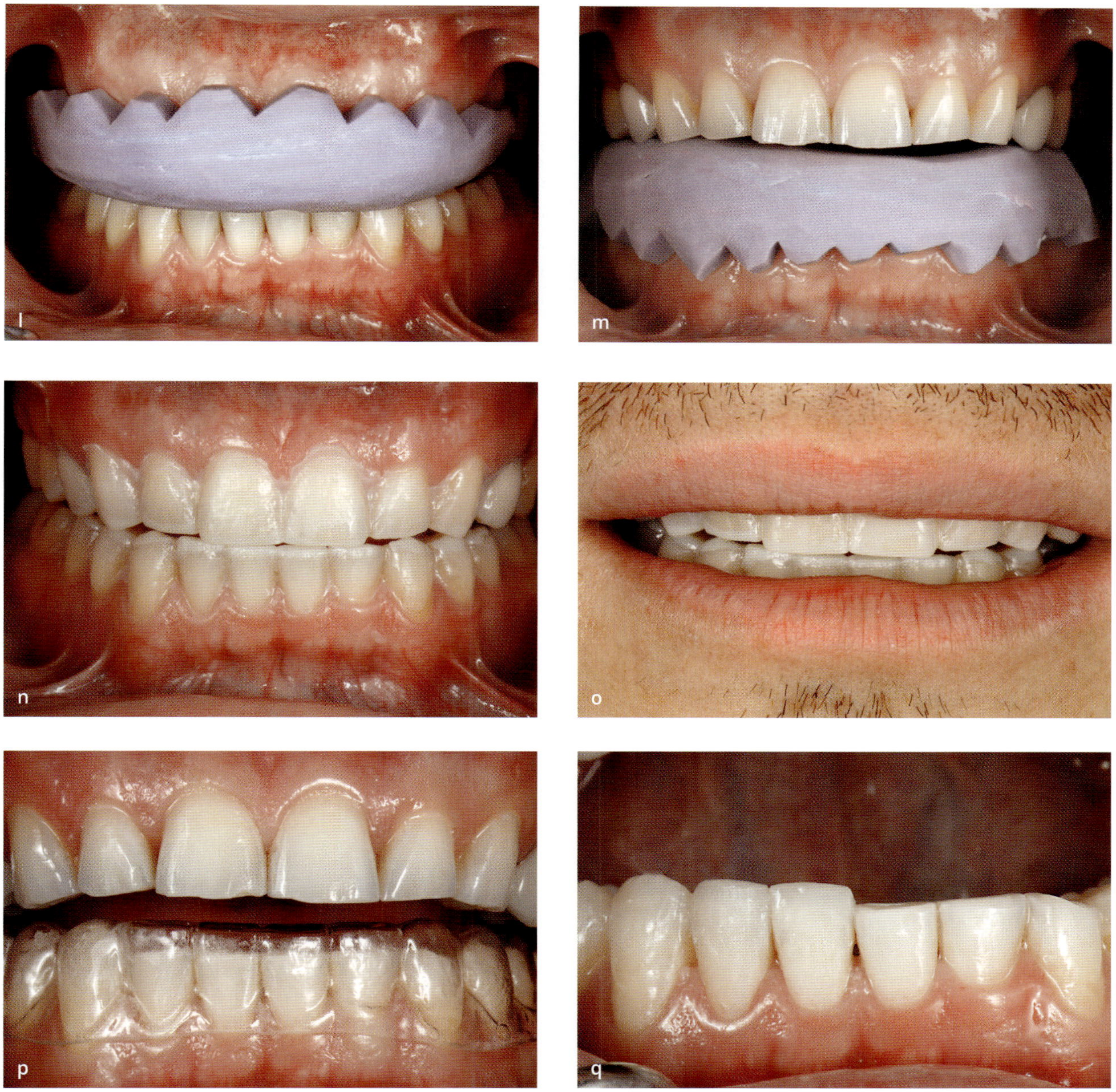


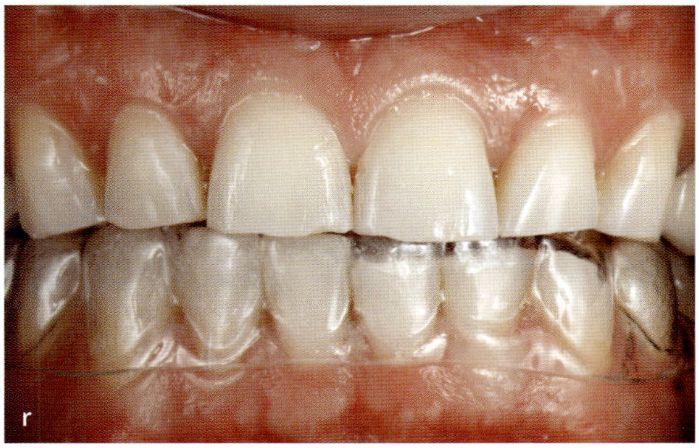


**Fig 6-20** *(continued)* A silicone index is used to transport acrylic resin onto the maxillary and mandibular teeth (l and m). A traditional mock-up is used as a previsualization tool (n and o). The dentist should be prepared for an initial patient reaction against the new smile, in particular the new length, as the pace at which teeth have been shortened has taken years, even decades, and patients are afraid of a sudden significant change. Whenever possible, as explained in chapters 4 and 5, the preferred sequence of restorative treatment starts with the buildup of the mandibular teeth first. Direct composites are performed in the mandibular teeth (Tetric EvoCeram, Ivoclar Vivadent). Checking the new length with the transparent Essix-like mouthguard facilitates the procedure (p to r). *(continued next page)*

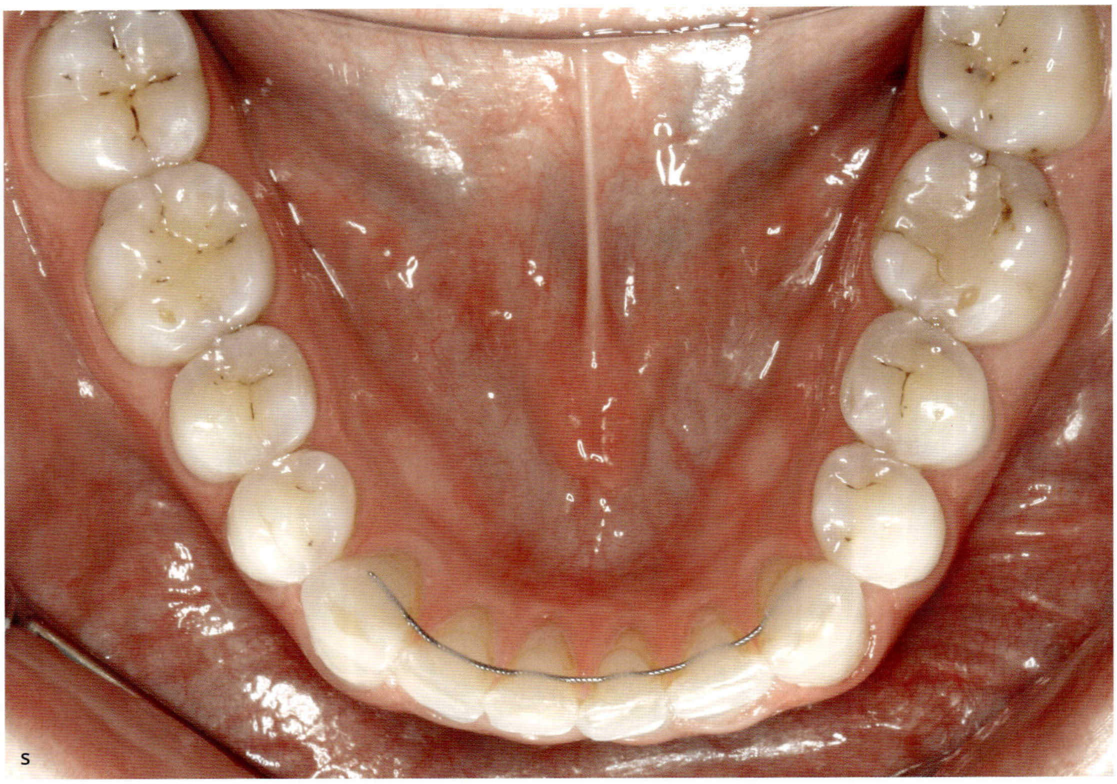

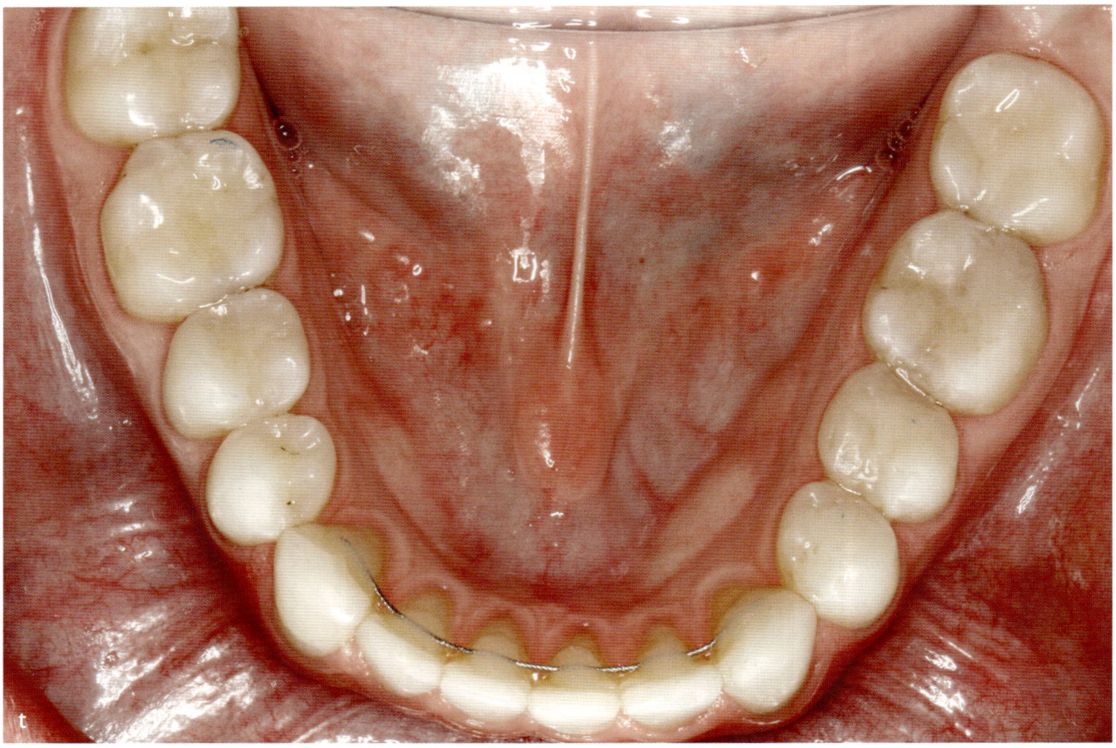

**Fig 6-20** *(continued)* Incisal restorations are performed with suction and relative isolation for humidity control and contamination prevention without the need for rubber dam. Most of the direct composite restoration can be done without anesthesia and with relative isolation as TW has not passed the contact points. Avoiding clamps when relative isolation is possible should facilitate a careful and controlled procedure (s and t).

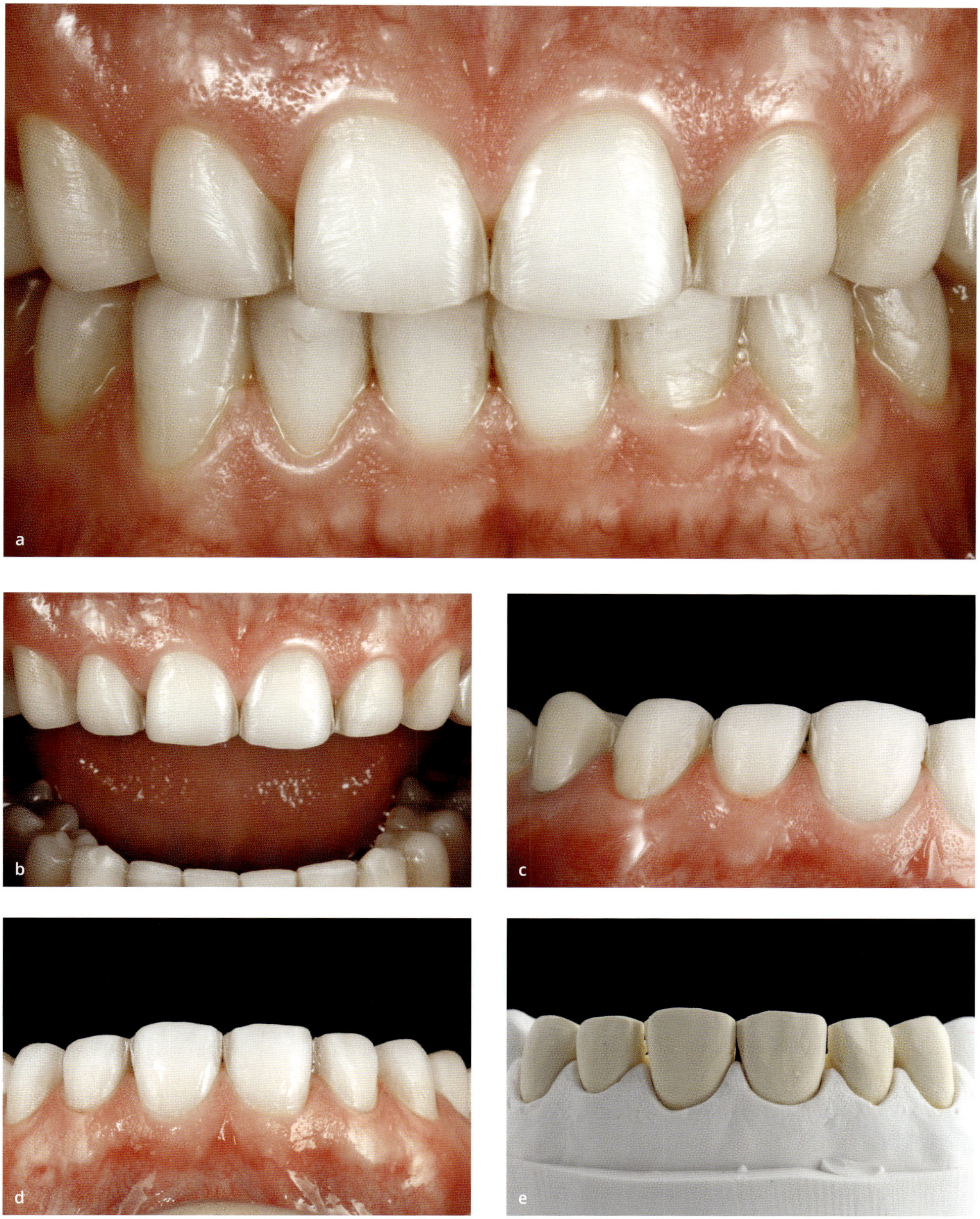

**Fig 6-21** Minimal preparation is preferred in cases where TW is present. The unwanted appearance of long-term postoperative sensitivity can be avoided with shallow roughening of the outer surface of the teeth to be veneered and rounding of the incisal platform. In contrast with what needs to be done in cases of loss of periodontal support and open embrasures, no interproximal reduction is made to open the contact point. Instead, a slight groove is made in the buccal surface both mesially and distally to avoid interproximal overcontouring and facilitate integration of the PLV. Also, when lightening of the tooth color with a lighter PLV is desired, this proximal notch-like groove enables a gentle transition between the porcelain and the tooth. Note that all gingival margins have been left supragingival (a to d). No retraction cord is used. In this case, an analog polyvinyl siloxane (PVS) impression is taken and sent to the lab technician, who will fabricate a Geller model (e). *(continued next page)*

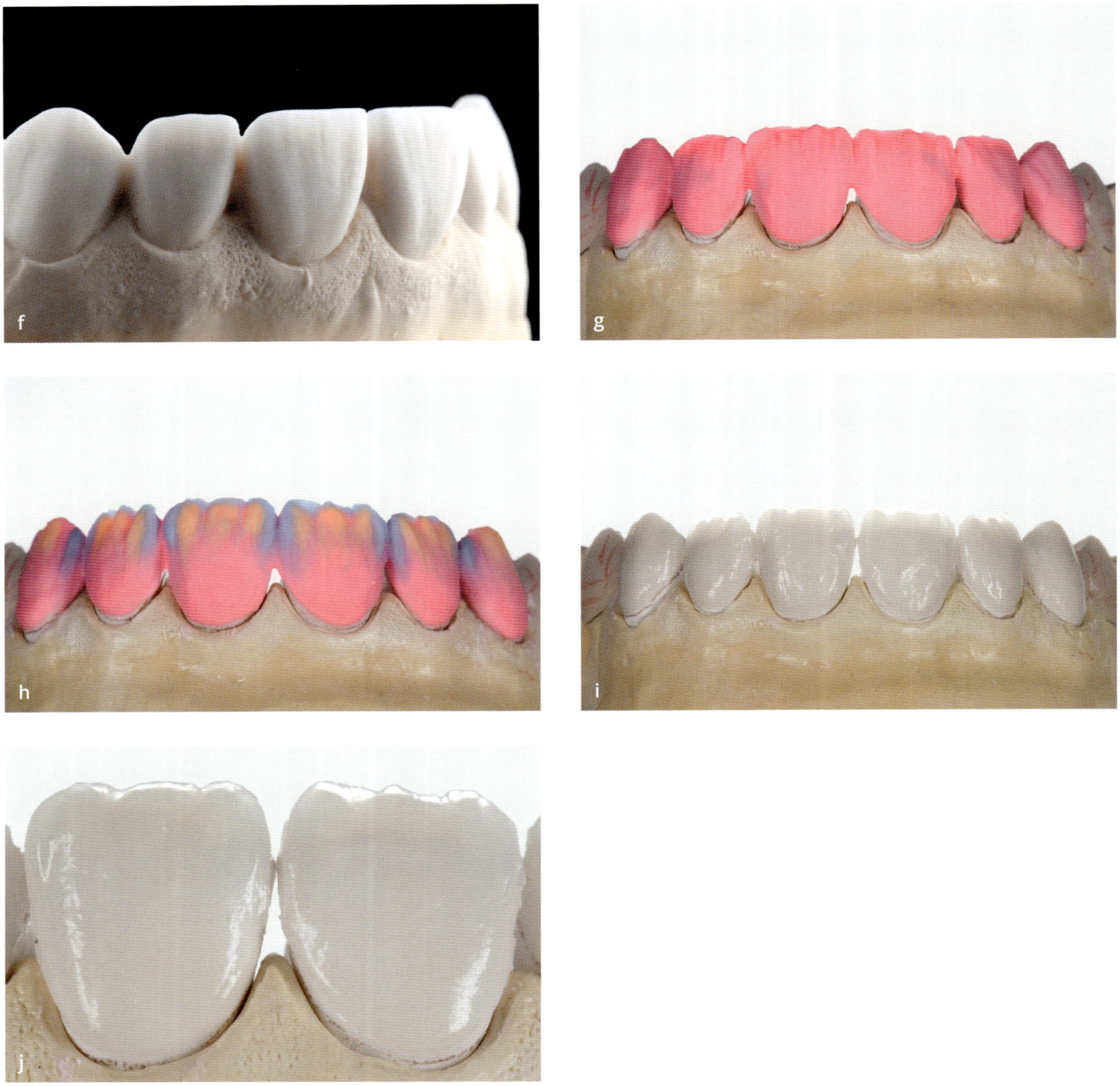

**Fig 6-21** *(continued)* It is advisable to do a fully detailed wax-up that resembles the approved (or retouched) mock-up (f). Traditional fabrication of the feldspathic PLV is done on a refractory die in a Geller model. The analog manufacturing procedure performed by the lab technician is highly sophisticated and requires a great deal of expertise. Sequential dentin, translucent, enamel, and fluorescent layering is covered by coats of porcelain and finally a thin gold layer to discriminate surface texture before the PLVs are delivered to the dental office (g to p). Some authors prefer the use of a platinum foil to avoid the intricacies of separating the finished PLV form the refractory model once baked; however, the intaglio of the PLV receives an advantageous coarse inner surface from the refractory texture. In any case, the PLVs should be chemically etched with 9% hydrofluoric acid (Ivoclar) for 2 minutes, washed with water for at least 30 seconds, and then dried before adhesion is performed.

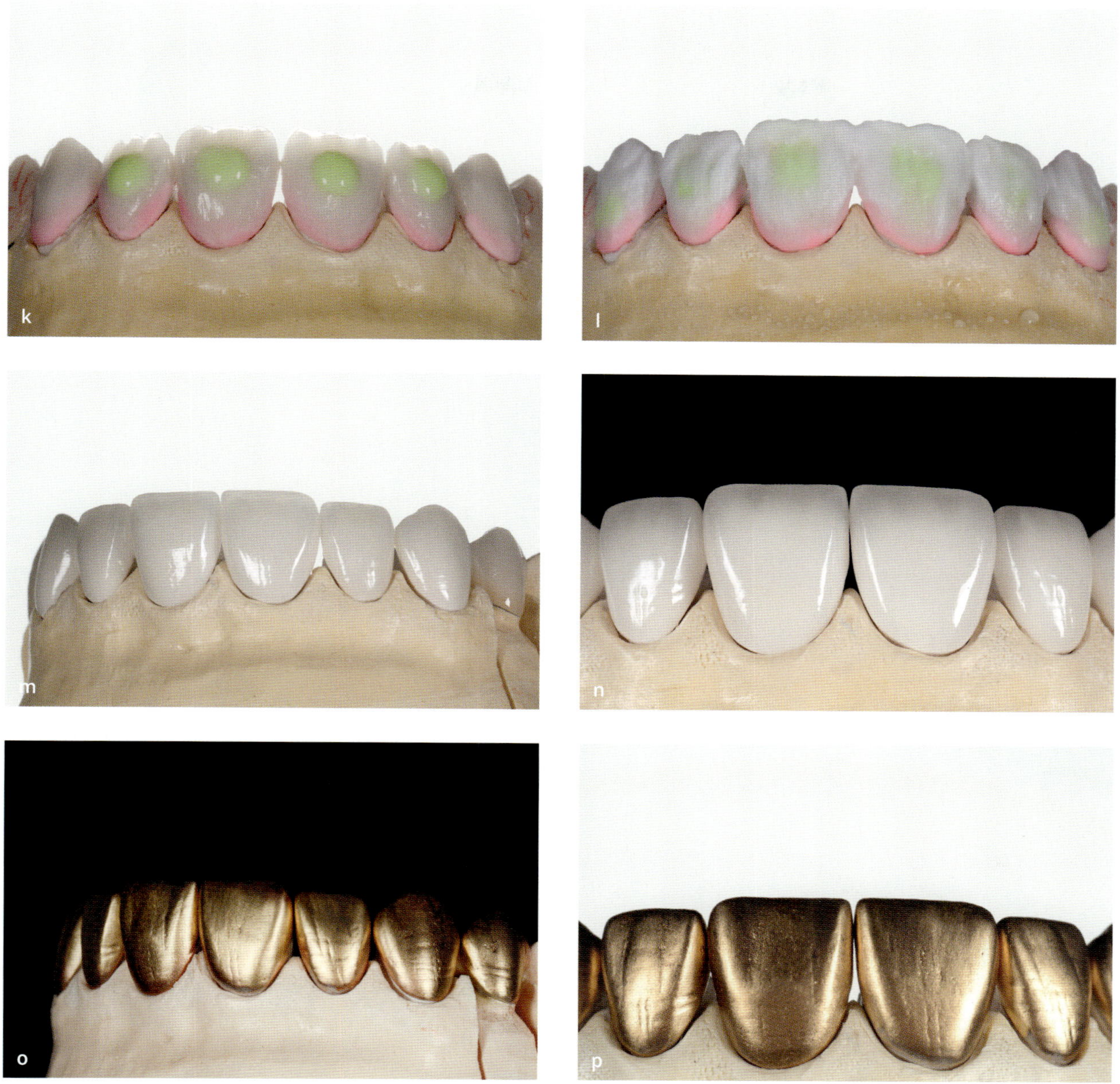


**Fig 6-21** *(continued next page)*

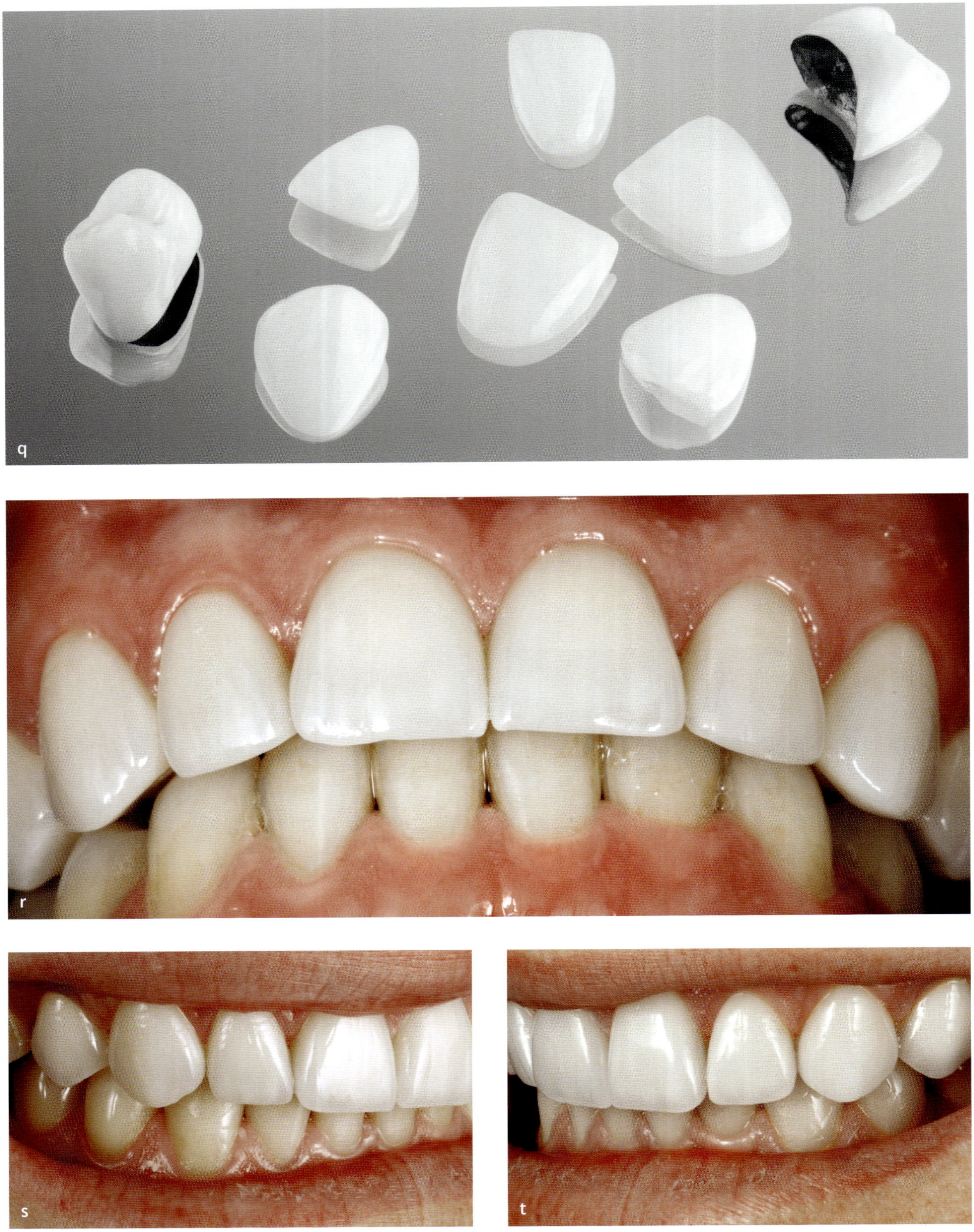


**Fig 6-21** *(continued)* Feldspathic PLVs manufactured by the expert hands of a lab technician offer the unequivocal appearance of healthy natural enamel. In addition, the recovered tooth anatomy provides effective anterior guidance as well as an ideal smile line and improved lip support (q to t). Feather-edge PLVs integrate optimally with the soft tissue. Minimal preparation ensures maximum enamel preservation, predictable adhesion values, and increased tooth endurance. The biomimetic effect achieved is not to be underestimated (u and v). Details of the extra-thin PLVs made from feldspathic porcelain have been copied from the analog wax-up (w). Note the average 0.5-mm thickness and the feather-edge emergence profile with the anatomy designed to perform during function and with the final volume contoured facially (x and y).

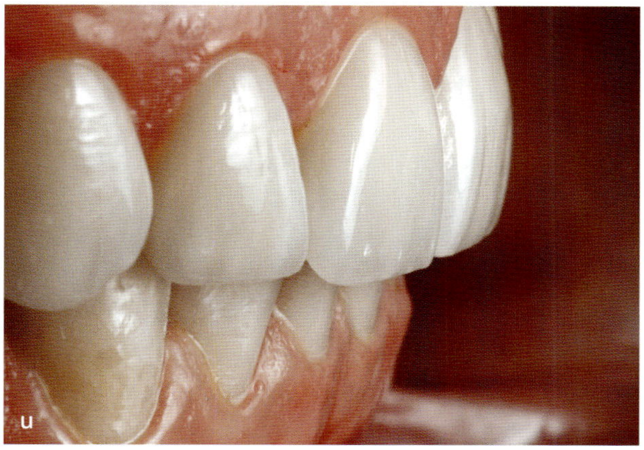

u

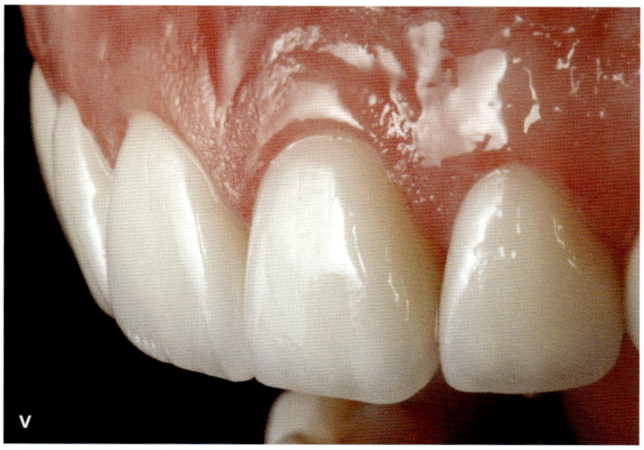

v

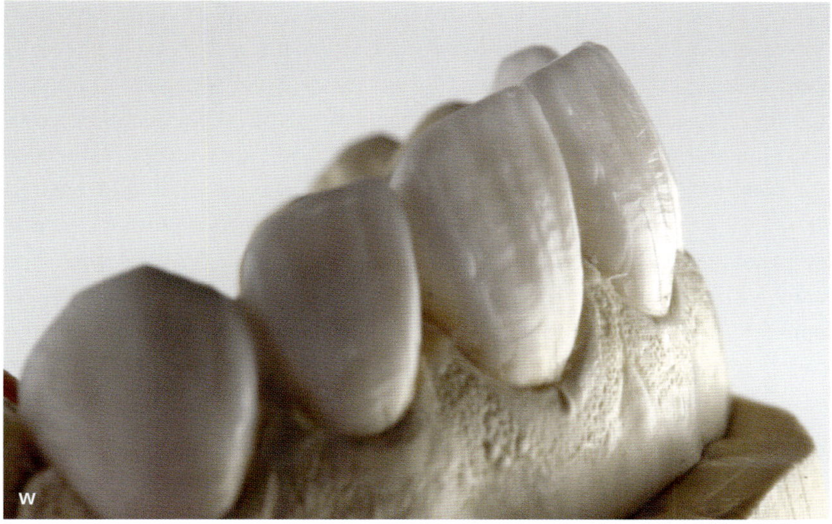

w

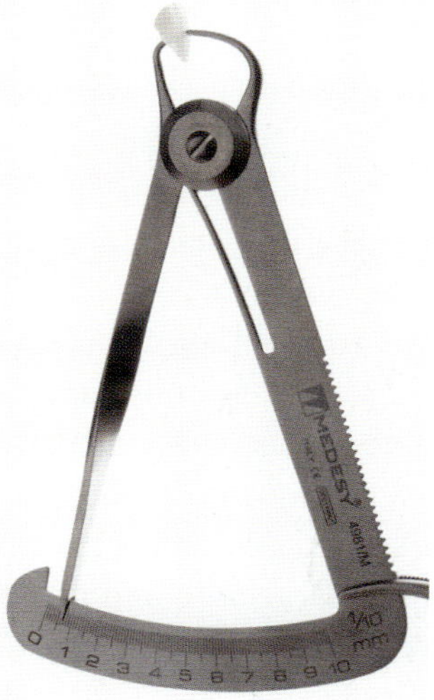


x

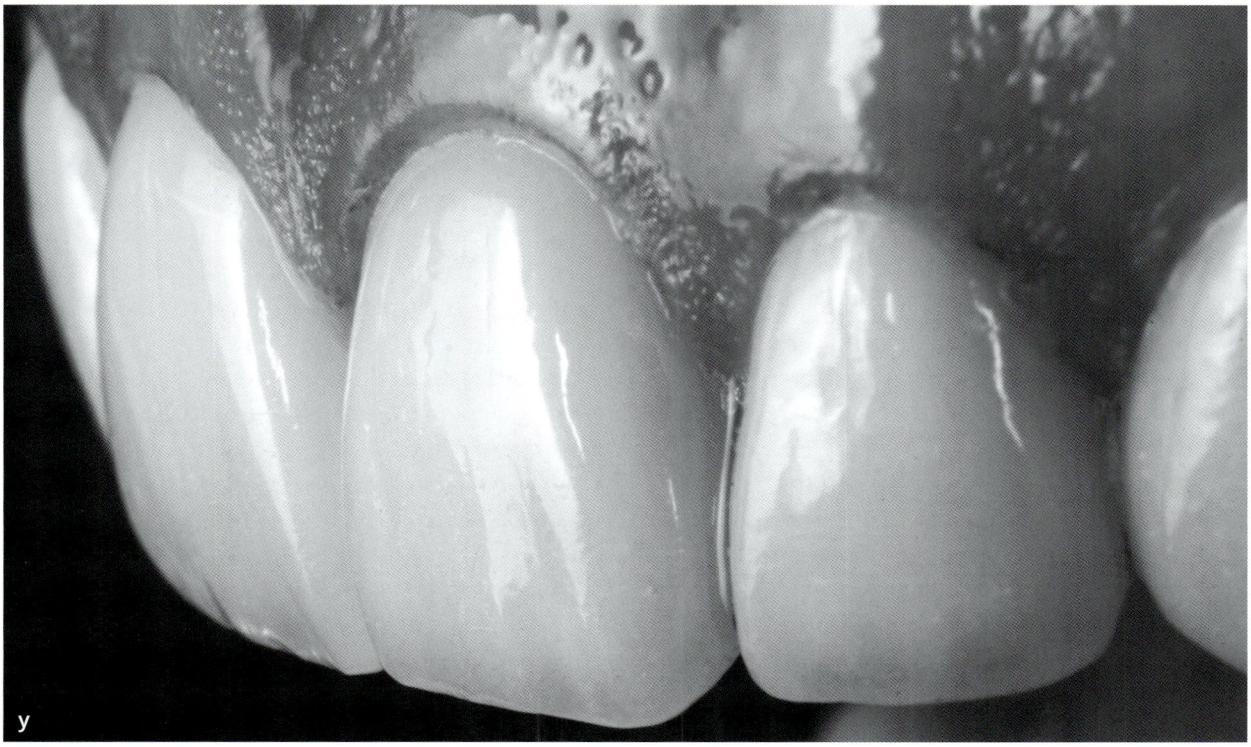

y

## 6. Increasing VDO: A Tool More Than a Target

In young patients, moderate wear may still only be localized in the anterior zone. Depending on the origin of TW and the dentoskeletal condition, providing space for the required restorations in order to offer both protection and restoration of the dentition is often a challenge.

The Dahl principle, which combines forced intrusion of anterior teeth and overeruption of posterior segments through the delivery of anterior restorations at an increased VDO, could still be an option today in cases in which orthodontic treatment is rejected and posterior occlusal anatomy is well maintained. However, in severe TW cases it is not uncommon to find multiple restorations. This might be a contraindication for intrusion as the periodontal tissue response to artificial materials would create permanent inflammation or a need for further treatment.

The Dahl approach should be carefully evaluated versus today's digital orthodontics that can simplify and facilitate the restorative portion of the treatment.[52]

Orthodontic treatment in advance of restorative work helps in safeguarding tooth structure while creating the necessary space and a beneficial occlusal scheme for years to come (see more in chapter 8). However, some dentoskeletal conditions make it impossible to exclusively resolve the compensatory lack of interocclusal space with orthodontic therapy. In these cases, an augmented VDO is also needed.

Occlusal restorations will be delivered at the original VDO or an augmented VDO depending on criteria for existing restorative space for both arches, applying the principle of tooth structure preservation. The determinants and indications for the feasibility of increasing the VDO to provide restorative space for the worn dentition are well understood.[53] Nevertheless, before deciding on a change in vertical dimension, a conscious and detailed analysis of the effect an increase of the VDO will have on both maxillomandibular and interdental relationships needs to be done. It should be taken into consideration that, whatever the VDO, contact should exist between the maxillary and mandibular anterior teeth. This is necessary for the stability of the occlusal plane as well as esthetics, phonetics, and function in anterior protection of the posterior dentition, otherwise known as anterior guidance. If a preview of an increase of VDO shows that the restoration of the anterior relationship would not be adequate, an orthodontic evaluation of the possible benefits of an orthodontic intervention is highly recommended.[54,55]

Controversy around the concept of increasing the VDO has occupied clinicians worried about the effects on the patient's muscles and TMJ. Originating with the fathers of occlusion and pioneers in cephalometrics and orthodontics, much has been written about VDO. In addition, when TW also has affected the posterior sector, the restorative team needs to foresee choosing from restoring in maximal intercuspal position (MIP) or centric relation (CR).[56,57] Nowadays there is extensive evidence about the good tolerance patients show to an increase of VDO up to a maximum of 5 mm.[53] The concept of there being a certain amount of VDO that should not to be exceeded is obsolete, and there is generally no need for intermediate transitional reconstructions to test certain increments of height except in patients with a history of TMJ symptoms. As in any other restorative procedure, causes of a TMJ disorder should be treated first, and only when patients are asymptomatic should they be considered candidates for TW treatment. It is important to keep in mind that most patients with TW do not experience TMJ problems. It would seem that the degradation of the occlusal anatomy is well accepted by the musculoskeletal system, which adapts to the occlusal changes that occur as has been cleverly described by some clinicians. These adaptations include the well-known overeruption of the dentition, which compensates for the amount of TW and reestablishes occlusal contact with the antagonist teeth, as well as overeruption of the supporting tissues, periodontium, and bone. The compensatory adaptation happens in both the sagittal (vertical compensatory eruption) and the frontal planes (mesial drift), with a decrease in arch length in the most advanced cases of TW. Interestingly, vertical dimensions do not show a significant difference as would be expected, probably as a result of this continuous eruption of the dentoalveolar complex together with postural and muscle adaptation.[58,59]

Nevertheless, occlusal restorations in the TW patient, with or without an increase of the VDO, should follow a newly redefined occlusal plane that contributes to the overall facial harmony, but principally provides occlusion with antagonist teeth as well as posterior support to appropriately distribute posterior loads (Figs 6-22 and 6-23).

When addressing the restorative phase of a TW patient, one may ask oneself whether to initially proceed with the mandibular or the maxillary arch. First mandibular and posterior and then maxillary and anterior, or vice versa?

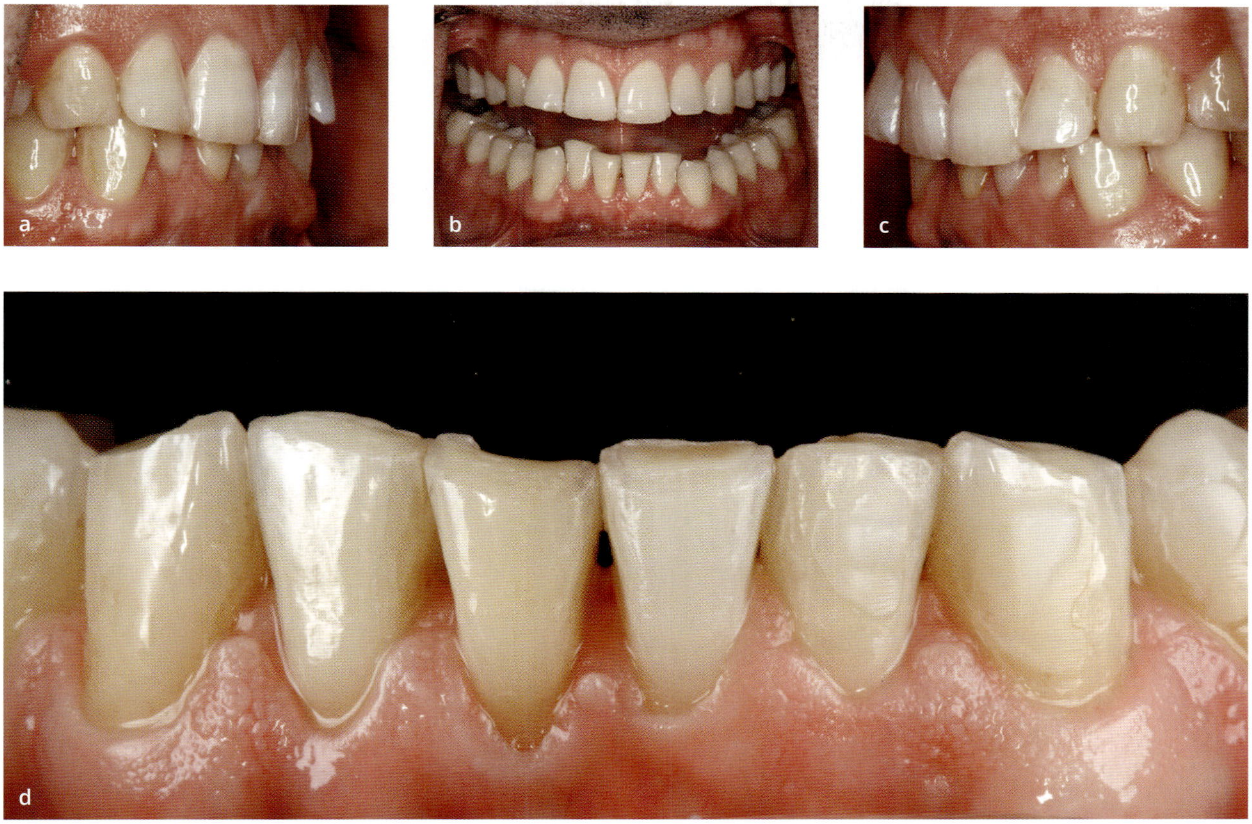


**Fig 6-22** Multifactorial moderate erosive and attrition TW in a male patient in his fourth decade of life. Malocclusion and interocclusal space distribution issues indicate pre-restorative orthodontic treatment, which is performed with clear aligners (Invisalign) (a to d). Nonsurgical periodontal treatment is performed to diminish inflammation and improve plaque control. *(continued next page)*

Those who have come to the TW field from the prosthodontic realm will have deeply incorporated the fully edentulous protocols in which anterior teeth are placed first. In most cases of TW, treating all mandibular teeth first, then maxillary posterior teeth, and finally maxillary anterior teeth supports a minimally invasive approach. Moderate TW often affects both the anterior and posterior dentition of both arches to a different extent, depending whether the origin of the wear factors is mechanical or chemical. TW of parafunctional eccentric origin usually flattens first the incisal plane of the six anterior teeth before spreading to the posterior region, eventually destroying the occlusal anatomy and occlusal planes of all or most of the arch. In moderate TW, changes in the smile line are followed by alteration of the curve of Spee with an overall flattening. Choosing an orthodontic path may prove helpful in optimizing the final occlusal scheme and saving tooth structure.

Finally, VDO is not a fixed figure or number, but a relative and dynamic approximation of both arches when in contact. There is a wide variability of acceptable VDO not only between patients but also within one patient, as long as the patient is comfortable and has good phonetic performance. An orthodontic path does not exclude the need for a restorative phase with or without an increase of the VDO.

Provided anatomical references have remained unaltered such as palatal ruggae, vestibular soft tissues, papillae, and other teeth in the arch, digital cross-mounting is a great tool in moderate and severe TW cases. The lab has the potential to perform digital cross-mounting, which provides a level of accuracy that analog cross-mounting does not. Also, with this technology, transmission of information to the lab technician becomes easier. Last but not least, the precision that can be obtained is very noticeable, reducing the need for occlusal adjustments that otherwise might be necessary upon completion of the treatment.

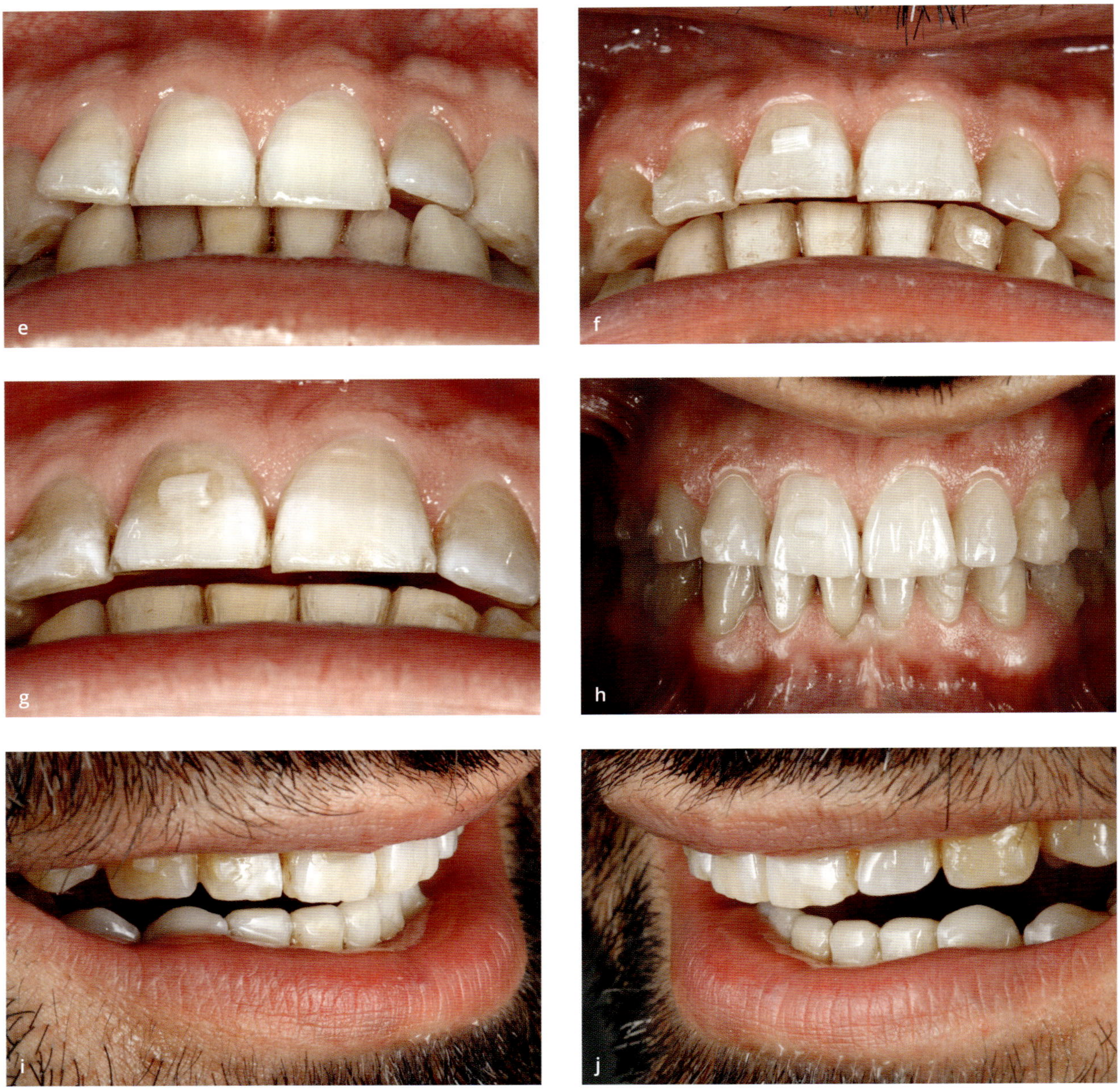


**Fig 6-22** *(continued)* The moderate TW mostly affects the anterior teeth in this patient with TW caused by attrition overlapped with episodes of acid challenge from intrinsic origin. The interocclusal space is compromised due to Class II malocclusion, compression, and crowding. The lack of interocclusal space is the primary reason, together with space distribution and crowding issues, for orthodontic treatment. Note the evolution of the overjet and interdental space in the occlusal anterior plane from the start of the orthodontic therapy to the end (e and f). As explained previously, more space would have been available in CR, but the retrognathic mandible discouraged this approach as it was not compatible with natural tooth form (see Fig 6-3). Instead, by restoring the mandibular dentition with direct composite in the worn areas, an increase of 0.5 mm was obtained in the VDO, creating space for restoration of anterior and canine guidance (g). In relation to orthodontic improvement, note the broadening of the arches as well as tooth alignment, which will be key to sparing tooth structure when preparing for PLVs (h to j).

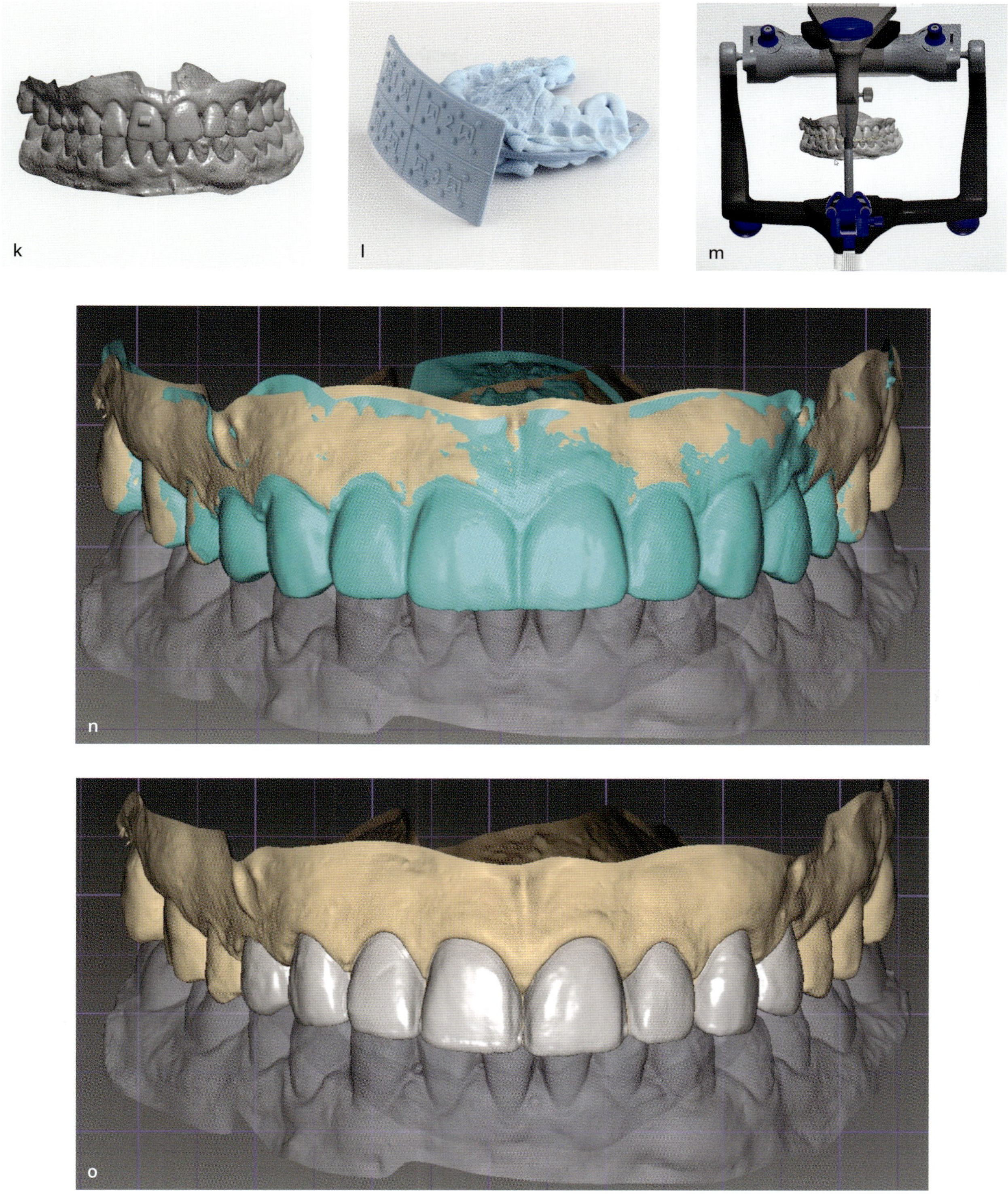

**Fig 6-22** *(continued)* At this stage, a traditional or a digital workflow offer different opportunities but should reach the same goal. In the traditional protocol, throughout the whole procedure, the different models are manipulated, and referential positioning of the dentition is transferred by a facebow, on a semi-adjustable articulator (by which models can be interchanged). In the digital workflow the work load is transferred to the CAD/CAM station, where the different acquisitions can be easily virtually superimposed, which is a very advantageous characteristic of the digital workflow. The digital workflow is able to provide a virtual try-in to test the anterior and canine guidance in the virtual articulator using virtual restorations that should almost be identical to the final computer-manufactured pieces. All digital models are matched with the specifications of the lab software, and communication back and forth with the dental team is done online without delays or misplacements. In this case, a digital workflow was chosen (k to m). Cross-mounting of all the digital data, including intraoral (n) and facial (o) scanning, together with the intraoral scanning of the accepted in vivo mock-up and the final digital acquisition of the arch is possible in the digital workflow. *(continued next page)*

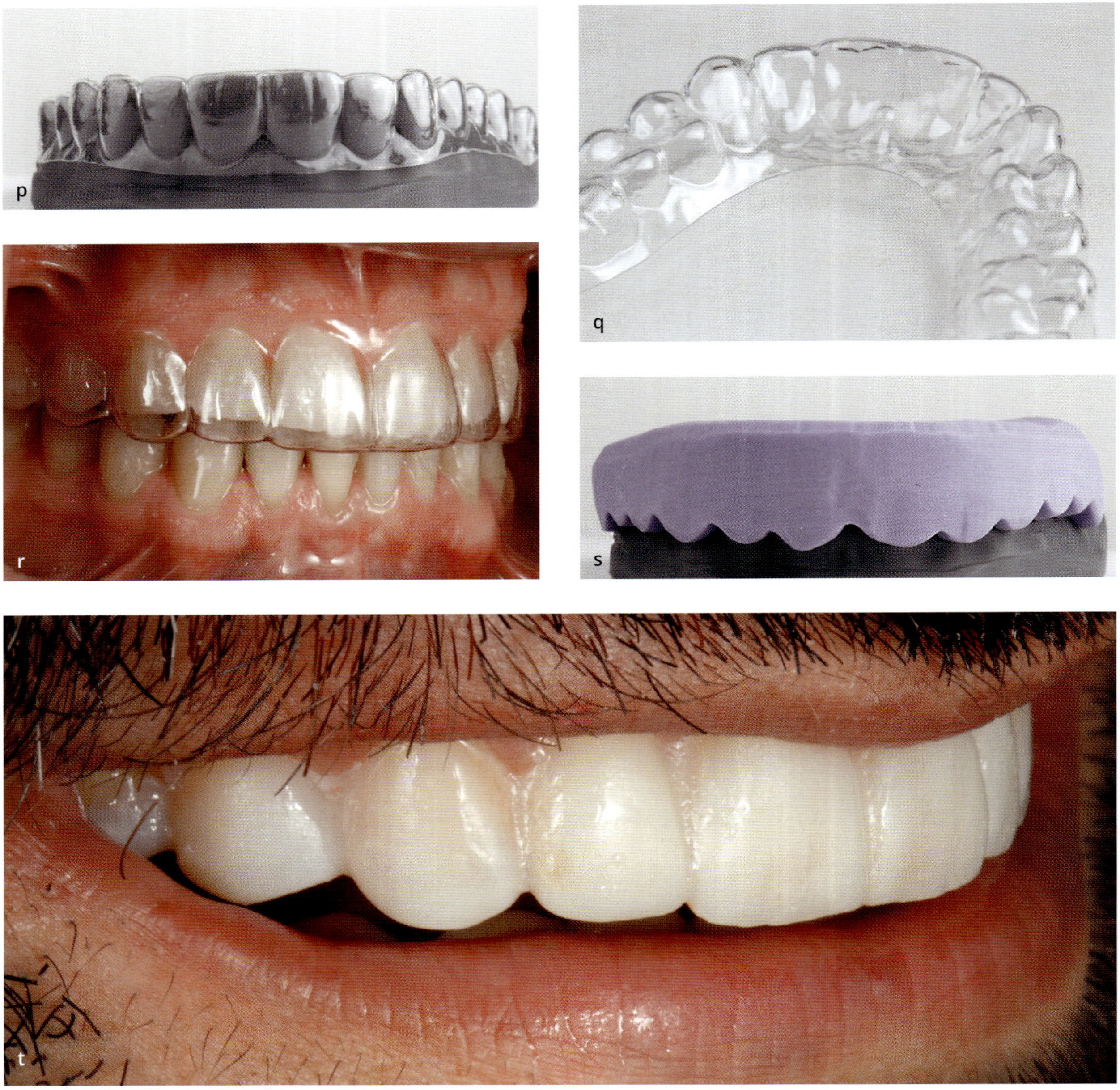


**Fig 6-22** *(continued)* The transparent Essix-like mock-up facilitates dentist-patient communication (p to r). Some patients may need to test-drive the new length with family and friends and get positive feedback, which is helpful at this stage as many TW patients experience difficulty and even anxiety when the final anatomy is rehabilitated at full length. The mock-up should be tested for length and function because modifications to the mock-up do not have any drawbacks. Modifications ideally should not be done at the final treatment delivery but before (s and t).

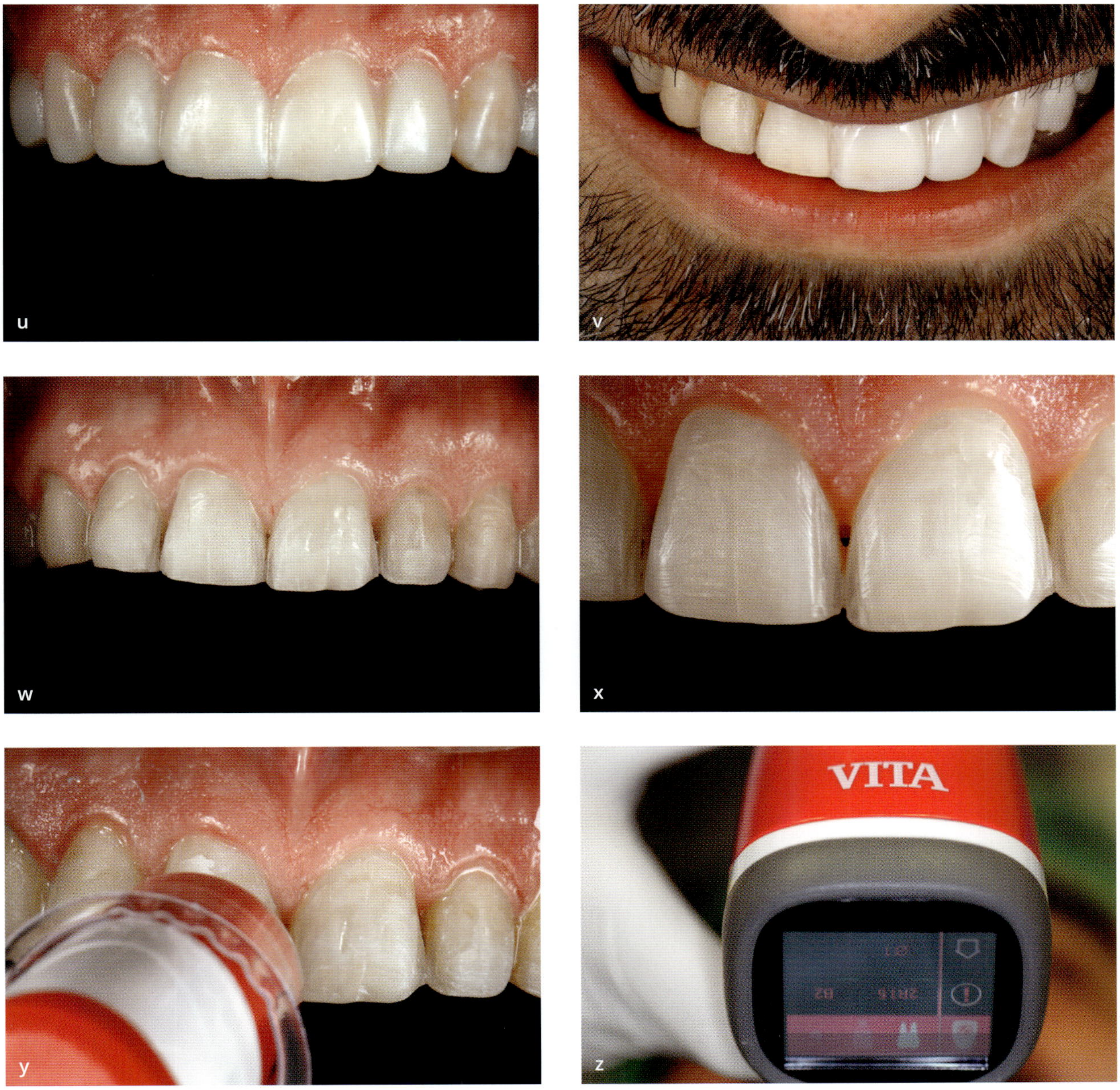


**Fig 6-22** *(continued)* Any modification should respect the minimum requirements necessary for anterior protection of the rest of the teeth. By all means, the absolute limitation should be the remaining tooth structure as the treatment plan guidelines and principles should be to restore and not to replace. The so-called "no-prep approach" can be deemed indicated in cases where TSL has already "prepared" the tooth, even though nowadays the trend is to perform a minimal preparation to avoid overcontouring as well as enhance natural esthetics. A shallow preparation through the acrylic mock-up leaves adequate space for the PLV and cement. Digital color acquisition (in the figure, VITA Easyshade) is a predictable way to transmit the tooth color to the lab, especially in cases where tooth color is not the same in all teeth (u to z).

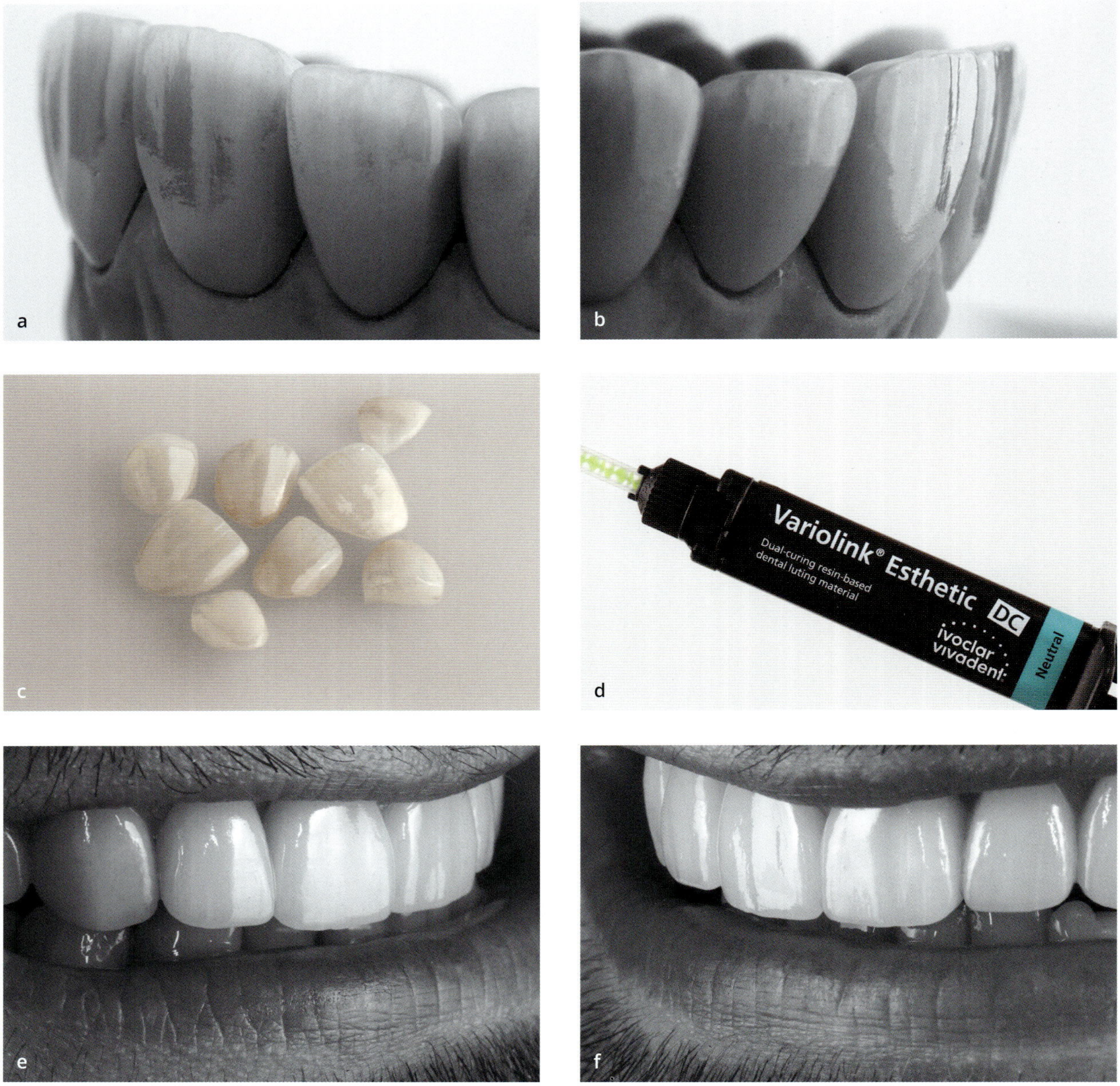


**Fig 6-23** A shallow preparation respectful of the interproximal areas should not prevent a smooth transition between the tooth and the porcelain. The gingival finishing line is clearly in a juxtagingival position. Vestibular enamel is present and preserved in a generous manner (a and b). The value of the final outcome will be determined by the combination of all three factors: tooth structure, composite, and PLV. In preserving as much enamel as possible, the natural tooth color will contribute to the final outcome, especially if the PLVs are not thick (ranging from 0.4 to 0.7 mm). If a lighter result is desired, the value of the composite cement should be lighter than that of the natural tooth (eg, Variolink Veneer, Ivoclar Vivadent). The shade of the porcelain laminate can also contribute to a lighter final outcome if needed (c to f).

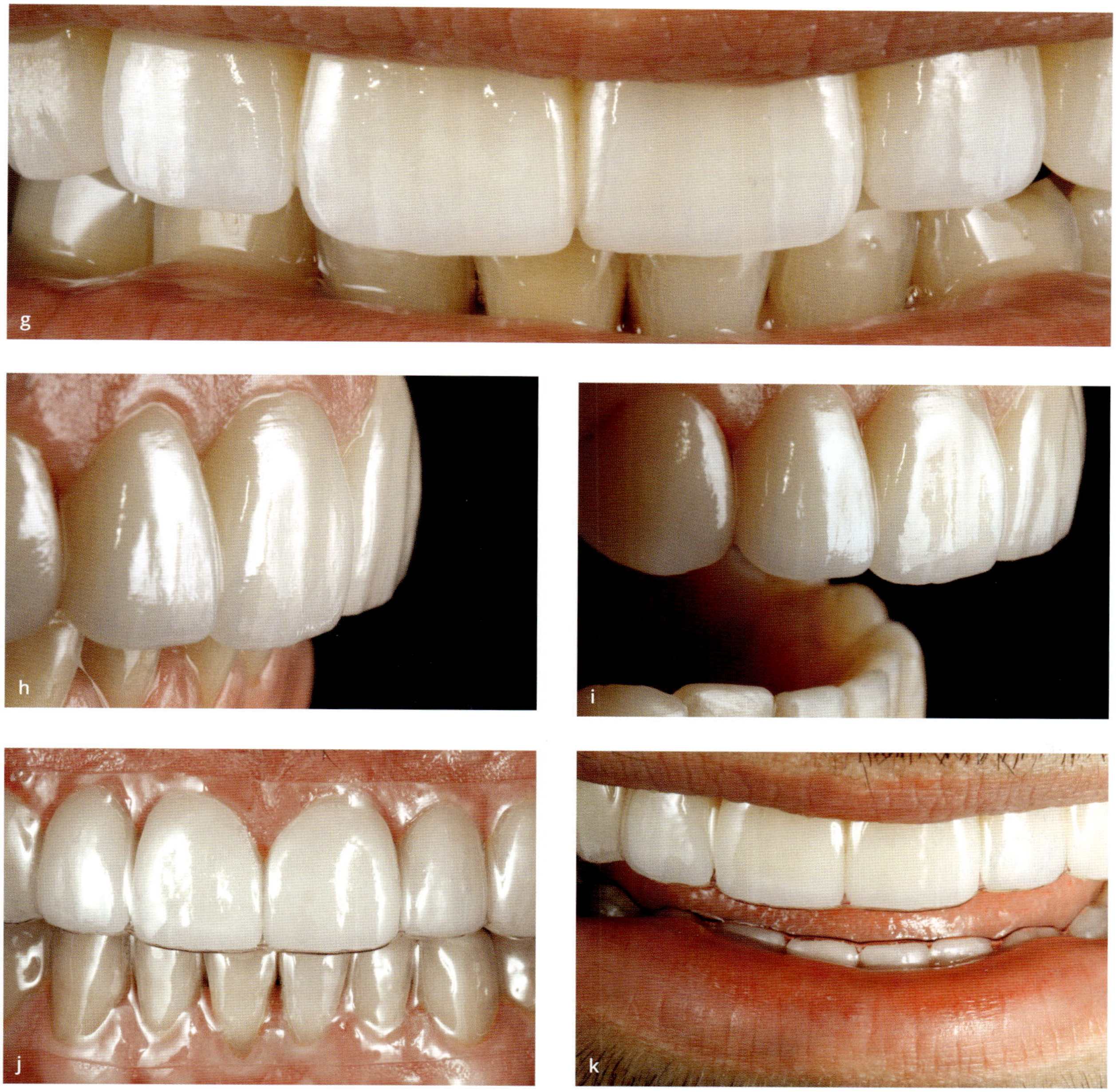

**Fig 6-23** *(continued)* CAD/CAM milled ceramics can be made from a feldspathic ceramic block (eg, VITABLOCS Mark II, VITA) or alternatively a lithium disilicate ceramic material that can be used both for pressed ceramic technology or CAD/CAM systems (eg, IPS Empress CAD, Ivoclar Vivadent). Excellent esthetic outcomes are possible, although some may agree that the traditional laboratory procedure, provided the lab technician has good expertise, offers superior esthetic results. The lithium disilicate ceramic has physical properties that may have potential in severely worn dentitions or in demanding situations. However, adhesively cemented porcelains, whichever type, benefit from the natural tooth mechanical properties and clinically behave well in cases in which minimal preparation is done. Digital workflows offer the benefit of a predictable outcome that matches the pre-evaluation mock-ups. The gingival-porcelain interface is easily accessed for composite removal as the gingival margin is fully respected. The eight thin, computer-manufactured PLVs help in preserving enamel while restoring the anatomy of natural dentition (g to i). A checklist of treatment goals should be done at the end of the treatment. Enamel has been widely preserved with the aid of orthodontic expansion and alignment. The non-constricted occlusal scenario provided by the orthodontic treatment provides the required space to rehabilitate both the posterior and anterior dentition. Adhesive additive restorations with a minimum tooth preparation have been done directly on the posterior teeth, with a VDO increase of 0.5 mm. PLVs have been milled after the blueprint of a digital and analog mock-up. Anterior and canine guidance will act as safeguards, while other TW risk factors will have to be monitored during the years to come. Once the treatment has been finished, a PPP (personalized preventive program) will be implemented. The use of a soft Essix-like guard is highly recommended. These can be worn in both arches during the day as they are barely noticeable and protect restorations from initial accidents. Lifestyle habits are readdressed toward TW risk control, along with a topical oral care regimen to ensure saliva stimulation. The PPP has been agreed upon by the patient, who complies with mouthguard use and regular checkups with hygiene at 4-month intervals. Any repair or refurbishment will be done as soon as the need for it is detected (j and k).

## 7. Non-carious Cervical Lesions

Non-carious cervical lesions (NCCLs) are seen in patients exhibiting TW in association with abrasion mechanisms in an already damaged enamel shield. Although there is controversy about whether a concomitant mechanism of tension or load excess is able to cause superficial fractures of the enamel at the cervical third, so-called abfraction lesions are frequent and require a clinical evaluation of the occlusal forces exerted on the teeth. Dentinal hypersensitivity might be a symptom in early stages of NCCLs, and its noninvasive interceptive treatment is desirable whenever possible.

Prevalence of NCCLs shows a large variation, from 5% to 85%.[60] It has been proven that NCCLs increase with age due to anatomical and biologic events occurring with the passing of the years, such as gingival recessions followed by root exposures and impairment of saliva secretion resulting in a decrease in its protective power.[61] Although any tooth can be affected by this kind of lesion, studies have pointed out that premolars are their most common location.[62]

The topography and shape of these lesions may help in assessing the probable origin (Fig 6-24). Broad, extended, and shallow lesions without clear margins are likely to be created by acid impact. Sharp margins and striated-like scratches point to an abrasive impact, such as that produced by improper toothbrushing. Wedge-shaped lesions, ie, the so-called abfraction lesions, are predominant in occlusal loading problems.

In the same manner as with TW in general, a multifactorial, combined etiology and varied appearance of NCCLs are normally the case, with overlapping of different types of NCCL[63] (Figs 6-25 and 6-26).

### Treatment Approach to NCCLs

Treatment strategies for NCCLs start with preventive measures in order to delay progression of the existing defects. The patient's toothbrushing technique should be modified if abrasion is the issue, while nutritional coaching and medical consultation in cases of erosive diets or medical conditions such as GERD or EDs are desirable. Dentinal hypersensitivity might be a symptom in early stages of NCCLs, and its noninvasive treatment is desirable whenever possible.

There is an ongoing debate regarding whether any type of occlusal therapy should be established in patients in whom overloading may be behind abfraction lesions. Occlusal adjustments requiring tooth structure elimination should be limited and only performed by professionals with occlusal expertise with the aim of preventing further progress of lesions from occlusal imbalance.[64] Occlusal splints are a much more conservative approach, although there is not sufficient support to demonstrate their efficacy in this type of lesion.[65] One study proved rapid progression in deeper V-shaped wedge lesions when compared with shallower U-shaped defects.[66]

Restorative treatment with direct composite restorations will be ideal when there are no other structural issues.[64] Minimal or no preparation whenever possible, with the election of a suitable adhesive system in the hands of a careful operator, will provide excellent longevity of the restoration. Soft tissue recessions should also be addressed through the implementation of periodontal procedures.[67–70] In cases where NCCLs coexist with other structural defects or special esthetic requirements, other therapies such as indirect porcelain laminate veneers or onlays might be a better option.

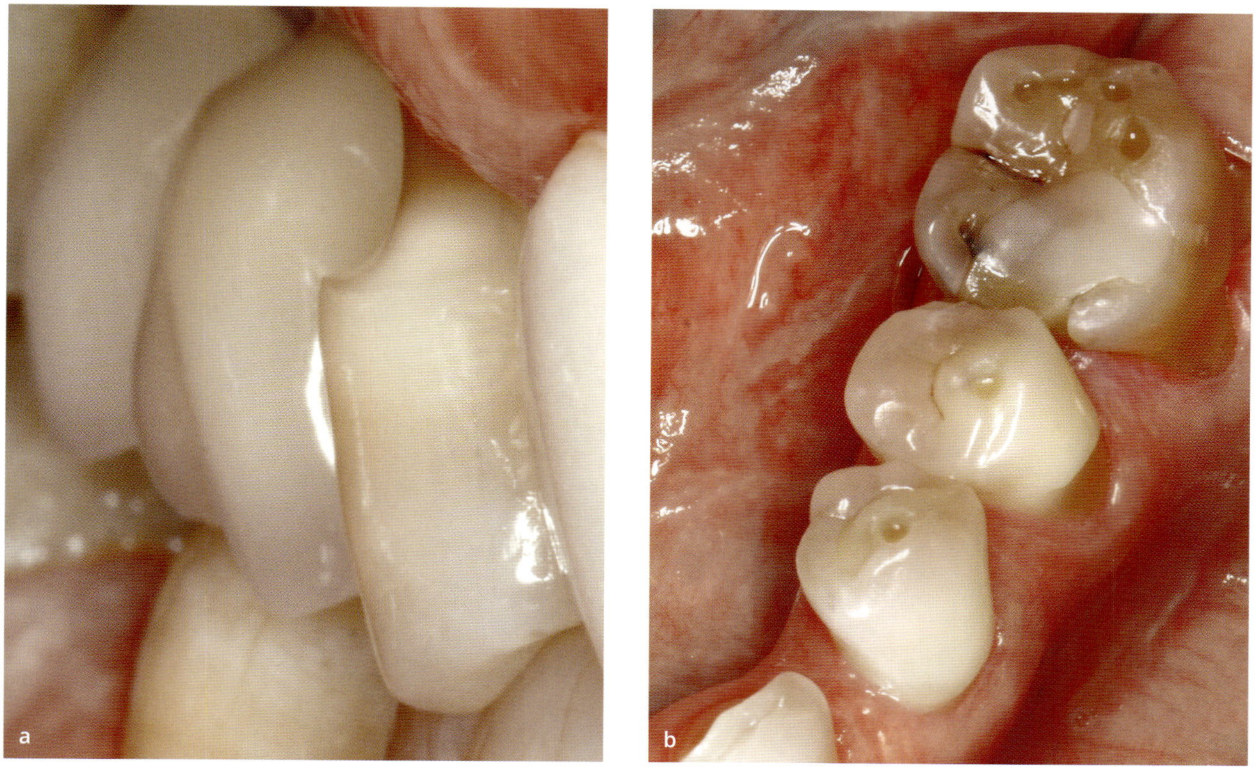


**Fig 6-24** Non-carious cervical lesions (NCCLs) appear as a loss of hard tissue at the cementoenamel junction. They are the consequence of lifestyle and nutritional habits combined with other factors, such as erosion, abrasion, and occlusal stress (a and b).

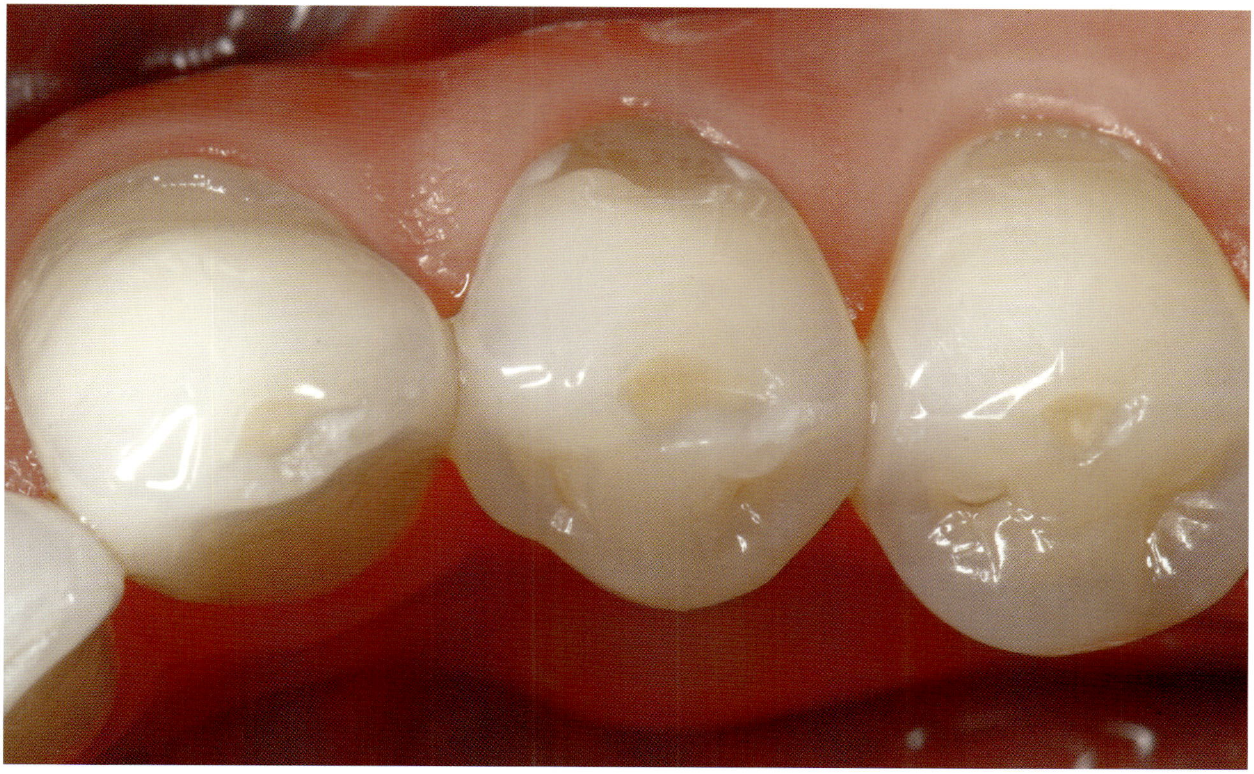

**Fig 6-25** Multifactorial TW in a young athletic patient. The concomitant presence of erosion multiplies the destructive capacity of TW.

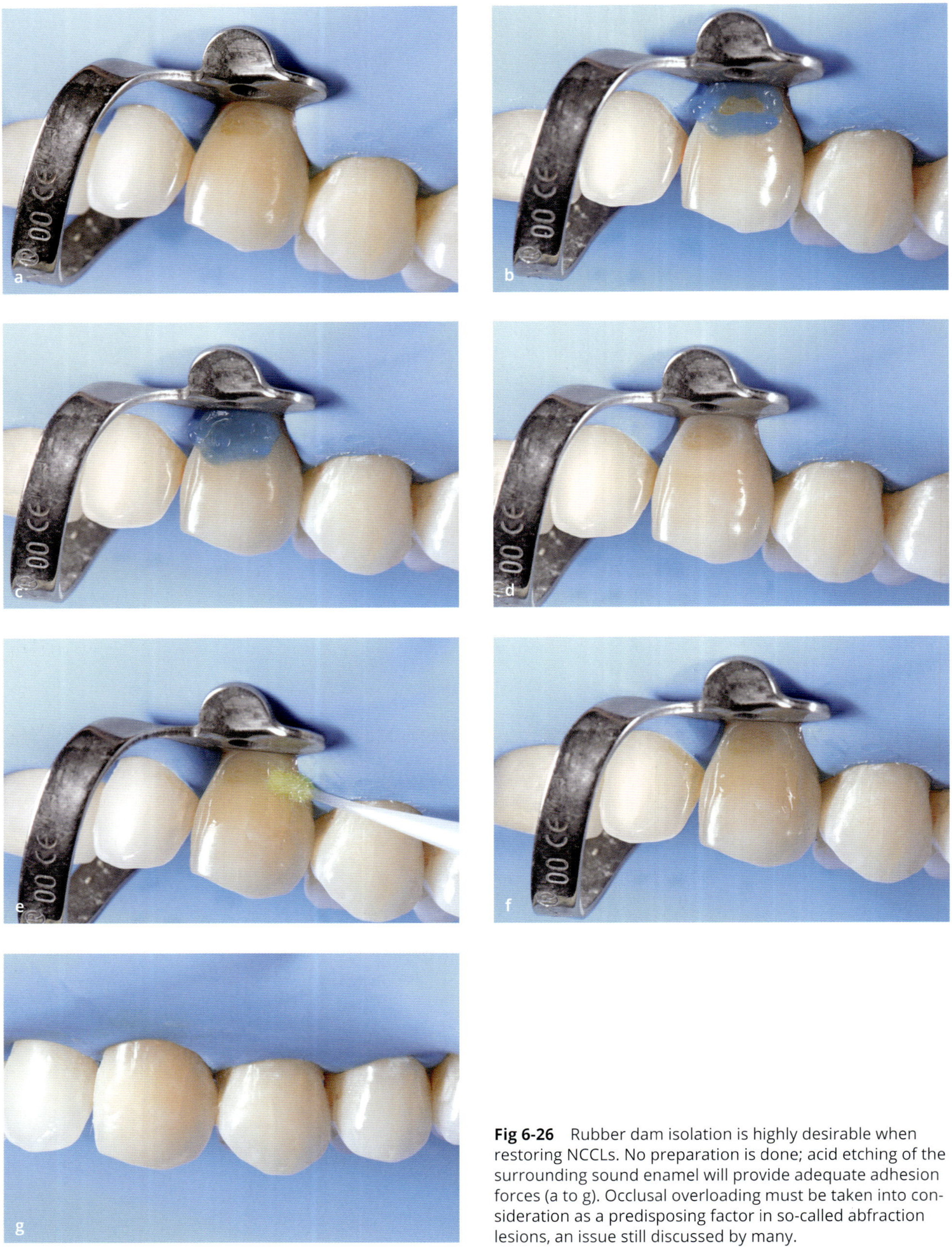


**Fig 6-26** Rubber dam isolation is highly desirable when restoring NCCLs. No preparation is done; acid etching of the surrounding sound enamel will provide adequate adhesion forces (a to g). Occlusal overloading must be taken into consideration as a predisposing factor in so-called abfraction lesions, an issue still discussed by many.

## 8. Key Points: Decision Making in Moderate/Severe TW

**Table 6-1** Decision making in moderate/severe TW.

| | |
|---|---|
| There is interocclusal space: TW mainly of attrition origin that has damaged mostly anterior sector. | Decide between MIP and CR after evaluation of posterior occlusal contacts:<br>▪ Restore mandibular posterior worn dentition first, then maxillary posterior worn dentition; check occlusal contacts.<br>▪ Restore maxillary anterior worn dentition; check occlusal scheme. |
| There is no interocclusal space: TW usually from erosive origin with damage to anterior, palatal, and posterior surfaces. | 1. The space is found in CR.<br>2. Dentoskeletal discrepancy or patient's profile impedes using CR for restorative planning:<br>▪ Orthodontics will expand and improve overbite and overjet with or without subsequent increase of VDO at restorative phase.<br>3. Orthodontic path:<br>▪ The space is found after treating the malocclusion with orthodontics.<br>4. Restorative path:<br>▪ The space is found after restoring posterior dentition (and mandibular anterior dentition) as a result of an augmented VDO.<br>5. Combination of the above is also possible. |
| PPP (TW risk reduction, counseling, mouthguard). | 1. Transparent thin splints if erosive origin.<br>2. Michigan mouthguard if attrition origi3.<br>3. Combination of the two. |

## References


1. Magne P, Kim TH, Cascione D, Donovan TE. Immediate dentin sealing improves bond strength of indirect restorations. J Prosthet Dent 2005;94:511–519.
2. Mallat E. ¿Qué detalles de la adhesión son de interés en los casos de desgaste dentario? Rev Int Protes Estomatol 2020;22(3):70.
3. Shimada Y, Tagami J. Effects of regional enamel and prism orientation on resin bonding. Oper Dent 2003;28(1):20–27.
4. Deari S, Wegehaupt FJ, Tauböck TT, Attin T. Influence of different pretreatments on the microtensile bond strength to eroded dentin. J Adhes Dent 2017;19(2):147–155.
5. Sawlani K, Lawson NC, Burgess JO, et al. Factors influencing the progression of non-carious cervical lesions: A 5-year prospective clinical evaluation. J Prosthet Dent 2016;115:571–577.
6. Tay FR, Pashley DH. Resin bonding to cervical sclerotic dentin: A review. J Dent 2004;32(3):173–196.
7. Kwong SM, Cheung GS, Kei LH, et al. Micro-tensile bond strengths to sclerotic dentin using a self-etching and a total-etching technique. Dent Mater 2002;18:359–369.
8. Tsai YL, Nakajima M, Wang CY, Foxton RM, Lin CP, Tagami J. Influence of etching ability of one-step self-etch adhesives on bonding to sound and non-carious cervical sclerotic dentin. Dent Mater J 2011;30:941–947.
9. Yoshiyama M, Sano H, Ebisu S, et al. Regional strengths of bonding agents to cervical sclerotic root dentin. J Dent Res 1996;75:1404–1413.
10. Devoto W, Pansecchi D. Composite restorations in the anterior region: Clinical and aesthetic performances. Pract Proced Aesthet Dent 2007;19(8):465–470.
11. Chikawa H, Inai N, Cho E, et al. Effect of incremental filling technique on adhesion of light-cured resin composite to cavity floor. Dent Mater J 2006;25:503–508.
12. Attin T, Filli T, Imfeld C, Schmidlin PR. Composite vertical bite reconstructions in eroded dentitions after 5.5 years: A case series. J Oral Rehabil 2012;39(1):73–79.
13. Schmidlin PR, Filli T, Imfeld C, Tepper S, Attin T. Three-year evaluation of posterior vertical bite reconstruction using direct resin composite—A case series. Oper Dent 2009;34(1):102–108.
14. Vajani D, Tejani TH, Milosevic A. Direct composite resin for the management of tooth wear: A systematic review. Clin Cosmet Investig Dent 2020;12:465–475.
15. Terry DA, Geller W, Tric O, Anderson MJ, Tourville M, Kobashigawa A. Anatomical form defines color: Function, form, and aesthetics. Pract Proced Aesthet Dent 2002;14(1):59–67.
16. Devoto W, Saracinelli M, Manauta J. Composite in everyday practice: How to choose the right material and simplify application techniques in the anterior teeth. Eur J Esthet Dent 2010;5(1):102–124.
17. Dietschi D. Free-hand bonding in the esthetic treatment of anterior teeth: Creating the illusion. J Esthet Dent 1997;9(4):156–164.
18. Terry DA, Powers JM. A predictable resin composite injection technique, Part I. Dent Today 2014;33(4):96,98–101.
19. Terry DA, Powers JM, Mehta D, Babu V. A predictable resin composite injection technique, Part 2. Dent Today 2014;33(8):12.
20. Ammannato R, Ferraris F, Marchesi G. The "index technique" in worn dentition: A new and conservative approach. Int J Esthet Dent 2015;10(1):68–99.
21. Dietschi D, Saratti CM. Interceptive treatment of tooth wear: A revised protocol for the full molding technique. Int J Esthet Dent 2020;15(3):264–286.
22. Ferraris F, Conti A. Superficial roughness on composite surface, composite-enamel and composite-dentin junctions after different finishing and polishing procedures. Part II: roughness with diamond finishing and differences between enamel composite vs body composite. Int J Esthet Dent 2014;9(2):184–204.
23. Loomans B, Opdam N, Attin T, et al. Severe tooth wear: European consensus statement on management guidelines. J Adhes Dent 2017;19(2):111–119.
24. Veneziani M. Posterior indirect adhesive restorations: Updated indications and the morphology driven preparation technique. Int J Esthet Dent 2017;12(2):204–230.
25. Wilson NH, Lynch CD. The teaching of posterior resin composites: Planning for the future based on 25 years of research. J Dent 2014;42:503–516.
26. Ruiz LF, Nicoloso GF, Franzon R, Lenzi TL, de Araujo FB, Casagrande L. Repair increases the survival of failed primary teeth restorations in high-caries risk children: A university-based retrospective study. Clin Oral Investig 2020;24(1):71–77.
27. Lynch CD, Hayashi M, Seow LL, Blum IR, Wilson NH. The management of defective resin composite restorations: Current trends in dental school teaching in Japan. Oper Dent 2013;38:497–504.
28. Cho E, Chikawa H, Kishikawa R, et al. Influence of elasticity on gap formation in a lining technique with flowable composite. Dent Mater J 2006;25:538–544.
29. Terry DA. Restoring with Flowables. Chicago: Quintessence, 2017.
30. Blum IR, Lynch CD, Wilson NH. Teaching of the repair of defective composite restorations in Scandinavian dental schools. J Oral Rehabil 2012;39:210–216.
31. Blum IR, Lynch CD, Wilson NH. Teaching of direct composite restoration repair in undergraduate dental schools in the United Kingdom and Ireland. Eur J Dent Educ 2012;16(1):e53–e58.
32. Lynch CD, Blum IR, McConnell RJ, Frazier KB, Brunton PA, Wilson NHF. Teaching posterior resin composites in UK and Ireland dental schools: Do current teaching programmes match the expectation of clinical practice arrangements? Br Dent J 2018;224:967–972.
33. Hayashi M, Haapasalo M, Imazato S, et al. Dentistry in the 21st century: Challenges of a globalising world. Int Dent J 2014;64:333–342.

34. Spyrou M, Koliniotou-Koumpia E, Kouros P, Koulaouzidou E, Dionysopoulos P. The reparability of contemporary composite resins. Eur J Dent 2014;8:353–359.
35. Kitasako Y, Sasaki Y, Takagaki T, Sadr A, Tagami J. Age-specific prevalence of erosive tooth wear by acidic diet and gastroesophageal reflux in Japan. J Dent 2015;43:418–423.
36. Kitasako Y, Sasaki Y, Takagaki T, Sadr A, Tagami J. Erosive tooth wear among different tooth types and surfaces in Japanese adults 15 to 89 years old. Oral Health Prev Dent 2017;15:357–364.
37. Ionta FQ, Alencar CRB, Val PP, et al. Effect of vegetable oils applied over acquired enamel pellicle on initial erosion. J Appl Oral Sci 2017;25:420–426.
38. Vailati F, Belser UC. Full-mouth adhesive rehabilitation of a severely eroded dentition: The three-step technique. Part 3. Eur J Esthet Dent 2008;3:236–257.
39. Vailati F, Belser UC. Full-mouth adhesive rehabilitation of a severely eroded dentition: The three-step technique. Part 2. Eur J Esthet Dent 2008;3:128–146.
40. Vailati F, Belser UC. Full-mouth adhesive rehabilitation of a severely eroded dentition: The three-step technique. Part 1. Eur J Esthet Dent 2008;3:30–44.
41. Gulamali AB, Hemmings KW, Tredwin CJ, Petrie A. Survival analysis of composite Dahl restorations provided to manage localised anterior tooth wear (ten year follow-up). Br Dent J 2011;211(4):E9.
42. Ash M. Freedom in centric. A practical occlusion concept [in German]. Phillip J Restaur Zahnmed 1987;4(1):7–14.
43. Thompson JR. The free-way space and the passivity of the teeth. CDS Rev 1981;74(1):31–34,36.
44. Mangani F, Cerutti A, Putignano A, Bollero R, Madini L. Clinical approach to anterior adhesive restorations using resin composite veneers. Eur J Esthet Dent 2007;2(2):188–209.
45. Magne P. Noninvasive bilaminar CAD/CAM composite resin veneers: A semi-(in)direct approach. Int J Esthet Dent 2017;12(2):134–154.
46. Liu M, Gai K, Chen J, Jiang L. Comparison of failure and complication risks of porcelain laminate and indirect resin veneer restorations: A meta-analysis. Int J Prosthodont 2019;32:59–65.
47. Magne P, Douglas WH. Additive contour of porcelain veneers: A key element in enamel preservation, adhesion, and esthetics for aging dentition. J Adhes Dent 1999;1(1):81–92.
48. Ferraris F, Conti A. Superficial roughness on composite surface, composite enamel and composite dentin junctions after different finishing and polishing procedures. Part I: Roughness after treatments with tungsten carbide vs diamond burs. Int J Esthet Dent 2014;9(1):70–89.
49. Montanaro L, Campoccia D, Rizzi S, et al. Evaluation of bacterial adhesion of *Streptococcus mutans* on dental restorative materials. Biomaterials 2004;25:4457–4463.
50. Patel SB, Gordan VV, Barrett AA, Shen C. The effect of surface finishing and storage solutions on the color stability of resin-based composites. J Am Dent Assoc 2004;135:587–594.
51. Edelhoff D, Sorensen JA. Tooth structure removal associated with various preparation designs for anterior teeth. J Prosthet Dent 2002;87:503–509.
52. Dahl BL, Krogstad O, Karlsen K. An alternative treatment in cases with advanced localized attrition. J Oral Rehabil 1975;2(3):209–214.
53. Abduo J, Lyons K. Clinical considerations for increasing occlusal vertical dimension: A review. Aust Dent J 2012;57(1):2–10.
54. Gracis S. Clinical considerations and rationale for the use of simplified instrumentation in occlusal rehabilitation. Part 2: setting of the articulator and occlusal optimization. Int J Periodontics Restorative Dent 2003;23(2):139–145.
55. Gracis S. Clinical considerations and rationale for the use of simplified instrumentation in occlusal rehabilitation. Part 1: Mounting of the models on the articulator. Int J Periodontics Restorative Dent 2003;23(1):57–67.
56. Magne P, Magne M, Belser UC. Adhesive restorations, centric relation, and the Dahl principle: Minimally invasive approaches to localized anterior tooth erosion. Eur J Esthet Dent 2007;2(3):260–273.
57. Vailati F, Belser UC. Classification and treatment of the anterior maxillary dentition affected by dental erosion: The ACE classification. Int J Periodontics Restorative Dent 2010;30:559–571.
58. d'Incau E, Rouas P, Couture-Veschambre C. Tooth wear and compensatory modification of the dentoalveolar complex in a Nubian sample. J Craniomandib Funct 2015;7:315–336.
59. Murphy, T., Compensatory mechanisms in facial height adjustment to functional tooth attrition. Aust Dent J 1959;4(5):312–323.
60. Telles D, Pegoraro LF, Pereira JC. Prevalence of noncarious cervical lesions and their relation to occlusal aspects: A clinical study. J Esthet Dent 2000;12(1):10–15.
61. Bartlett DW, Shah P. A critical review of non-carious cervical (wear) lesions and the role of abfraction, erosion, and abrasion. J Dent Res 2006;85:306–312.
62. Borcic J, Anic I, Urek MM, Ferreri S. The prevalence of non-carious cervical lesions in permanent dentition. J Oral Rehabil 2004;31(2):117–123.
63. Michael JA, Townsend GC, Greenwood LF, Kaidonis JA. Abfraction: Separating fact from fiction. Aust Dent J 2009;54(1):2–8.
64. Soares PV, Grippo JO (eds). Noncarious Cervical Lesions and Cervical Dentin Hypersensitivity: Etiology, Diagnosis, and Treatment. Chicago: Quintessence, 2017.
65. Peumans M, Politano G, Van Meerbeek B. Treatment of noncarious cervical lesions: When, why, and how. Int J Esthet Dent 2020;15(1):16–42.
66. Sugita I, Nakashima S, Ikeda A, et al. A pilot study to assess the morphology and progression of non-carious cervical lesions. J Dent 2017;57:51–56.
67. Zuhr O, Hürzeler M, Plastic-Esthetic Periodontal and Implant Surgery: A Microsurgical Approach. London: Quintessence, 2012.
68. Zucchelli G. Mucogingival Esthetic Surgery. Milan: Quintessence, 2013.
69. Gil A, Bakhshalian N, Min S, Nart J, Zadeh HH. Three-dimensional volumetric analysis of multiple gingival recession defects treated by the vestibular incision subperiosteal tunnel access (VISTA) procedure. Int J Periodontics Restorative Dent 2019;39:687–695.
70. Zadeh HH. Minimally invasive treatment of maxillary anterior gingival recession defects by vestibular incision subperiosteal tunnel access and platelet-derived growth factor BB. Int J Periodontics Restorative Dent 2011;31:653–660.

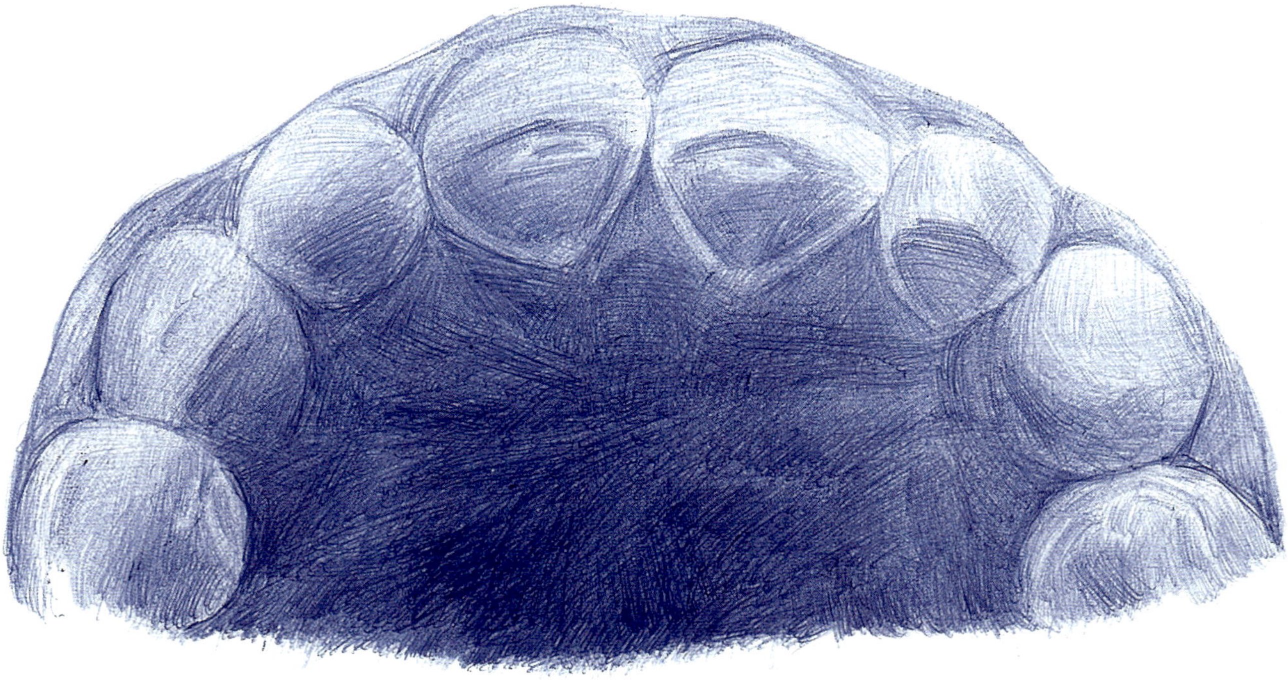

*Hope for the best, expect the worst. Life is a play. We are unrehearsed.*

—Mel Brooks, American director, writer, comedian, and actor

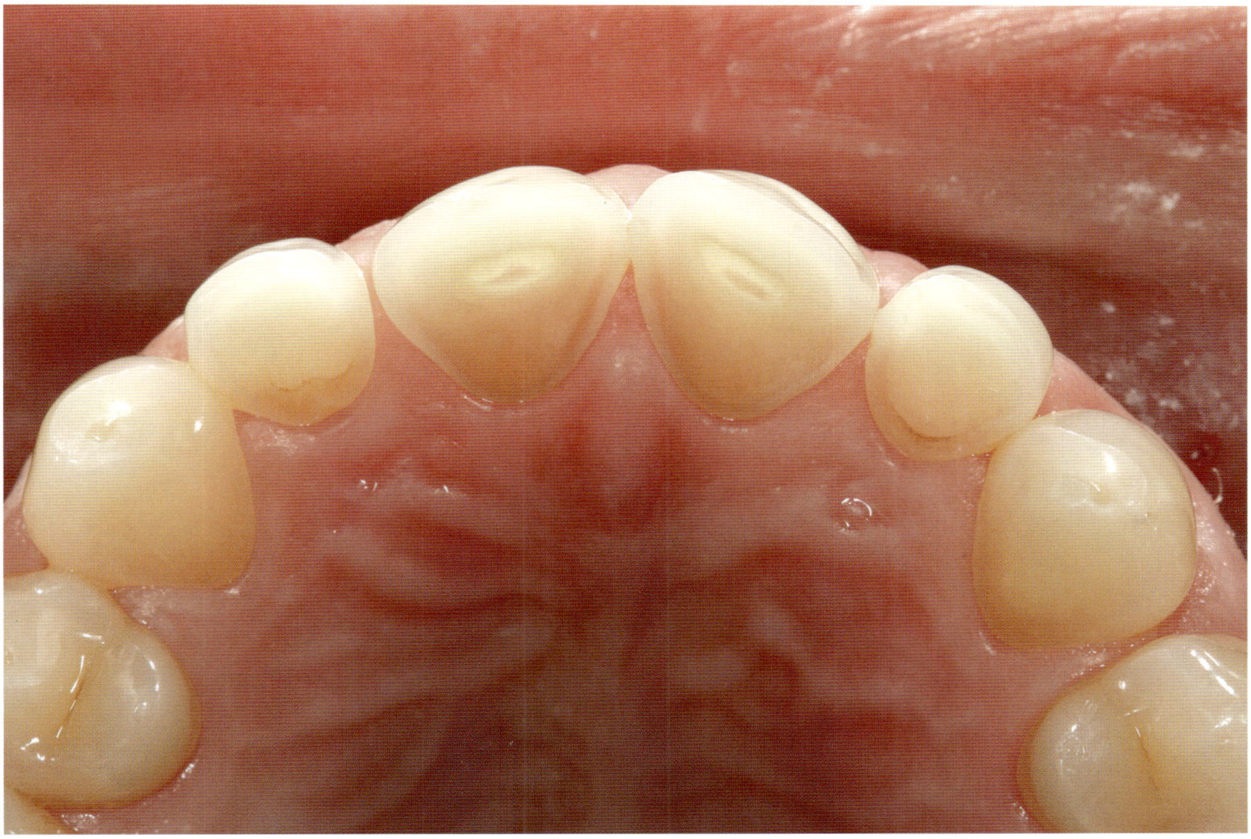

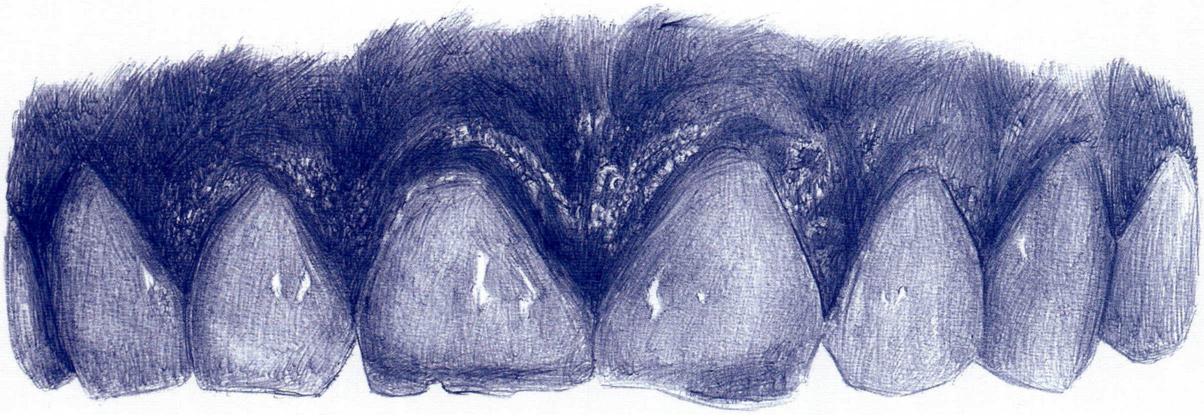

*Have no fear of perfection, you'll never reach it.*

—Salvador Dalí

CHAPTER 7

# SEVERE TOOTH WEAR: TREATMENT STRATEGIES

The treatment of a patient with severe TW is a complex and demanding three-dimensional process; in many cases, it is an authentic challenge. Minor direct composite restorations are the first line of treatment for patients with minor or incipient tooth wear and can still be of use in cases of advanced TW. Nevertheless, a thorough 3D evaluation of all aspects of the teeth, including when they are in function, will dictate the extent of the restorative treatment as well as the indication for improvement of the anterior and canine guidance. This is already relevant in a patient with moderate TW displaying damage to the anterior sector and essential in cases of severe TW.

In cases of severe damage to the hard tissues, the impact to the vertical dimension needs to be taken into consideration, and a proper strategy to regain height must be established from the beginning, whether it is restorative, orthodontic, or a combination of both. The timing and type of therapy will be key to the extent and invasiveness of the treatment applied.

In severe TW, the damage to the dentition can be so profound that there is no barrier between the management of the worn dentition and what is understood as a prosthodontic full-mouth rehabilitation. However, the difference lies in the presence or absence of TW risk factors that will inevitably challenge the survival of the restorations.

Particularly in the presence of erosive etiology, a thorough general health anamnesis and lifestyle discussion is needed for risk assessment and to mitigate further damage.

## 1. From Moderate to Severe Tooth Wear

The wait-and-see approach and the reluctance of the patient to undergo interceptive treatment while asymptomatic can lead to major tooth loss, even in patients that regularly attend the dental office. It is difficult to anticipate the rate of progression at which the TW damage will occur and when the patient will seek treatment again.[1] On the other hand, there is evidence to suggest that the amount of tooth structure remaining has a direct correlation with the duration of the restoration.[2]

In addition, age is not a reliable indicator of severe TW. As per some extensive reviews and international consensus, TW is already a concern in children and young adults[3–5] (Fig 7-1). Furthermore, by the time patients experience either pain or functional impairment, the damage is already intense, affecting deep layers of dentin and even pulp (Fig 7-2). All of these facts may serve to explain why dentists today are confronted with an avalanche of patients with moderate to severe TW.

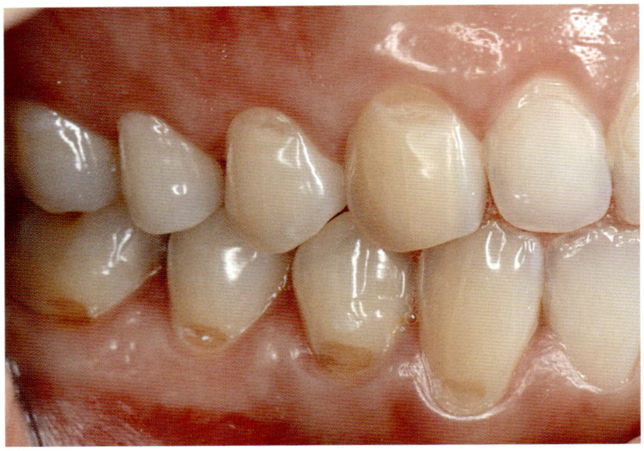

**Fig 7-1** Dentin exposure in a female patient in her early 20s as a consequence of TW of a combined erosion, attrition, and abfraction/abrasion origin. Note the cervical NCCLs as well as the flattening of the canine cusp.

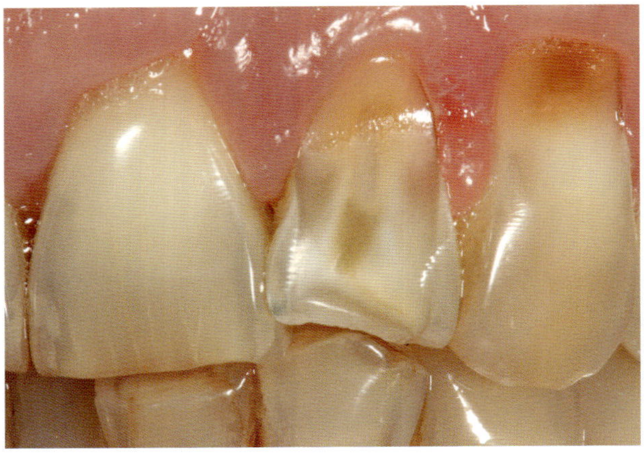

**Fig 7-2** A 59-year-old female patient presented with multifactorial severe TW with pulp transparency and disappearance of all labial tooth anatomy in her maxillary right lateral incisor. The Class II division 2 malocclusion, and the resulting abrasion caused by tooth brushing and lip friction occurred on already severely acid-softened buccal enamel, especially in the lateral incisors. The adjacent teeth have suffered to a lesser degree because of their retroclination. The NCCL on the canine indicates there is a mechanical component aside from the chemical imbalance. The patient was asymptomatic, with the abnormal appearance of her teeth as her major concern.

## Three-Dimensional Thinking in Severe TW

When confronting a severe TW case, it should be expected to find a substantial loss of tooth structure with dentin exposure and therefore significant loss of the clinical crown. Subsequent collapse may not be apparent as compensatory dentoskeletal adaptation may have happened, hiding the loss in the three dimensions of space. Therefore, a strategy to recuperate the lost space should be established from the beginning.

Esthetic damage is clearly perceived, and function is impaired in severe TW. However, if other factors such as age, the rate of progression, or the etiology are taken into consideration, cases with a lesser amount of tooth structure loss also might be considered severe. As previously discussed, the finding of any one of the following factors elevates the severity of TW by one grade (see the Wear Aggravating Severity Scale [WASS] in chapter 4):

- Young patient
- Active TW present at the time of evaluation
- Etiologic factor, such as GERD or polymedication, present at the time of evaluation
- Erosive dietary pattern (eg, soft drinks, fruit juices, food intolerances, vegetarian diet)
- Malocclusion
- Mouth breathing, sleep apnea
- Etiology of TW is not clear
- Generalized TW affecting more than one group of teeth
- Rate of progression is rapid
- General health conditions present
- Salivary dysfunction, hyposalivation, xerostomia
- Parafunctional habits (eg, lip, nail, cheek biting)

The WASS is meant to be a practical, dynamic assessment index that helps categorize patients chairside by any member of the team. It is intended to avoid tooth-oriented static evaluation in an otherwise dynamic and challenging condition.

For instance, a 25-year-old woman with wear mostly in the anterior sector would be diagnosed as having moderate wear using the Wear Easy Clinical Classification (WECC) index. However, the aggravating factors of a Class III occlusion and a skeletal open bite with mouth breathing and a lacto-ovo-vegetarian diet make this a severe case (Figs 7-3 and 7-4).

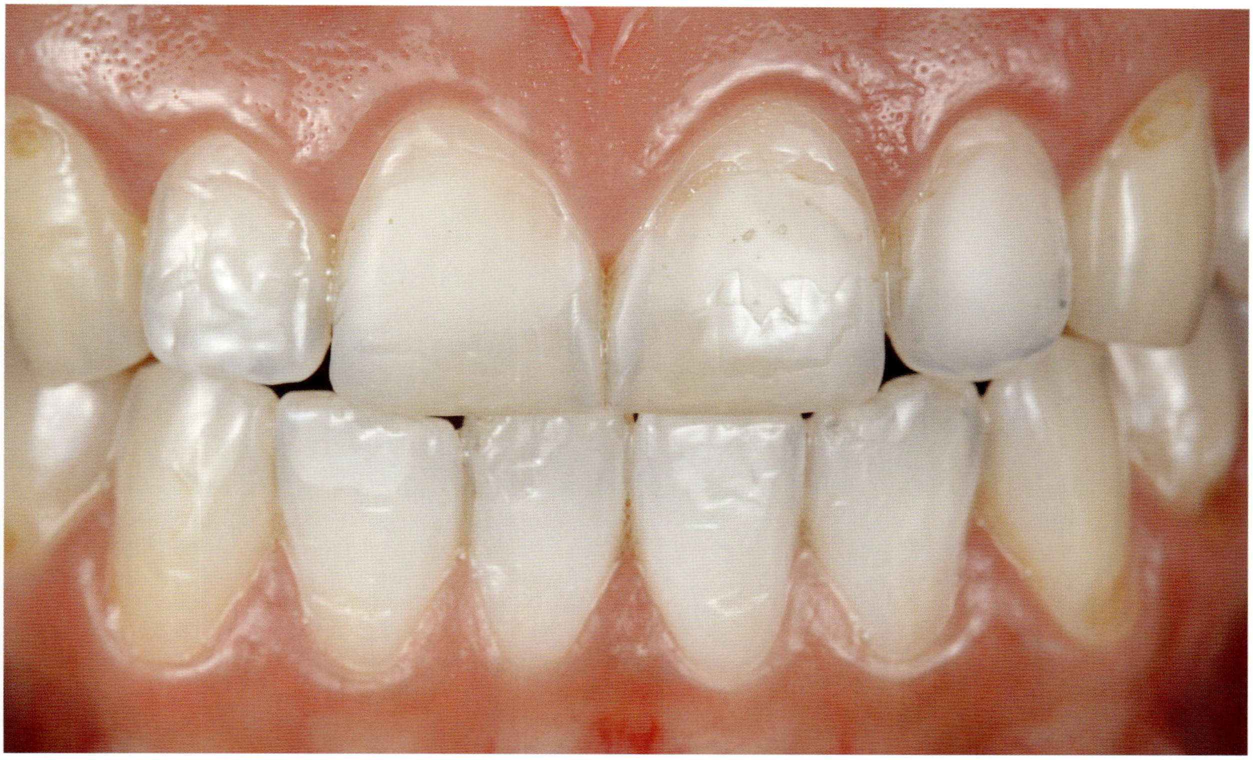

**Fig 7-3** The vestibular enamel is partially covered by inadequate composite restorations with fragments of exposed dentin still visible. The patient's awareness of the damage to her teeth had caused her to seek cosmetic treatment that unfortunately had failed to address her anterior open bite mouth breathing. The oral cavity appears desiccated, with inflammation of the soft tissues. The mouth breathing and skeletal open bite along with a restricted dietary pattern rich in acids are considered risk factors for TW progression and elevate the diagnosis from moderate to severe TW.

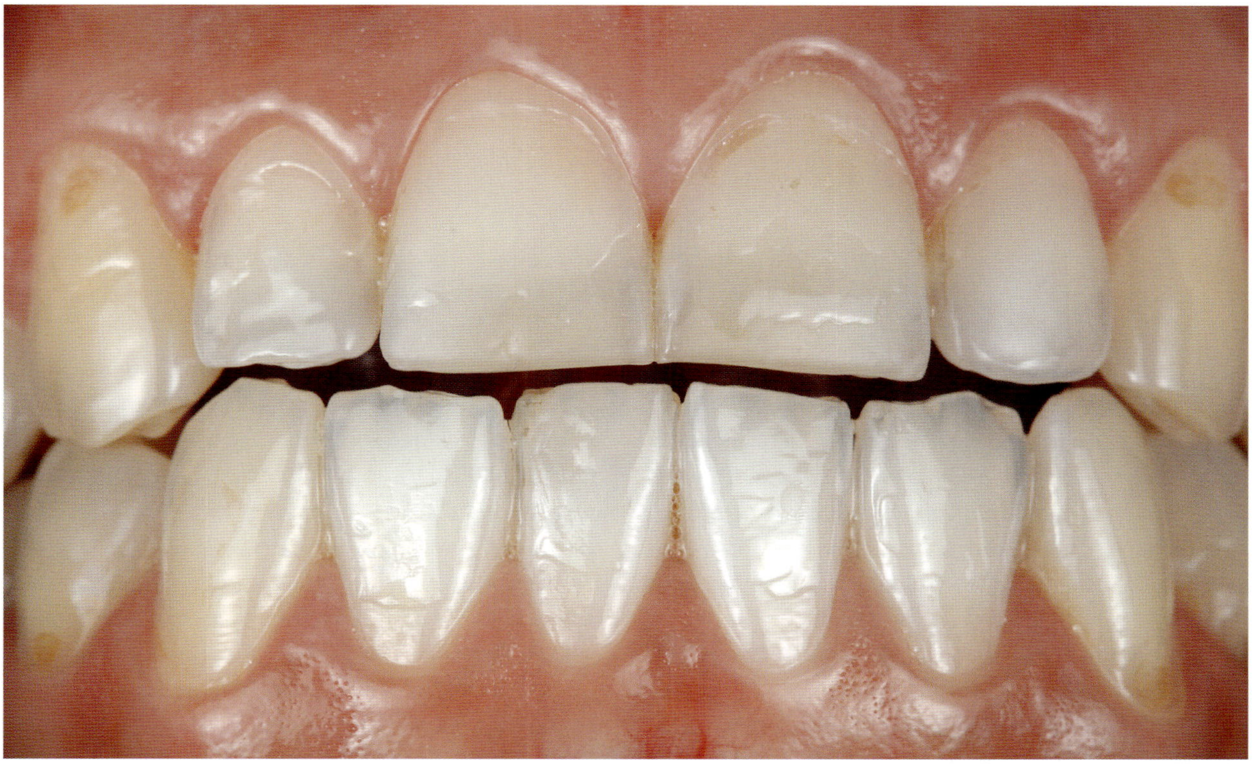

**Fig 7-4** Tooth proportion and tooth position are altered because of the skeletal pattern and malfunctioning of the upper respiratory apparatus. The environmental changes of the mouth breathing habit have changed the oral pH, and this acidity together with an erosive diet have facilitated tooth erosion.

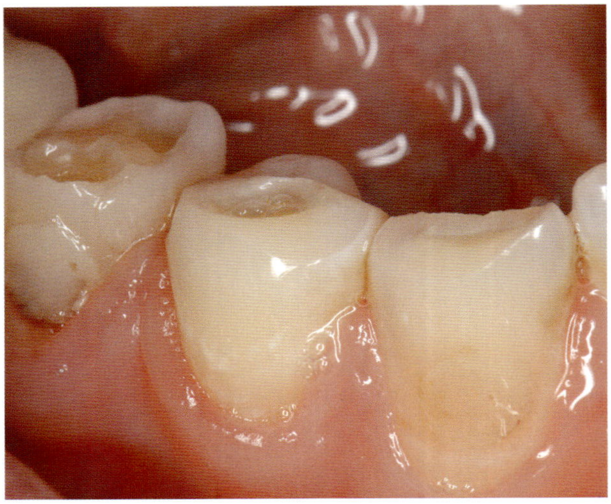

**Fig 7-5** Erosive blurring of the anatomy of cusps, ridges, and fossae and the appearance of concave occlusal anatomies.

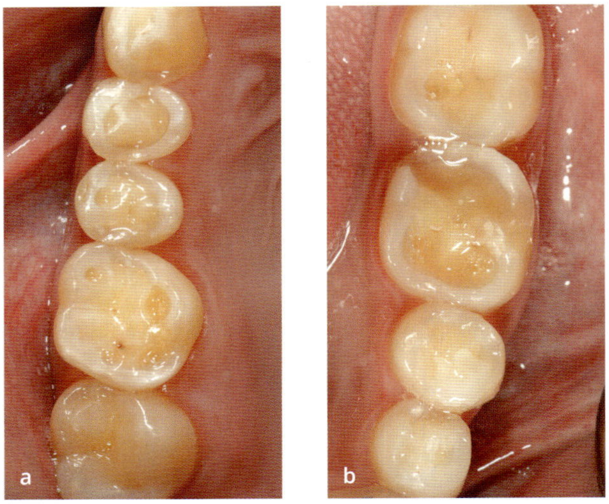


**Fig 7-6** Erosive severe TW in the maxillary molars and premolars of a compulsive soft drink consumer (a). The damage of extrinsic acids is usually more evident in the mandibular teeth, which act as natural reservoirs for liquids (b).

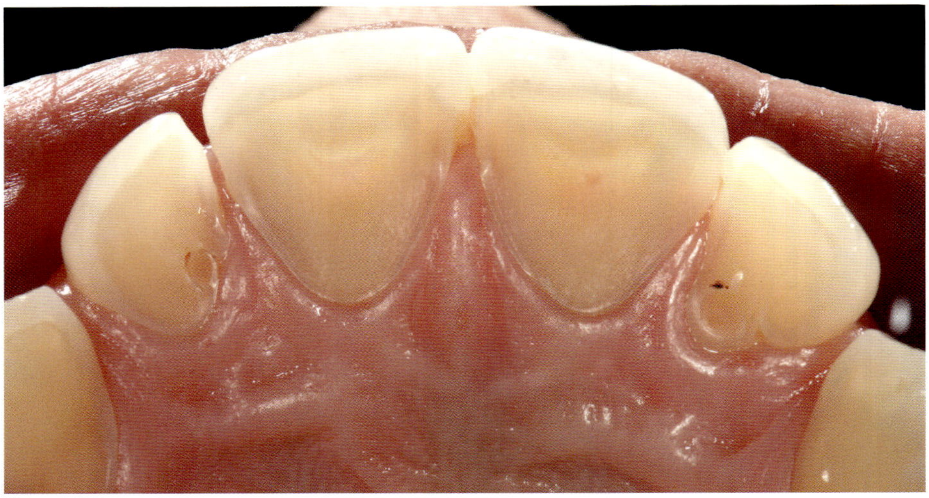

**Fig 7-7** Repeated exposure to gastric content has erased the palatal enamel of all four anterior teeth, causing pulp transparency. The patient was treated with PLVs 11 years before because of the esthetic damage done to the anterior teeth, but the palatal pathway of the acidic fluid was left unprotected.

## Erosive Factors in Severe TW

The literature supports that clinicians should be alerted to an increased risk of erosion in the general population.[6,7] In fact, gastroenterology specialists have seen a shift toward an increasing number of intolerance-related inflammatory conditions of the digestive tract in younger patients as well as an exponential growth of dyspepsia and reflux of digestive liquids to the oral cavity in adults.[8]

On the other hand, eating disorders (EDs) as well as demanding lifestyles are also behind cases of severe TW.[9,10] Hyperconnectivity and overworking are also behind stress, microbiome changes, and hyposalivation that have been related to rapid TW progression in executive-level entrepreneurs.

Severe TW not only affects the cusps of the posterior dentition but also the whole of the occlusal surface, erasing the morphology of all, or most, of the posterior teeth as well as other aspects like the labial and palatal surfaces of the anterior dentition[11,12] (Figs 7-5 to 7-7). This disruption of the occlusal plane and/or the incisal plane may even be visible in the rest position (Fig 7-8).

Furthermore, the collapse of the vertical dimension of occlusion is not always accompanied by an augmented vertical rest dimension, as the space that has developed from the loss of hard tissue may be taken up by compensatory eruption (mostly of the mandible teeth). This is one of the biggest challenges that the restorative team faces: providing the required space for occlusal restorations[13] (Fig 7-9)

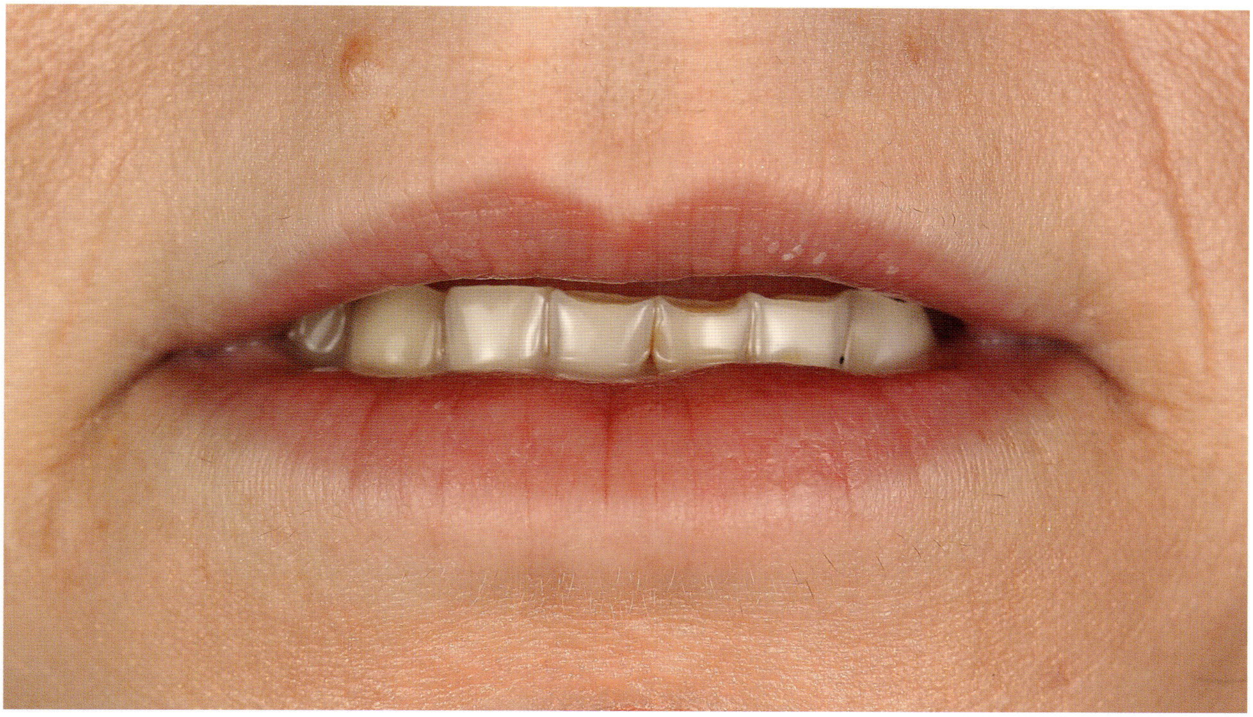

**Fig 7-8** Showing mostly mandibular anterior teeth when talking is a common finding in compensatory eruption in cases of severe TW.

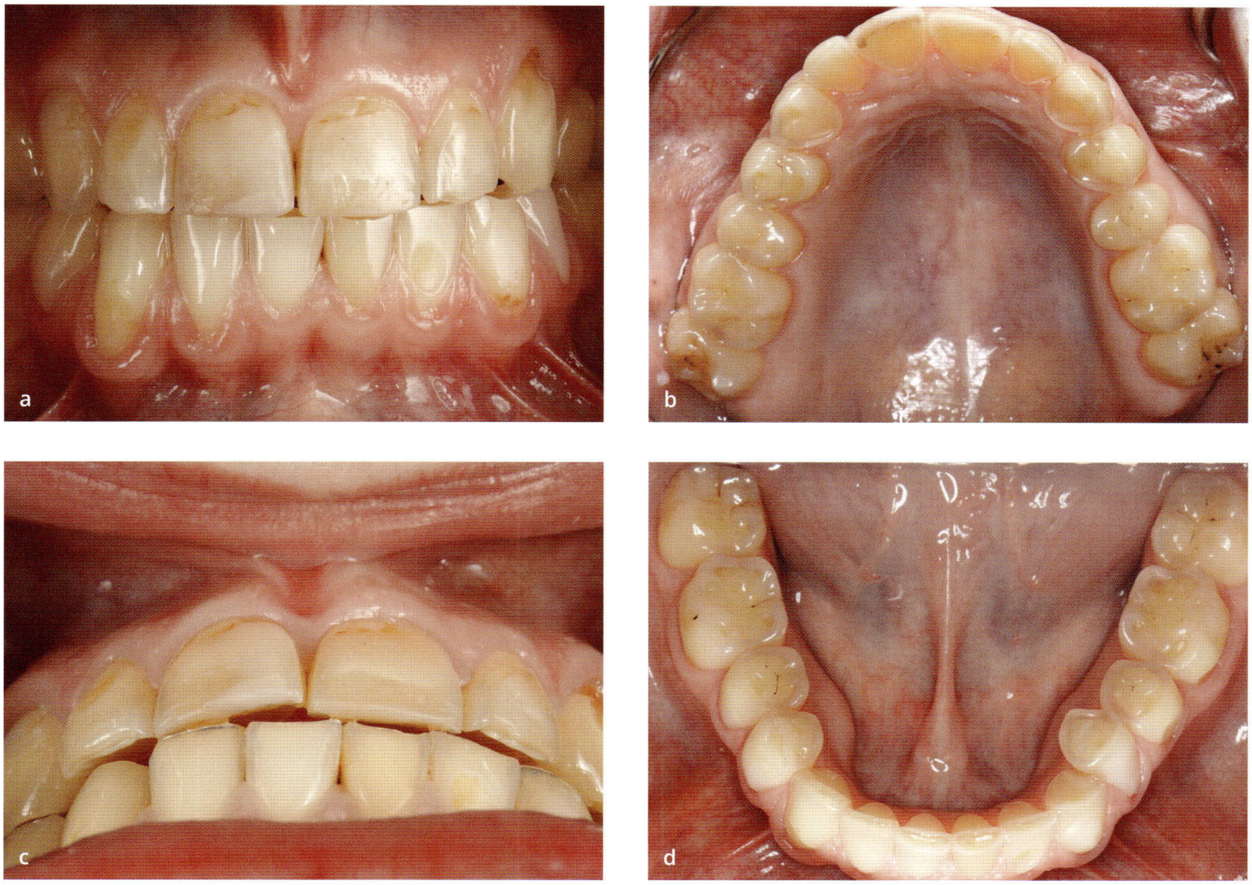

**Fig 7-9** The erosive challenge has caused severe damage to the integrity of these teeth. The 3D challenge resides in finding the least invasive restorative approach to provide the needed interocclusal space (a to d).

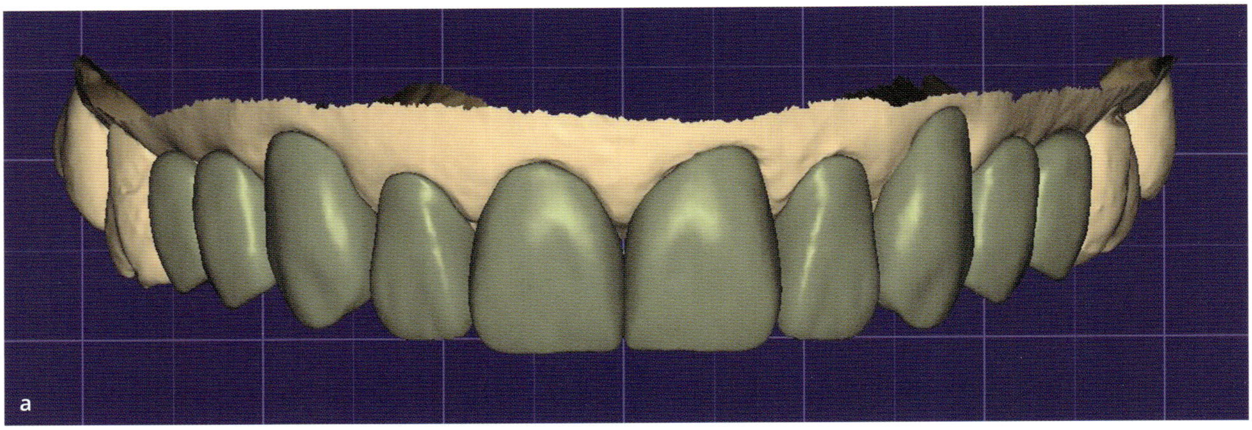


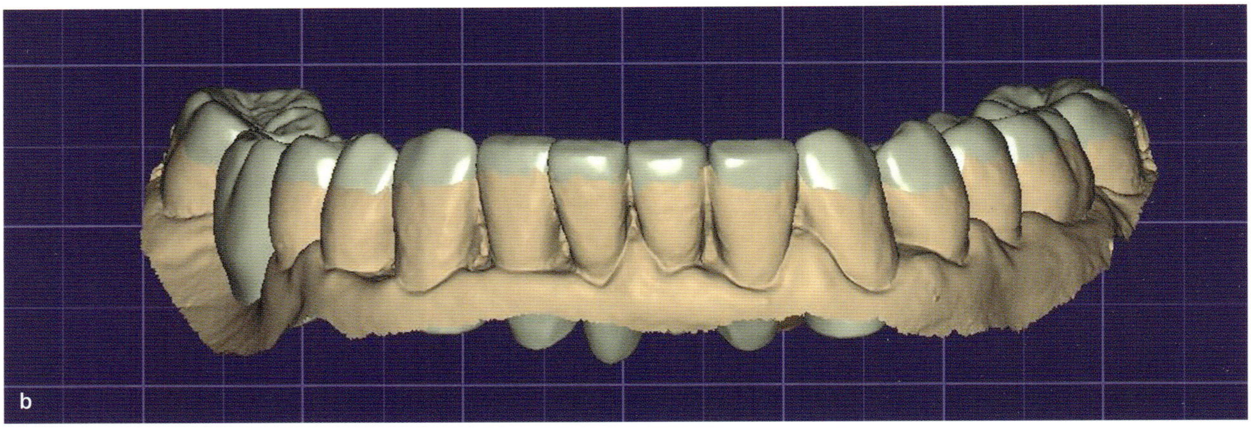


## 2. Wax-Up: The Blueprint

Adhesion and adhesive restorative dentistry have enabled modern dentistry to address TW lesions that would have been impossible to restore with traditional restorations.[14] The morphology of the TW lesion is totally different from a caries lesion. Also, the remaining tissue is not suspected of being contaminated in the wear patient, and therefore no further removal of dentin is needed nor desired. In cases where damage is incipient or moderate, a defect-oriented approach is sufficient as the anatomical landmarks may still be present.[15]

In cases of severe damage, the restorative team should be guided by a wax-up, be it analog or digital. Clinical or virtual transfer of the wax-up to the patient's mouth allows assessment of most of the classic prosthodontic and esthetic parameters (Fig 7-10). However, phonetic evaluation can only be done in a clinical try-in, not in a virtual analysis.

In severe TW, efficient anterior and canine guidance together with a maximum number of occlusal contacts (ideally in centric relation) and sufficient occlusal support should guide the team from the very beginning of the conceptualization and manufacturing of the wax-up. Once the wax-up is transfered to the mouth, a thorough functional evaluation follows, as severe TW is a devastating condition with high risk of failure and premature tooth loss not only because of restoration leakage or further erosion but because of an inappropriate occlusal scheme.[16]

Consequently, there is a need for 3D planning and a fabrication of a blueprint, be it analog or digital, which is mandatory for the rehabilitation of the worn dentition.[17]

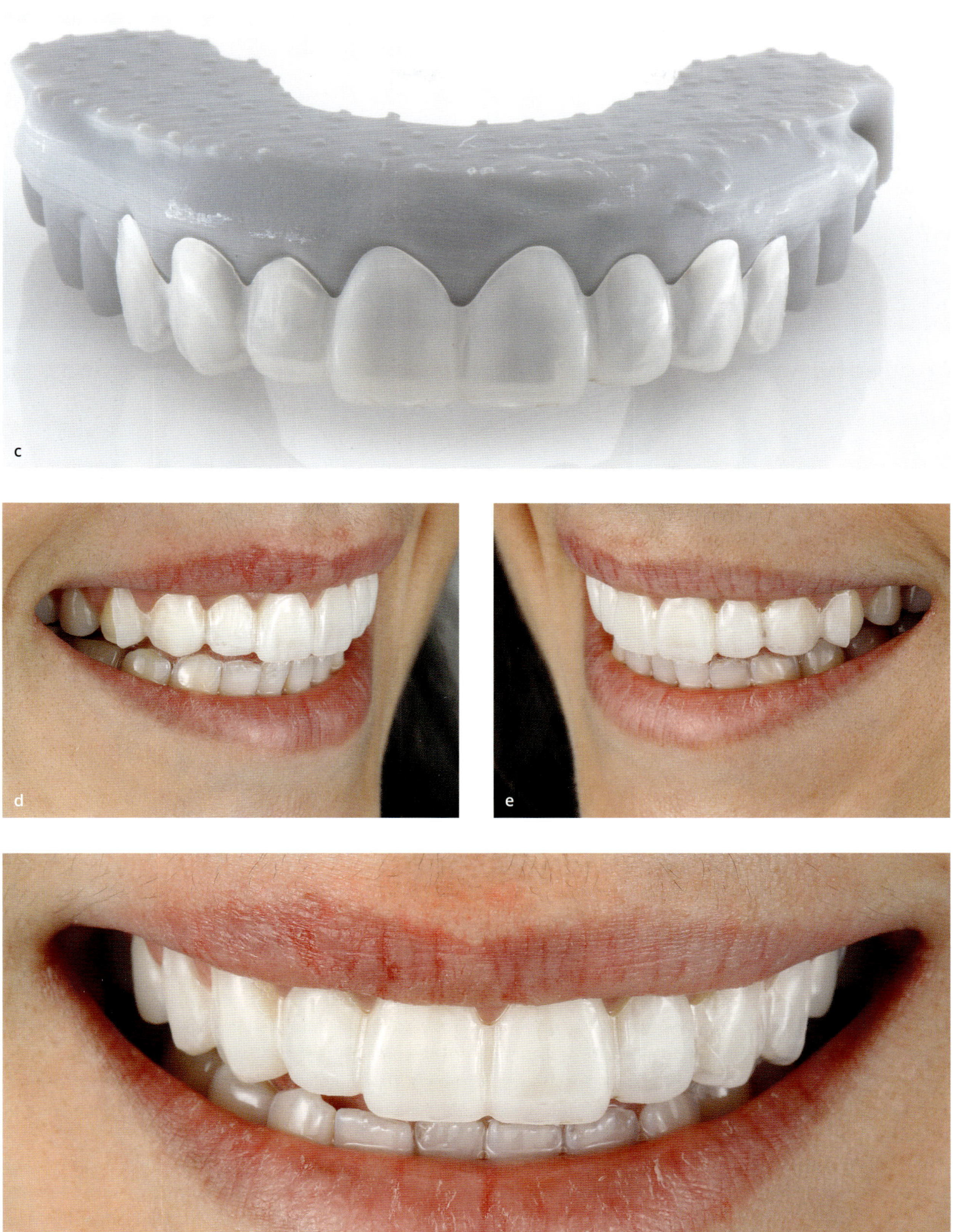

**Fig 7-10** Digital scanning is followed by a digital wax-up of all of the affected maxillary and mandibular teeth (a and b). A thin shell-type mock-up is transferred to the mouth, and changes are made digitally if needed (c to f).

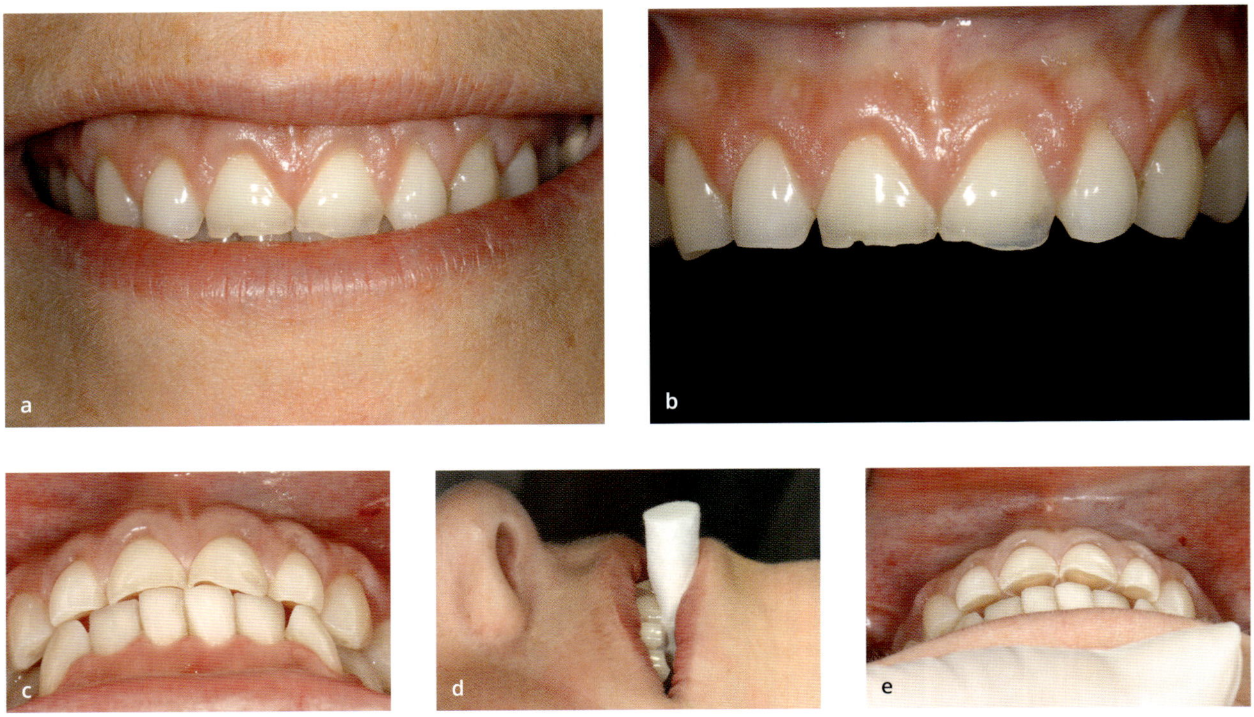

**Fig 7-11** Severe erosive TW in a very young professional swimmer and athlete, extensively affecting the anterior region of the mouth (a and b). Interocclusal space was lacking, but a manipulation in CR was productive in finding the necessary space to prevent further reduction. A shallow interference was eliminated, and no need for further adjustment was needed (c to e). An analog flow is chosen, with traditional model mounting with a facebow for restoration with six anterior "V" veneers and two posterior onlays made with feldspathic porcelain (f to k). A minimal preparation protocol is applied, and once the anterior and canine guidance is achieved, the patient is checked for final occlusion and asked to wear a protective transparent mouthguard while practicing sports (l to q).

## 3. Additive Approach with Porcelain Laminate Veneers for Anterior Guidance

In the majority of severe TW cases, reducing tooth structure leaves the dentition at even more extreme risk of failure, with a shortening of the life cycle of not only the restoration but also the teeth. Additive techniques that preserve as much enamel as possible for increased adhesion have been documented to be a safe and predictable means of restoration.[18,19] Occlusal equilibration of gross interferences and establishment of centric relation (CR) are appropriate parameters in full-mouth rehabilitation. Patients with severe TW can have an anterior position of the mandible in the aim to seek more contact points and compensate for the changes they experience. An easy chairside manipulation to check CR and evaluate the improvement of occlusal contacts is recommended. Using an additive approach rather than adjusting prematurities through reduction can be highly satisfactory in providing the needed interocclusal space in severe TW[20] (Figs 7-11a to 7-11g).

Severe TW also compromises self-esteem as it hinders attractiveness and a young-looking smile.[21] Severe or even moderate cases of TW require improvement of the appearance and predominance of the smile. Moreover, severe TW affects functional aspects of the dentition, such as anterior and canine guidance, and therefore restoration of the anatomy and function of the anterior teeth is required in most cases.[22]

A minimally invasive approach resides in keeping as much of the remnant tooth structure as possible while adding back substance to the damaged dentition and increasing the vertical dimension of occlusion.[23] Hence, the traditional reductive approach with PFM crowns or more recently metal-free all-ceramic crowns has given way to porcelain laminate veneers, porcelain onlays, and most recently CAD/CAM milled onlays[14,24–27] (Figs 7-11h to 7-11t).

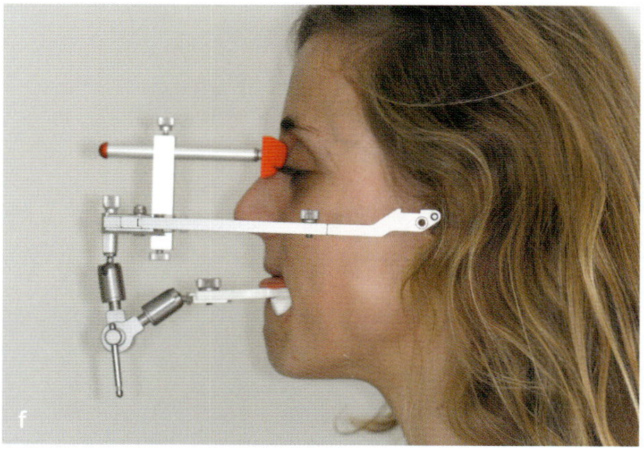
f

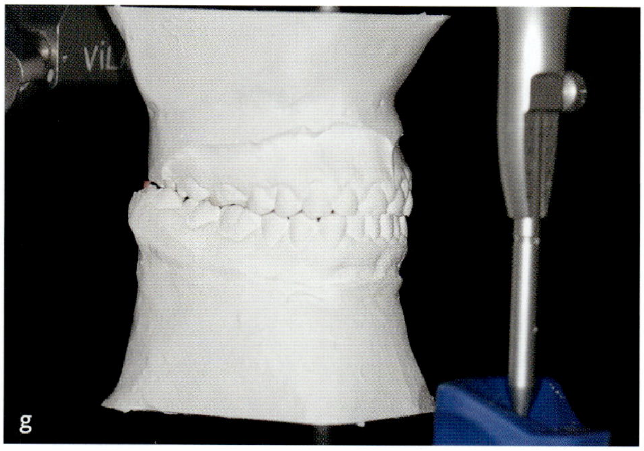
g

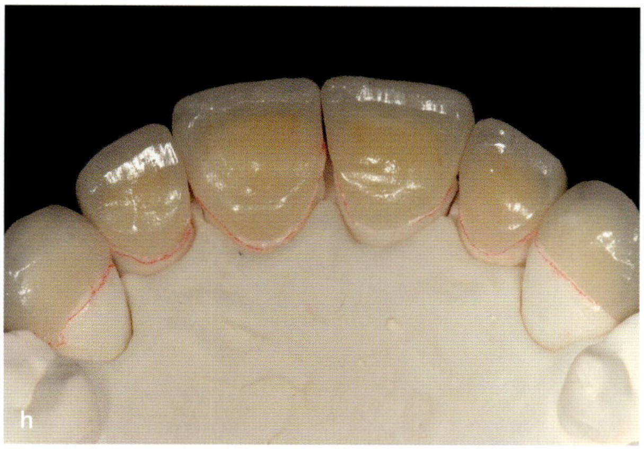
h

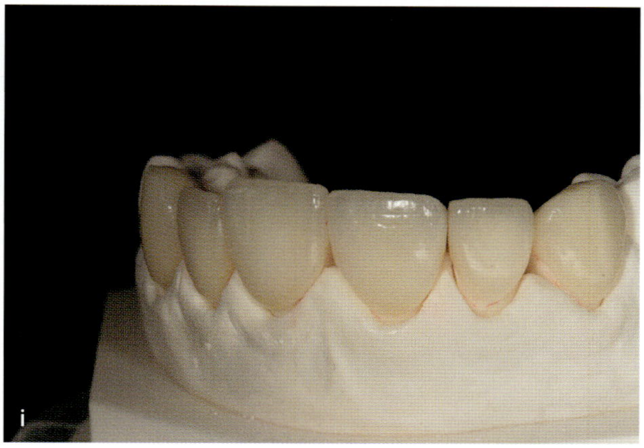
i

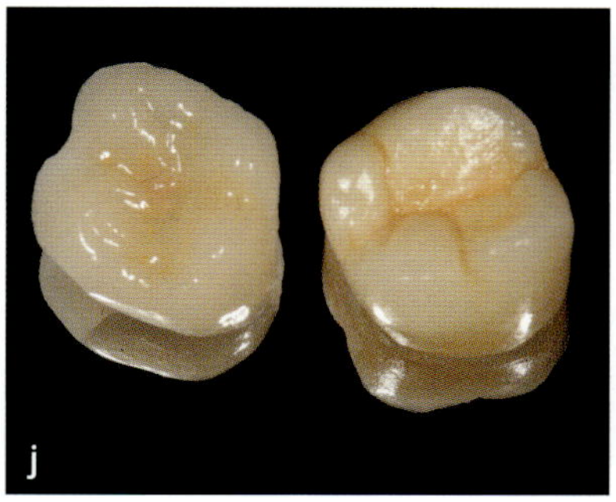
j

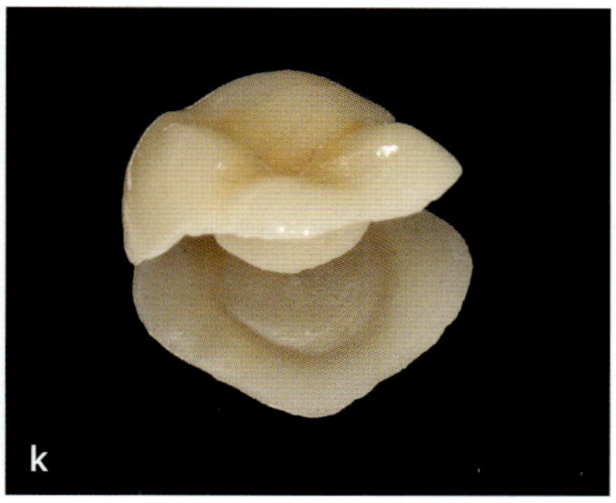
k

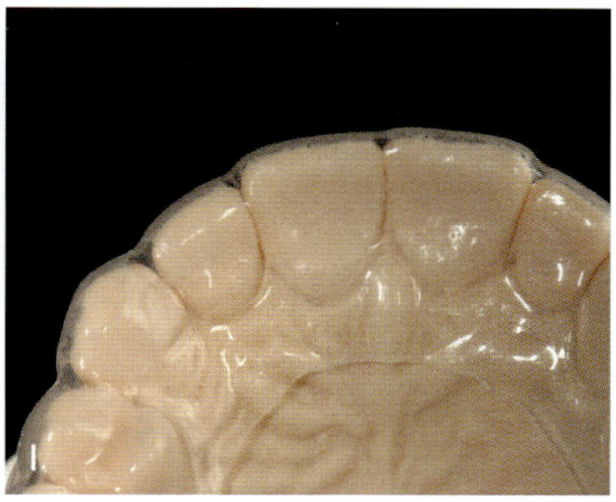
l

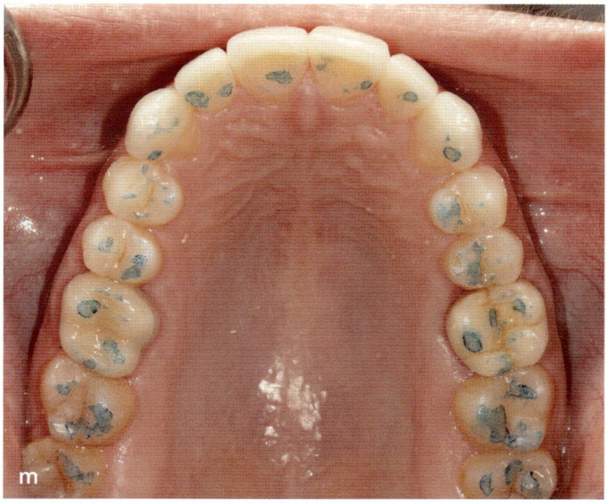
m

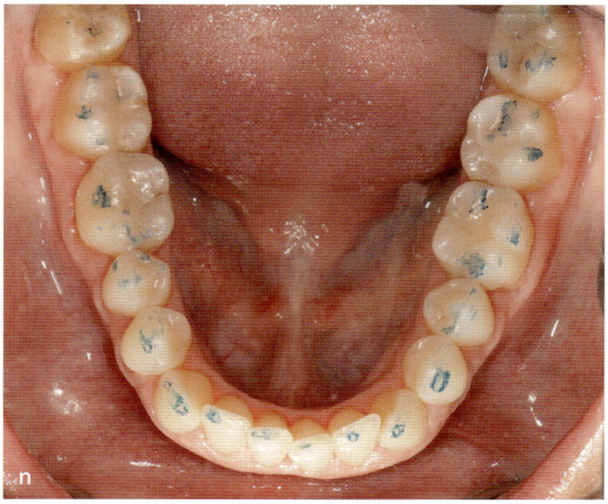
n

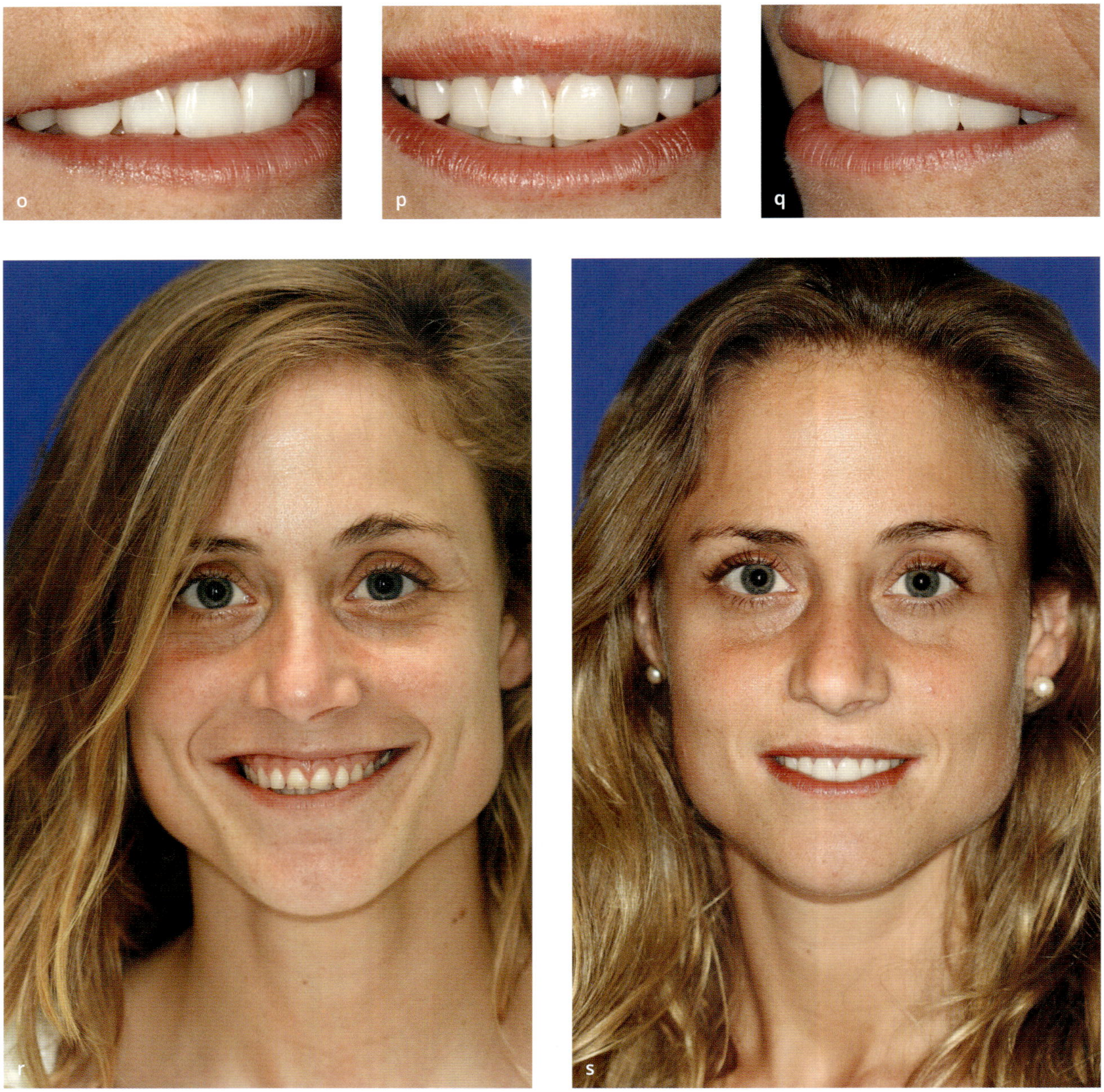


**Fig 7-11** *(continued)* The demanding profession of the patient should be counteracted with a PPP and regular checkups to help the patient in the prevention of further damage. Pictures of the patient at age 16 (r), 30 (s), and 35 (t) show that the prevention and counseling measures agreed upon with the patient may prove a safeguard for restoration survival and a good patient-dentist relationship.

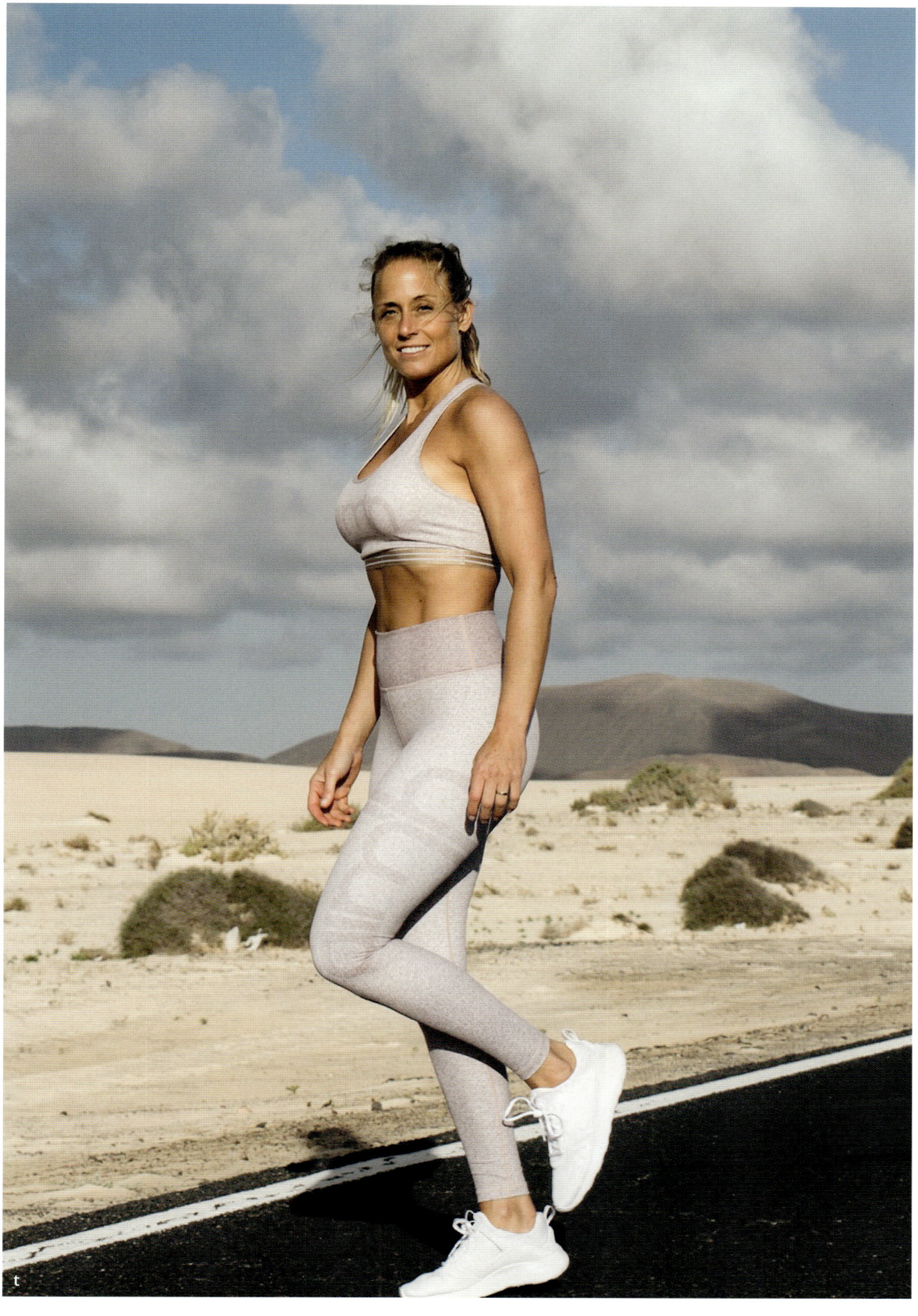
t

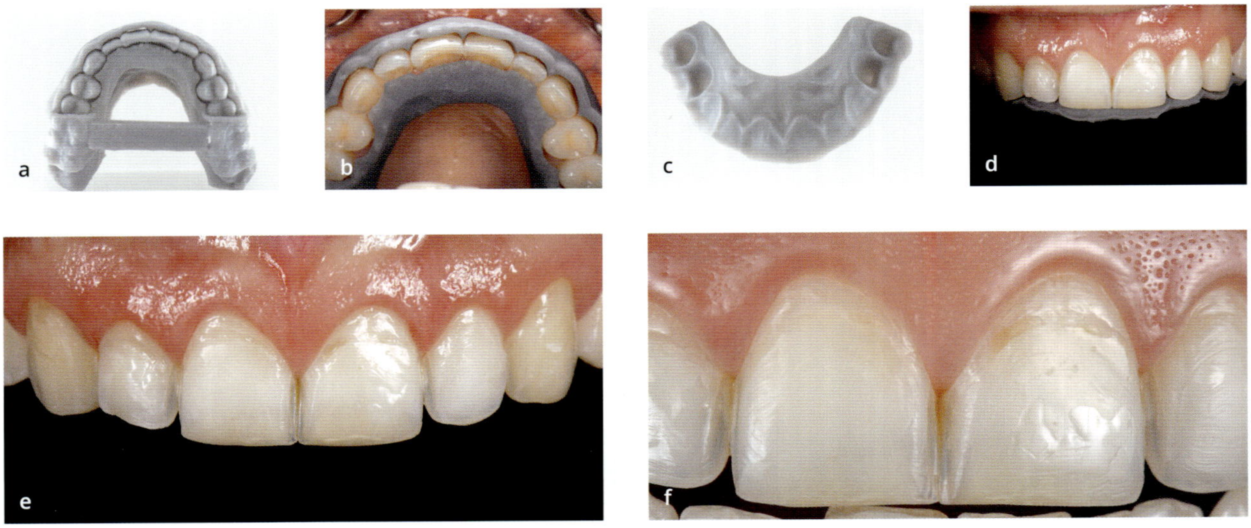


## Indirect Additive Versus Subtractive Approach in Severe TW

The direct restorative approach is primarily appropriate for incipient and moderate TW as the remaining tooth structure guides the restorative dentist, who will be steered by the adjacent anatomy in a similar way to someone restoring a work of art. Nonetheless, there should always be space for direct composite restorations, even in severe cases, as TW damage is not homogeneous, even within the same patient. Direct additive composites are convenient and require no tooth sacrifice at all.

Currently, an additive approach is much preferred to a subtractive one because maintaining as much of the tooth structure as possible is a desirable goal for the TW restorative team.[28] Yet, indirect restorations are needed in cases where tooth structure is not sufficient or when the esthetic and functional requirements of the worn dentition are clearly in excess of what the physical and optical properties of direct restorations can deliver. The patient should understand that this option is not exempt from complications and that minimally invasive additive restorations will deteriorate after some years.[29] Providing stronger restorations that will withstand the passage of time could be regarded in principle as the ideal treatment of choice. However, it has been demonstrated that a 70% reduction of tooth structure is expected when choosing a crown, while partial restorations require a noticeably smaller reduction of 45%, and a PLV only requires a 15% reduction.

At the same time, the improvements in adhesion science, together with the documented long life span of partial restorations such as PLVs, have resulted in a great option for severe TW patients: a combination of direct composite restorations in areas of little destruction, indirect polymer-infiltrated ceramic network (PICN) or glass-ceramic restorations in posterior areas with severe damage, and PLVs in the anterior region of the mouth where esthetic and functional demands are extremely high.[30] PLVs, originally belonging only in the esthetic realm, today have been acclaimed as the treatment of choice for restoring function of the anterior teeth and for good biologic integration (Fig 7-12).

Today, feldspathic porcelain veneers are the gold standard for anterior restorations, not only for their undisputable beauty and translucency but also because of their evidence-based performance provided the correct occlusal scheme is developed. PLVs meet the goal of preserving as much tooth structure as possible when compared to more conventional prosthodontics. However, PLVs can be even more conservative in cases of severe TW since the intrinsic loss of enamel in some of these cases allows for a much shallower enamel preparation. Such is the case when the volume of vestibular enamel has already been thinned as a consequence of exposure to an acidic environment for long periods of time. In fact, 3D planning in such cases needs to take into consideration the ideal morphology and surface characteristics of sound enamel, which varies in depth between individuals, and avoid as much as possible reducing the remaining tooth structure.

The minimally invasive procedure for PLV preparation should always keep in mind enamel preservation whenever possible. Optimal adhesion, lack of sensitivity, and increased strength of the final treated dentition are some of the paradigmatic benefits of minimal tooth reduction. The wax-up is the driving force, together with digital or analog preparation guides. The concept of the additive approach is well demonstrated in the paradigmatic shift in terminology from *adhesive restorations* to *additive restorations* (Fig 7-13).

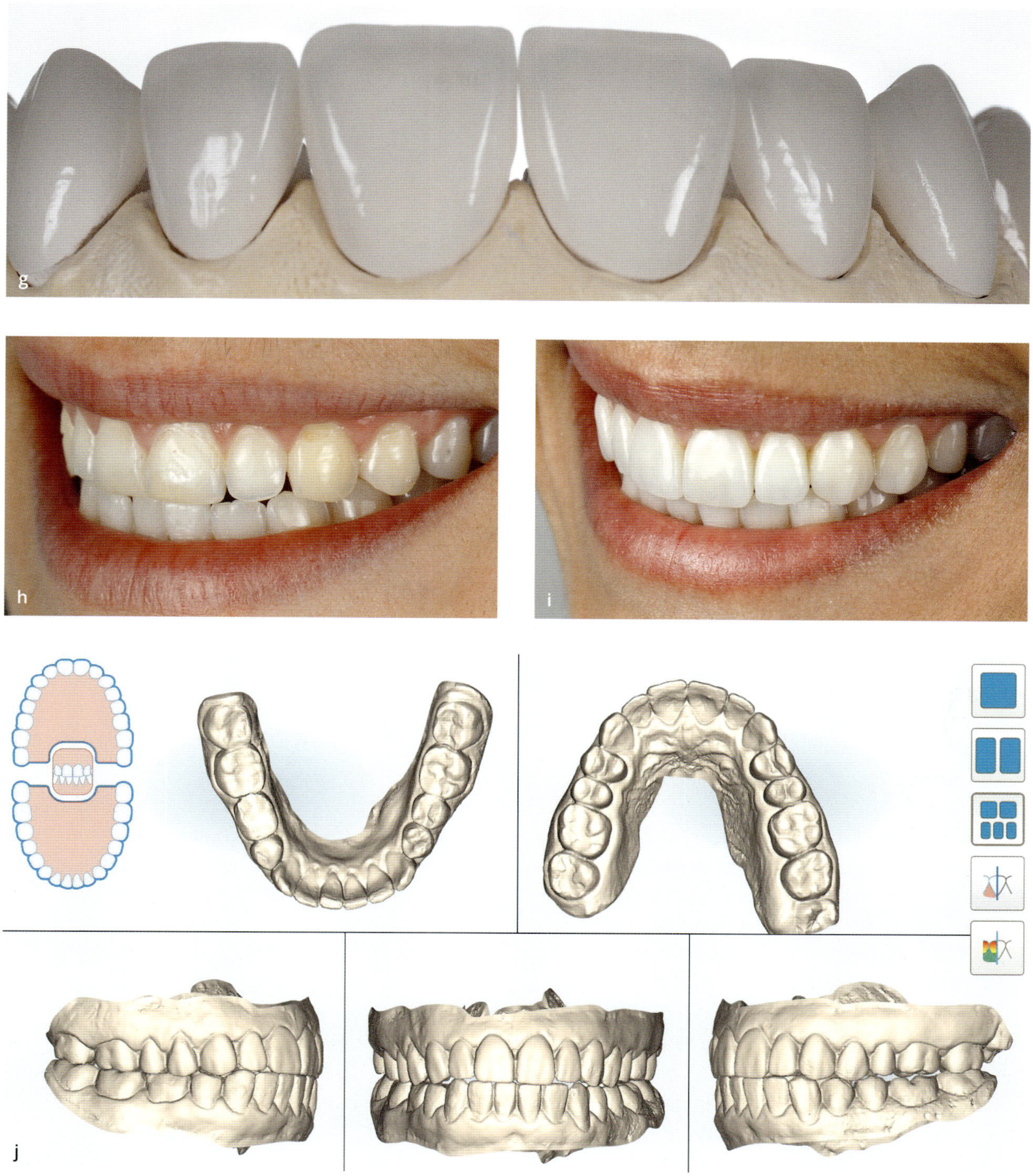

**Fig 7-12** Minimally invasive preparation for PLVs in a severe TW case. Occlusal view of the printed PLV preparation templates (a). After an additive wax-up is approved, a set of printed vestibular (b) and occlusal (c and d) reduction guides are tried in before the teeth are prepared. The figures show there is almost no need for tooth reduction, neither in volume nor in length, as the PLVs are going to add onto the worn teeth. Once prepared, the teeth are ready for impressions (e). Neither anesthesia nor a retraction cord is used because, as explained in chapter 6, the margin will be placed supragingivally. Shallow proximal finish line preparation enables precise placement during the delivery phase, and no interproximal reduction is done (f). It will be followed by a minimal facial reduction if sufficient space is not already available. Usually in severe TW enamel volume has already been reduced by the wear condition. Feather-edge termination of PLVs can be achieved both using a feldspathic refractory model workflow or using CAD/CAM-milled felspathic porcelain. Both workflows should be compatible with tooth structure preservation and final integration (g to i). Success is achieved when the final restoration blends in with the existing tooth structure, ideally with minimal tooth reduction whenever possible. Whatever the workflow—analog, digital, or a hop-on, hop-off combination—it is advisable to record the end result in order to facilitate the monitoring of potential relapse or progression of TW. In this case it was decided to do intraoral scanning with digital tools (j).

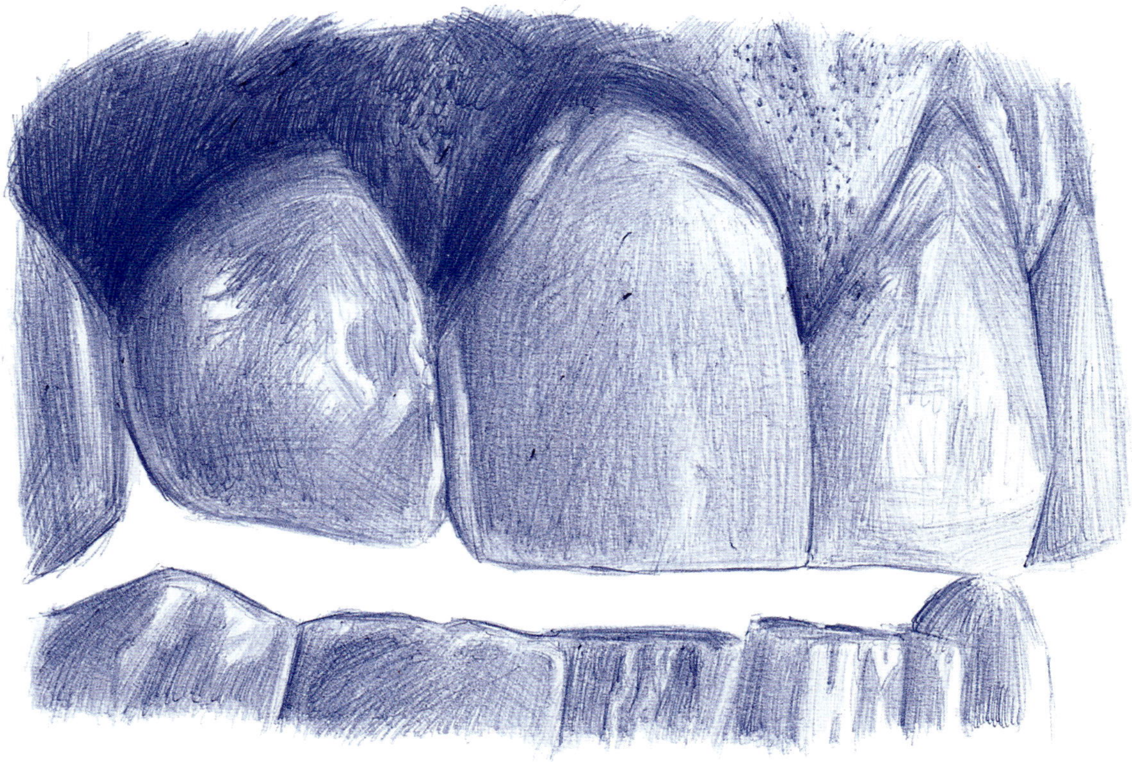

*Less is more.*

—Ludwig Mies van der Rohe, German-American architect

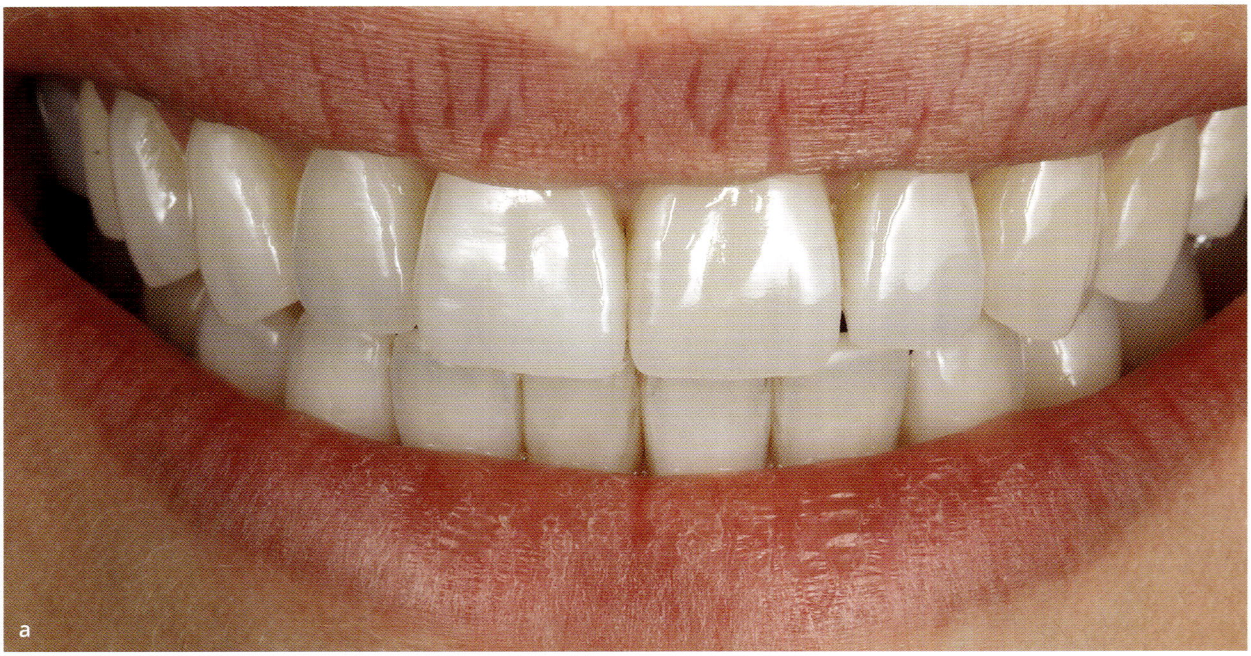


**Fig 7-13** The shallow preparation in this erosive case involves merely a slight notch on the distal and mesial of every tooth receiving a PLV with a delicate rounding of the incisal edges and a roughening of the buccal aspects (a). The final restorarions in the mouth help to restore the lost volume (b).

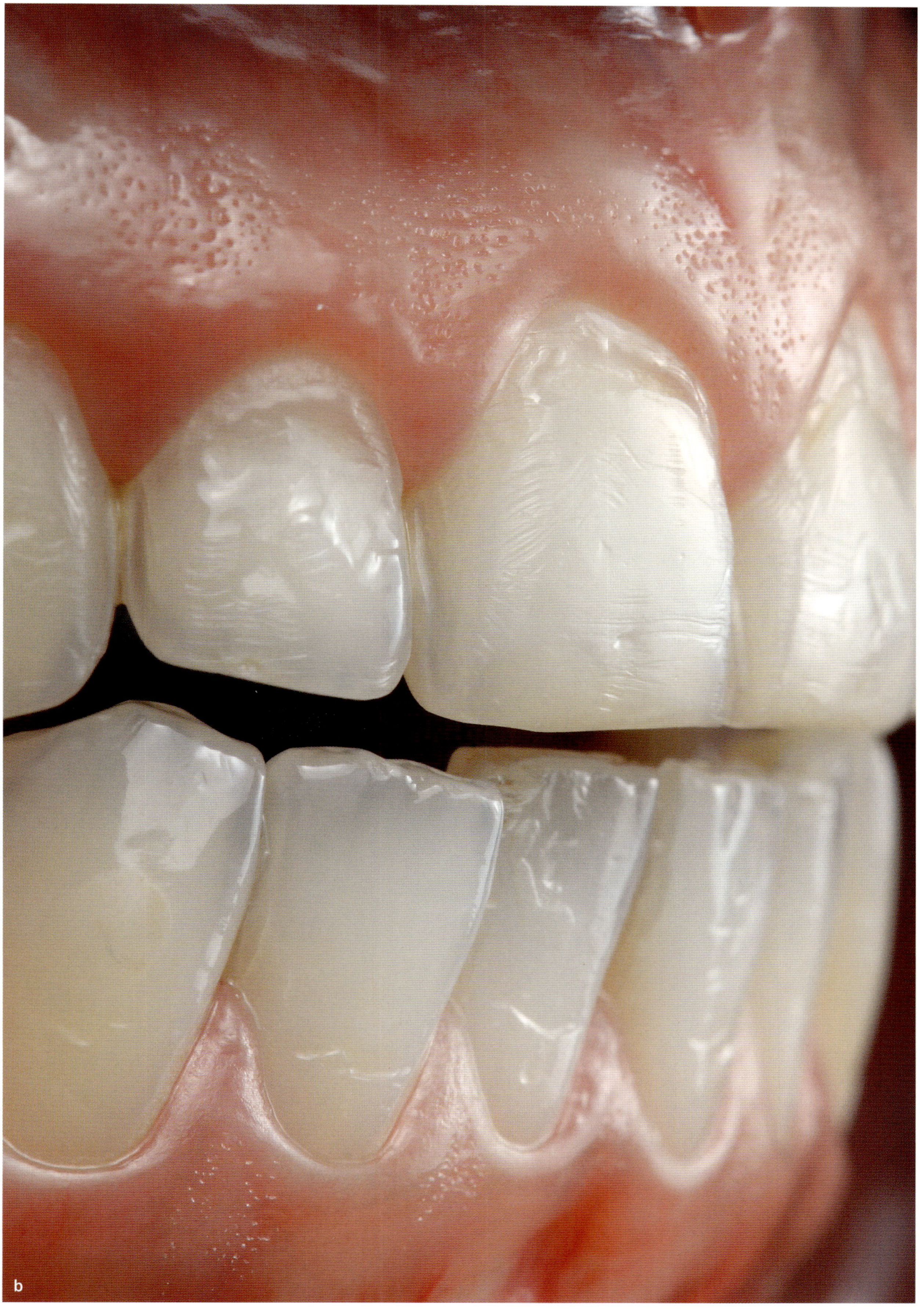
b

## 4. Occlusal Scheme: Vertical Dimension of Occlusion and Centric Relation

In young patients, severe wear may still only be localized in the anterior zone of the maxillary teeth. Providing space for the restorations required to offer both protection and restoration of the dentition is often a challenge.

As mentioned in chapter 6, the Dahl principle of combining forced intrusion of anterior teeth with over eruption of posterior segments through the delivery of anterior restorations at an increased VDO could be considered when orthodontic treatment is rejected and posterior occlusal anatomy is well maintained. However, it should be carefully evaluated against the more predictable 3D positioning of anterior teeth possibly through digital orthodontics.[31] Moreover, in severe TW cases it is not uncommon to find preexisting multiple restorations, which might be a contraindication for intrusion due to a potential adverse reaction of the periodontal tissue to the artificial materials (see chapter 6, section VI).

In recent decades, orthodontic treatment in advance of any restorative procedure has proven very effective and efficient in safeguarding tooth structure while creating the necessary space and a beneficial occlusal scheme for years to come. Experienced authors and clinicians on TW have advocated for treating patients in MIP independently of a VDO alteration, especially if the restoration is going to be performed one quadrant at a time.[32] However, by exploring the CR of a patient, a new restorative space can appear without the need to increase VDO (see chapter 6). This is especially important if the posterior teeth (second molars and sometimes the distal aspect of the first molars) do not need to be treated, ie, they have intact anatomy.

Similarly, any attempt to restore the worn dentition has to incorporate adequate anterior and canine guidance (or group function) and provide sufficient posterior disocclusion. There are no exact guidelines as to how much the VDO should be augmented or even what type of maxillomandibular relationship should be achieved when closing and during function. We should treat our TW patient individually and as a whole person, not only based on a specific tooth size or position. Notwithstanding that, the possibility of maintaining a stable, reproducible, nonforced posterior position (CR) with a precise VDO has been clinically proven to be a safe and effective alternative in the hands of an experienced prosthodontist. Whatever the preference is, when TW has severely attacked both anterior and posterior sectors, the restorative team needs to evaluate the advantages for the patient of restoring in MIP or CR[33] (Fig 7-14).

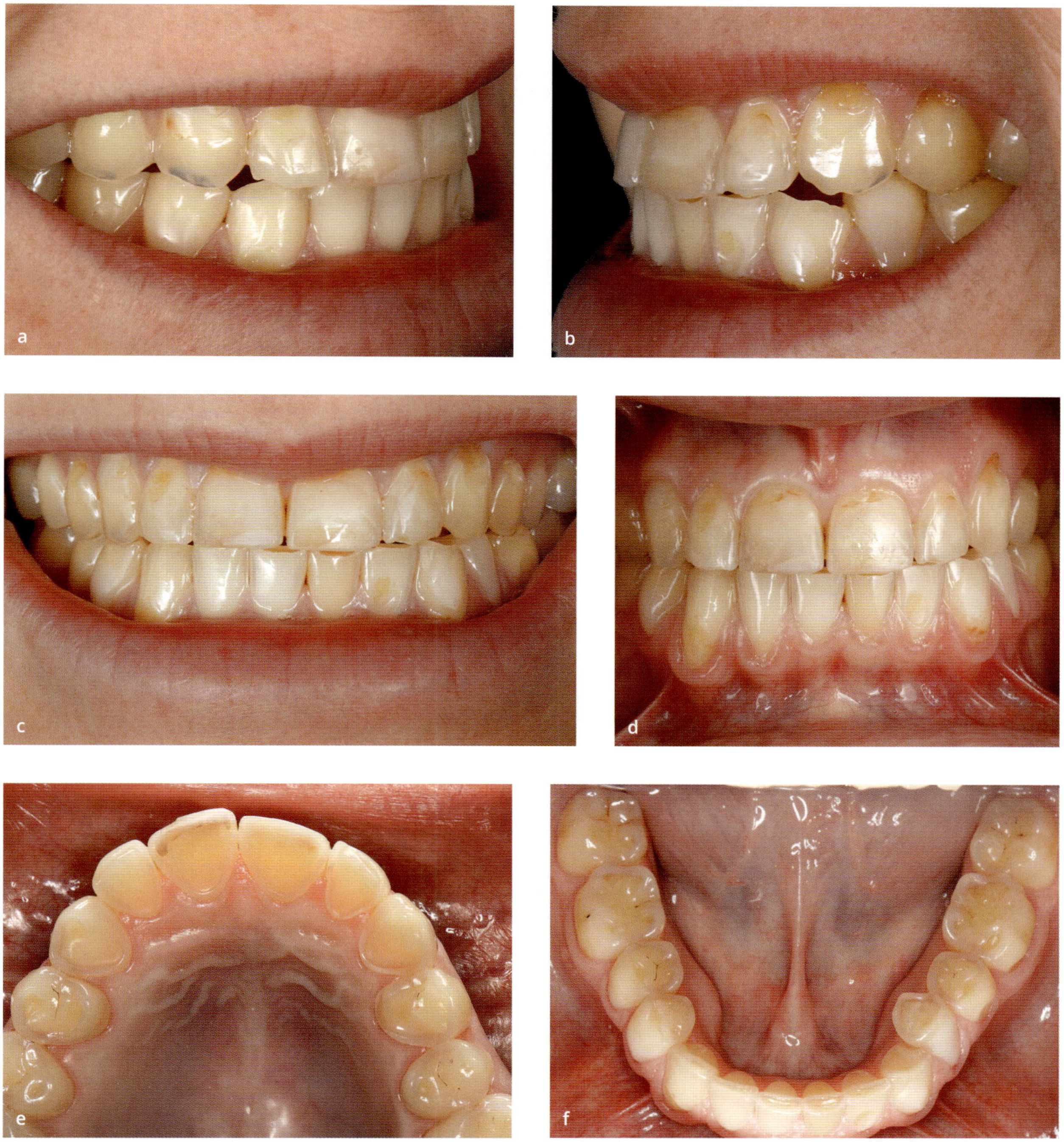


**Fig 7-14** At her first visit, a young, diet-conscious woman under constant stress complains of hypersensitivity, especially in her fourth quadrant. She has not yet been diagnosed with TW but has received treatment for non-carious lesions in several teeth. She reports episodes of reflux and that she much favors vegetables and fruits in her diet. The severe TW affects almost all teeth except the maxillary second molars and barely the first molars (a to d). The maxillary palatal (e) as well as the occlusal and labial surfaces of teeth in both arches, especially the mandible (f), are also severely damaged. The patient also says she has undergone orthodontic treatment in the past. *(continued next page)*

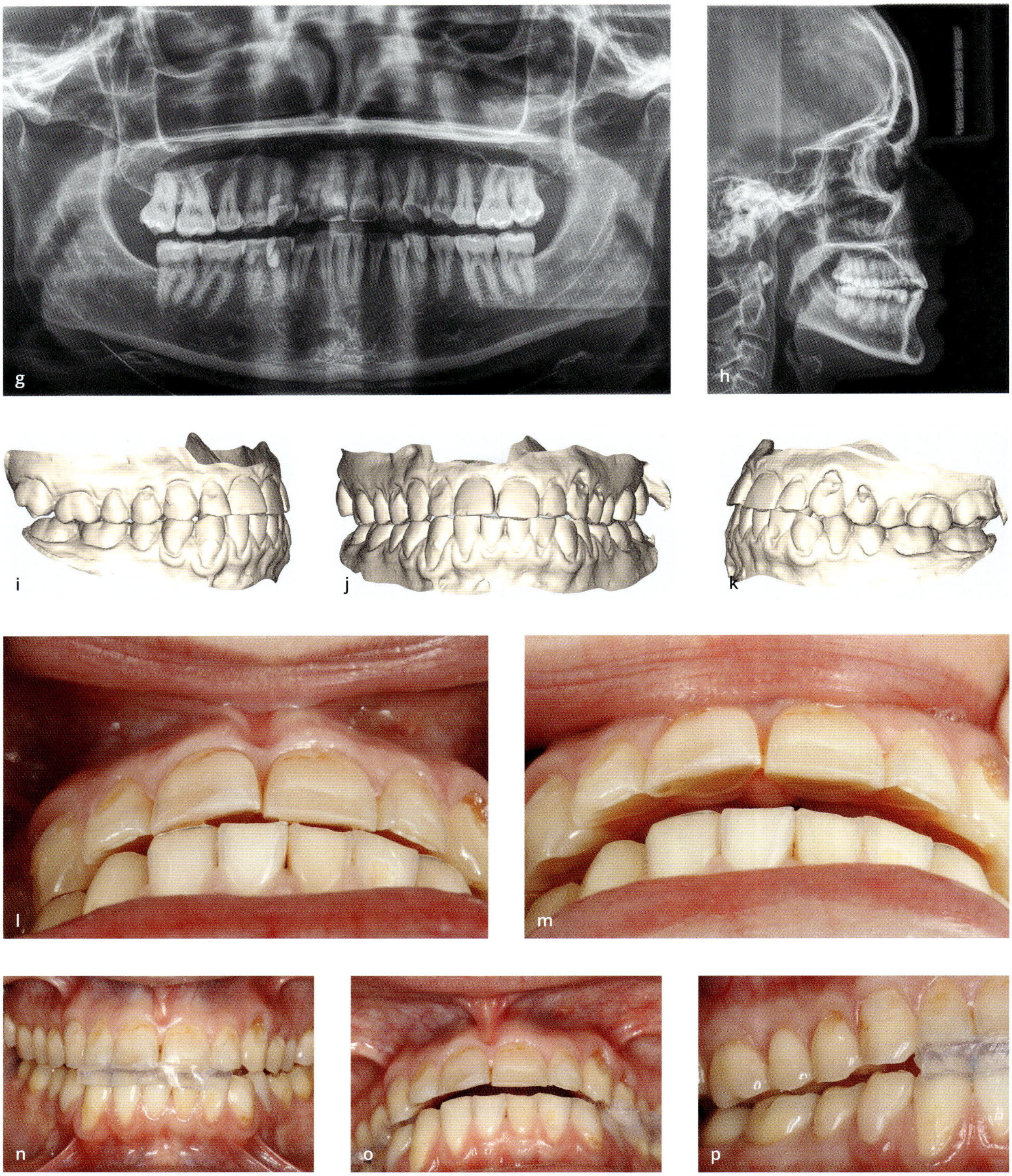

**Fig 7-14** *(continued)* The radiographs show that she has had no major dental treatments so far (g), while the lateral radiograph depicts a dentoskeletal Class III occlusion (h). The study of the STL virtual models shows Class III occlusion at the molars and right canine (i and j) and Class I occlusion at the left canine (k). The vertical collapse in this case is evident, affecting anterior and posterior areas. Also, and most importantly, the edge to edge anterior relationship (l) should be noted as an added difficulty for a minimally invasive approach if anterior teeth are going to be reconstructed in a safe and stable manner. An otherwise hidden space arises as a result of chairside CR manipulation with posterior contact (m). This space naturally occurs as the mandible moves posteriorly as there are still contacts at the distal aspects of the first and second molars, which have been relatively spared from the erosion. This space in CR will be useful for the reconstruction of the worn palatal surfaces of the anterior teeth as well as anterior and canine guidance. Three jigs are made chairside in CR with a transparent, quick-setting silicone (Elite Glass, Zhermack) to help stabilize the CR position at three points: anterior (n) and posterior bilaterally (o). The three separated jigs can be removed one by one when the intraoral scan is capturing that area without the need to remove the others, guaranteeing an accurate CR acquisition (p to r). Note that the distal aspect of the first molars as well as the second molars are the only teeth in contact in CR (s).

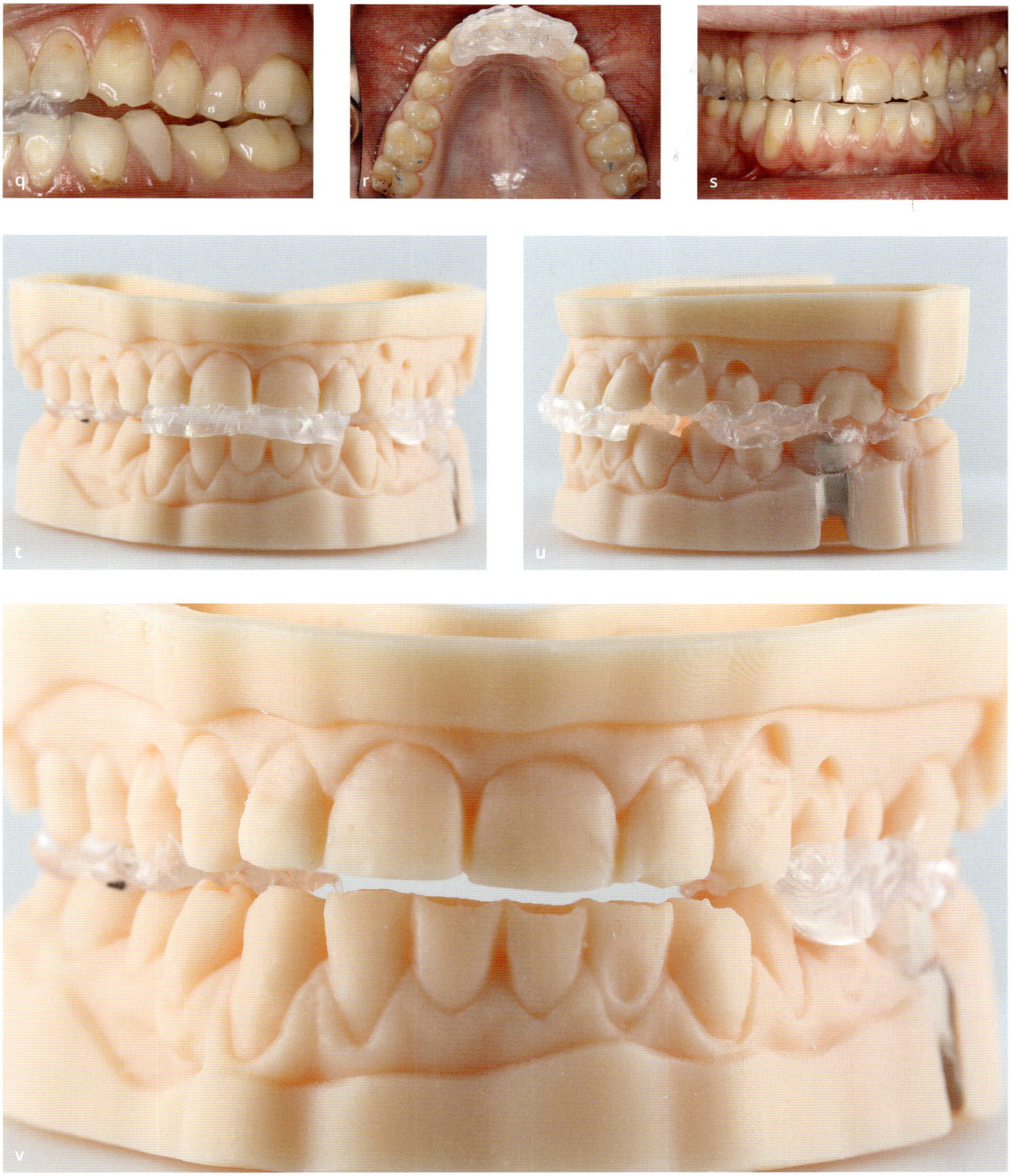


**Fig 7-14** *(continued)* STL of the intraoral acquisitions is used to create an exact printed copy in which the three silicone jigs can be precisely placed (t to v). An ideal individualized virtual wax-up of the full arch except for the occlusodistal aspect of the first molars and occlusal aspect of the second molars is printed (w). Two transparent splints, maxillary (x) and mandibular, are vacuum-formed over the wax-up models. The two transparent mock-ups are placed on the baseline models to communicate with the patient and the restorative team and provide a preview of the restorations (y and z). Using the unrestored second molars as a reference for a transfer guide may be helpful in some cases. Also, in a majority of cases the occlusal surface of the second molars, more often in the maxilla, have been spared the erosive attack as they are apical to the level of acid as a result of the curve of Spee. In this case, a combination of indirect onlays and partial direct freehand composite restorations are going to be created without the use of a mold. *(continued next page)*

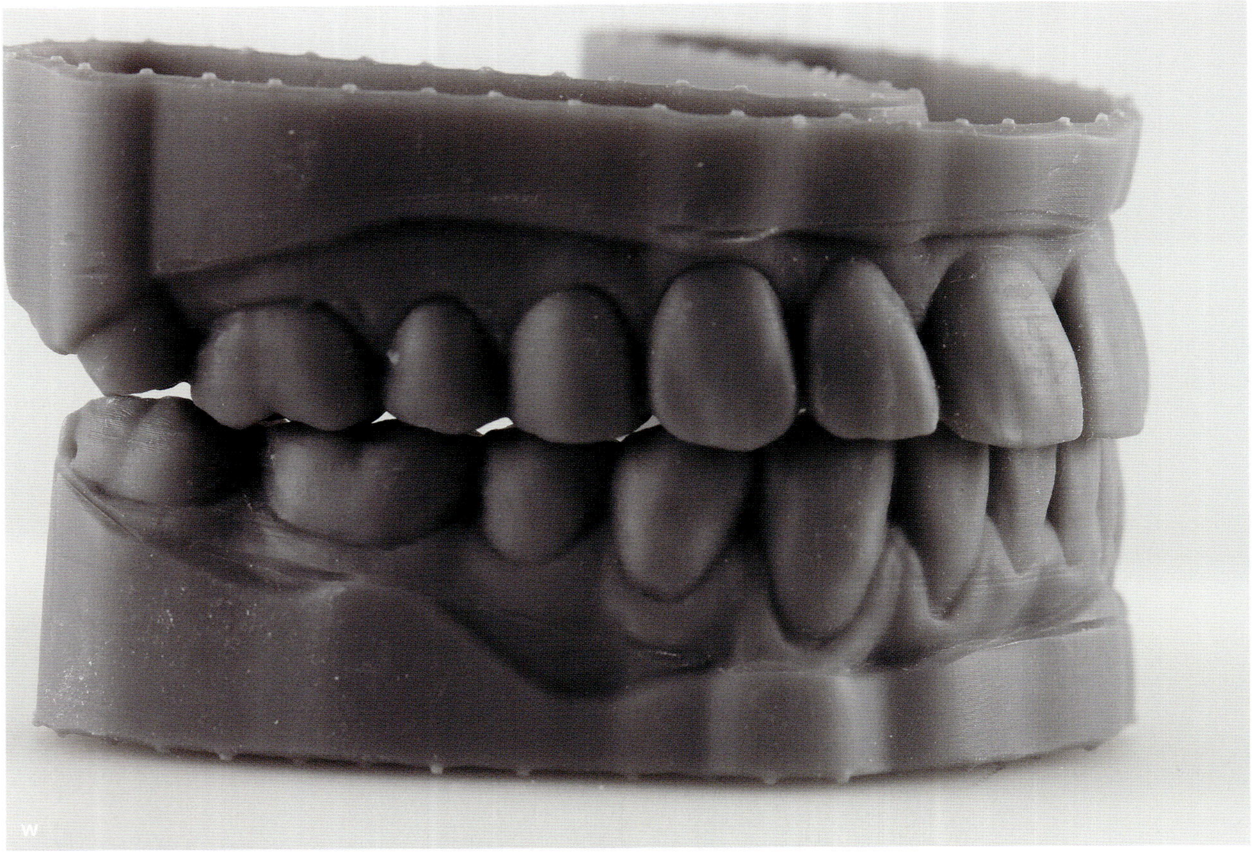

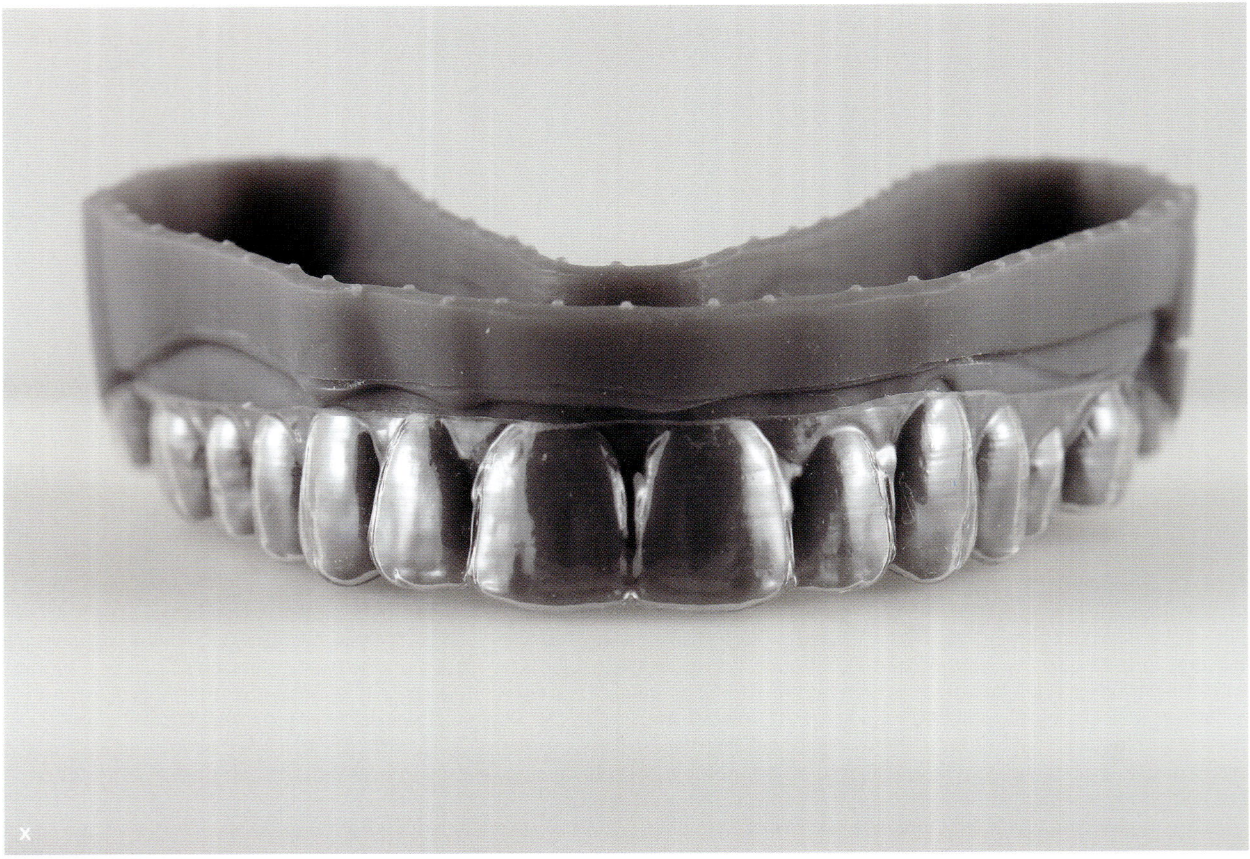

**Fig 7-14** *(continued)*

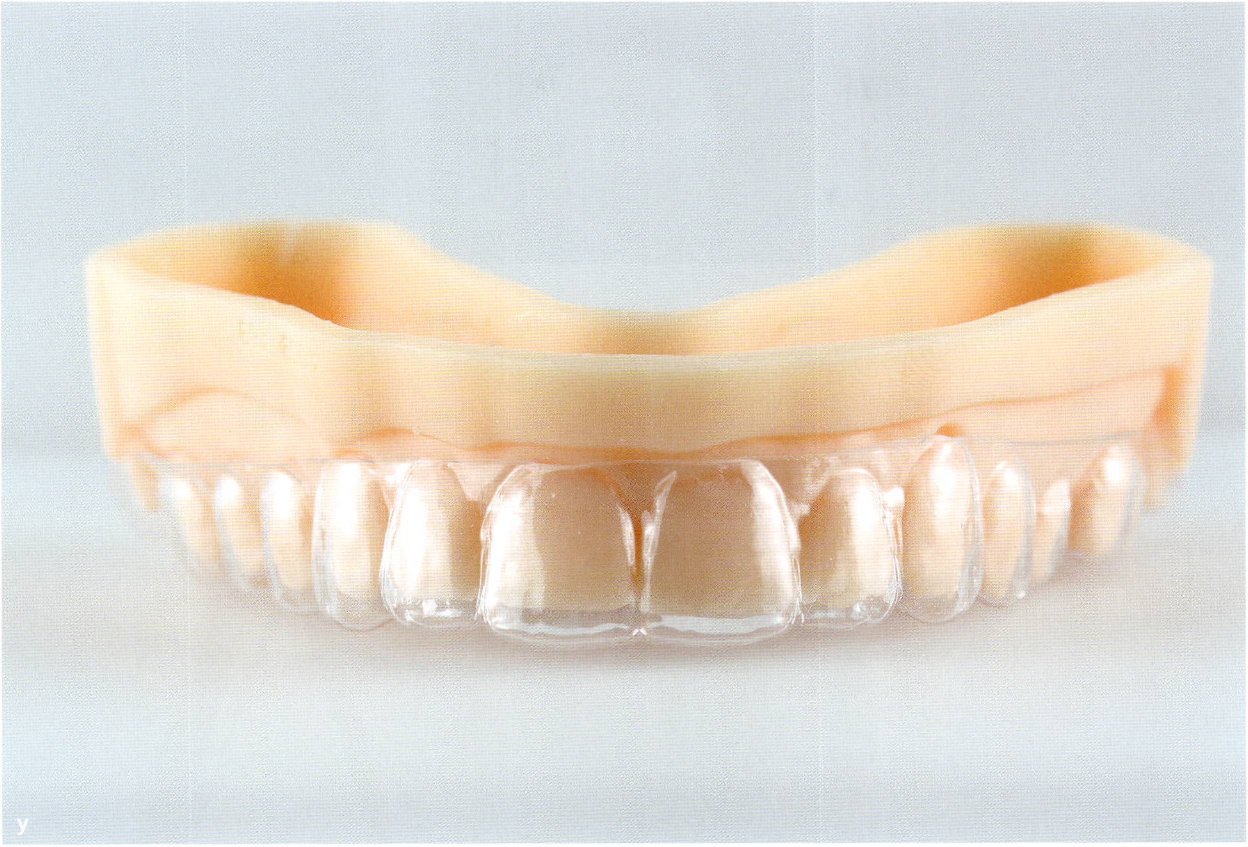

y

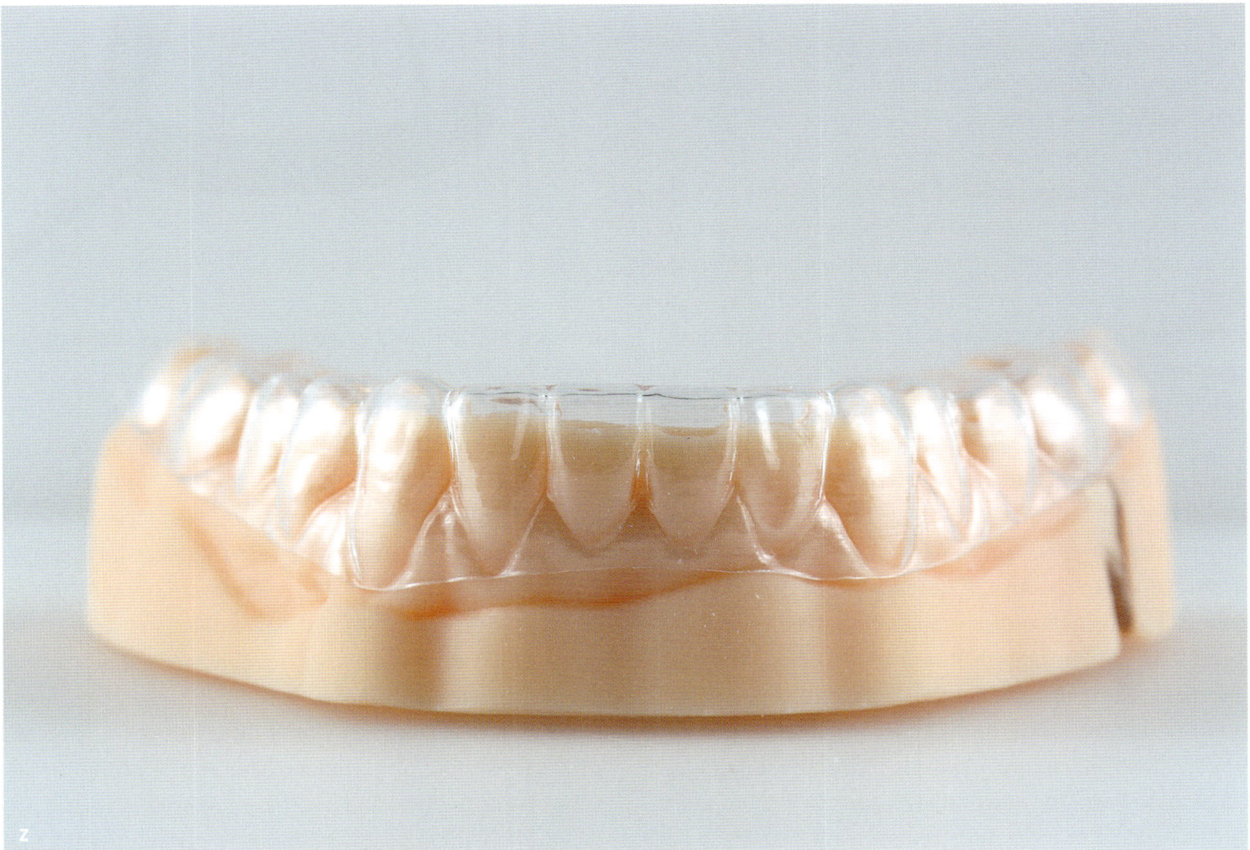

z

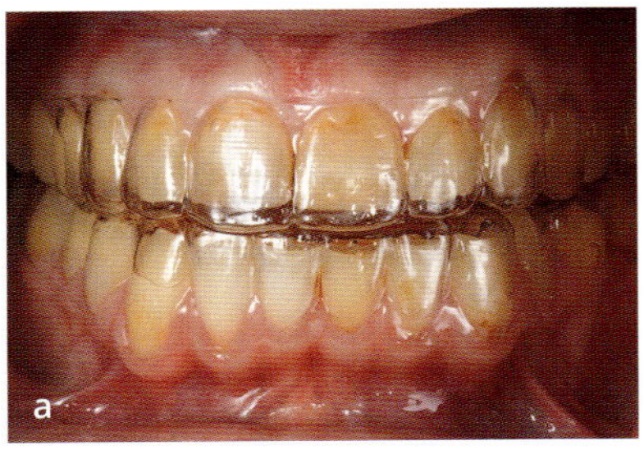

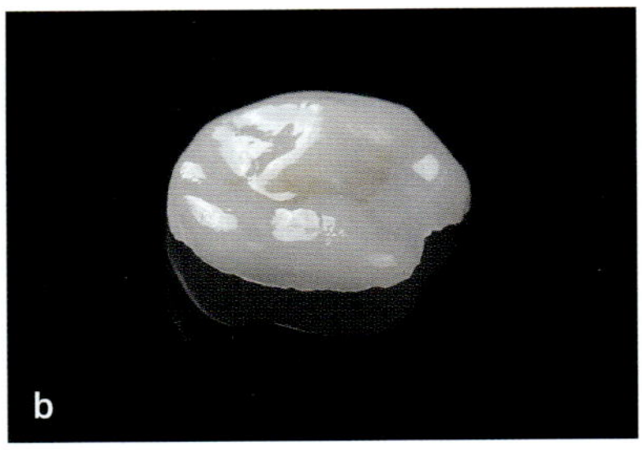

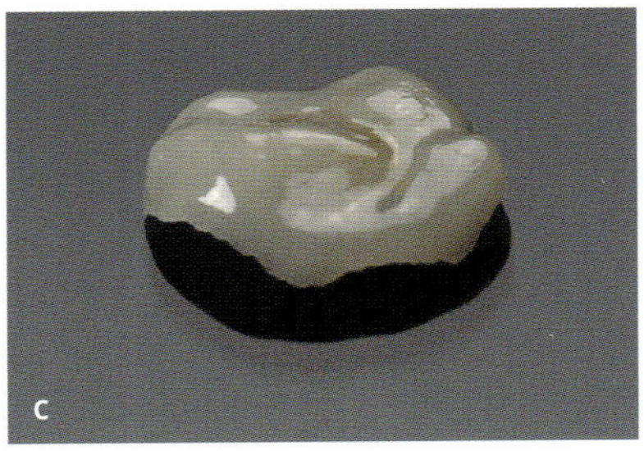

In cases where there is no possibility of finding space nor the adequate skeletal anatomy to restore in CR, another option is to increase the VDO. For many years the VDO was considered an absolute figure that could not be altered. The fear of changing the VDO and triggering TMJ symptoms is not supported by the literature, and in fact today we know that VDO can be safely increased and tolerated well by the patient, provided there is a correct occlusal scheme and a comfortable, uncompromised rest space.

The decision regarding how much to increase the VDO relies strongly on the expertise of the dentist and involves functional and esthetic parameters as there is not a unique and univocally adequate VDO[20,23,34] (Fig 7-15).

On the other hand, multiple previous restorations in the posterior sector might offer an opportunity as they can be replaced with an implicit increased VDO to encompass the new anatomy of the restored dentition. The VDO refers to the distance between two marked points in maximal intercuspal position. The VDO increase provides the opportunity for improvement of overbite, overjet, and lip support, among others, while enabling a less invasive additive approach in many patients. In cases of previous extractions with a shortened arch, further support for correct arch form and occlusion is ideally provided through implant therapy.[34]

In some patients with TW, dental fear is a barrier to seeking treatment. Patients with severe TW may have experienced sensitivity, even pain, prior to any treatment. Any tooth reduction is a risk factor for permanent pain in severe TW cases. Also, if deep layers of dentin are exposed, an alternative to the additive-adhesive approach should be contemplated. Performing gentle, minimally invasive treatment whenever possible facilitates commitment and compliance. In addition, the digital approach enables a virtual setting in which space and volume can be assessed and the restorative approach evaluated in a virtual articulator before restorations are manufactured, allowing the apprehensive patient to spend less time in the dental chair. This is another advantage of the digital workflow.

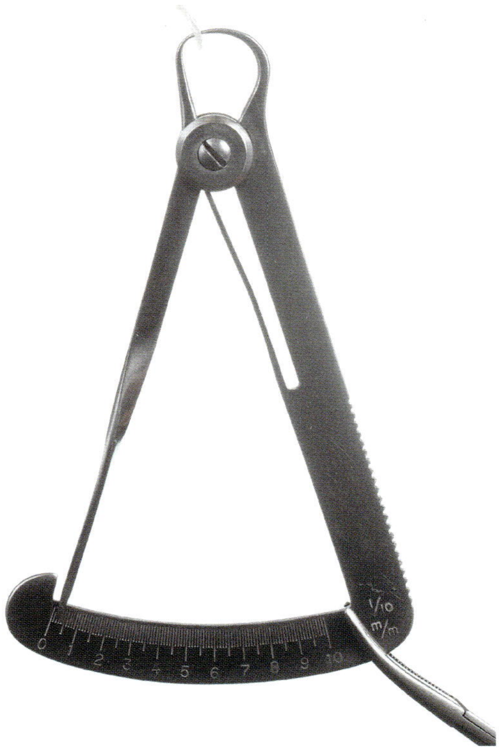

d

In cases where there is a severe erosive attack from intrinsic origin such as in EDs or severe GERD, the damage to the palatal aspect of anterior teeth has sometimes totally dissolved the palatal anatomy, leaving a yellowish, jelly-like dentin as the first defense against further TW. The diminished resistance to tearing and bending forces will often cause chipping of the enamel in the incisal third but also in the cervical area, recognized as non-carious cervical lesions (NCCLs).

Restoring both anatomy and function can be achieved without preparation of teeth. The proper occlusal scheme, overjet, and overbite, together with and anterior and canine guidance, helps to reduce the risks of further destruction (Figs 7-16 to 7-18).

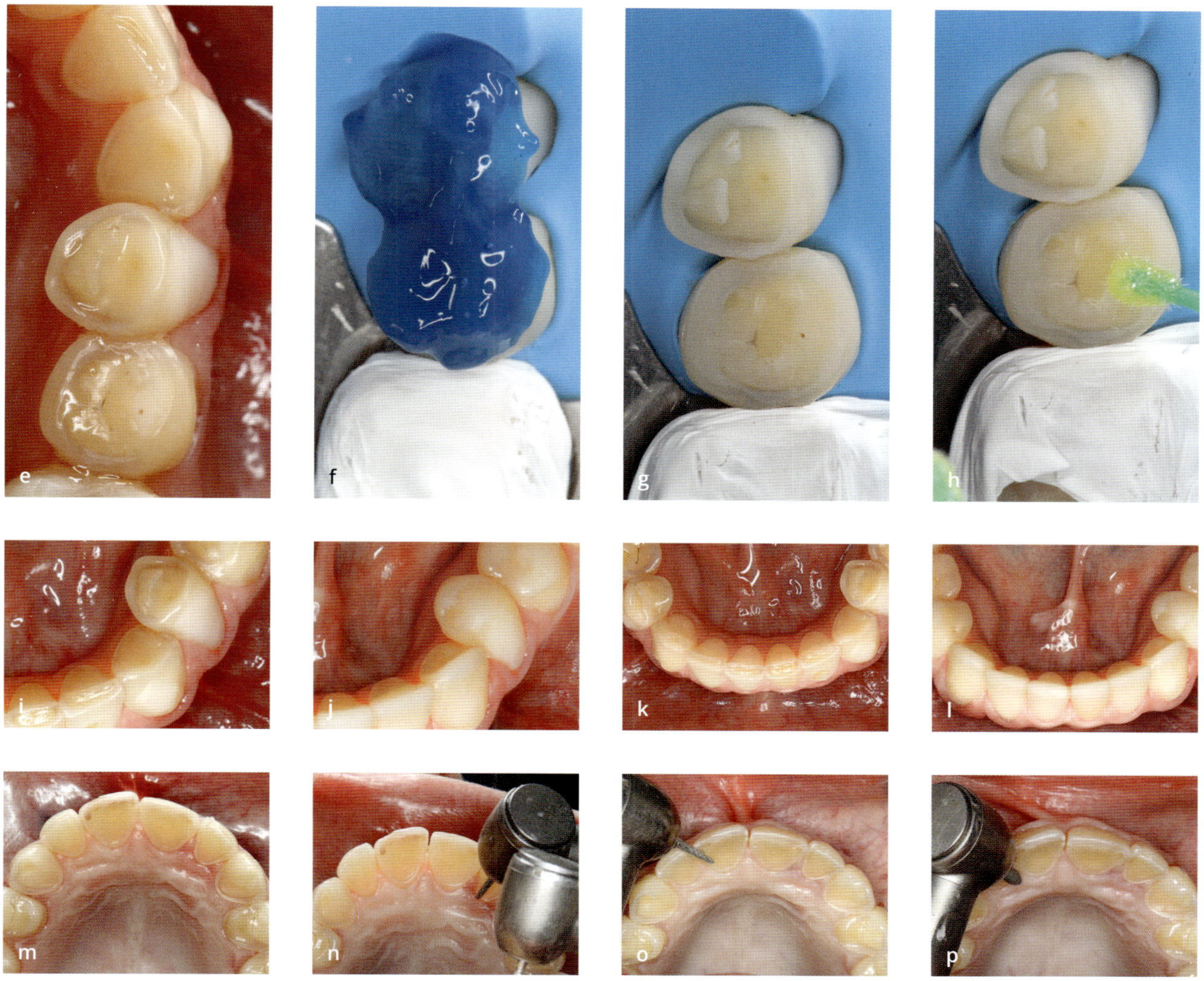

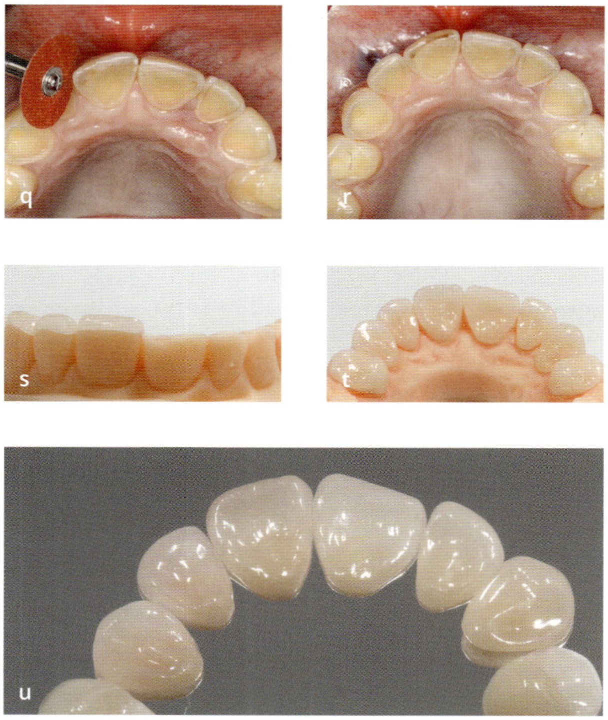

**Fig 7-15** Occlusal overlays were milled from PICN (Enamic, VITA) at the chosen CR (a and b). In this case (continued from Fig 7-14), a totally additive approach is elected, and the protocols are adapted as needed. All exposed dentin was sealed, with deeply excavated concave lesions filled with flowable composite, following a meticulous adhesion protocol. Then a digital impression was taken. The thin pieces (less than 0.5 mm; c and d) were adhesively cemented to the mandibular premolars, which were treated without tooth preparation as the patient had claimed to have sensitivity and even pain during the first visits (e to h). Attending to the timeline already described, the mandibular anterior teeth were also treated at this stage, as were the NCCLs with direct composite (i to l). The patient experienced a gradual reduction in her pain soon after. Only the narrow remaining collar of enamel was roughened gently with the use of a fine diamond bullet bur and a fine diamond chamfer, and sharp edges were rounded with a soft disk (Sof-Lex, 3M; m to r). Airborne-particle abrasion is not considered as the proximity to the gingiva and the thin enamel margin would have provoked unnecessary gingival irritation and bleeding. As explained before, the length of the palatal overlays will be such that they reproduce the final length of the planned restoration. Therefore, the eight overlays will cover the original incisal edge or, in the case of the first premolars, buccal axial aspects (s to u).

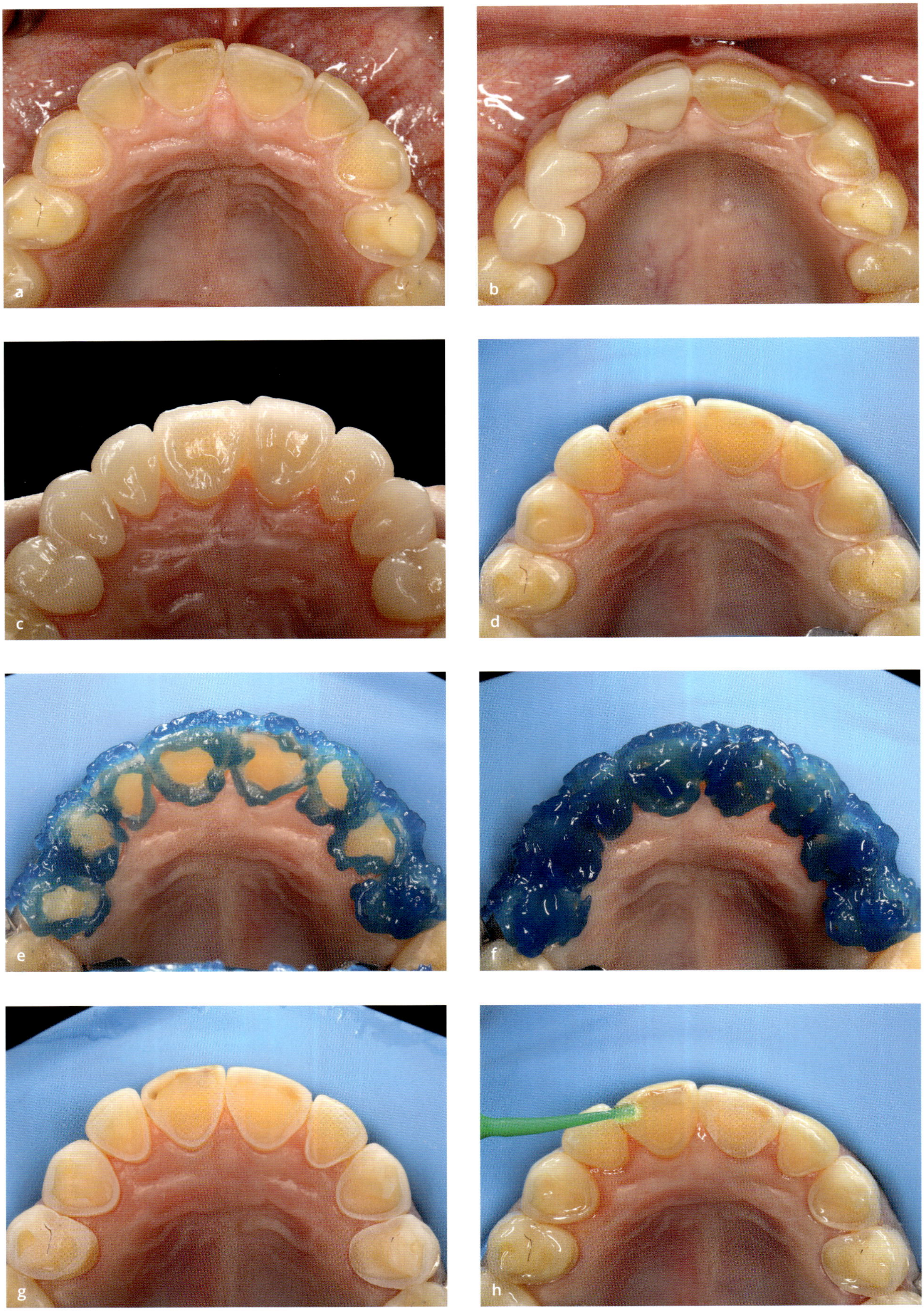
a
b
c
d
e
f
g
h

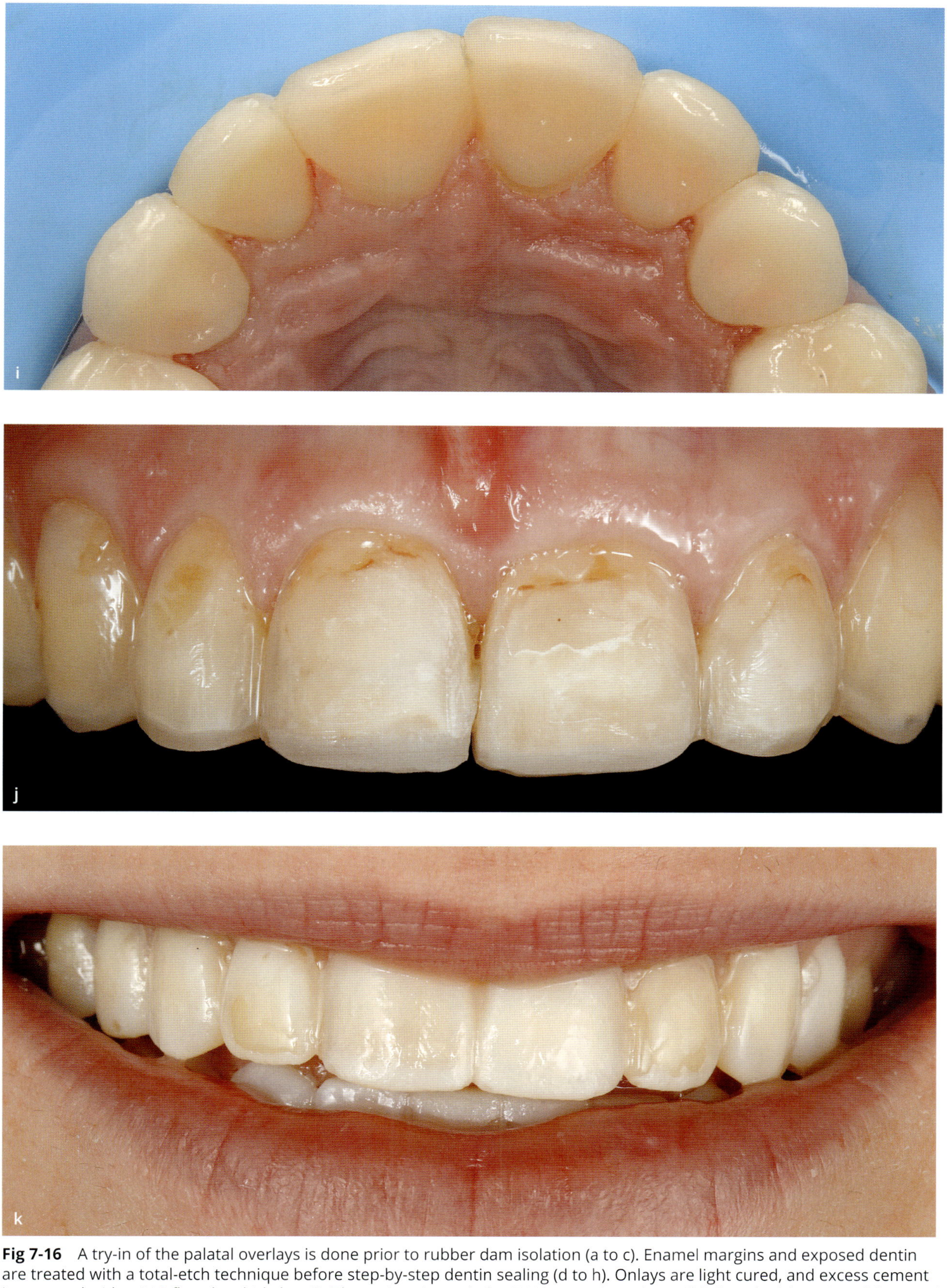

**Fig 7-16** A try-in of the palatal overlays is done prior to rubber dam isolation (a to c). Enamel margins and exposed dentin are treated with a total-etch technique before step-by-step dentin sealing (d to h). Onlays are light cured, and excess cement is removed with a #12 fluted carbide bur (i). The patient is ready for PLV impressions that will follow the blueprint of the initial wax-up and mock-up, which can be used as a preparation guide as previously explained (j and k). An impression was taken traditionally to benefit from an analog flow, another example of a hop-on, hop-off work flow.

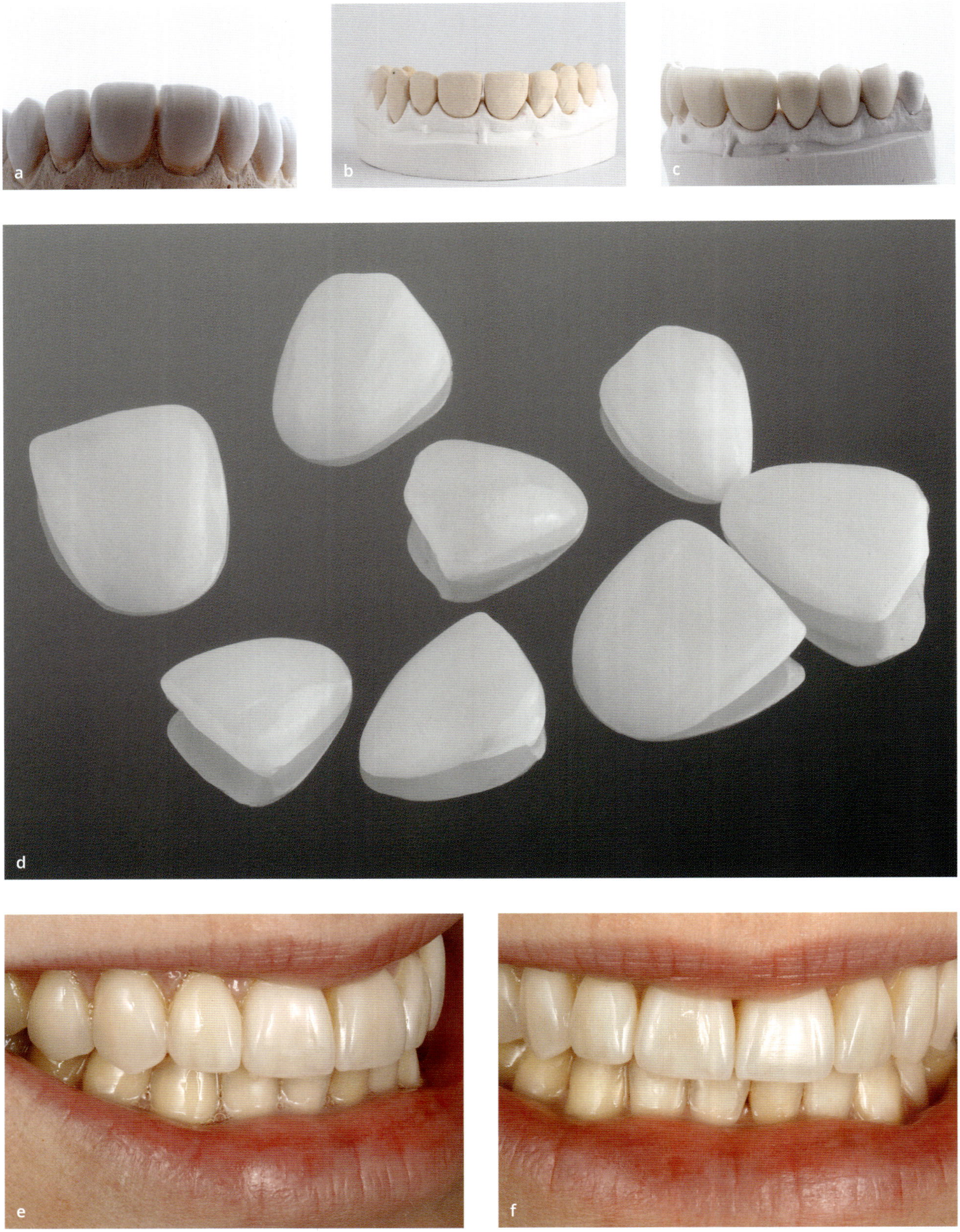


**Fig 7-17** Eight feldspathic PLVs are made (a to d). Highly demanding cases might benefit from a new wax-up at this point. The integration of the final restorations depends on many factors, one of them the articulation of the different steps and alignment of the TW team (e to l).

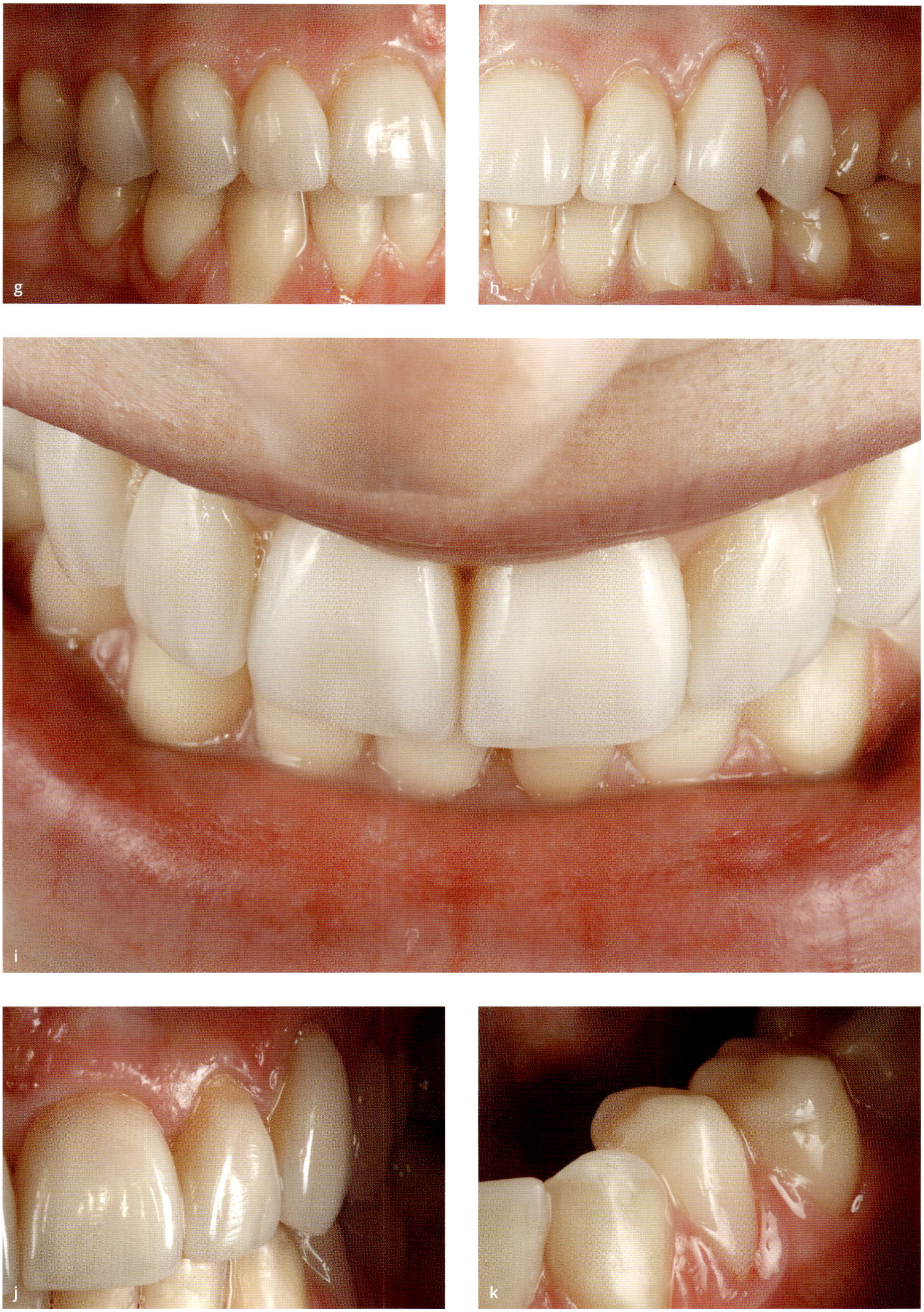
g
h
i
j
k

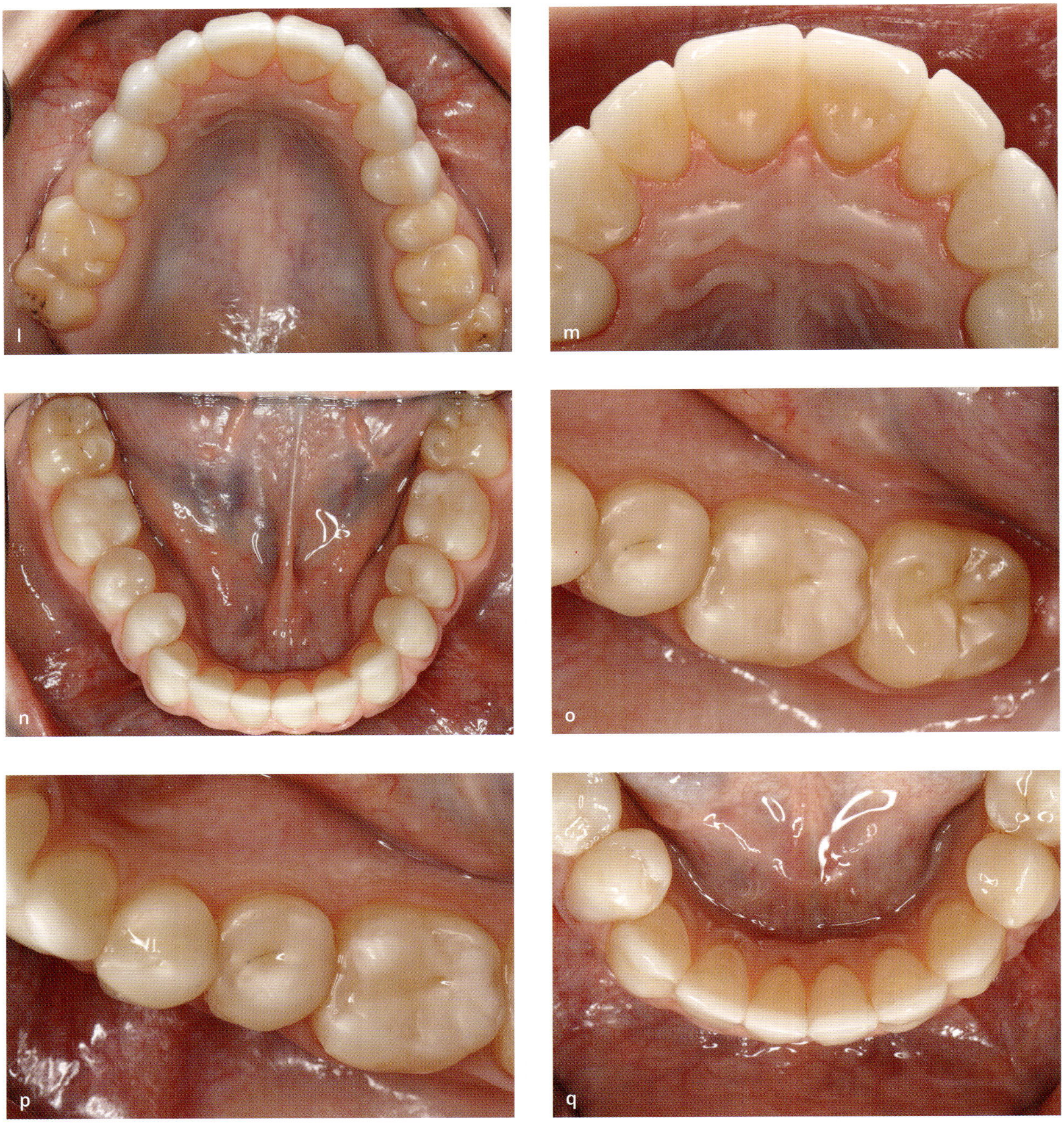


**Fig 7-17** *(continued)* In severe TW the principle of enamel preservation might be critical for restorative stability. Therefore, some compromises need to be anticipated (m to q). The combination of direct and indirect and traditional and digital approaches might be complicated in the beginning, but keeping the patient's interests at the center of the decisions will help in the decision chain.

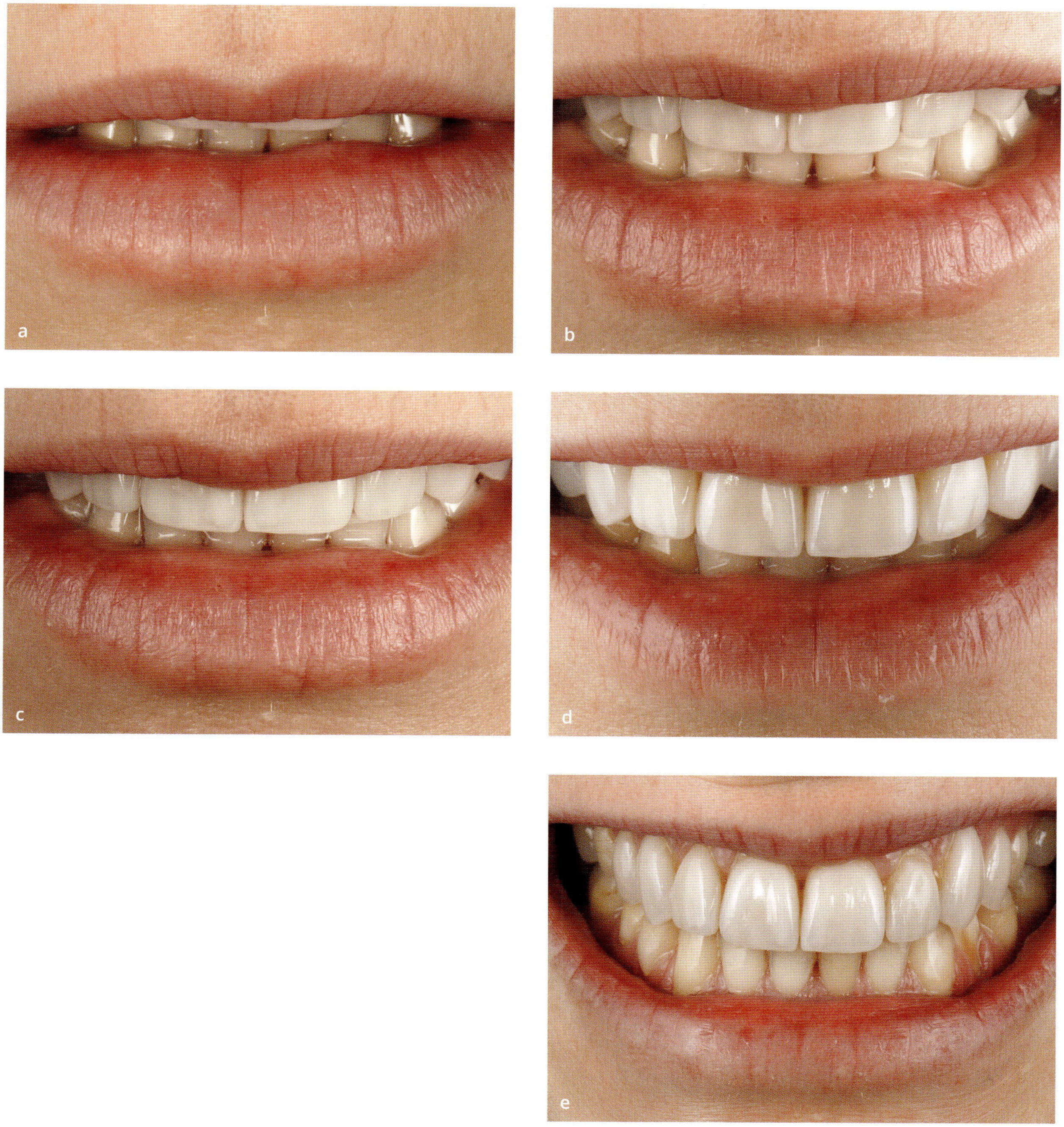


**Fig 7-18** In this young woman (case continued from Figs 7-14 to 7-17), the high esthetic prerequisites together with the high sensitivity are indications for the intervention of the expert lab technician in order to aim at the best outcome possible. Feldspathic porcelain veneers are chosen for their outstanding beauty and excellent clinical performance. Biologic integration coronal to the visible cementoenamel junction demands thin, feather-edge gingival margins that integrate biologically without postoperative polishing. Minimal preparation is done in order to facilitate the path of insertion, which is a combination of facial and incisal. The more prominent anatomy is gently reduced, taking special care to ensure the labial aspects of the incisors do not lose convexity. This is important to maintain lip support and arch volume as well as for long-term survival of the porcelain laminate. The sharp incisal edges are smoothed, and no interproximal reduction is done if the contact point is correct, the enamel is intact, and a healthy papilla is present. All cement excess is removed with the aid of a brush gently impregnated in liquid resin before light polymerization, which is performed first from the palatal and then from the labial. After cement hardening, a blade is used with short concise movements parallel to the tooth axis to eliminate the remains of hard resin and cement. Sometimes the patient with severe TW needs to learn to smile again as it takes time to adjust to the new length and volume (a to r). The PPP is implemented immediately after the delivery of the restorations, for which a digital new acquisition, mouthguards, and regular checkups are essential (see chapter 10).

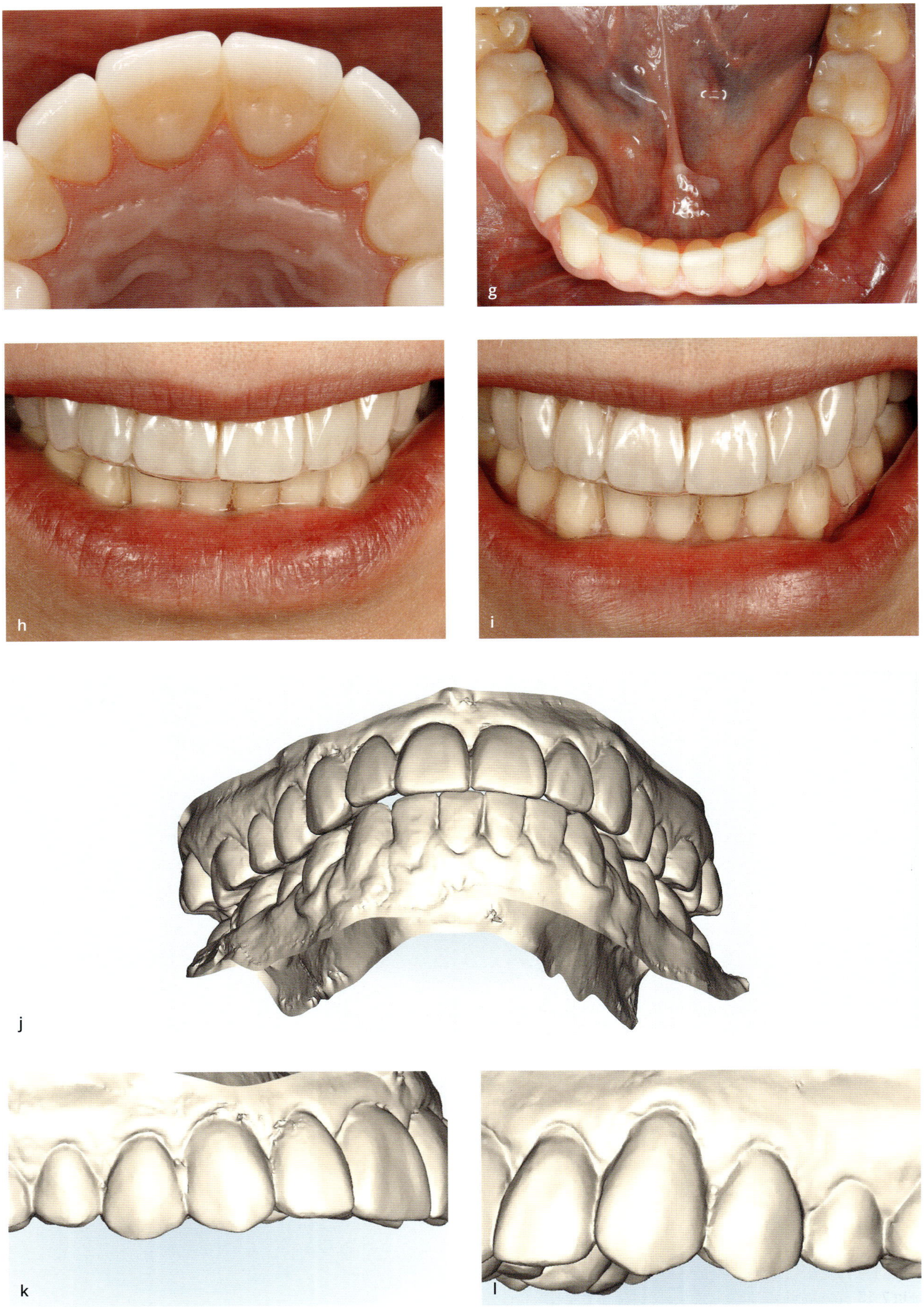
f
g
h
i
j
k
l

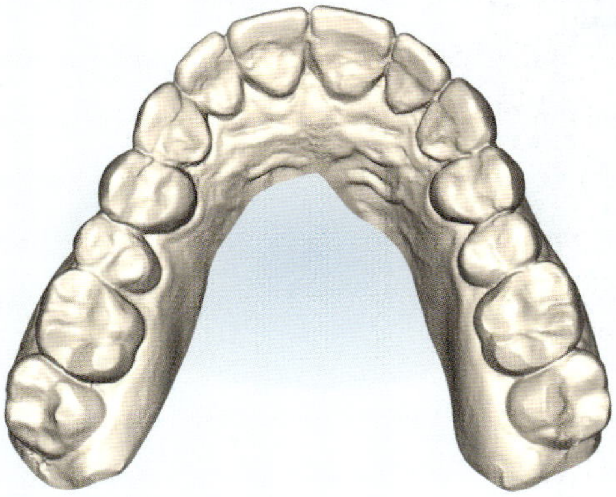

m

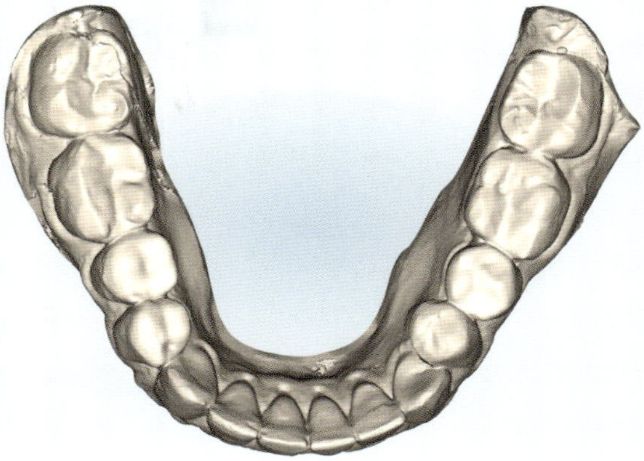

n

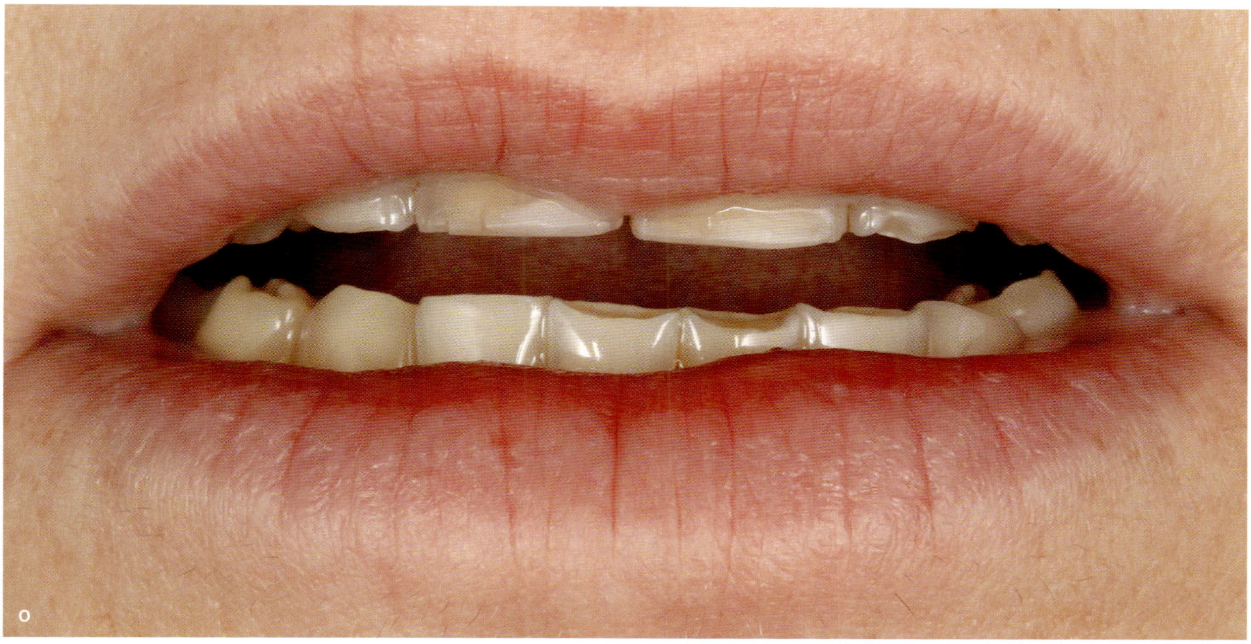

o

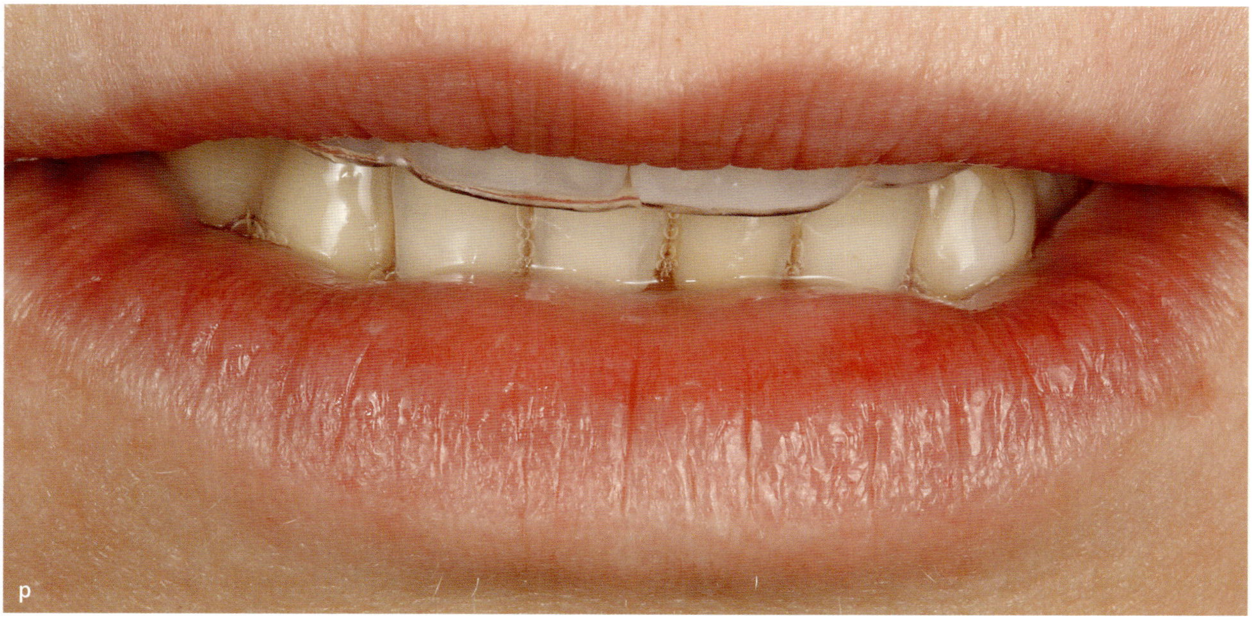

p

**Fig 7-18** *(continued)*

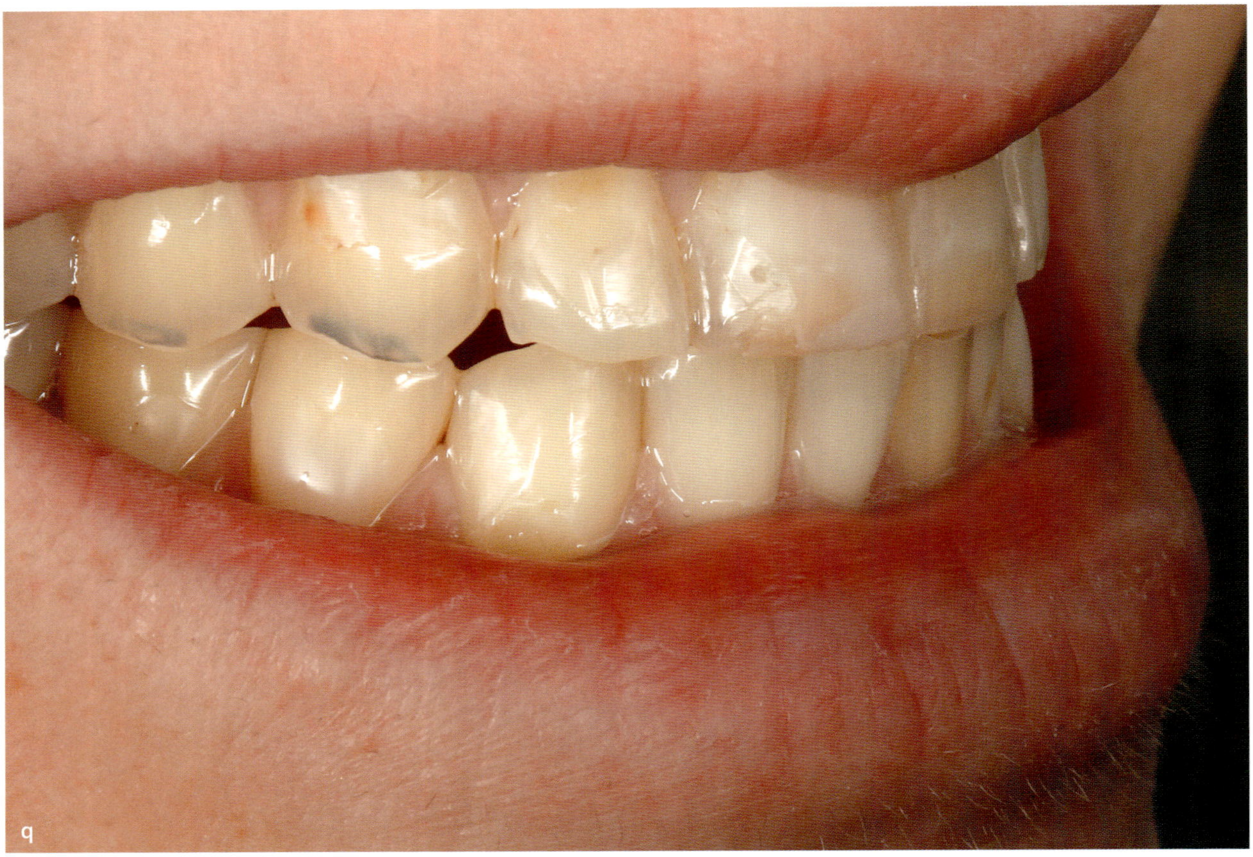

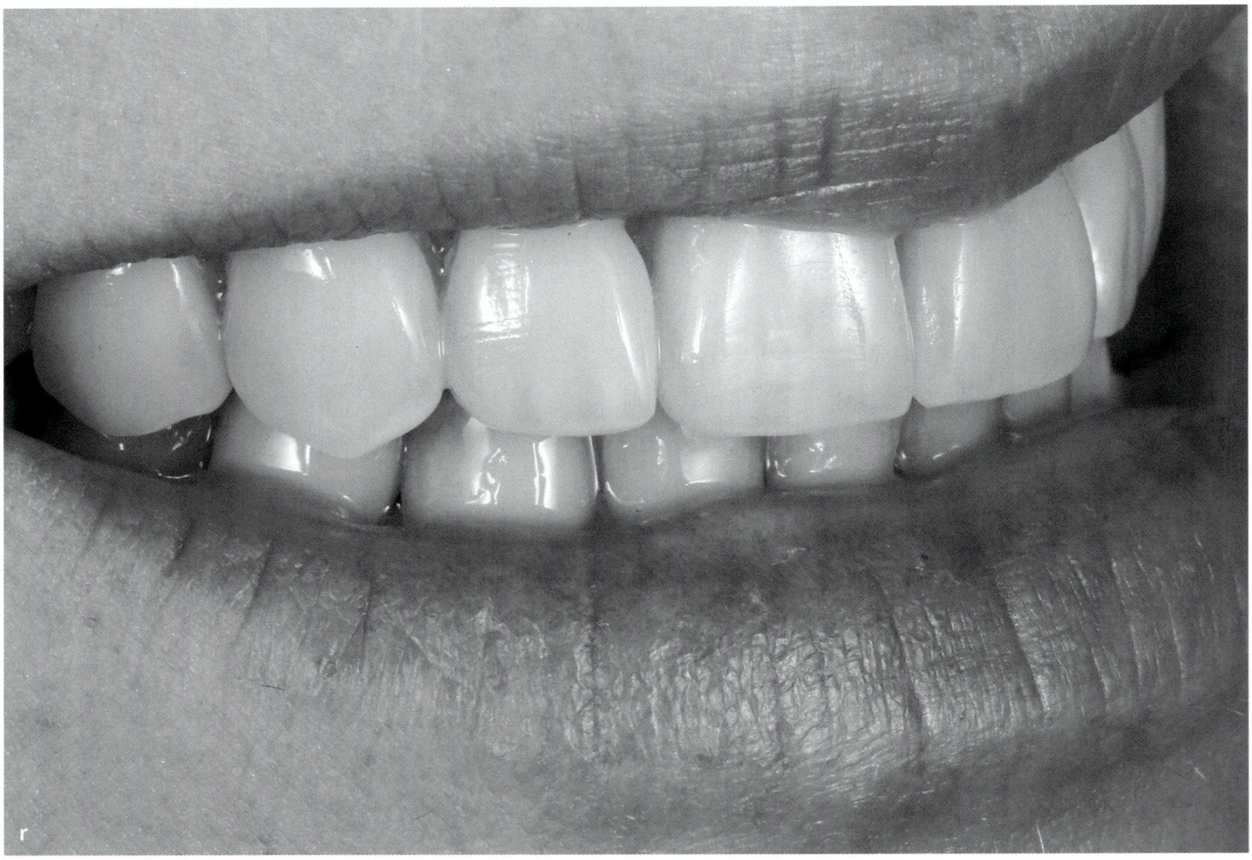

**Fig 7-18** *(continued)*

## 5. Indirect Bonded Inlays/Onlays

In moderate to severe TW cases, especially when VDO needs to be augmented, indirect bonded onlays or inlays may be an appropriate treatment modality to restore posterior segments. There is ample variation in decision making, be it CAD/CAM versus conventional manufacturing or choosing from among composite, ceramic, or the new polymer-infiltrated ceramic network (PICN; eg, Enamic) materials.

Tooth structure conservation should be kept in mind, and credit should be given to the authors who developed the concepts and protocols for adhesive inlays and onlays.[19] Implementation of dual bonding and immediate dentin sealing (IDS) should be performed before impressions and provisionalization to protect dentin and enhance adhesion.[35–40]

A cavity design preparation with a liner to protect dentin, guarantee harmonious geometry of the cavity, and ensure a homogeneous and relatively limited thickness of the restoration is ideal.[36,37] The deep margin elevation (DME) procedure provides the ability to place the margin supragingivally in cases that would otherwise have a deep or intracrevicular margin with the associated challenges of performing adequate impression and cementation procedures.[36,41] Finally, the use of light-curing composites offers, among other advantages, extended working time.[42,43]

An average thickness varying from 1.0 to 1.5 mm is recommended. Even if thicker restorations are known to be stronger, the tissue sacrifice required may not be recommended.[44–46] On the other hand, extremely thin restorations do have their limitations and should only be considered if monolithic materials are chosen. Cusp coverage has been indicated when wall thickness is 1 mm or thinner.[47,48]

Taking all of the above into consideration, in severe TW the thickness limitations are oftentimes not a problem, with the strongest limitation being the presence of preoperative sensitivity. Therefore, the recommendation is to build up with flowable composite and exchange the more traditional partial restoration preparation for roughening with a round diamond bur.

## 6. Partial and Full Crowns for Single-Tooth Restorations: Occlusal Adjustment and Polishing

Unlike the majority of patients with conventional restorative treatment derived from infectious diseases and their sequelae, only a small percentage of patients with TW will fit into the category of needing a full-mouth rehabilitation. The young age at which TW might already affect the dentition, the patient's life expectancy, and the economic burden of a conventional full-mouth rehabilitation can keep the patient with TW from seeking treatment.

Porcelain restorations, mainly feldspathic or lithium disilicate for partial anterior restorations, but also new hybrid materials such as PICN show huge potential for TW patients. Today zirconia, especially in tooth-colored monolithic CAD/CAM form, is a valid option for a severely destroyed tooth, showing high fracture load resistance even with a thickness as small as 0.5 mm, provided a good preparation and adhesion/cementation protocol is followed.

Zirconia implant-supported restorations are a valid option and especially useful in a fully digital work flow. Flawless conventional restorations such as monolithic zirconia full crowns may please not only the patient but also the prosthodontist, but when taking into consideration the preservation principle, the alternatives should be thoroughly weighed when selecting the material, treatment approach, and the type of preparation.[49,50]

The preservation of tooth structure implies the minimum restoration thickness possible. It is feasible today to deliver full monolithic zirconia crowns with a 0.5-mm thickness in a predictable manner. However, it is also true that surface adjustment of these restorations after cementation may be a wear factor for the antagonist.[51] This is even more critical in the patient with TW, in whom the smoothness of the prosthetic surfaces is needed to protect the opposing teeth. Therefore, a strict chairside protocol for polishing the adjusted restoration should be followed, provided the total exposed zirconia surface does not exceed 1 $mm^2$, as the needed reduction should preferably not be done on sound teeth in a patient with wear risk. In minor adjustments, a series of finishing polishes with a finer coarse bur has shown good results. Otherwise, it is preferable to send the crown back to the lab for glazing to eliminate any roughness. The same principles apply for an implant-retained crown or partial denture.[52–60]

## 7. Key Points: Decision Making in Severe TW

**Table 7-1** Decision making in severe TW.

| | |
|---|---|
| There is no interocclusal space: TW of multifactorial origin that has damaged both anterior and posterior dentition | 1. Decide between MIP and CR for the TW rehabilitation project. Dentoskeletal discrepancy and/or patient's profile may impede using CR for restorative planning.<br>2. Orthodontic path: Orthodontics will expand and improve overbite and overjet with or without subsequent increase of VDO at restorative phase.<br>3. Restorative path: The space is found after restoring the dentition and increasing VDO.<br>4. Restorative treatment timeline:<br>▪ First: Restore mandibular dentition and then maxillary posterior teeth and check occlusal contacts.<br>▪ Second: Restore maxillary anterior dentition and check occlusion.<br>▪ Third: Implant restorations should be delivered at final VDO.<br>5. Orthodontic and restorative approaches can be combined. |
| PPP (TW risk reduction, counseling, mouthguard) | 1. Transparent thin splints to be worn during the day and/or night.<br>2. Michigan nightguard if night bruxism or sleep disorders are present.<br>3. Combination of the two is also possible. |
| Follow-up visits at periodic intervals with:<br>▪ Radiographs<br>▪ Pulp vitality monitoring<br>▪ Intraoral scanning comparison | Repairs should be implemented as soon as possible whenever necessary. |

## References


1. Kullmer O, Benazzi S, Fiorenza L, Schulz D, Bacso S, Winzen O. Technical note: Occlusal fingerprint analysis: Quantification of tooth wear pattern. Am J Phys Anthropol 2009;139:600–605.
2. Alhamdan MM, Knowles JC, McDonald A. Digital image correlation and strain gauges to map and compare strain in teeth with different quantity and quality of remaining tooth structure. Int J Prosthodont 2019;32:82–90.
3. Loomans B, Opdam N, Attin T, et al. Severe tooth wear: European consensus statement on management guidelines. J Adhes Dent 2017;19:111–119.
4. Mouatt RB. Children's dental health in the United Kingdom 1983—A review. Health Bull (Edinb) 1986;44:283–285.
5. Smithers G, Gregory JR, Bates CJ, Prentice A, Jackson LV, Wenlock R. The National Diet and Nutrition Survey: Young people aged 4–18 years. Nutr Bull 2000;25(2):105–111.
6. Johansson AK, Omar R, Carlsson GE, Johansson A. Dental erosion and its growing importance in clinical practice: from past to present. Int J Dent 2012;2012:632907.
7. Järvinen VK, Rytömaa II, Heinonen OP. Risk factors in dental erosion. J Dent Res 1991;70(6):942–947.
8. Guo J, Reside G, Cooper LF. Full-mouth rehabilitation of a patient with gastroesophageal reflux disease: A clinical report. J Prosthodont 2011;20(Suppl 2):S9–S13.
9. Milosevic A, Dawson LJ. Salivary factors in vomiting bulimics with and without pathological tooth wear. Caries Res 1996;30:361–366.
10. Smink FR, van Hoeken D, Hoek HW. Epidemiology of eating disorders: Incidence, prevalence and mortality rates. Curr Psychiatry Rep 2012;14:406–414.
11. Fissore B. A clinical case of a patient with a history of anorexia nervosa restored with all-ceramic restorations. Int J Esthet Dent 2016;11:287–290.
12. Lifante-Oliva C, López-Jornet P, Camacho-Alonso F, Esteve-Salinas J. Study of oral changes in patients with eating disorders. Int J Dent Hyg 2008;6(2):119–122.
13. Gargari M, Ceruso FM, Prete V, Pujia A. Prosthetic-restorative approach for the restoration of tooth wear. VDO increase, rehabilitation of anatomy and function and aesthetic restoration of anterior teeth. Case report. Oral Implantol (Rome) 2012;5(2-3):70–74.
14. Edelhoff D, Ahlers MO. Occlusal onlays as a modern treatment concept for the reconstruction of severely worn occlusal surfaces. Quintessence Int 2018;49:521–533.
15. Veneziani M. Posterior indirect adhesive restorations: Updated indications and the morphology driven preparation technique. Int J Esthet Dent 2017;12:204–230.
16. Legaz J, Karasan D, Fehmer V, Sailer I. The 3D-printed prototype: A new protocol for the evaluation and potential adaptation of monolithic all-ceramic restorations before finalization. Quintessence Int 2020;51:538–544.
17. Teich S. Three-dimensional thinking—It is just a matter of time. Quintessence Int 2018;49:519–520.
18. Dietschi D, Argente A. A comprehensive and conservative approach for the restoration of abrasion and erosion. Part II: Clinical procedures and case report. Eur J Esthet Dent 2011;6:142–159.
19. Dietschi D, Argente A. A comprehensive and conservative approach for the restoration of abrasion and erosion. Part I: Concepts and clinical rationale for early intervention using adhesive techniques. Eur J Esthet Dent 2011;6:20–33.
20. Kois JC, Phillips KM. Occlusal vertical dimension: Alteration concerns. Compend Contin Educ Dent 1997;18:1169–1174,1176–1177.
21. Bronstrup MB, Palmeiro MR, Shinkai RS. Impact of prosthetic rehabilitation on quality of life in patients with significant dental and orofacial tissue loss: A mixed-methods study. Int J Prosthodont 2019;32:32–35.
22. Edelhoff D. Innovative treatment concepts in the rehabilitation of the worn dentition—Clinical strategies outside the box. Int J Esthet Dent 2017;12:272–273.
23. Fradeani M, Barducci G, Bacherini L. Esthetic rehabilitation of a severely worn dentition with minimally invasive prosthetic procedures (MIPP). Int J Periodontics Restorative Dent 2012;32:135–147.
24. Del Curto F, Saratti CM, Krejci I. CAD/CAM-based chairside restorative technique with composite resin for full-mouth adhesive rehabilitation of excessively worn dentition. Int J Esthet Dent 2018;13:50–64.
25. Magne P. Noninvasive bilaminar CAD/CAM composite resin veneers: A semi-(in)direct approach. Int J Esthet Dent 2017;12:134–154.
26. Rayyan MR, Alauti RY, Abanmy MA, AlReshaid RM, Bin Ahmad HA. Endocrowns versus post-core retained crowns for restoration of compromised mandibular molars: An in vitro study. Int J Comput Dent 2019;22(1):39–44.
27. Strasding M, Sebestyén-Hüvös E, Studer S, Lehner C, Jung RE, Sailer I. Long-term outcomes of all-ceramic inlays and onlays after a mean observation time of 11 years. Quintessence Int 2020;51:566–576.
28. Vailati F, Carciofo S. CAD/CAM monolithic restorations and full-mouth adhesive rehabilitation to restore a patient with a past history of bulimia: The modified three-step technique. Int J Esthet Dent 2016;11:36–56.

29. Gresnigt M, Magne M, Magne P. Porcelain veneer post-bonding crack repair by resin infiltration. Int J Esthet Dent 2017;12:156–170.
30. Gracis S, Marinello C. Selecting the ideal esthetic restorative material: Some clinical aspects and suggestions. Int J Esthet Dent 2016;11(2):260–263.
31. Dahl BL, Krogstad O, Karlsen K. An alternative treatment in cases with advanced localized attrition. J Oral Rehabil 1975;2(3):209–214.
32. Grütter L, Vailati F. Full-mouth adhesive rehabilitation in case of severe dental erosion, a minimally invasive approach following the 3-step technique. Eur J Esthet Dent 2013;8:358–375.
33. Magne P, Magne M, Belser UC. Adhesive restorations, centric relation, and the Dahl principle: Minimally invasive approaches to localized anterior tooth erosion. Eur J Esthet Dent 2007;2:260–273.
34. Reich S, Hartkamp O, Reiss B. A chairside concept for increasing the vertical dimension of occlusion in the maxilla and mandible. Int J Comput Dent 2019;22(1):81–98.
35. Dietschi D, Herzfeld D. In vitro evaluation of marginal and internal adaptation of class II resin composite restorations after thermal and occlusal stressing. Eur J Oral Sci 1998;106:1033–1042.
36. Dietschi D, Spreafico R. Adhesive Metal-Free Restorations: Current Concepts for the Esthetic Treatment of Posterior Teeth. Chicago: Quintessence, 1997.
37. Dietschi D, Spreafico R. Current clinical concepts for adhesive cementation of tooth-colored posterior restorations. Pract Periodontics Aesthet Dent 1998;10(1):47–54.
38. Magne P. Immediate dentin sealing: A fundamental procedure for indirect bonded restorations. J Esthet Restor Dent 2005;17:144–154.
39. Magne P, Kim TH, Cascione D, Donovan TE. Immediate dentin sealing improves bond strength of indirect restorations. J Prosthet Dent 2005;94:511–519.
40. Paul SJ, Schärer P. The dual bonding technique: A modified method to improve adhesive luting procedures. Int J Periodontics Restorative Dent 1997;17:536–545.
41. Magne, P. and R.C. Spreafico, Deep margin elevation: A paradigm shift. Am J Esthet Dent, 2012. 2(2): p. 86-96.
42. Besek M, Mörmann WH, Persi C, Lutz F. The curing of composites under Cerec inlays [in German]. Schweiz Monatsschr Zahnmed 1995;105:1123–1128.
43. Dietschi D, Marret N, Krejci I. Comparative efficiency of plasma and halogen light sources on composite micro-hardness in different curing conditions. Dent Mater 2003;19:493–500.
44. Beier US, Kapferer I, Burtscher D, Giesinger JM, Dumfahrt H. Clinical performance of all-ceramic inlay and onlay restorations in posterior teeth. Int J Prosthodont 2012;25:395–402.
45. Fennis WM, Kuijs RH, Kreulen CM, Verdonschot N, Creugers NH. Fatigue resistance of teeth restored with cuspal-coverage composite restorations. Int J Prosthodont 2004;17:313–317.
46. Rocca GT, Rizcalla N, Krejci I, Dietschi D. Evidence-based concepts and procedures for bonded inlays and onlays. Part II. Guidelines for cavity preparation and restoration fabrication. Int J Esthet Dent 2015;10:392–413.
47. Rocca GT, Krejci I. Crown and post-free adhesive restorations for endodontically treated posterior teeth: from direct composite to endocrowns. Eur J Esthet Dent 2013;8(2):156–179.
48. Stappert CF, Abe P, Kurths V, Gerds T, Strub JR. Masticatory fatigue, fracture resistance, and marginal discrepancy of ceramic partial crowns with and without coverage of compromised cusps. J Adhes Dent 2008;10(1):41–48.
49. Güth JF, Wallbach J, Stimmelmayr M, Gernet W, Beuer F, Edelhoff D. Computer-aided evaluation of preparations for CAD/CAM-fabricated all-ceramic crowns. Clin Oral Investig 2013;17:1389–1395.
50. Güth JF, Stawarczyk B, Edelhoff D, Liebermann A. Zirconia and its novel compositions: What do clinicians need to know? Quintessence Int, 2019;50:512–520.
51. Lohbauer U, Reich S. Antagonist wear of monolithic zirconia crowns after 2 years. Clin Oral Investig 2017;21:1165–1172.
52. Bateli M, Kern M, Wolkewitz M, Strub JR, Att W. A retrospective evaluation of teeth restored with zirconia ceramic posts: 10-year results. Clin Oral Investig 2014;18:1181–1187.
53. Fehmer V, Mühlemann S, Hämmerle CH, Sailer I. Criteria for the selection of restoration materials. Quintessence Int 2014;45:723–730.
54. Koutayas SO, Vagkopoulou T, Pelekanos S, Koidis P, Strub JR. Zirconia in dentistry: Part 2. Evidence-based clinical breakthrough. Eur J Esthet Dent 2009;4:348–380.
55. Mühlemann S, Benic GI, Fehmer V, Hämmerle CHF, Sailer I. Randomized controlled clinical trial of digital and conventional workflows for the fabrication of zirconia-ceramic posterior fixed partial dentures. Part II: Time efficiency of CAD-CAM versus conventional laboratory procedures. J Prosthet Dent 2019;121:252–257.
56. Sailer I, Balmer M, Hüsler J, Hämmerle CHF, Känel S, Thoma DS. 10-year randomized trial (RCT) of zirconia-ceramic and metal-ceramic fixed dental prostheses. J Dent 2018;76:32–39.
57. Sailer I, Fehér A, Filser F, et al. Prospective clinical study of zirconia posterior fixed partial dentures: 3-year follow-up. Quintessence Int 2006;37(9):685–693.
58. Sailer I, Mühlemann S, Fehmer V, Hämmerle CHF, Benic GI. Randomized controlled clinical trial of digital and conventional workflows for the fabrication of zirconia-ceramic fixed partial dentures. Part I: Time efficiency of complete-arch digital scans versus conventional impressions. J Prosthet Dent 2019;121(1):69–75.
59. Selz CF, Bogler J, Vach K, Strub JR, Guess PC. Veneered anatomically designed zirconia FDPs resulting from digital intraoral scans: Preliminary results of a prospective clinical study. J Dent 2015;43:1428–1435.
60. Strub JR, Malament KA. Do zirconia ceramics have a future in restorative dentistry? Int J Periodontics Restorative Dent 2013;33:259.

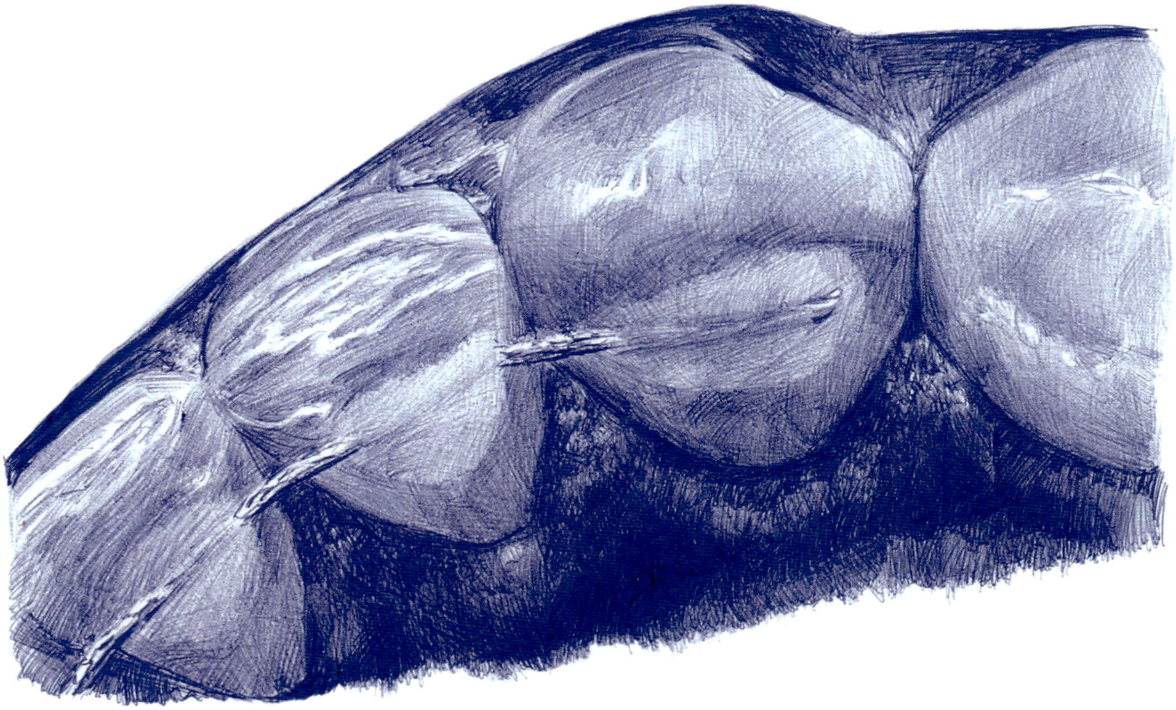

*If you're offered a seat on a rocket ship, don't ask what seat! Just get on.*

—Sheryl Sandberg, American economist, COO of Facebook, founder of Leanin.org

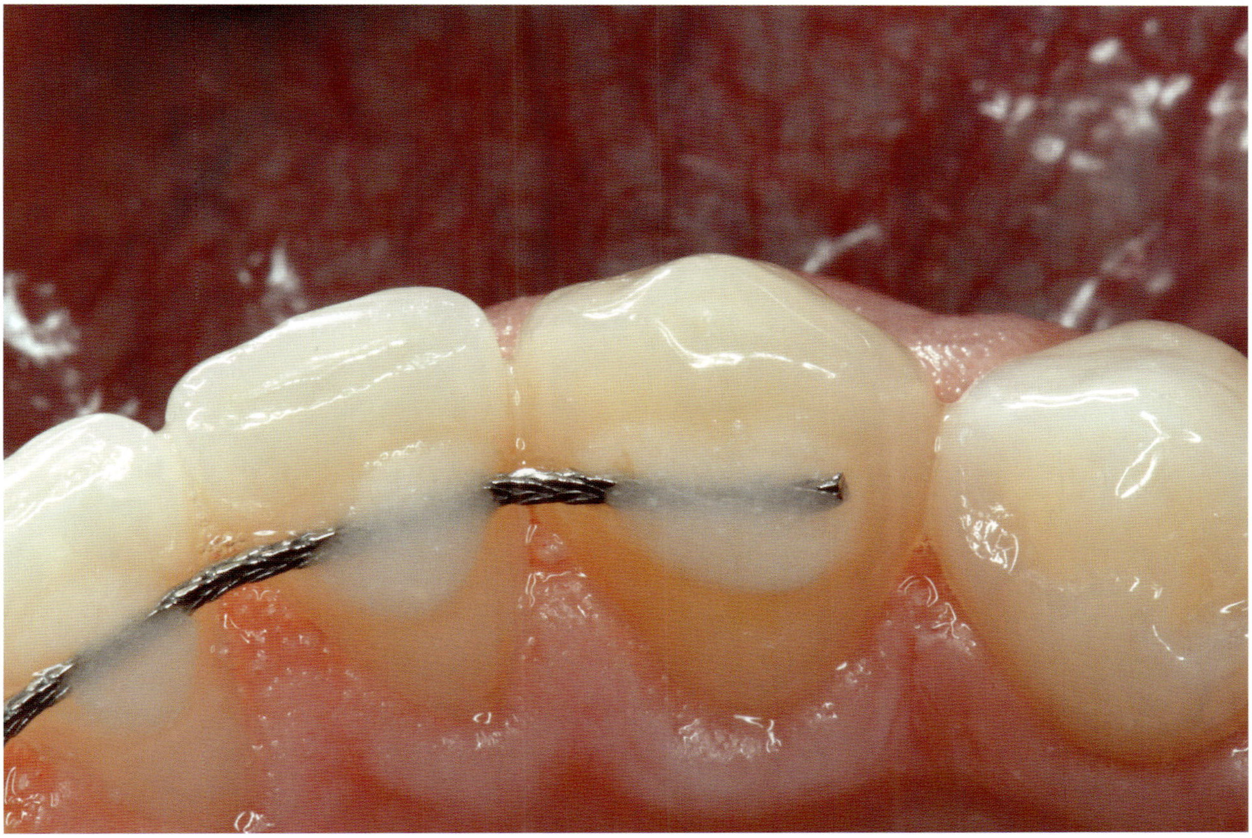

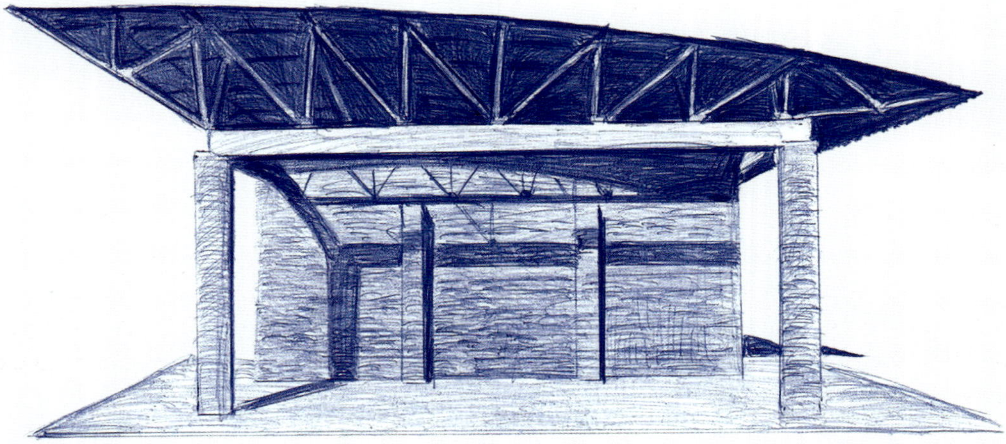

Primary school, Burkina Faso

*Architecture is not just about building. It's about improving people's quality of life.*

—Diébédo Francis Kéré, architect born in Burkina Faso, founder of Kere Architecture Berlin

CHAPTER 8

# ORTHODONTICS IN TOOTH WEAR TREATMENT

Orthodontics is an essential part of a multidisciplinary approach. Orthodontic therapy is the standard of care for patients affected with malocclusion, whatever the type and severity. During the last decades, orthodontics has become part of the routine treatment of adults in need of prosthetic, restorative, and/or implant therapy as well as for the correction of misalignment and crowding.

In young patients who still have growth potential, orthodontic therapy should also focus on the correction and improvement of malfunction of the upper respiratory and digestive systems, which are both implicated in the future onset of severe TW. The general recommendation of a thorough orthodontic evaluation in the early years has become habitual in the first world. The increasing prevalence of TW in children needs not to be forgotten as it may happen that TW will be first diagnosed by the orthodontist.

The digitalization and strong development of new CAD/CAM technologies started first in the discipline of orthodontics, which found in the ortho-specialist someone trained to visualize tooth volumes, profile, and setup prior to starting the treatment. This three-dimensional thinking, together with a facially driven treatment plan, is of paramount help in the TW team.

Furthermore, it is in the incipient, moderate, and severe cases of TW where the orthodontist may play a leading role. A well-planned team approach to orthodontic therapy will save tooth structure more than any other therapy. Failing to evaluate the patient with TW orthodontically may leave the restorative team in need of reducing more tooth structure.

## 1. Malocclusion and Tooth Wear

Orthodontics is understood as the dental specialty that includes the diagnosis, prevention, interception, guidance, and correction of malrelationships of developing and mature orofacial structures.[1] Malocclusions are a precipitating condition for TW.[2] This is not only because of the physical response to the lack of harmony between the masticatory components, but also because the fine balance between enamel protection and enamel loss requires ideal ororespiratory function. This is commonly endangered in individuals with a deviation in intra-arch and/or maxillomandibular relationships and/or from normal occlusion. Malocclusion has been shown to play an important role in the onset of tooth wear; however, little has been written about the advantages of orthodontic therapy in patients with TW.

Orthodontics plays a fundamental role not only in the development of the dentition but also in craniofacial growth. For many years orthodontic treatment was limited to children who had not finished growing to help achieve a better relationship between the maxilla and mandible. It is clear that orthodontic treatment has become a standard of care in young patients in whom orthodontics can intercept incipient cases that appear at a young age.[3]

The daily practice of an orthodontist consists of treating malocclusions in patients that, at a young age, still benefit from all their potential growth and a functional rehabilitation with little restorative treatment required adjunctive to the orthodontic therapy. In recent years the number of young and adult patients whose first diagnosis is loss of original tooth anatomy has changed orthodontic daily practice toward a comprehensive TW team approach. Orthodontic therapy to improve compression and overbite and regulate overjet is without a doubt an effective means of providing more space within the arch.

Malocclusion is one of the most common dental problems globally, together with caries, fluorosis, gingivitis, and periodontitis.

Our goal is not only to correct occlusal restriction and resolve crowding related to dentofacial esthetics, but also to eliminate possible interferences in oral function, such as mastication and swallowing; protect anterior and lateral guidance; and improve the patient's quality of life.[4] Tooth wear is a dynamic, insidious condition, by which occlusal adaptation and compensatory bone growth alter the original parameters.

Although the association between orthodontic treatment and dental health has been studied previously, no studies have hitherto investigated whether the need for, or the receipt of, orthodontic treatment leads to differences in tooth wear in the long term. The orthodontist and restorative dentist can work together to improve occlusion and esthetics for adult orthodontic patients seeking restoration of worn or abraded teeth.

All malocclusions have been linked to TW, with variations in severity and location in the mouth. While TW in Class I occlusion is said to affect both jaws equally, maxillary teeth are supposedly affected most in Class II malocclusion, and mandibular teeth are affected most in Class III malocclusion.[2,5]

Orthodontists should be prepared to diagnose whether there is an underlying orthodontic condition that would perpetuate the wear of the dentition in the coming years, and if so, take the correct measures to intercept further TW damage.

## TW in Class I Occlusion

TW is commonly associated with Class II and Class III malocclusions. However, TW also occurs in Class I occlusion and Class I malocclusion.

As part of the TW team, the orthodontist should analyze the occlusal scheme and the functional performance, in particular the canine and anterior guidance. Independently of the skeletal and dental class, an insufficient functional protection, namely a poor anterior and/or canine guidance, can happen as a consequence of the presence of parafunctional habits such as lip biting, nail biting, and bruxism and/or erosive challenges, among other factors (Fig 8-1).

In general, an erosive challenge, associated or not with an attrition-mechanical challenge, can be present in any type of occlusion, be it Class I, II, III, or in combinations thereof. Furthermore, TW itself, when advanced, can lead to malpositioning of teeth, anterior rotation of the mandible, vertical and horizontal collapse, and compensatory changes that may complicate the orthodontic diagnosis.

Clinical evidence shows that anterior growth of the mandible, compensatory eruption, and occlusal adaptation, such as so-called group function, all linked to TW, may disrupt the original skeletal and dental class of the TW patient. In principle, Class I, as an ideal scheme, protects teeth from excessive occlusal forces but not from parafunctional habits, such as nail biting, or from erosion-related TW.

In fact, in Class I compared to Class II cases, the finding of TSL can be linked to specific TW etiologic factors on the palatal aspects of maxillary teeth and incisal aspects of mandibular teeth, such as erosive challenges in the first location and grinding or bruxism in the second location (Figs 8-2 and 8-3).

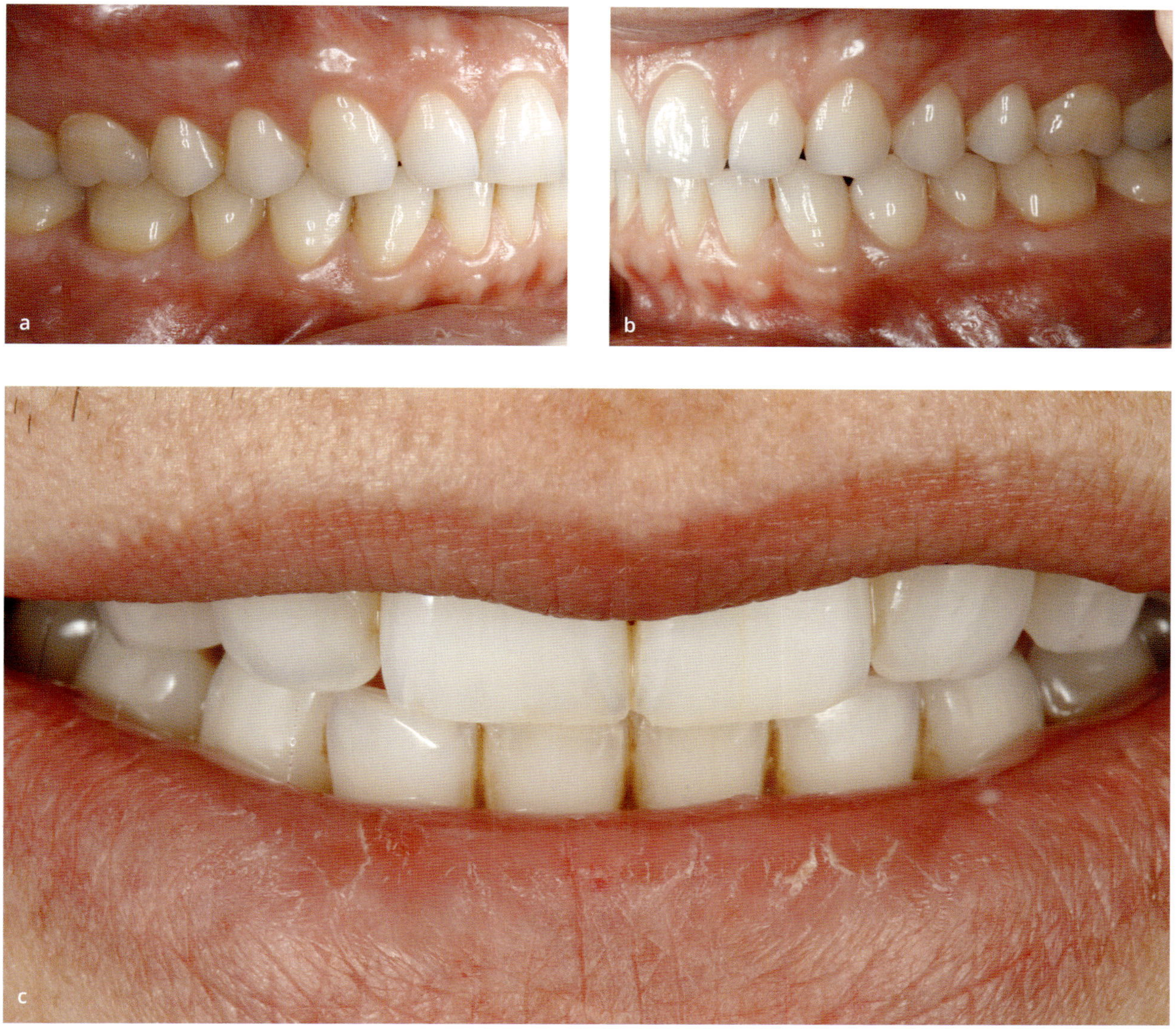

**Fig 8-1** Bilateral Class I (normal) occlusion at both the canine and molar has not stopped the patient from wearing the incisal edges and canine cusps due to parafunctional habits (a to c). *(continued next page)*

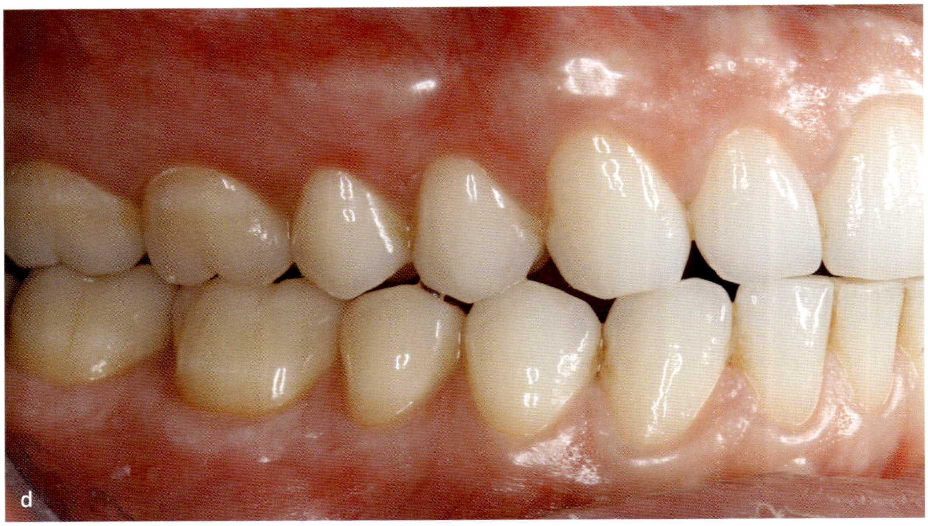

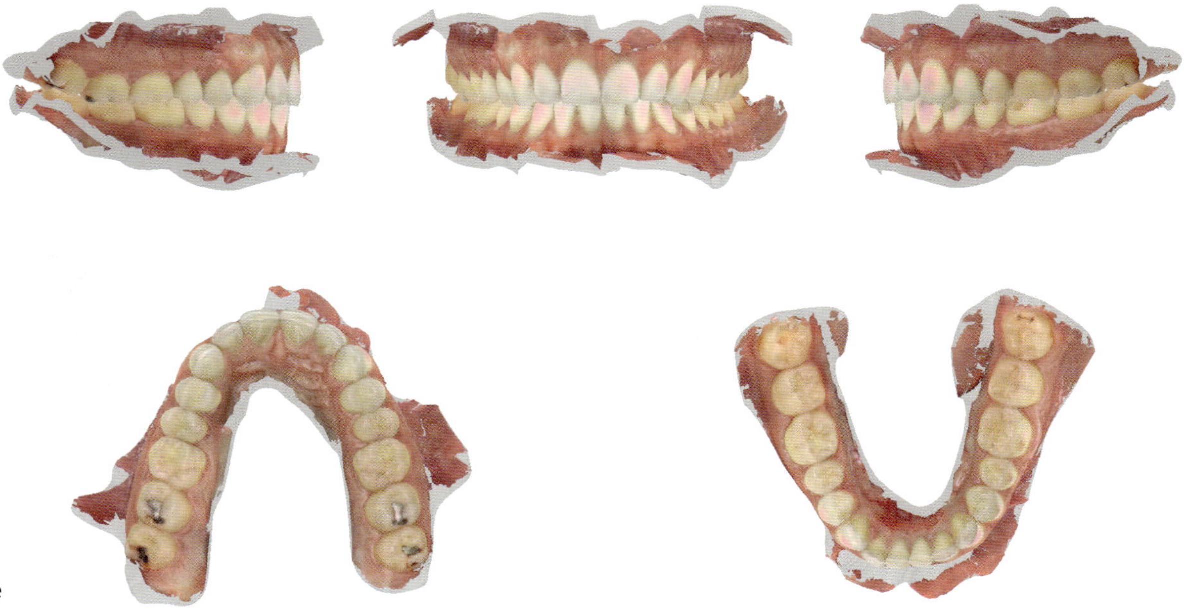

e

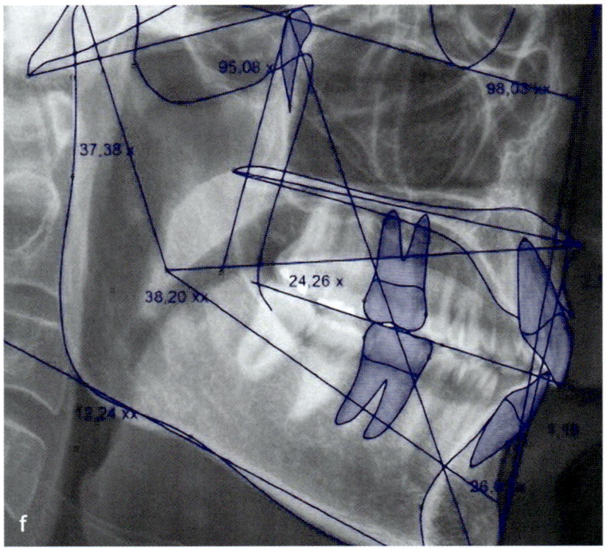


**Fig 8-1** *(continued)* Group function in the presence of anterior incipient TW is a risk factor and may well be the consequence of TW and not a naturally occurring occlusal scheme (d) (see chapter 10). Nevertheless, the orthodontic evaluation of a TW patient does not necessarily lead to an orthodontic therapy indication. In that case, a restorative alternative should be evaluated (see chapters 5 and 10). Once the patient was diagnosed of incipient TW, he was scheduled for orthodontic evaluation. Intraoral scanning shows correct arch form with symmetric arches and no crowding (e). The detailed outline in the cephalometric evaluation depicts a normal and correct interincisal relationship and angulation despite the somewhat dolichofacial pattern. Cephalometric analysis shows correct angulation with correct SNA and SNB angles, normal Class I occlusion, skeletal Class I, and Class I molar and canine relationships (f). No indication for orthodontic therapy is derived from this cephalometric evaluation.

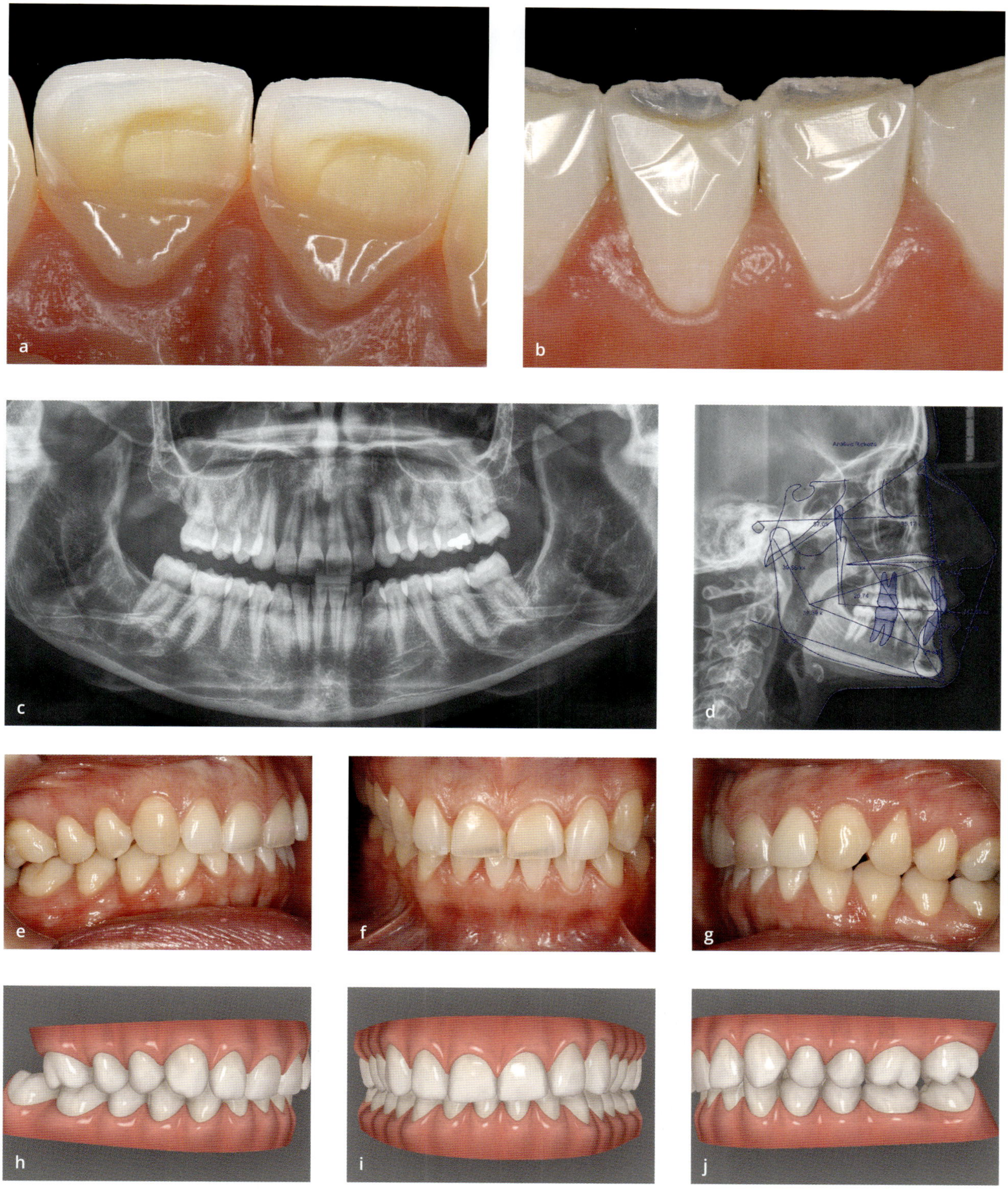

**Fig 8-2** In this patient an intrinsic erosive challenge and a grinding habit has occurred in a combined Class I on the right side and Class II on the left side at the time of diagnosis. The slight crowding and increased overbite have restricted the envelope of function in which the teeth need to function with an increased muscle response that has worn the teeth, especially the mandibular incisors. At the same time, the acidic environment has affected the palatal aspect of the maxillary incisors, which as a result have increased translucency and a shortened, irregular incisal edge (a). The mandibular incisors show clearly the type of combined erosive and attrition damage that arises as a consequence of the insidious character of TW (b). The panoramic radiograph shows the presence of almost intact posterior anatomy without signs of posterior TSL (c). The lateral radiograph shows the patient has an inadequate interincisal relationship with increased overbite and diminished overjet (d). The digital photographs and STL of the initial situation show the compensatory eruption has left the interocclusal restorative possibilities almost nonexistent except for reductive dentistry. The excessively vertical anterior disocclusion together with the softened enamel has rapidly worn the anterior sector of the dentition (e to p). *(continued next page)*

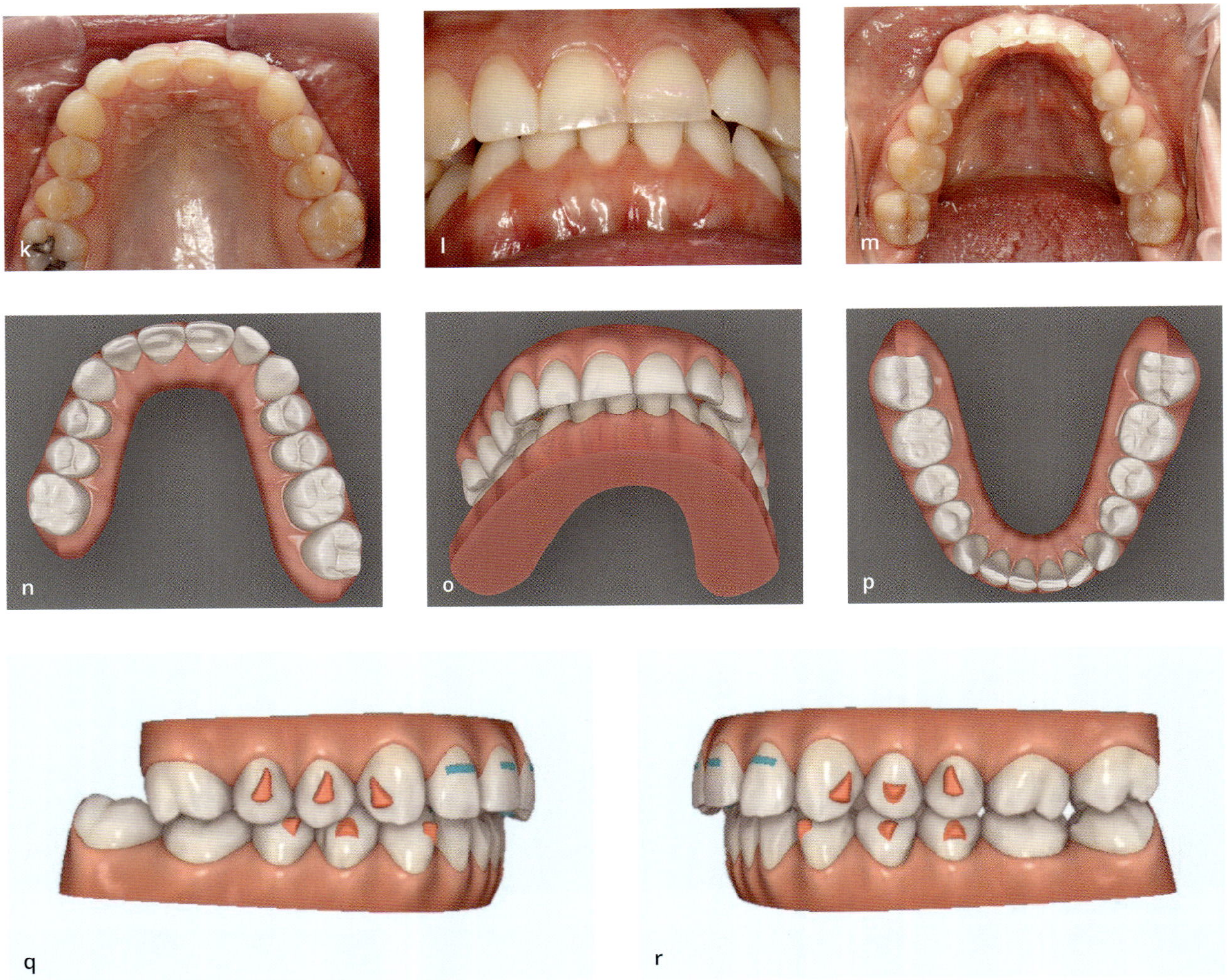

**Fig 8-2** *(continued)* The compression of both arches and slight crowding will also need to be addressed in order to prevent more tooth enamel loss. An orthodontic digital setup is done, including expansion and proclination of the teeth with a digital orthodontic therapy protocol to achieve a more favorable tooth relationship at the end of the orthodontic therapy (q and r). Moderate forces are used with clear aligners to be changed at 3-week intervals. Moderate expansion of posterior teeth and proclination of anterosuperior teeth result in broader maxillary and mandibular arches and creation of a new restorative space where most needed. Worn teeth are aligned respectful of their gingival margin. Note the design of the optimized attachments to control not only the mesiodistal crown movement but also the tilting of the roots.

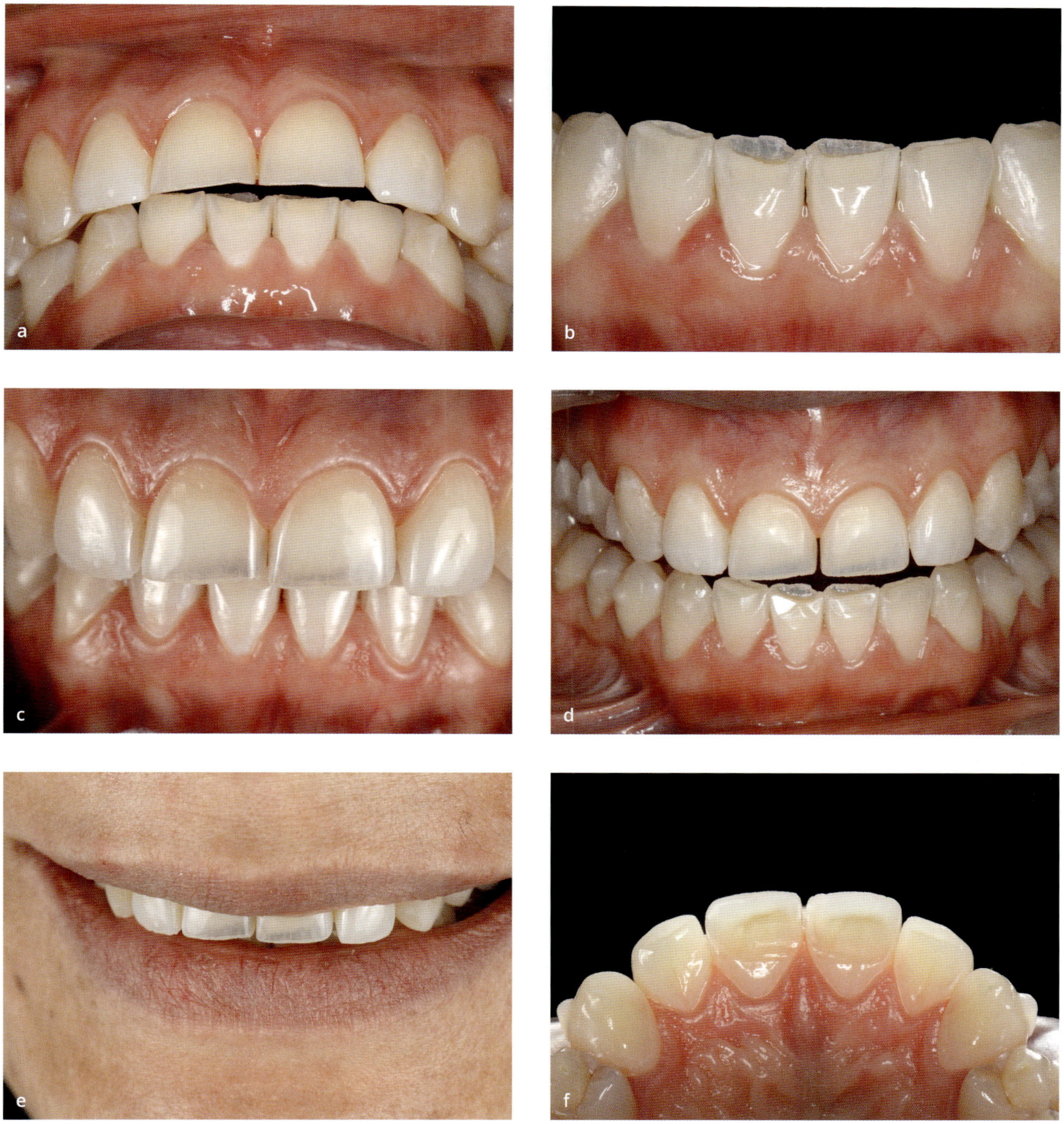

**Fig 8-3** The expansion and dental alignment has provided a broader smile. The combined direct composite in the mandibular incisors with an indirect protocol to restore the palatal aspect of the four maxillary incisors has been facilitated by the orthodontic therapy and can be done now without removing tooth structure at all (a to f). *(continued next page)*

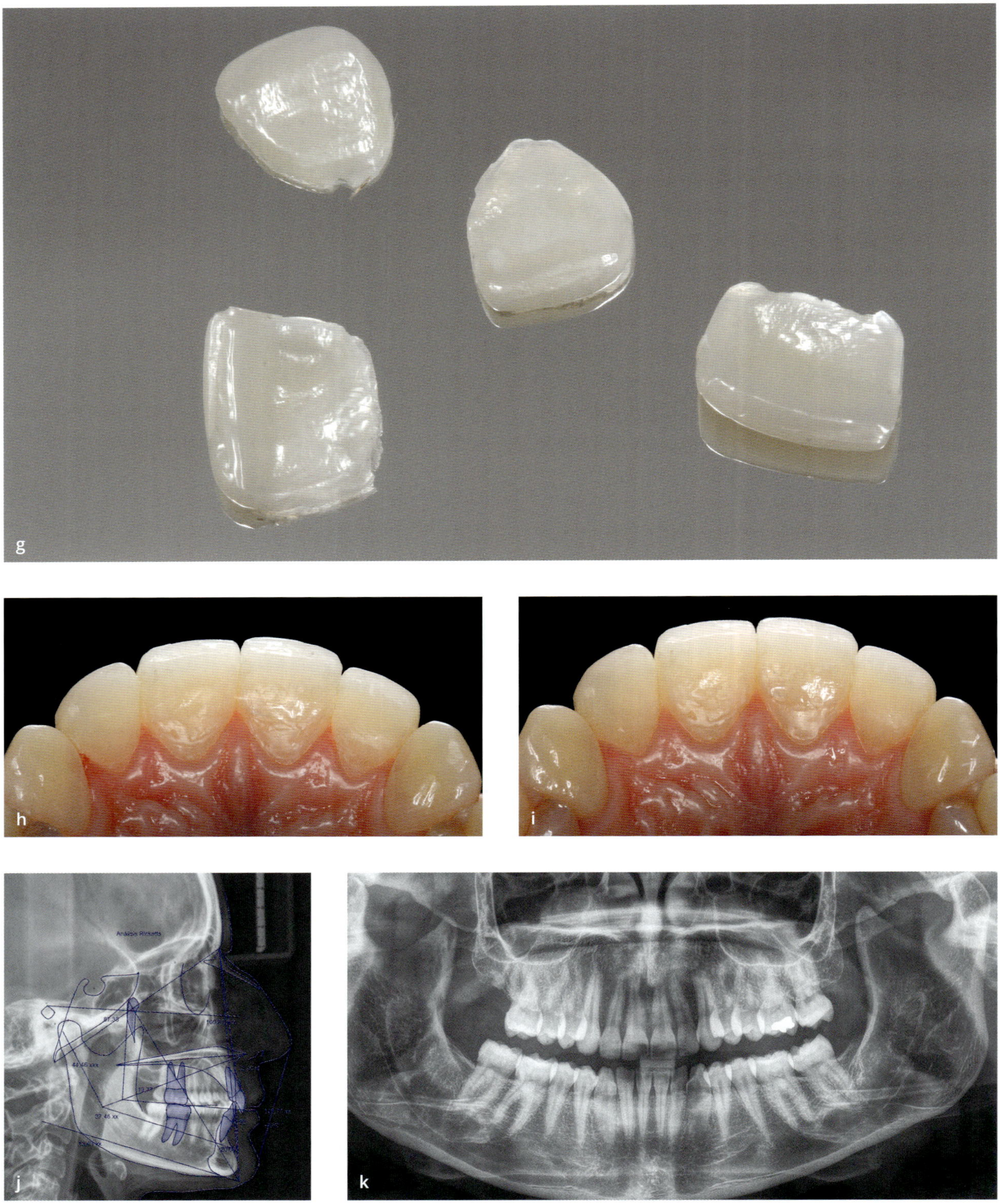

**Fig 8-3** *(continued)* The palatal onlays are handmade to the ideal length, guided by the tip of the well-preserved natural maxillary canine. The central incisors will receive a partial palatal onlay up until the remaining healthy gingival third, while the lateral incisors will receive a full palatal overlay as treatment of the arch has been esthetically driven, and the lateral incisors would otherwise remain out of occlusion (g to i). At the end of the treatment, new radiographic and intraoral images are acquired to enable TW control (j to q). The four onlays overlap the worn incisal edge and supplement the lost palatal and incisal anatomy (r and s). Note that no labial masking or restoration has been done to hide the interface between the natural labial enamel and the palatal composite onlay at this stage (t). The mutually protected occlusal scheme and more freedom in function after decompressing and broadening are subsequent to the improvement of the three-dimensional interdental relationship and occlusal plane (u). The patient is given extra-thin maxillary and mandibular mouthguards and scheduled for checkups at 6-month intervals (v).

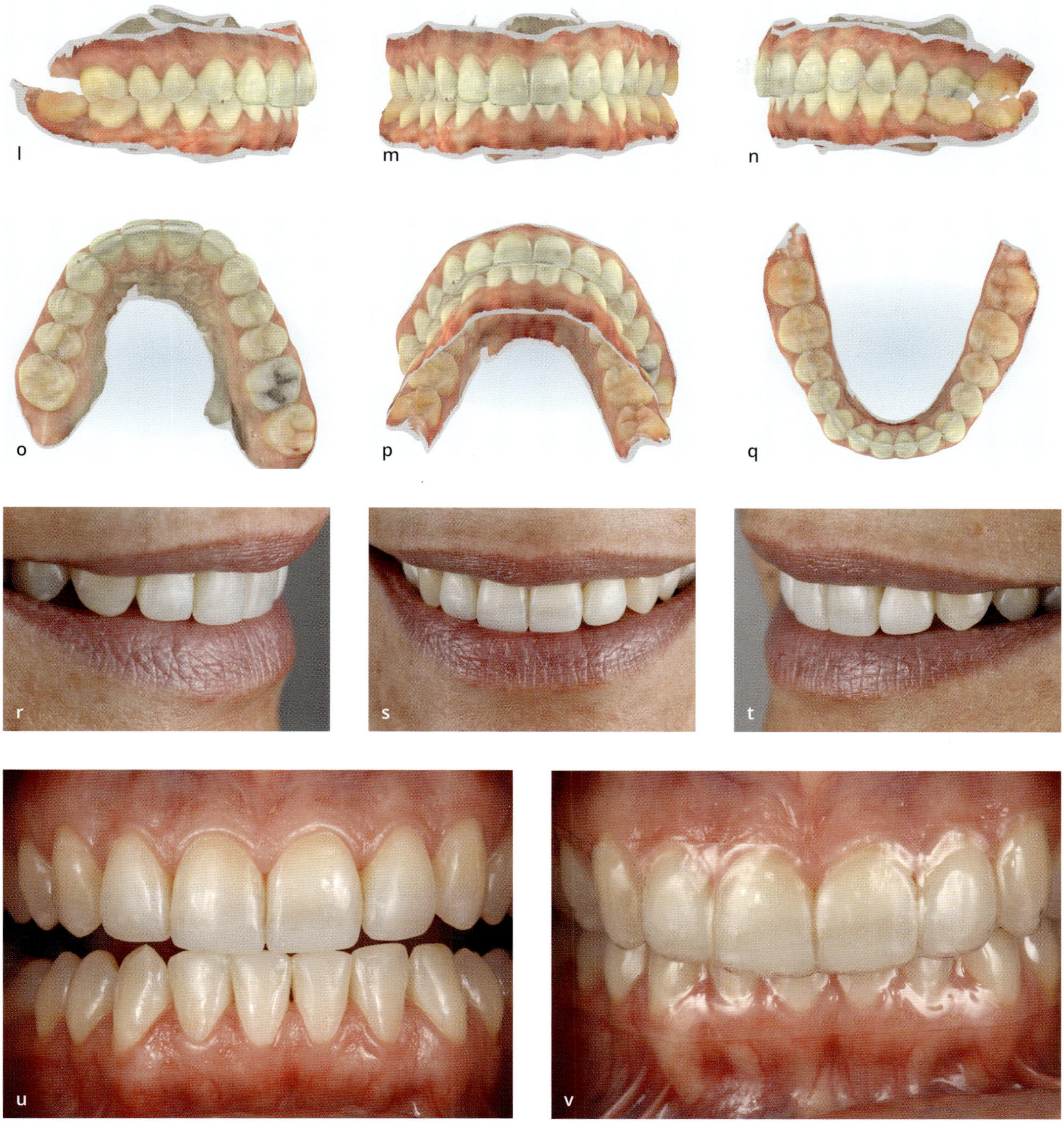
l
m
n
o
p
q
r
s
t
u
v

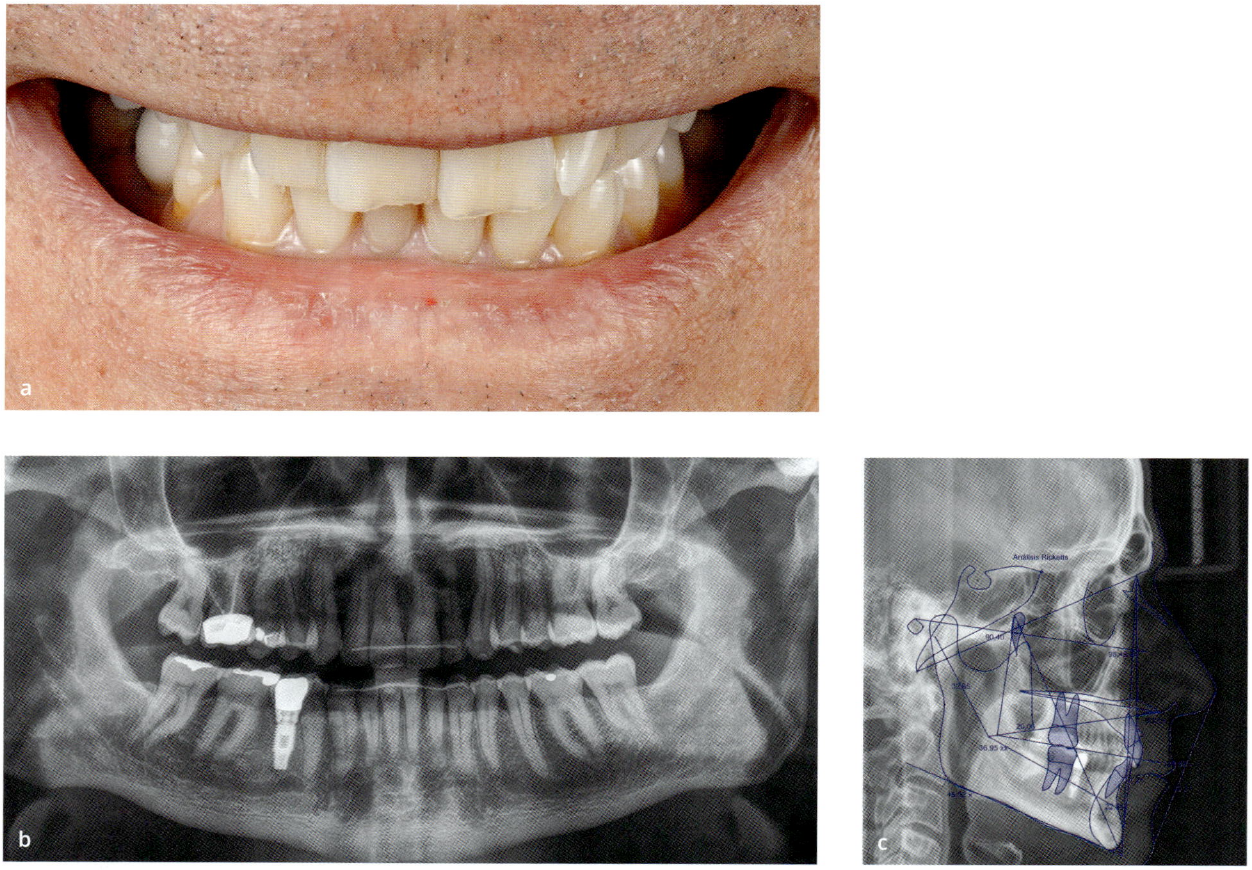


**Fig 8-4** This patient, in his sixth decade of life, has incipient TW along with an untreated Class II, division 1 malocclusion with augmented overbite and compressed arches. The esthetic appearance of the smile is affected by a slightly disharmonious incisal plane and tooth size discrepancy, accompanied by anterior crowding, narrow arches, misalignment, and unlevel, worn incisal edges (a). The radiographic and cephalometric evaluation demonstrates an adequate skeletal but compromised dental relationship, with crowding and a slight Class II relationship because of the retrognathic mandible (b and c). The interincisal relationship is not correct, with maxillary and mandibular incisors running in an almost parallel vertical plane, as seen in the lateral radiograph (c).

## TW in Class II Malocclusion

In general, TW in Class II cases has been explained as a mechanical consequence of the occlusal pattern and incorrectly considered nonpathological.[2,5] Yet, other conditions can be combined or associated with a narrow, compressed arch form, in particular, restricted masticatory and/or upper respiratory dysfunction that can eventually lead to a diminished protection from TW. Age does not always correlate with TW severity (see chapter 5). Therefore, upon a TW diagnosis all orthodontic possibilities should be discussed with the patient irrespective of the decade of life (Fig 8-4).

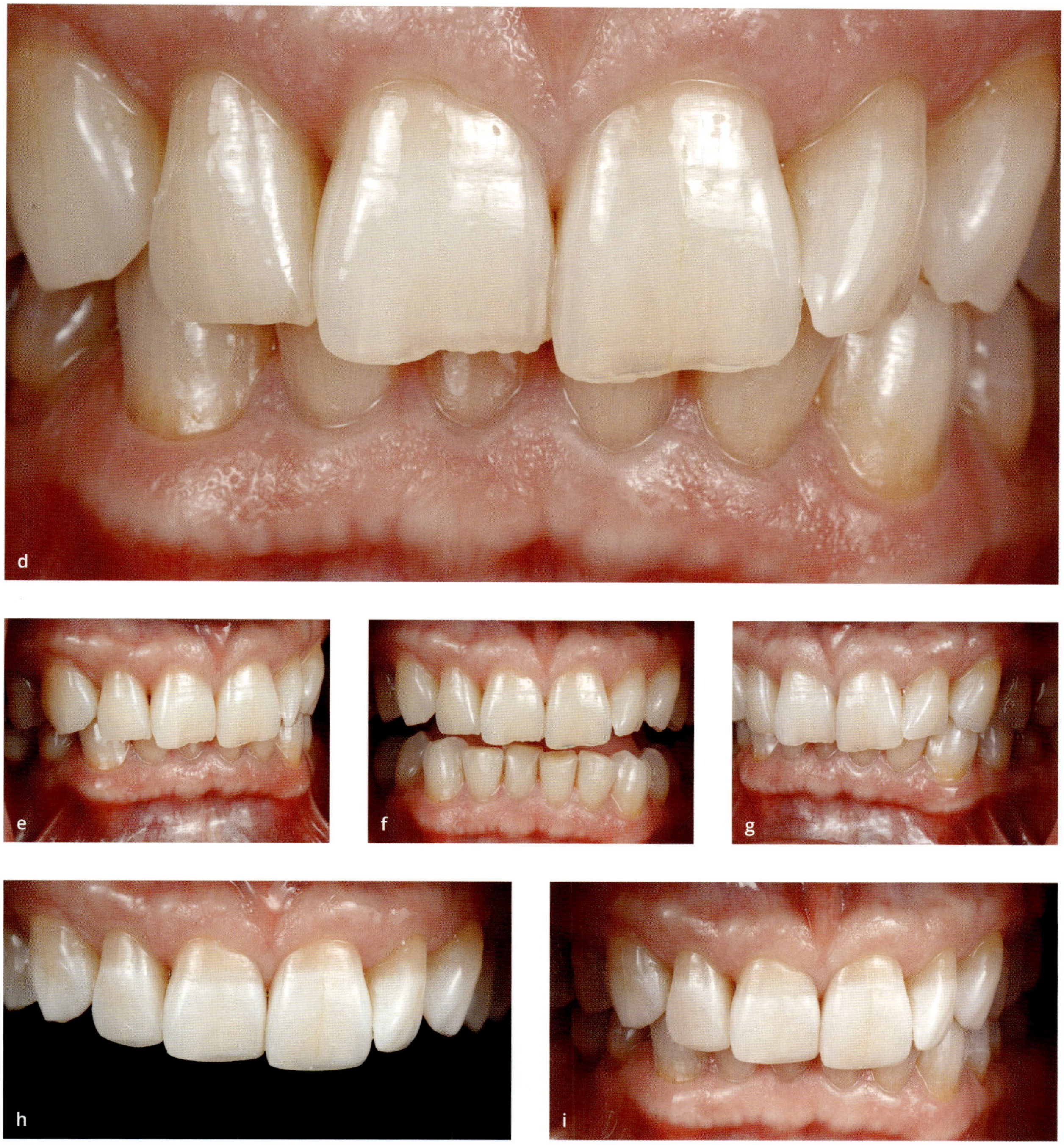

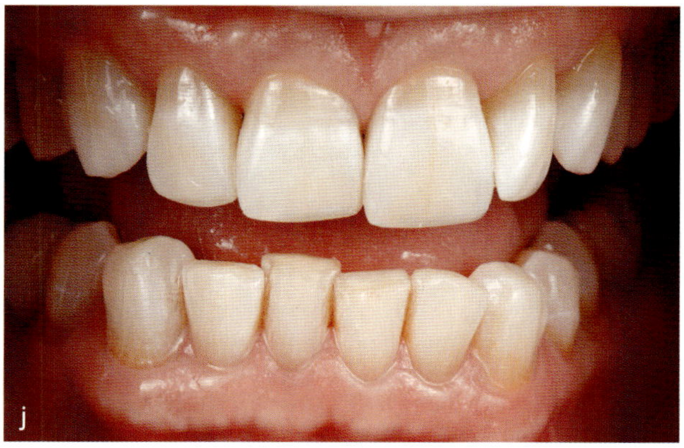

**Fig 8-4** *(continued)* Note the excessively curved incisal plane and anterior crowding (d to g). The patient does not want to have his teeth heavily restored. It is decided to do the restorative phase before the orthodontic phase. Tooth alignment is agreed to be addressed, respecting the congenital tooth size asymmetry both in length and width between the two central incisors. In this case it is decided to restore the incisal wear, attending to the remaining sound incisal edge within each tooth and ignore the length discrepancy between the two centrals, as this is matched with a different width between the two (h to j). The restoration is done with freehand composite before starting any tooth alignment, and the teeth are leveled respectful of their original gingival outline. *(continued next page)*

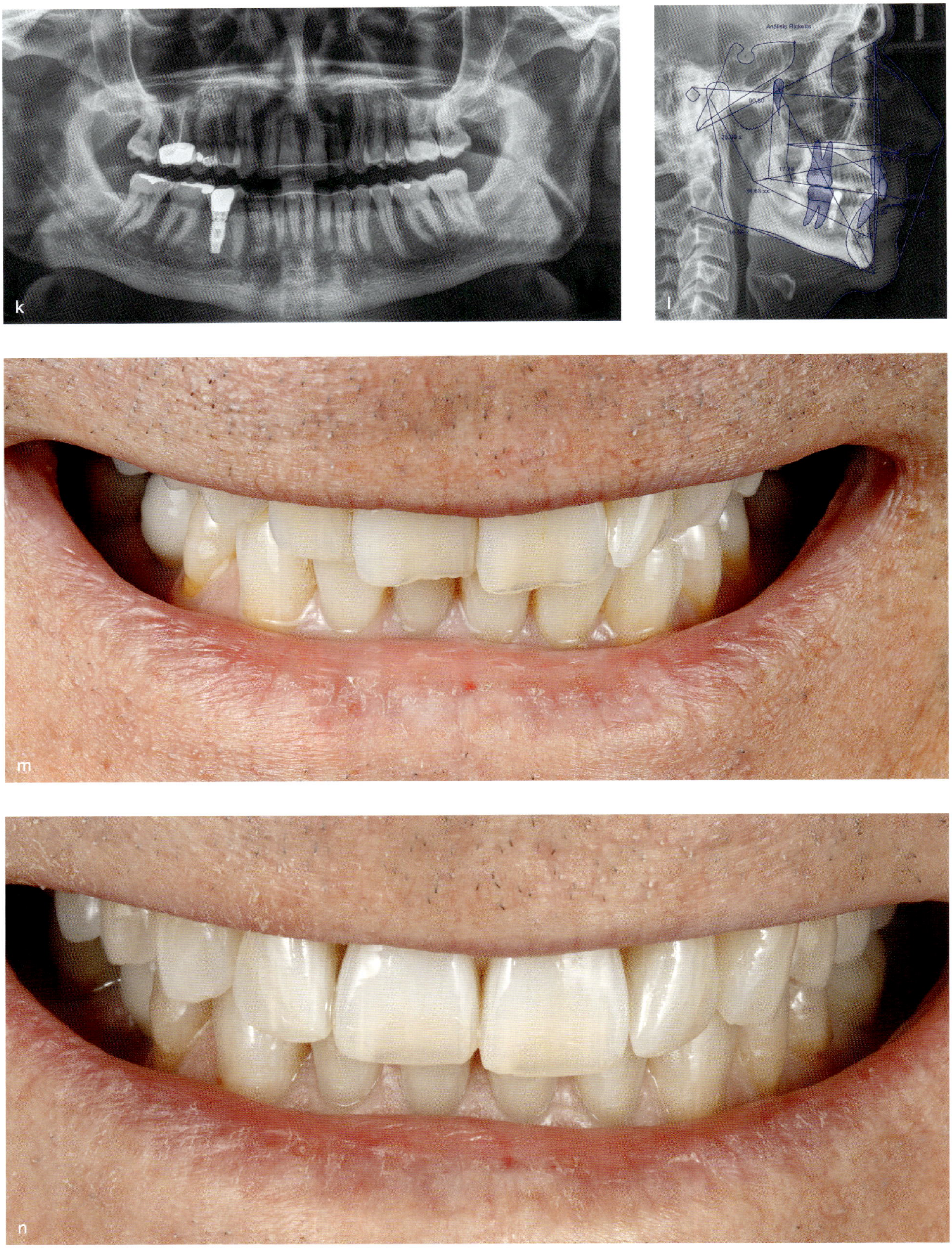


**Fig 8-4** *(continued)* The improvement of the curve of Spee and curve of Wilson along with the broadening of both arches is accompanied by a more appropriate overjet and overbite (k and l). The desire of the patient to avoid major restorations limits the closure of gingival embrasures related to long-term bone remodeling. The width and length discrepancy between the two central incisors had been anticipated and does not disturb the patient, who appreciates the restoration of the worn incisal edges when compared to the initial situation (m and n).

## TW in Class III Malocclusion

Malocclusion of all types complicates management of TW and may even worsen the course of this condition. It is in the moderate and severe cases of TW where the orthodontist may play a leading role. A well-planned team approach will save tooth structure.[6-8] Failing to orthodontically evaluate the patient with TW may leave the restorative team in need of reducing more tooth structure than desirable.[6]

Preprosthetic orthodontic treatment has traditionally provided a more conservative prosthetic outcome. Aligning the teeth first can reduce the amount of tooth preparation, and it can also improve oral hygiene and provide a healthier periodontium. Conversely, if orthodontics is not considered, in order to achieve ideal tooth form and function in severe malocclusions, more tooth structure has to be removed to compensate for the misalignment of the teeth.[9,10]

Likewise, when confronted with a patient with TW who has a severe malocclusion, not addressing the dentoskeletal condition will unequivocally mean more tooth reduction when teeth are restored. That being said, the special determinants of TSL in TW make it advisable to aim at accessible and rapid tooth protection, even if the orthodontic objectives have to be limited.

Integrated and articulated comprehensive treatment planning should include the objectives of all therapies—periodontal, orthodontic, restorative, surgical, and preventive—into one plan whenever possible.[9-12] The esthetically driven approach is well understood and appreciated by patients as self-esteem is hampered in severe TW and severe malocclusions. Yet it should come as no surprise that most of the patients with TW are asymptomatic and may not be aware of the TW.[13]

The origin of TW in these patients is usually multifactorial with a combination of abrasion, erosion, and parafunctional habits. The role of altered mastication together with dietary adaptation to the malocclusion has been mentioned in previous chapters.

Congenital conditions such as skeletal Class III can be accompanied by any other form of malocclusion such as open bite, crossbite, edge-to-edge bite, compressed arches, or altered eruption, to name the most common. Dental conditions such as agenesis, enamel hypoplasia, and ankylosis are findings that complicate the treatment timeline in these patients (Figs 8-5 and 8-6).

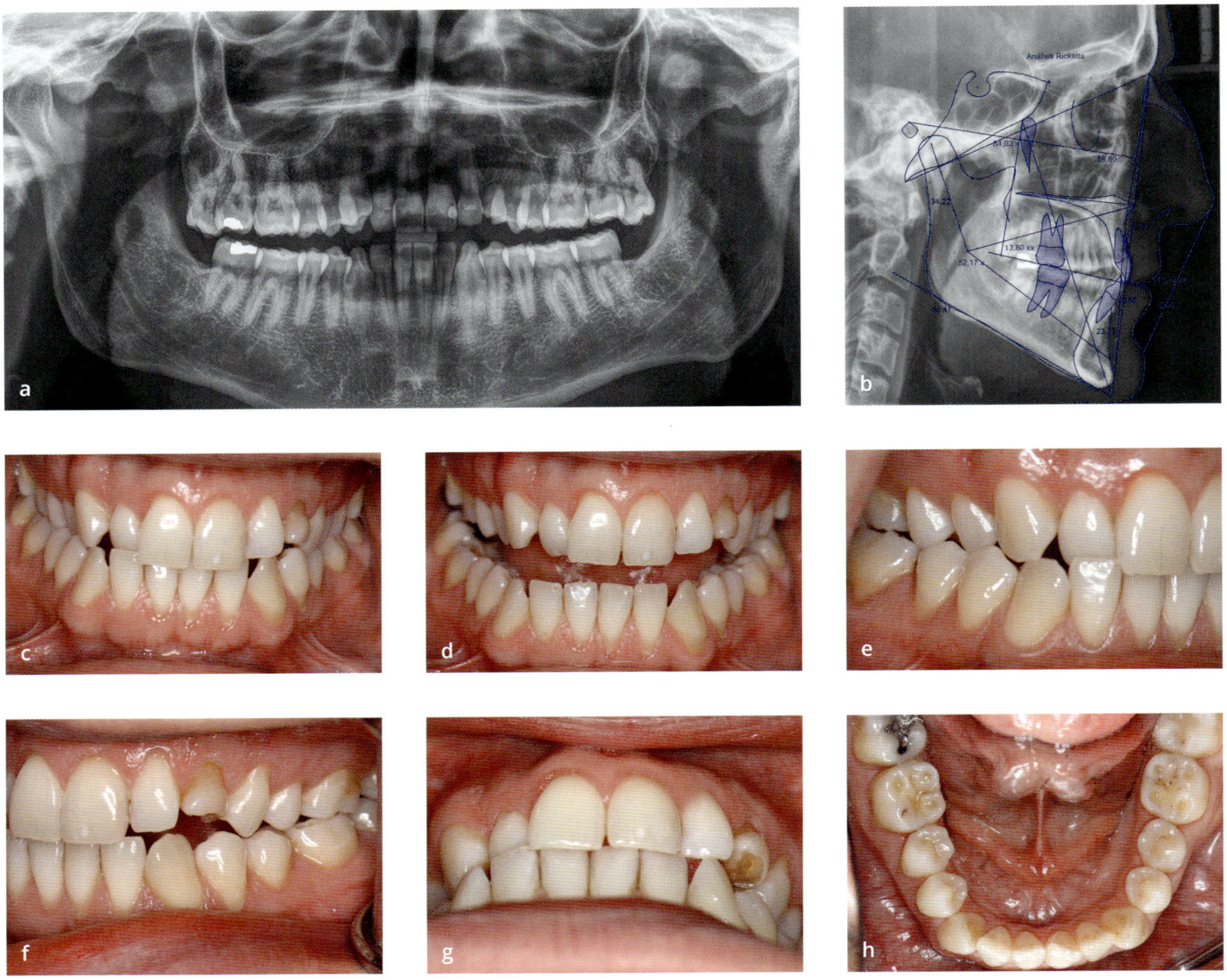

**Fig 8-5** A young entrepreneur is not conscious that the untreated Class III malocclusion may have had a negative impact in the combined attrition/erosion pattern that he has suffered since a young age, especially in his mandibular first molars. Agenesis of the maxillary left canine as well as anterior and posterior crossbite with unilateral open bite all have contributed to an altered occlusal scheme, compromising enamel integrity. The WECC (Wear Easy Clinical Classification) finding of incipient TW (despite the presence of dentin exposure, only a group of teeth have been affected so far) is advanced by the presence of malocclusion to moderate TW according to the WASS (Wear Aggravating Severity Scale), as explained in chapter 4 (a to h).

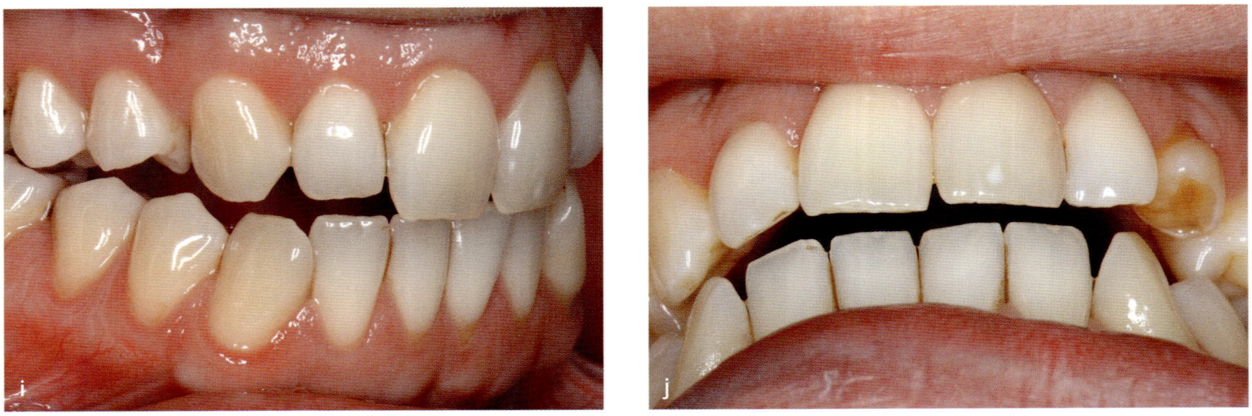

**Fig 8-5** *(continued)* The digitalization of the patient images assists in creating an esthetically driven treatment plan that starts with orthodontic expansion and includes implant replacement of the primary canine as well as restoration of the worn teeth. The first phase of orthodontic therapy consists of expansion with a fixed palatal quad-helix. Once the expansion has taken place, the open bite temporarily worsens (i to k). A second phase starts with clear aligners (Invisalign, Align Technology) to improve the anterior relationship, canine and anterior guidance, and posterior occlusion. The space for the implant is secured (l to n). The implant-retained crown (Nobel Active, Nobel Biocare) is delivered 4 months after the first surgery (o to q).

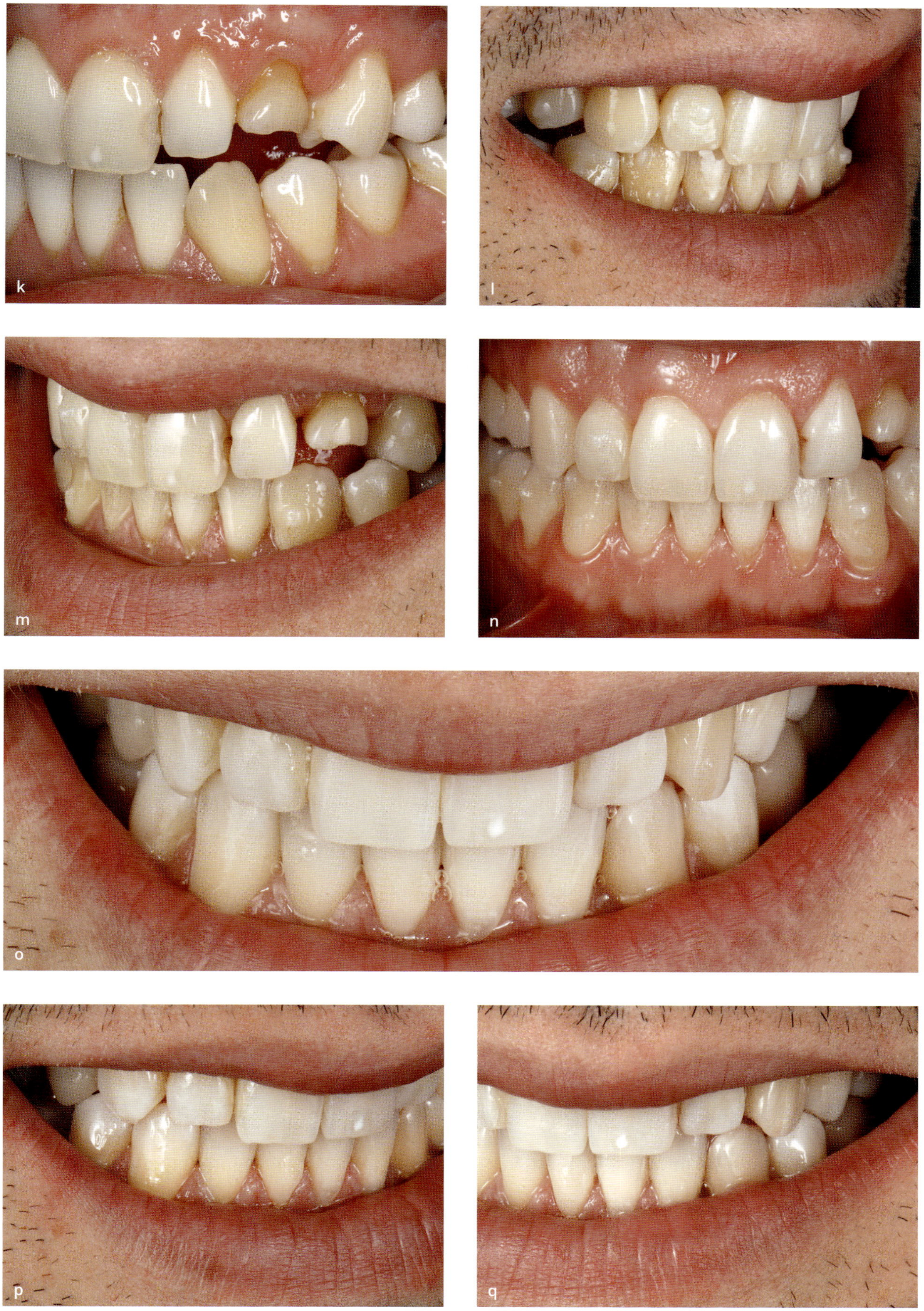
k
l
m
n
o
p
q

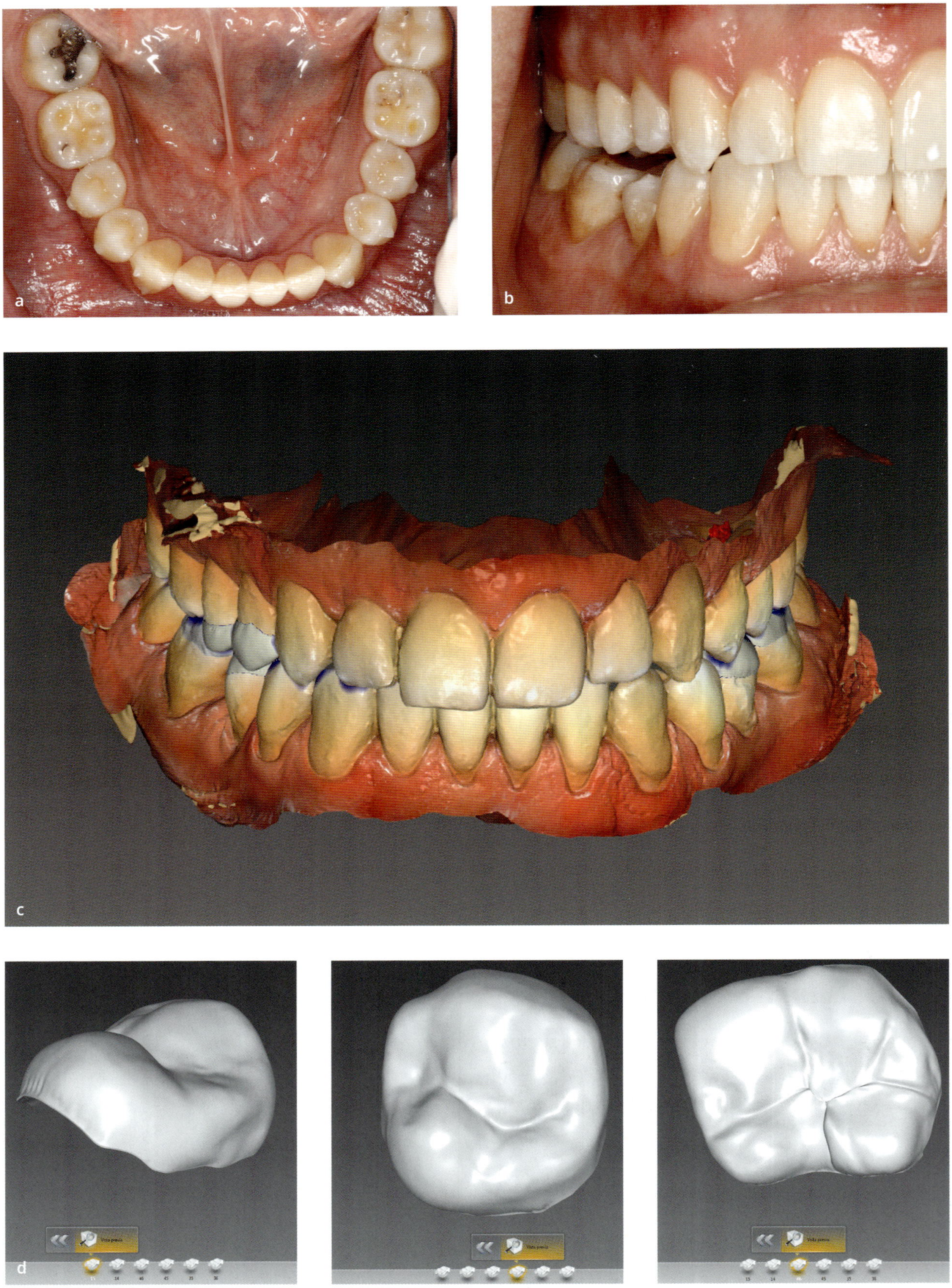

**Fig 8-6** Erosive damage in the same patient's posterior teeth, namely in the first molars, is planned to be restored with overlays. Adjacent and opposing teeth are aligned in regard to their gingival margin and will be occlusally restored with overlays. The six non-prep overlays are milled from a PICN block (Enamic, VITA) and adhered to the recipient teeth (a to y).

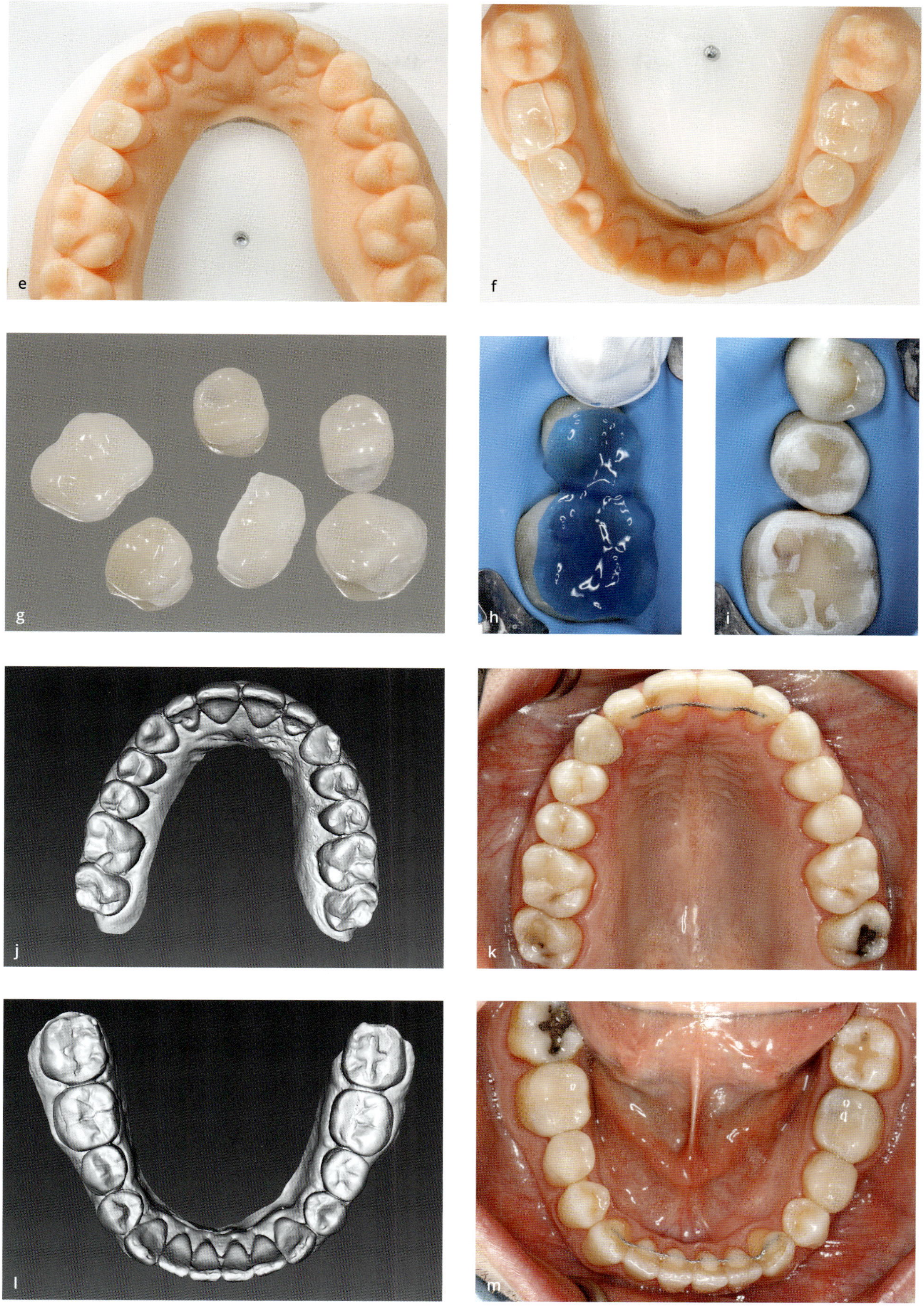
e
f
g
h
i
j
k
l
m

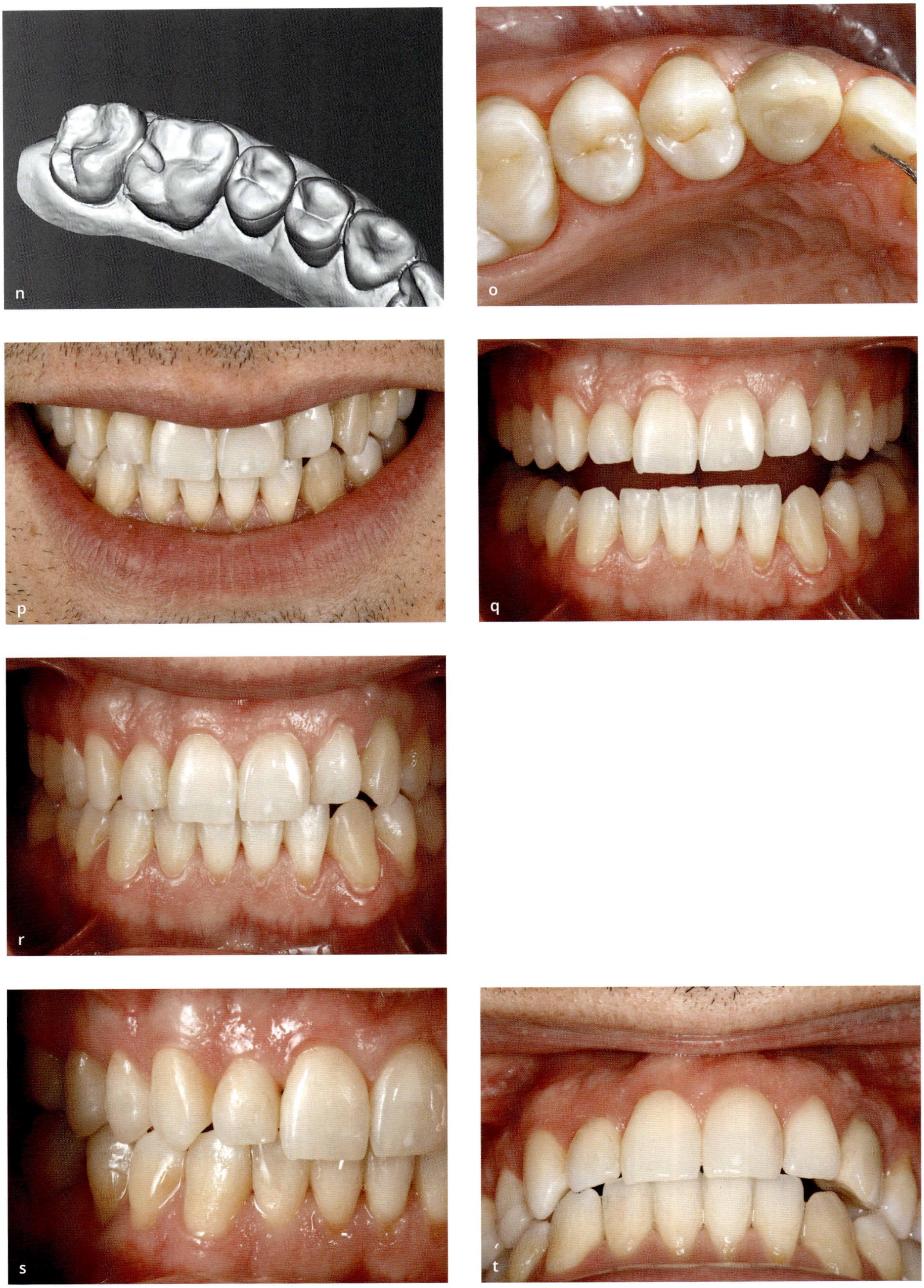


**Fig 8-6** *(continued)*

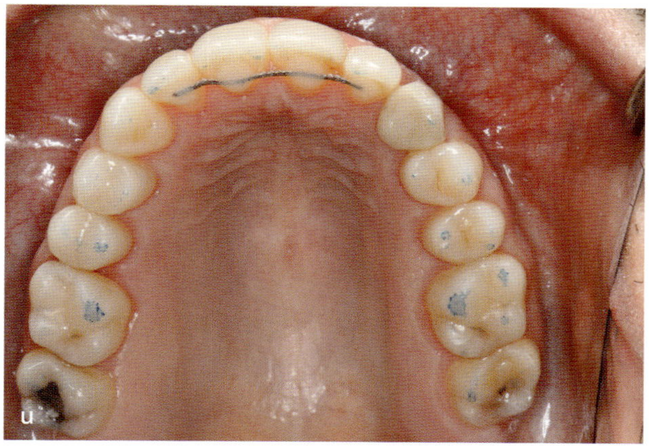
u

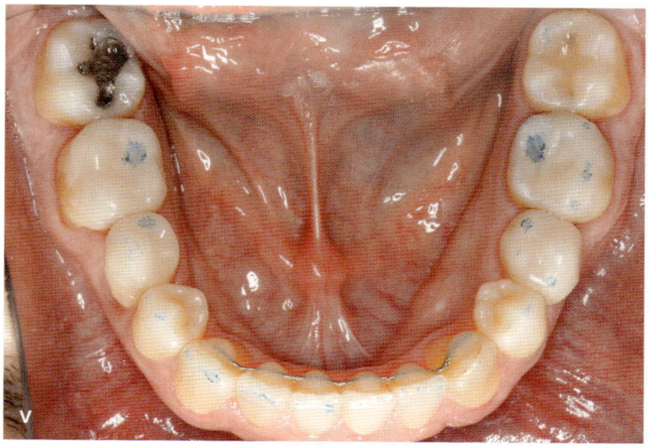
v

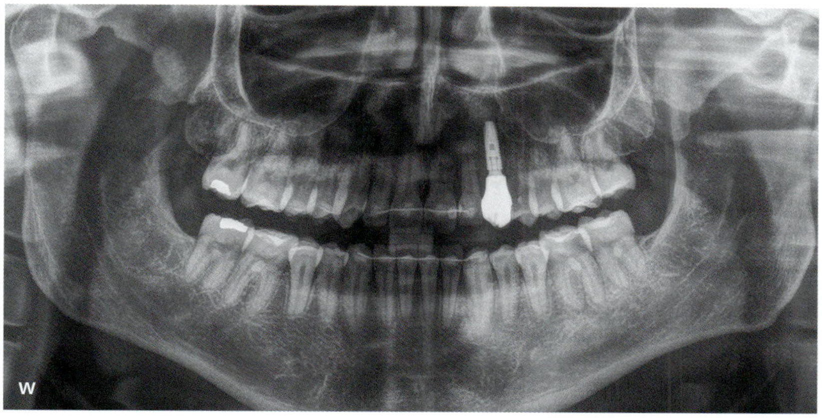
w

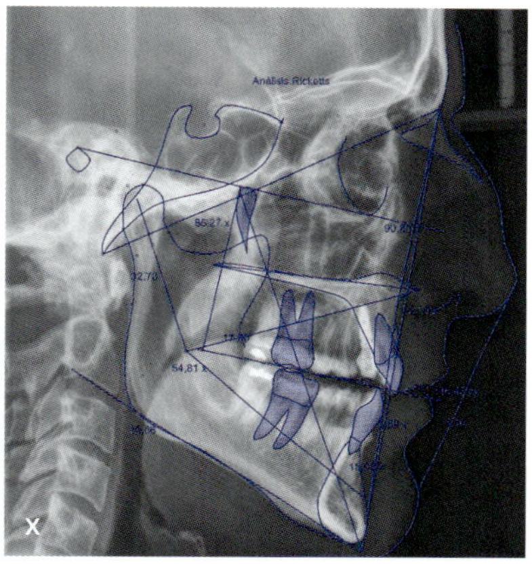
x

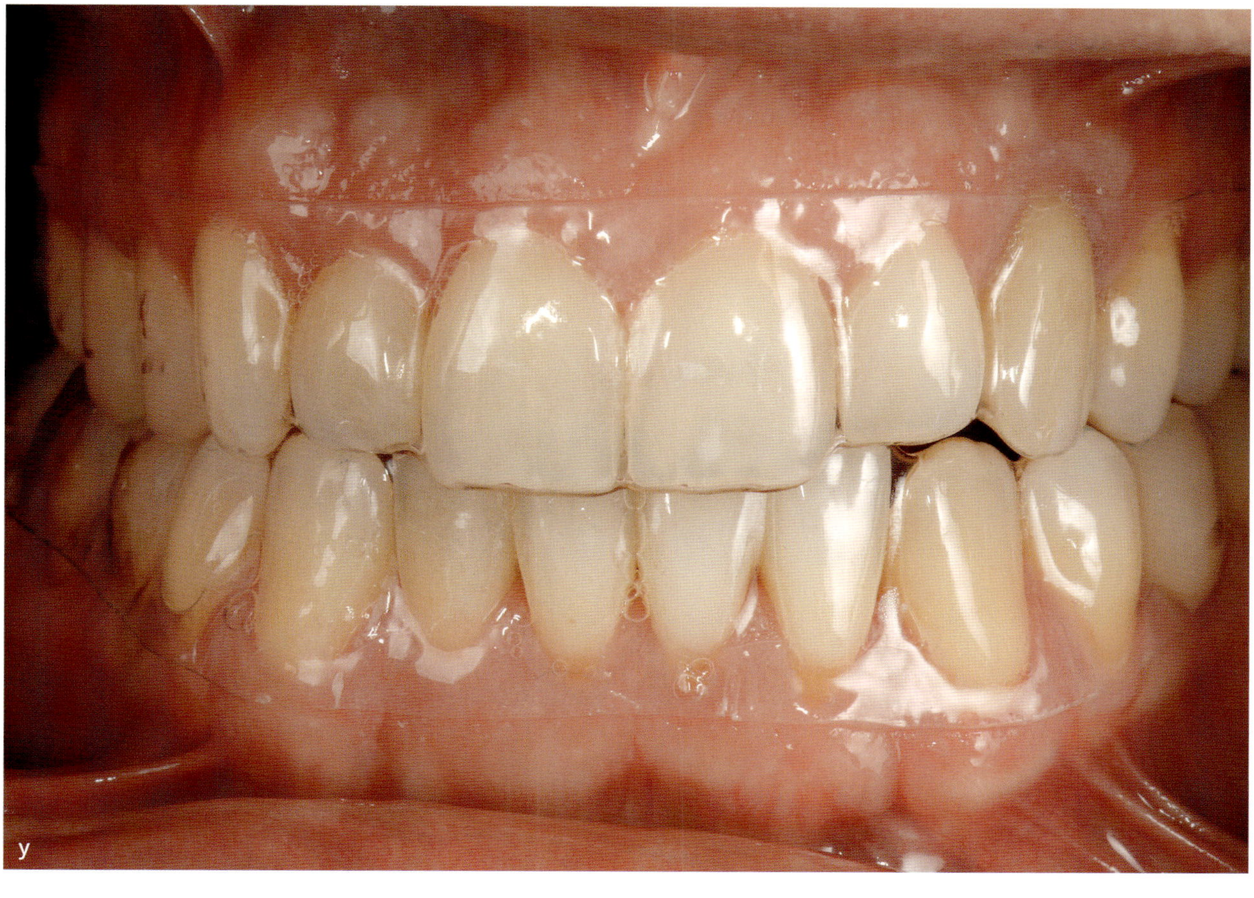
y

## 2. Orthodontics to Intercept Tooth Wear and Preserve Tooth Structure

Orthodontic therapy can cause a paradigm shift in intercepting incipient TW. There is no doubt that orthodontic evaluation is a prerequisite in cases of incipient TW.

Traditionally the absence of wear in the canine cusps in young children was regarded as problematic as the flattening of the primary dentition was thought to guide the mandible into a correct position, and hence wear of the canine cusps was desirable to achieve a correct occlusion. While this may be acceptable for the primary dentition, anatomical features such as the tips of the canines and incisal edges of the anterior teeth are key factors in the permanent dentition to protect the dentition throughout life. It now has been demonstrated that correcting the crossbite in the early dentition will help minimize future possible erosion or grinding in adult patients.[14]

Intercepting incipient TSL in malocclusions can save tooth structure and avoid the need for dental procedures that could have been considered necessary initially (Figs 8-7 and 8-8).

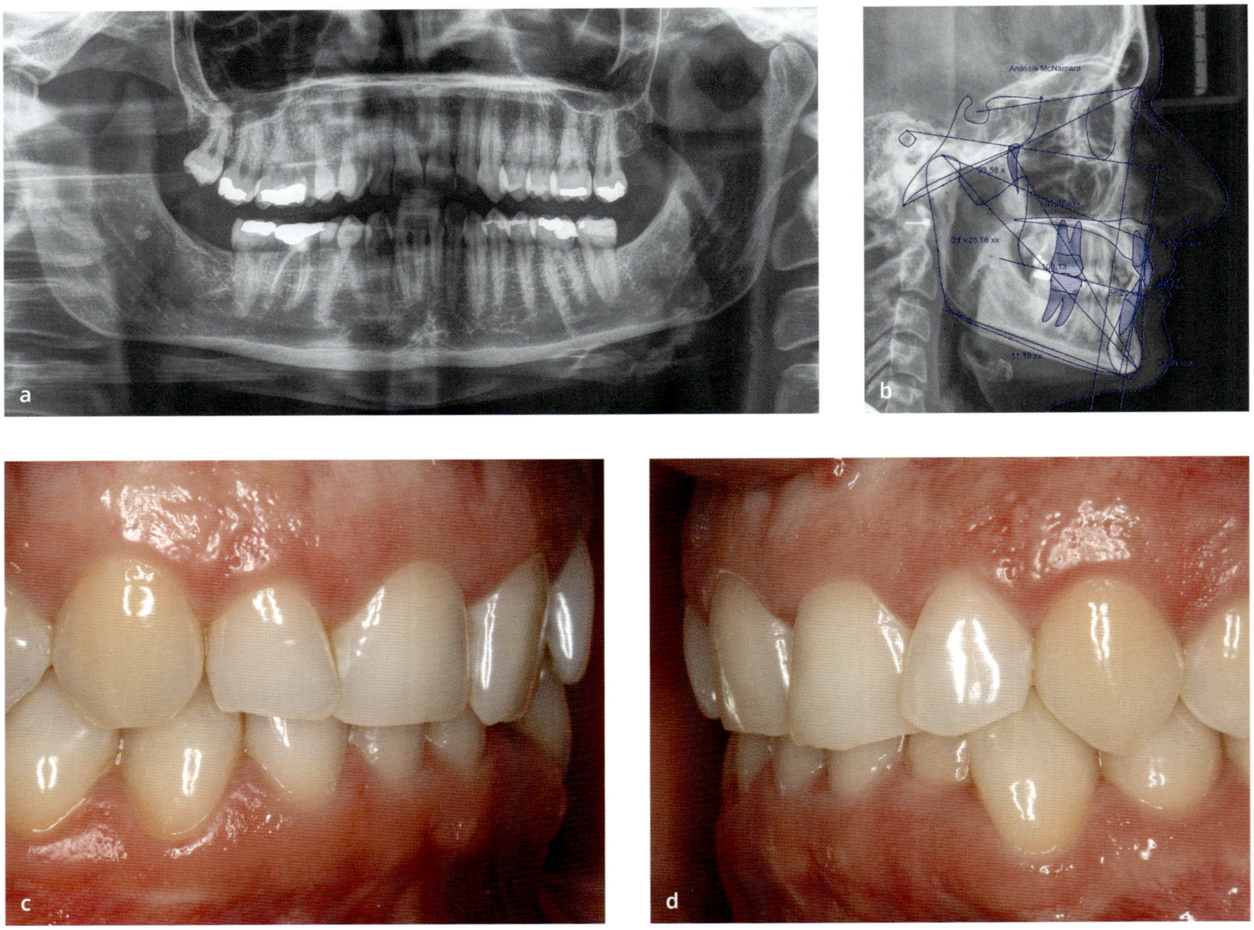

**Fig 8-7** This young woman presented to the office with the complaint that her teeth "have started to overlap and collapse." She is not conscious of her teeth wearing down and does not report any risk behavior or medical conditions. A diagnosis of incipient TW is made. The radiographic exam reveals no other findings of interest except for the disruption of the occlusal and incisal planes (a). The cephalometric analysis reveals an incorrect interincisal relationship in a normal Class I occlusion and a skeletal Class I relationship (b). The Class I compressed arches, crowding, and misalignment are behind the incipient TW that affects so far the six maxillary anterior teeth and the two mandibular central incisors (c to h).

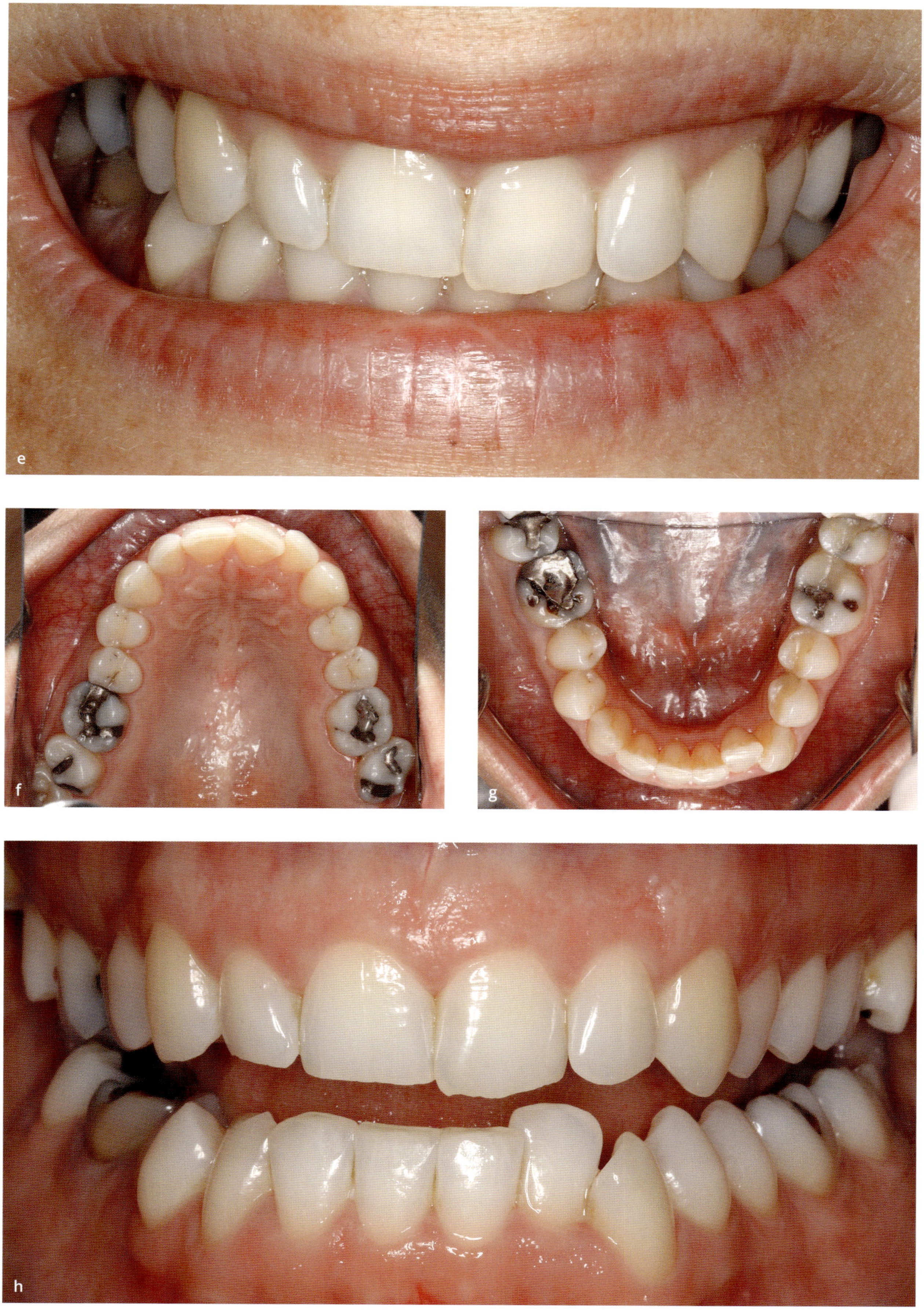

e
f
g
h

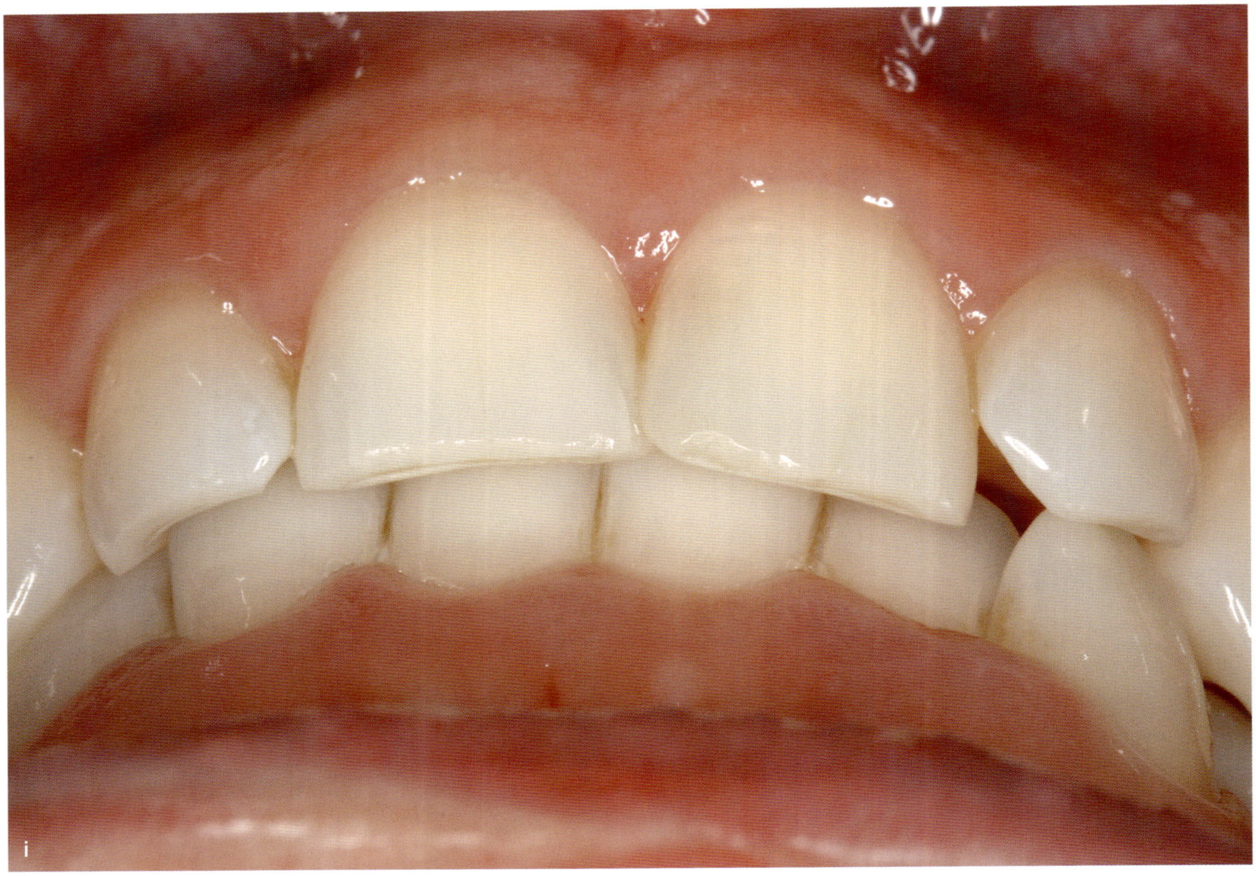

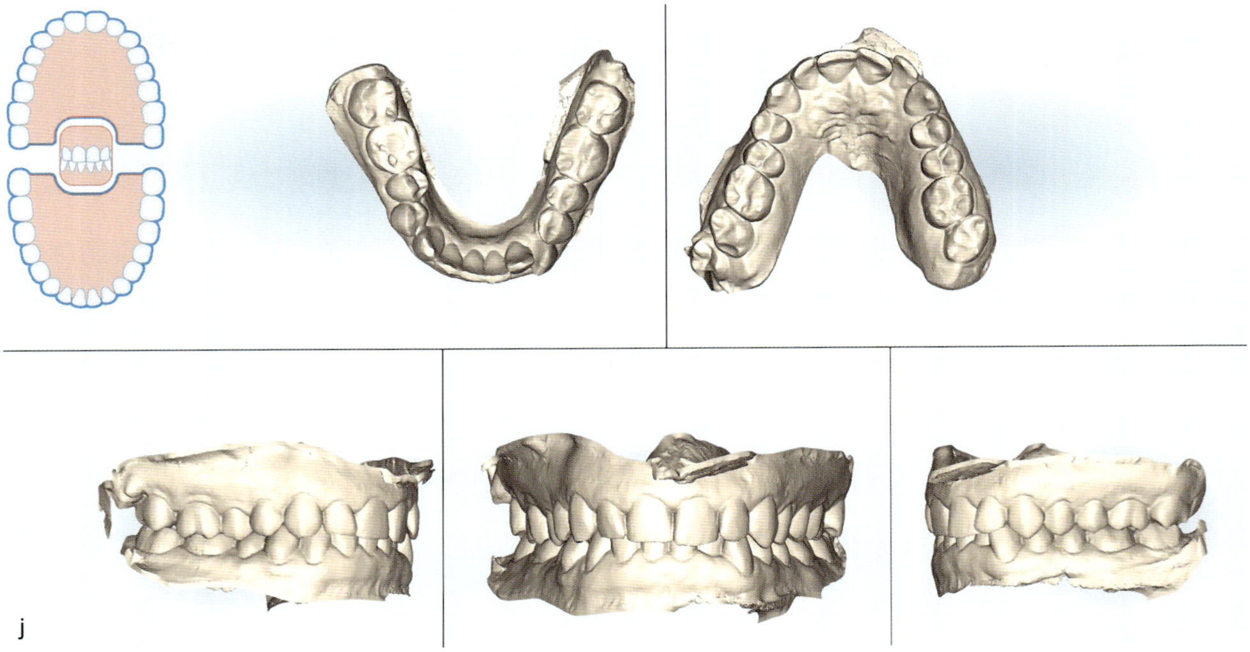

**Fig 8-7** *(continued)* The incisal compression with irregular wear relative to the incorrect relationship between the anterior teeth would make it impossible to adequately restore the worn teeth without orthodontic therapy (i). The intraoral digitalization (j) shows the above-mentioned findings and is shared with the team who plans to do the restorative treatment after the orthodontic therapy.

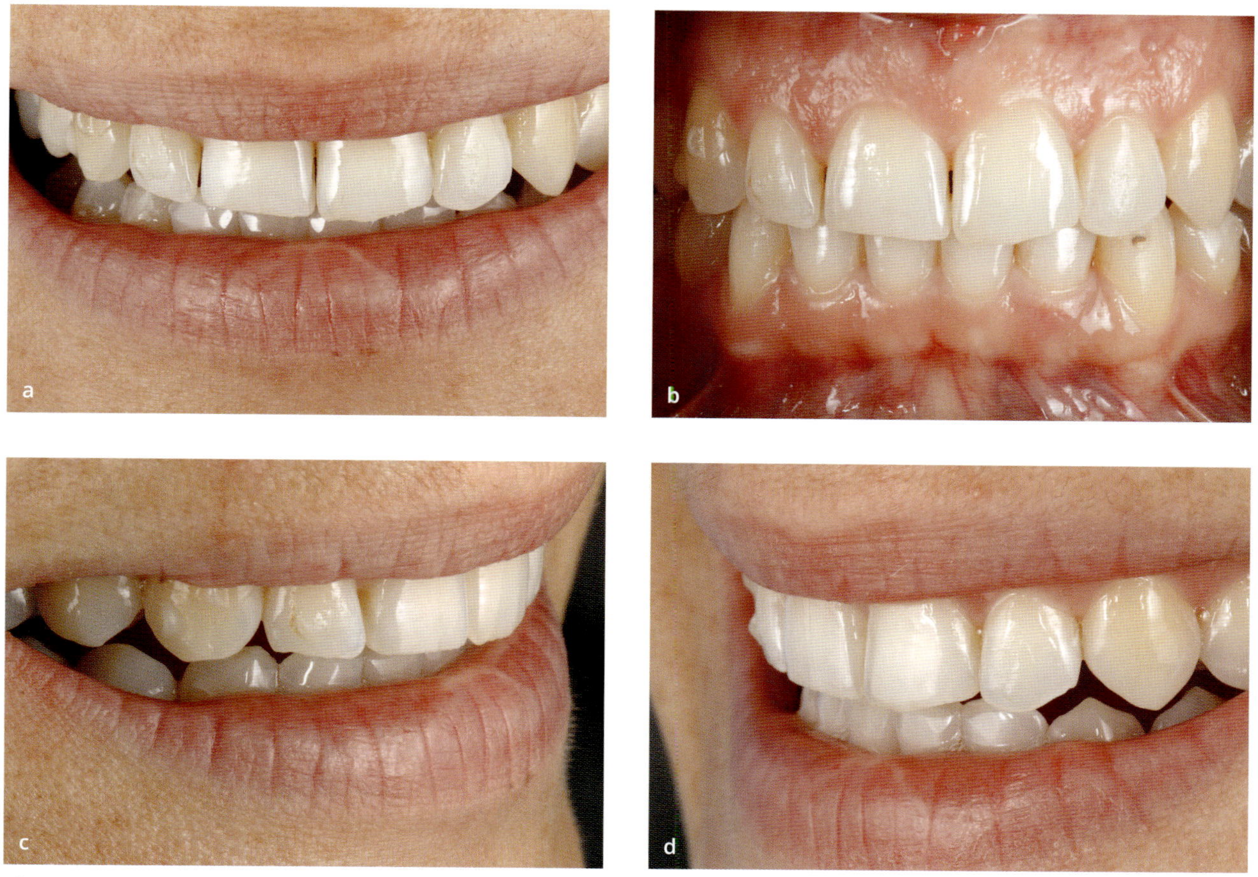

**Fig 8-8** The patient is started on a clear aligner (Invisalign) comprehensive treatment of both arches to decompress, align, and improve the anterior relationship. The slight discrepancy in width between the two lateral incisors is corrected in the digital wax-up but is not to be addressed until the end of the orthodontic treatment (a to d). *(continued next page)*

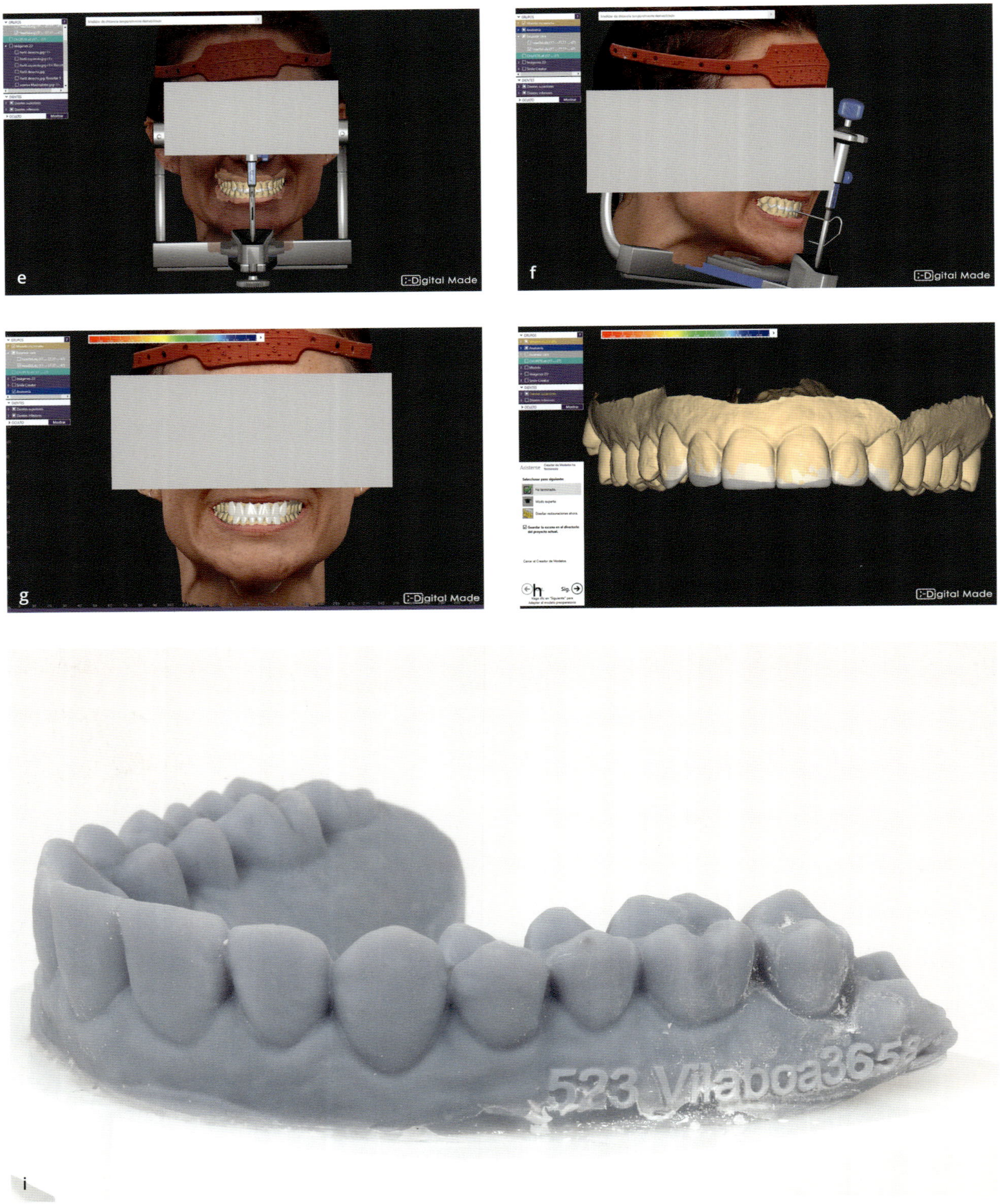

**Fig 8-8** *(continued)* A face scan is taken, and a virtual articulation of the virtual models is superimposed on a digital image of the patient's face to check all the wax-ups considering facial (e) and profile (f) views. If a face scan had been done before orthodontics, the new intraoral scan could be cross-mounted with the initial wax-up. The restorative plan is to reconstruct the worn incisal edges to rehabilitate the smile. Two wax-ups are done, and the less invasive option is chosen. The patient does not feel the need to receive porcelain laminate veneers at this stage (g and h). Instead, a printed model with the subtle incisal restorations serves as the blueprint for the restorative dentist (i).

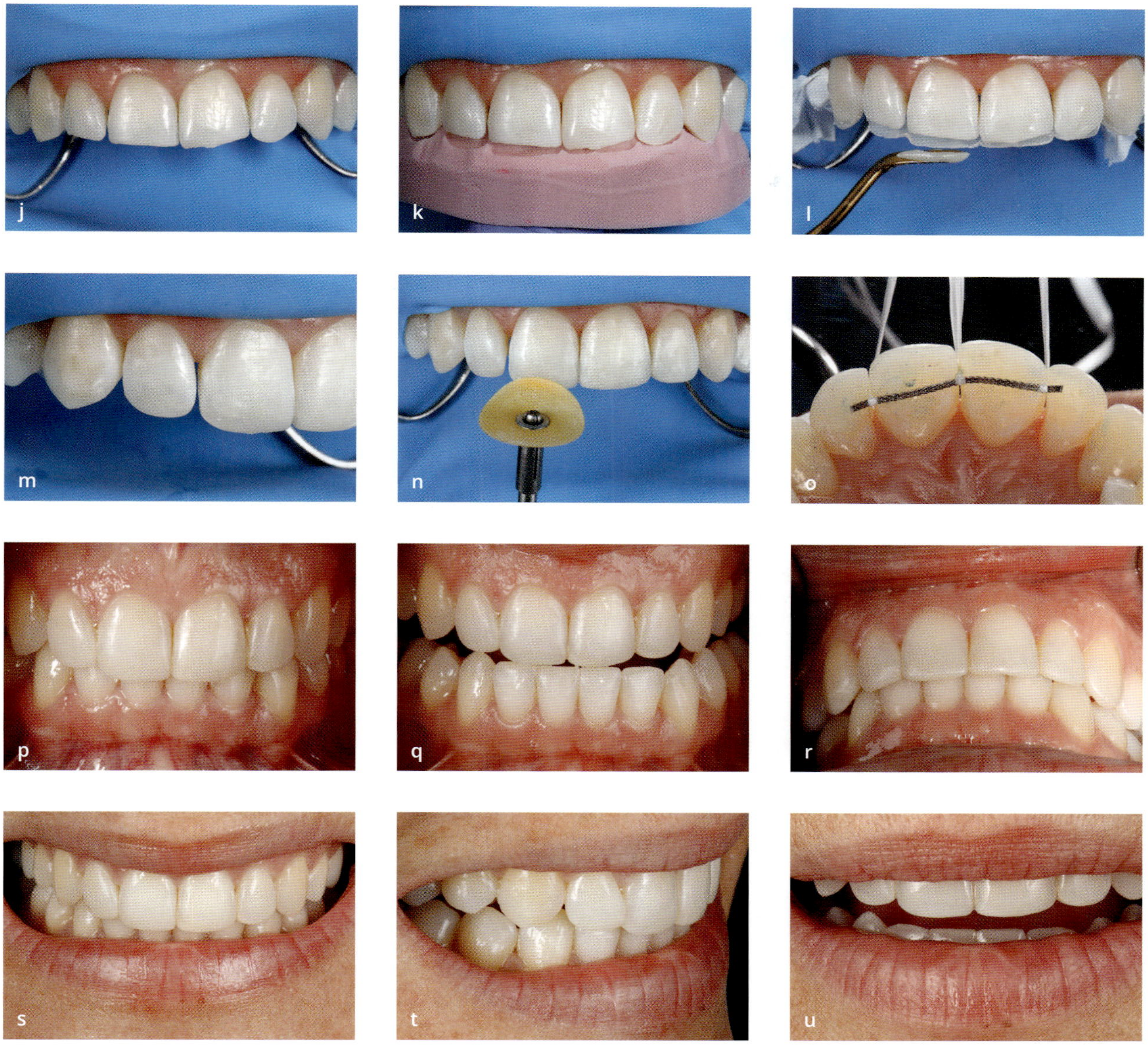

**Fig 8-8** *(continued)* The digital wax-up is the blueprint that will be copied with the aid of a silicone tray and a printed model (j and k). The restorative phase includes direct freehand composite (Inspiro, Edelweiss DR) in a semidirect protocol in the six maxillary teeth and two mandibular central incisors to restore the incipient wear and provide functional protection upon discursions (l to n). Also, the width discrepancy of the maxillary right lateral incisor will be addressed immediately before delivering the fixed retainer (o). Upon completion of the restorations (p to y), the patient is scanned intraorally and asked to come for regular checkups. *(continued next page)*

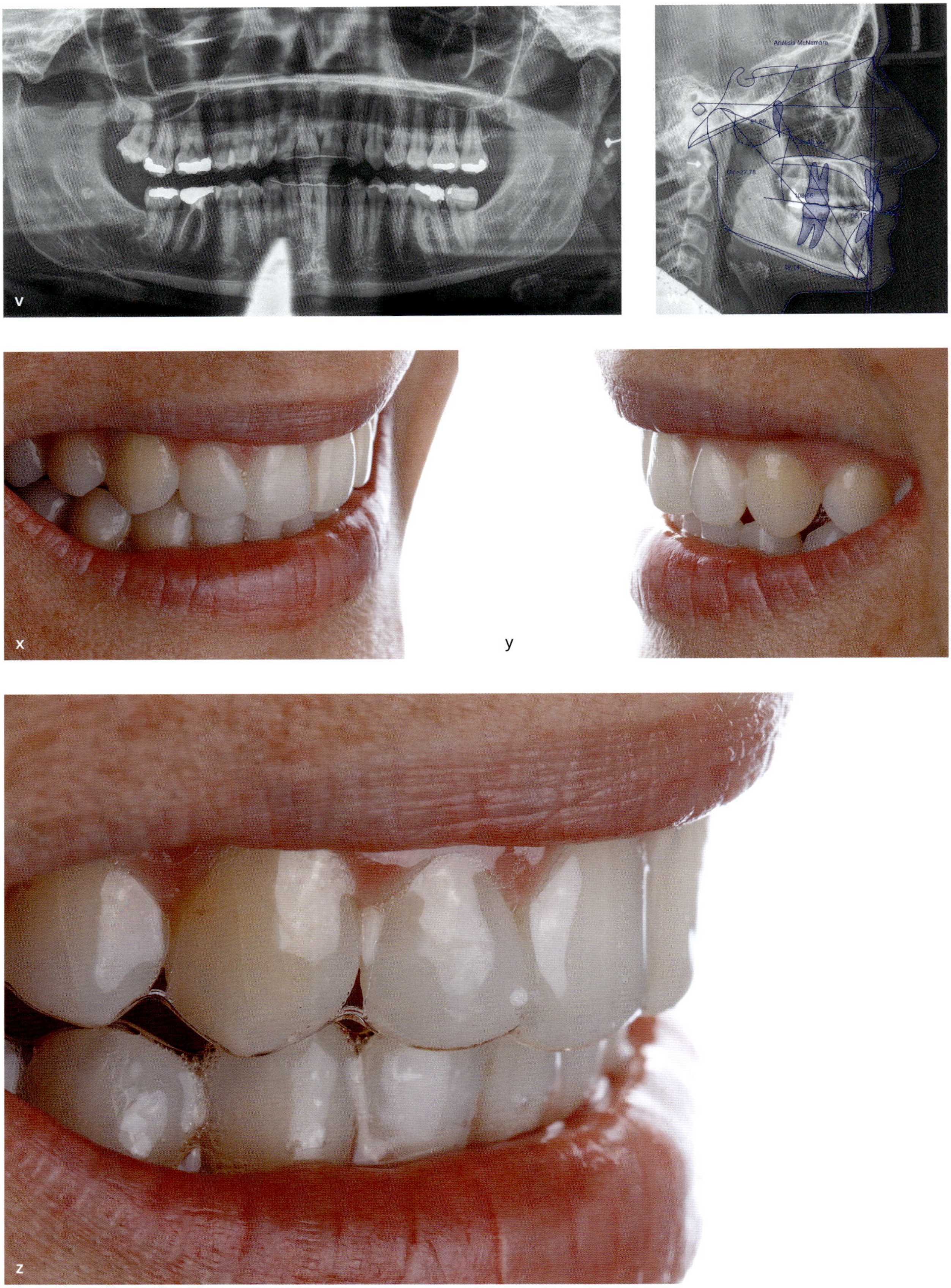

**Fig 8-8** *(continued)* The TW will be monitored with progressive scans in order to detect minor changes and prevent further wear. The patient is given a set of two transparent extra-thin splints to be worn at night and during exercise in the daytime (z).

TW has also been linked to mouth breathing caused by an obstruction of the upper airway, which can lead to bruxism and future tooth erosion, fracture, abfraction, and other lesions, as well as chronic gingival inflammation, causing periodontal disease.[15] In the presence of compressed arches in young patients with crowding, it should be investigated whether there is a concomitant compromised airway, which is an added risk factor for future TW.

There is a correlation between improvement in breathing, swallowing, speech, phonetics, and quality of life thanks to widening of the arches with orthodontic treatment, based on the expansion and improvement of the arch relationship, which will all protect tooth enamel or future restorations if needed.

There are several questions an orthodontist should address:

- Is there any limitation in the airflow through the upper airway, creating any disturbance of the maxilla or the positioning of the mandible?
- Has the patient had to compensate for the lack of proper breathing? Are there any postural, breathing, or tongue functions that have become habitual as a result?
- Are there any consequences of these compensations? Is there any physical external or facial proportion change? Are the jaws in the correct position?

Mouth breathing often courses together with compressed arches and a dolichofacial pattern. Ideally orthodontic correction should be done at a young age in order to prevent any form of TW and to improve the upper respiratory function (Figs 8-9 and 8-10).

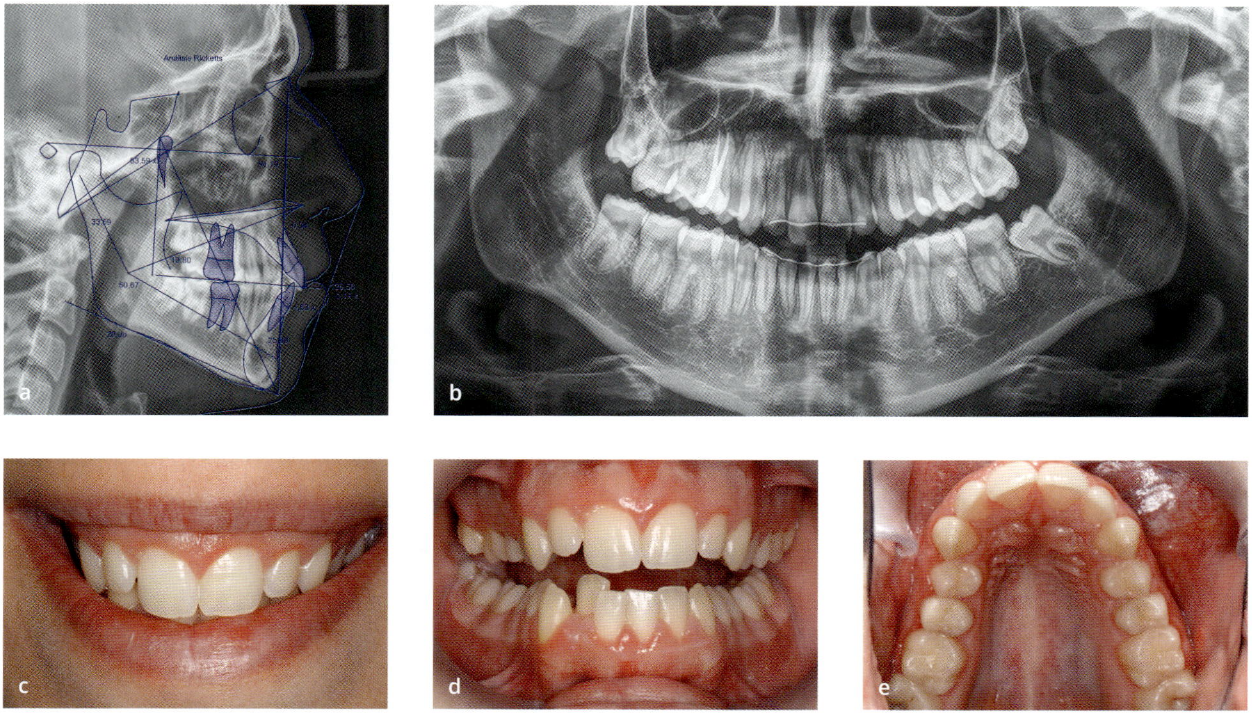

**Fig 8-9** This young patient shows no TW but complains of worsening gingivitis and reports that he has started to snore and wake up at night. A diagnosis of a dolichofacial pattern with skeletal and dental Class I relationships, severe arch compression, and severe lower crowding follows an intraoral as well as radiographic examination and intraoral scanning (a to h). *(continued next page)*

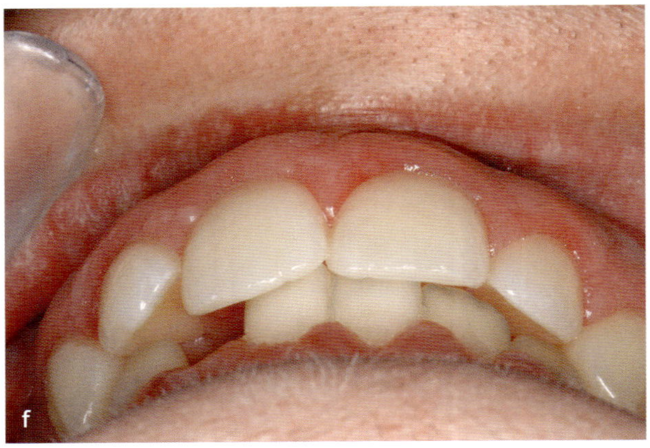


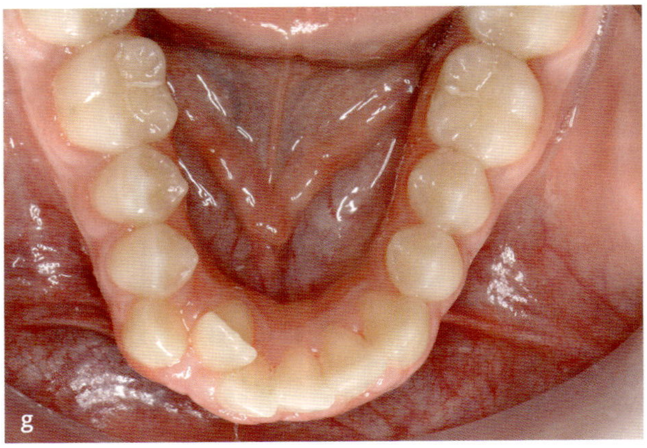


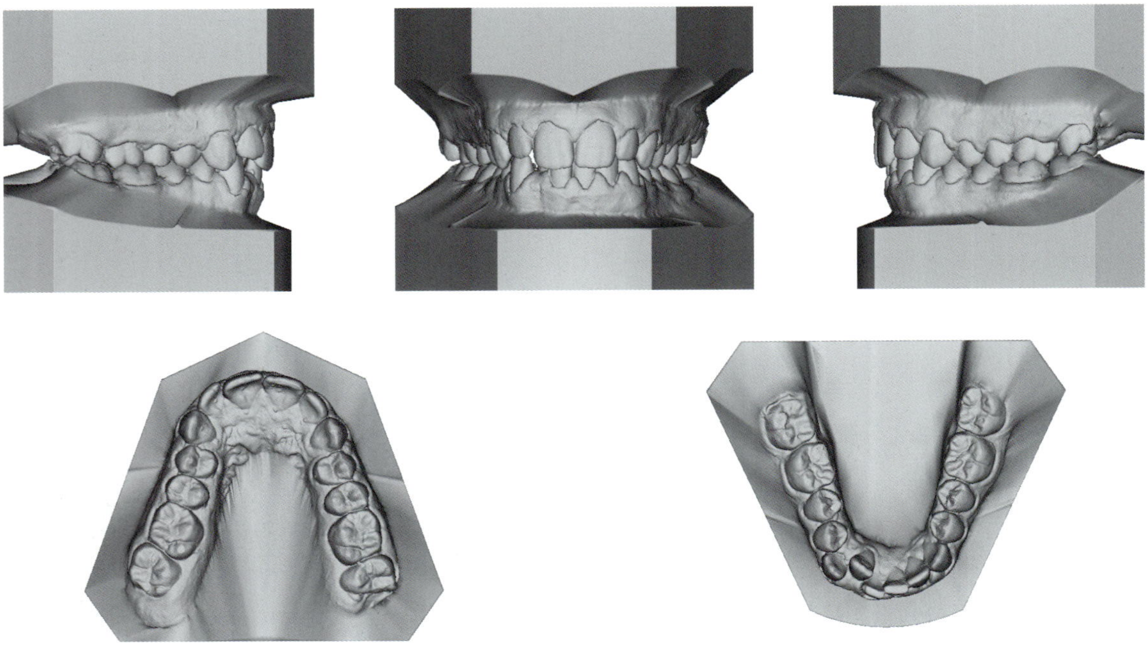

h

**Fig 8-9** *(continued)*

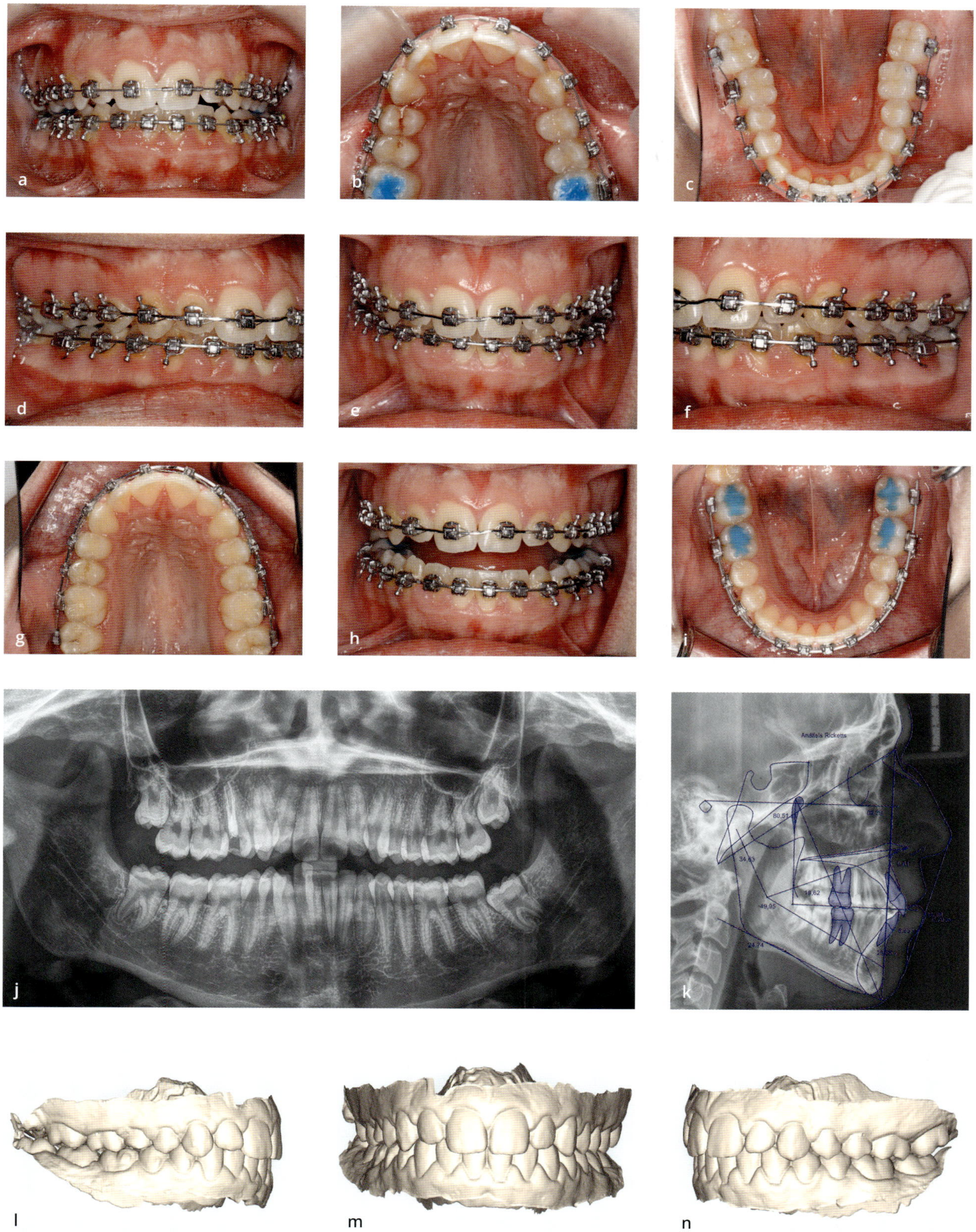

**Fig 8-10** Orthodontic therapy with a fixed orthodontic appliance is started in this case with a self-ligating bracket system and slow-force archwire using a slide mechanism that minimizes the friction and binding without the need for elastic bands, providing improved hygiene possibilities for the patient. This therapy was chosen for widening the arches by applying light, gentle forces (a to c). Gingival inflammation improved at the same pace as the arches were decompressed and the teeth aligned (d to i). The patient was intraorally scanned after the fixed appliances (Damon System, ORMCO) were removed, and the fixed retainers were delivered (j to t). *(continued next page)*

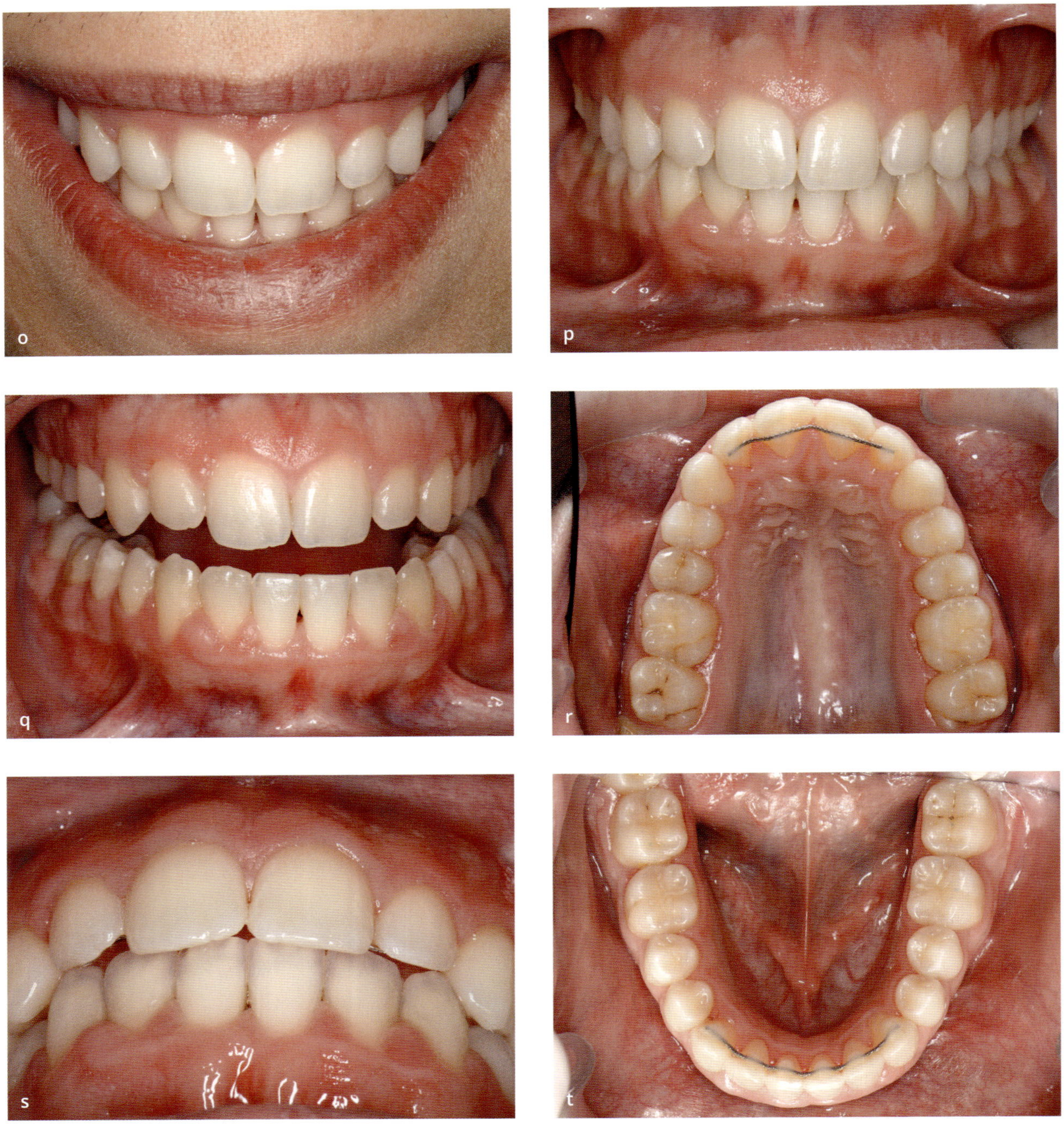


**Fig 8-10** *(continued)* The patient was given recommendations as to sleep hygiene and nutritional counseling.

# 3. Orthodontics to Provide Missing Space and Preserve Tooth Structure

It is in cases in which TW has damaged the anatomy of the teeth and altered the function of the masticatory system that orthodontic therapy needs to be used with specific objectives such as finding the space for restorations. Occlusal restorations can be delivered at the original VDO or at an augmented VDO depending on criteria for existing restorative space for both arches. The literature and clinical experience show extensive evidence on the feasibility of increasing the VDO enough to provide for restorative space in the worn dentition. If a restorative-only approach is chosen, the patient has to know that either more teeth will receive restorations at an augmented VDO, or alternatively some teeth will have to be reduced.[16] Moreover, the preventive benefits of orthodontic therapy will not be present. Choosing an orthodontic path adjunctively to the restorative path will save tooth structure and bring improvement of the occlusal scheme. In most adult cases the arches will be broadened, which will facilitate finding space for future restorations.

If orthodontics is not considered, patients with moderate to severe TW will probably require a more invasive approach. Orthodontic therapy will facilitate the restorative treatment as well as an assist in prevention management. The main goal of orthodontic therapy is to achieve an ideal maxillomandibular relationship within a healthy environment and overall facial harmony with a stable occlusion and a pleasing esthetic outcome. No efforts should be spared in obtaining an ideal mutual protective discursive pattern in which anterior teeth protect posterior teeth from lateral forces and posterior teeth safeguard anterior teeth from occlusal forces.[17]

Generally speaking, the number of adult patients who seek orthodontic treatment is currently increasing. Orthodontic treatment's main goal is to alleviate physical health problems. Adults that are treated orthodontically have shown that they are less susceptible to tooth decay, gingival disease, bone destruction, chewing and digestive difficulties, speech impairments, tooth loss, and other dental injuries.[18]

The challenges associated with the management of patients with TSL are increasing in every field in dentistry, and orthodontics is not an exception. Therefore, the treatment objectives in TW need to be considered. These are outlined in the following sections.

## Reestablishing Arch Width and Height

The TW effect on the sagittal and horizontal dimensions is such that the final dimensions of both arches in the patient with TW are narrower and flatter. In the vertical plane, a true collapse accompanies severe TW cases, calling for action from different specialties of dentistry, such as implants, prosthodontics, orthodontics, and restorative treatment. However, there is a window of opportunity for intercepting the incipient collapse of the worn dentition and thus avoiding the loss of references for anterior guidance, the occlusal plane, VDO, and facial esthetics.[16,19]

## Providing Restorative Space While Preserving Tooth Structure

### Preservation of tooth structure: The Dahl principle

The main goal of treating patients from an orthodontic point of view is to prevent tooth structure loss, as it was first presented in the Dahl concept traditionally associated with the management of worn teeth. The Dahl principle and Dahl appliance were first introduced to solve the situation caused by the lack of space in the anterior sector due to overeruption of the anterior segment (Class II, division 2 malocclusion) or due to compensatory eruption subsequent to tooth structure loss in the anterior sector (TW from intrinsic erosive attack). Originally described as a metal bite platform, the Dahl appliance created space where apparently no interocclusal height existed, provided this happened in a sector of the mouth.[19-22]

Traditionally thought to use the benefit of tooth axial intrusion movement consequent to either a removable appliance or fixed restorations placed in supraocclusion, it was accompanied by extrusion movements of the rest of the dentition. In principle, this can solve sectorial space problems in patients in whom compensatory eruption has used up all the space generated after the loss of TSL. The Dahl appliance, used for the management of interocclusal space loss subsequent to dentoalveolar compensation, alleviated the paradox of the restorative dentist wanting to protect teeth from TW but finding no other solution than reducing tooth structure to place a restoration in a conventional prosthodontic approach. At the same time as enabling the future restorations, this approach, which is still used today, has a secondary benefit of improving the outcome of the future restorations.[23]

However, the drawbacks are the limitations and contraindications of these techniques, together with the fact that they are technique-sensitive and their orthodontic outcomes are not fully predictable. Among the limitations is the fact that preexisting restorations with interfaces in the cementoenamel junction (CEJ) and implant-retained crowns cannot be intruded or extruded. Extruding a full quadrant, or even more four quadrants, in order to properly restore the anterior dentition is not practical as intrusion of the molars and premolars should be anticipated once the completed restorations are in occlusion.

### Expansion of the maxillary bones

This can only be done in the young dentition. In the adult dentition, a subsidiary broadening of the arches can be done by coronobuccal inclination of all or most of the teeth in the arch. Correction of malocclusions in adult and young patients is considerably different. In adults, correcting a skeletal anomaly can involve surgery or, on the other side of the scale, dental camouflage. In contrast to treatment of young or adolescent patients, growth modification appliances are not placed in adults. The movement that can be achieved in adults is purely dentoalveolar and is achieved by giving these teeth a different torque or inclination. Mild forces should be applied for optimal dental response. By doing this, supplementary space is gained that will serve the purpose of restoring without reducing tooth anatomy in TW patients who need a multiple restoration approach. As previously mentioned, this will help to improve function, facial esthetics, and psychologic confidence in adult patients.

### Improving overjet and overbite

The orthodontist will help to improve overjet and overbite in a minimally invasive manner. A special difficulty arises when there is erosive damage that has affected the palatal or incisal aspect of maxillary teeth. In this case, the orthodontist may also find space for additive restorations wherever needed. Modern orthodontics, digital dentistry, and digital/analog combined workflows help retain tooth structure and at the same time provide an ideal occlusal scheme (Figs 8-11 and 8-12).

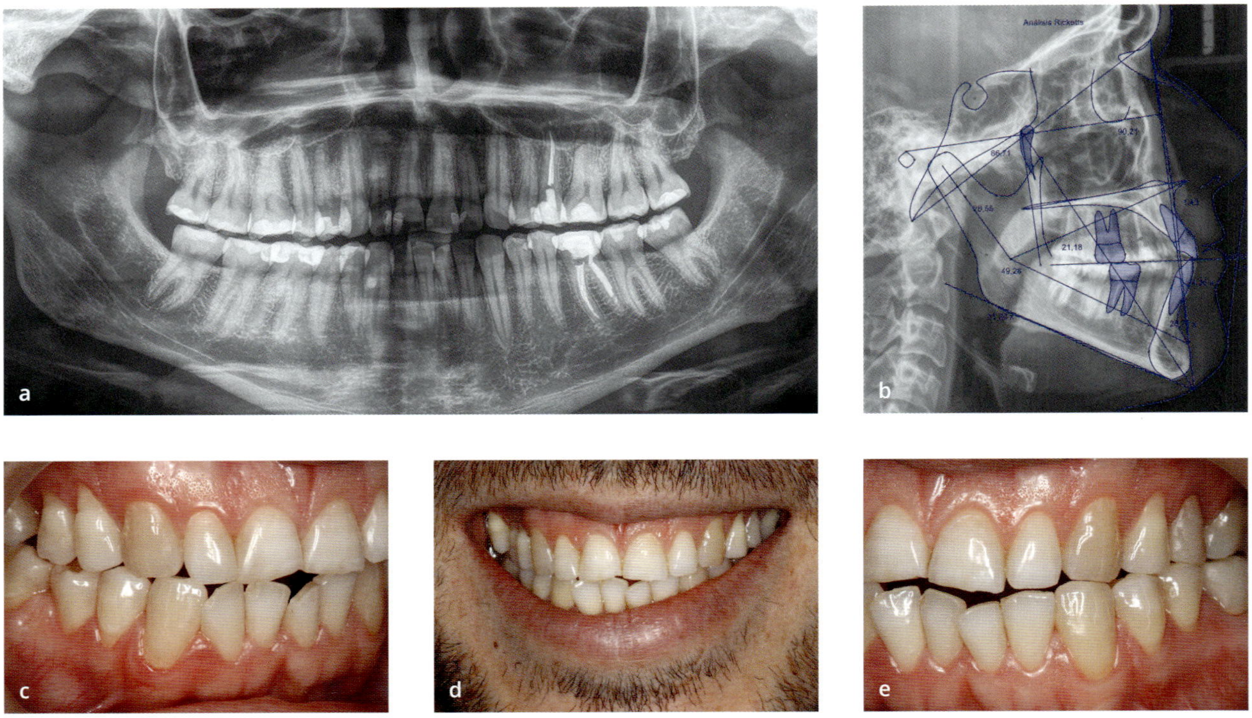

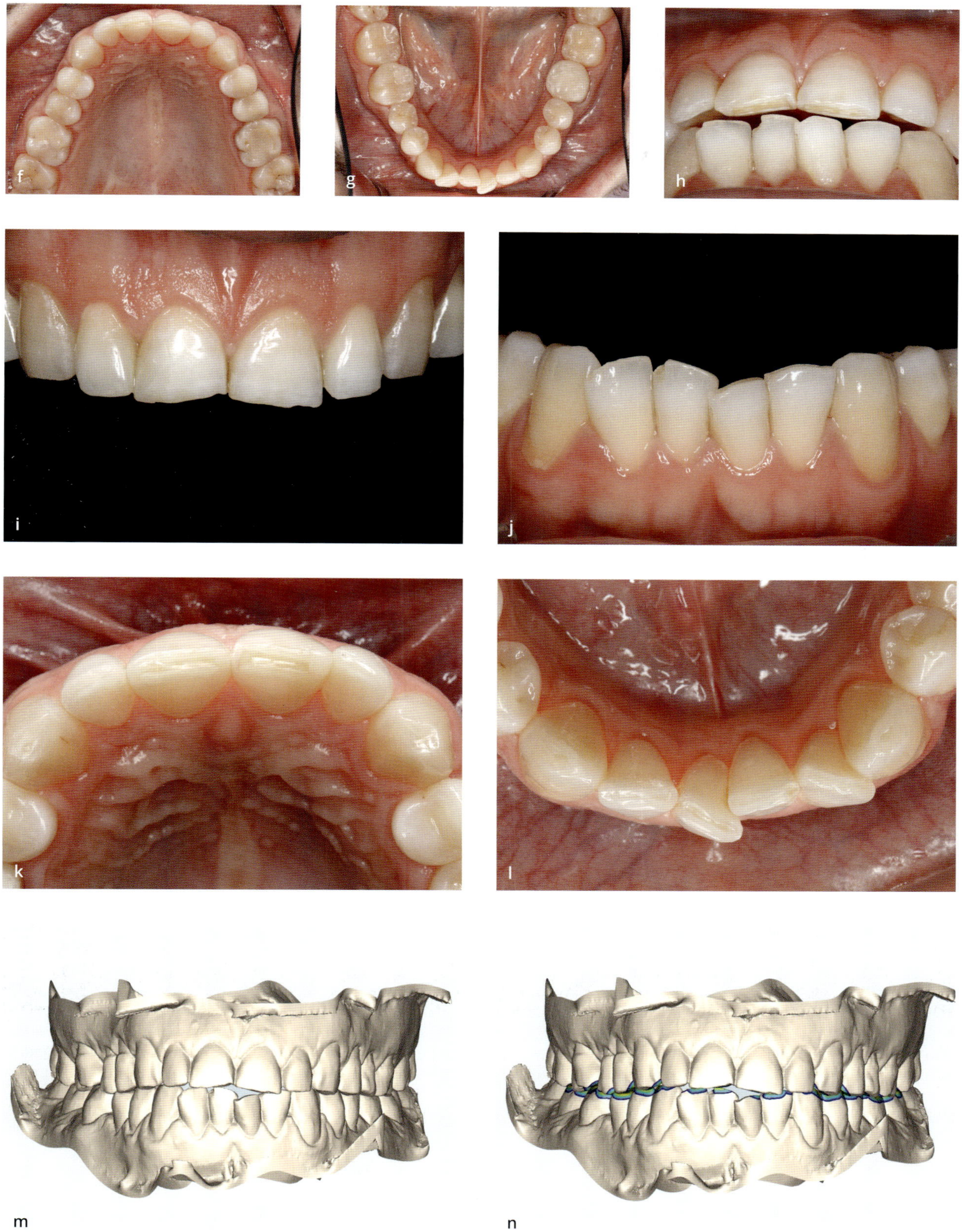


**Fig 8-11** Today's trend is for an esthetically driven orthodontic approach when treating adults. This vision, once possible only in the mind of the treatment director, now can be shared by all members of the team thanks to a digital work flow (a to n).

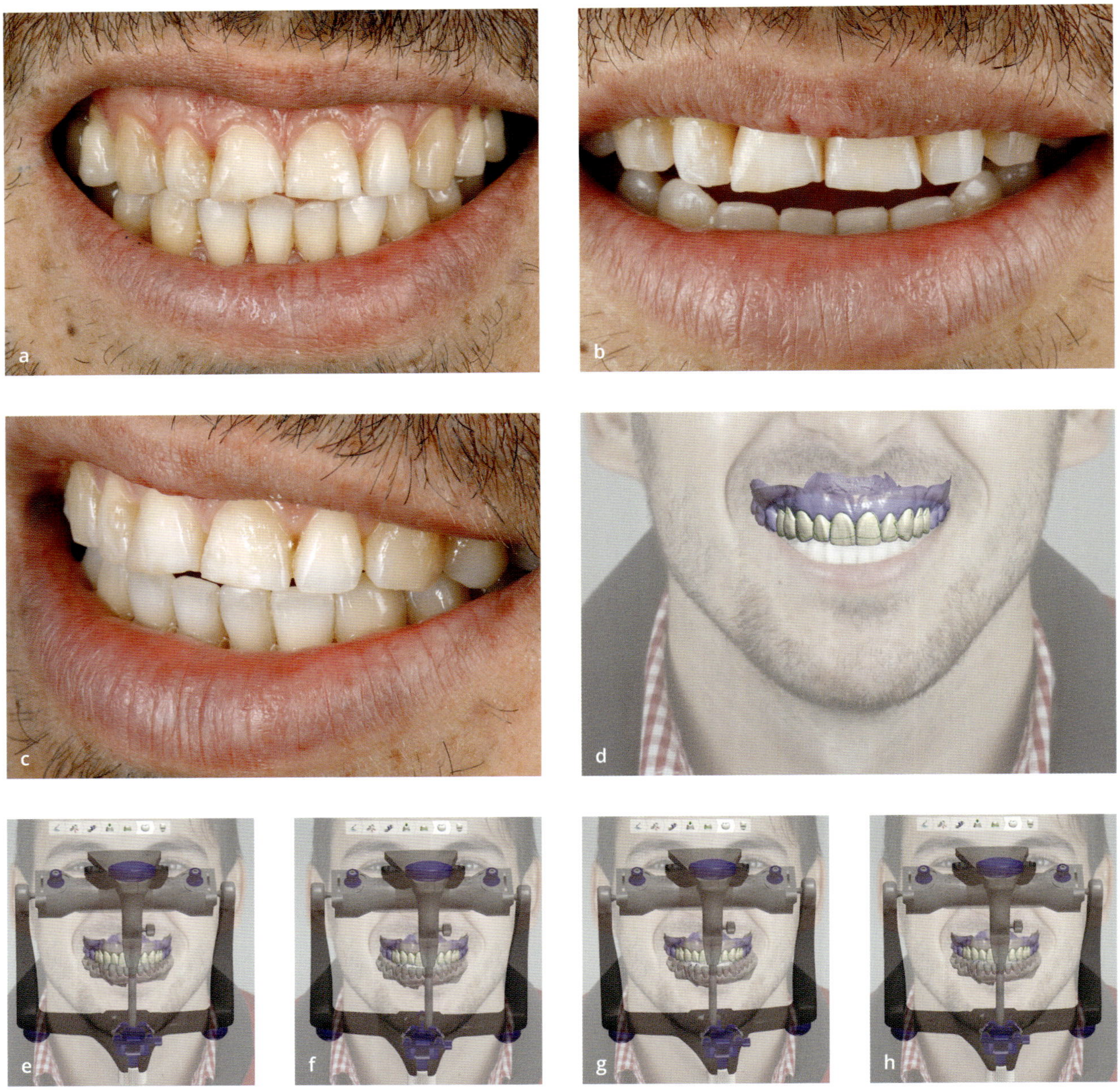

**Fig 8-12** Facial analysis, static and dynamic, with evaluation of incisal exposure in resting and smile positions, should be included in the ideal restoration, which should be respectful of the occlusal pattern that is thought to best protect the patient's teeth from future wear (a to c). In this case, the esthetic evaluation is followed by a digital functional dynamic evaluation (d to i). It is decided to restore the worn four maxillary incisors and two canines with PLV with a minimal preparation, for which a mock-up-guided tooth preparation is followed by a digital impression (j to o). This approach can be used in combination with direct freehand composites, which may be considered a better option for mandibular incisors that otherwise would require more tooth reduction or extension of the PLV to more posterior teeth to enable good integration (p to r).

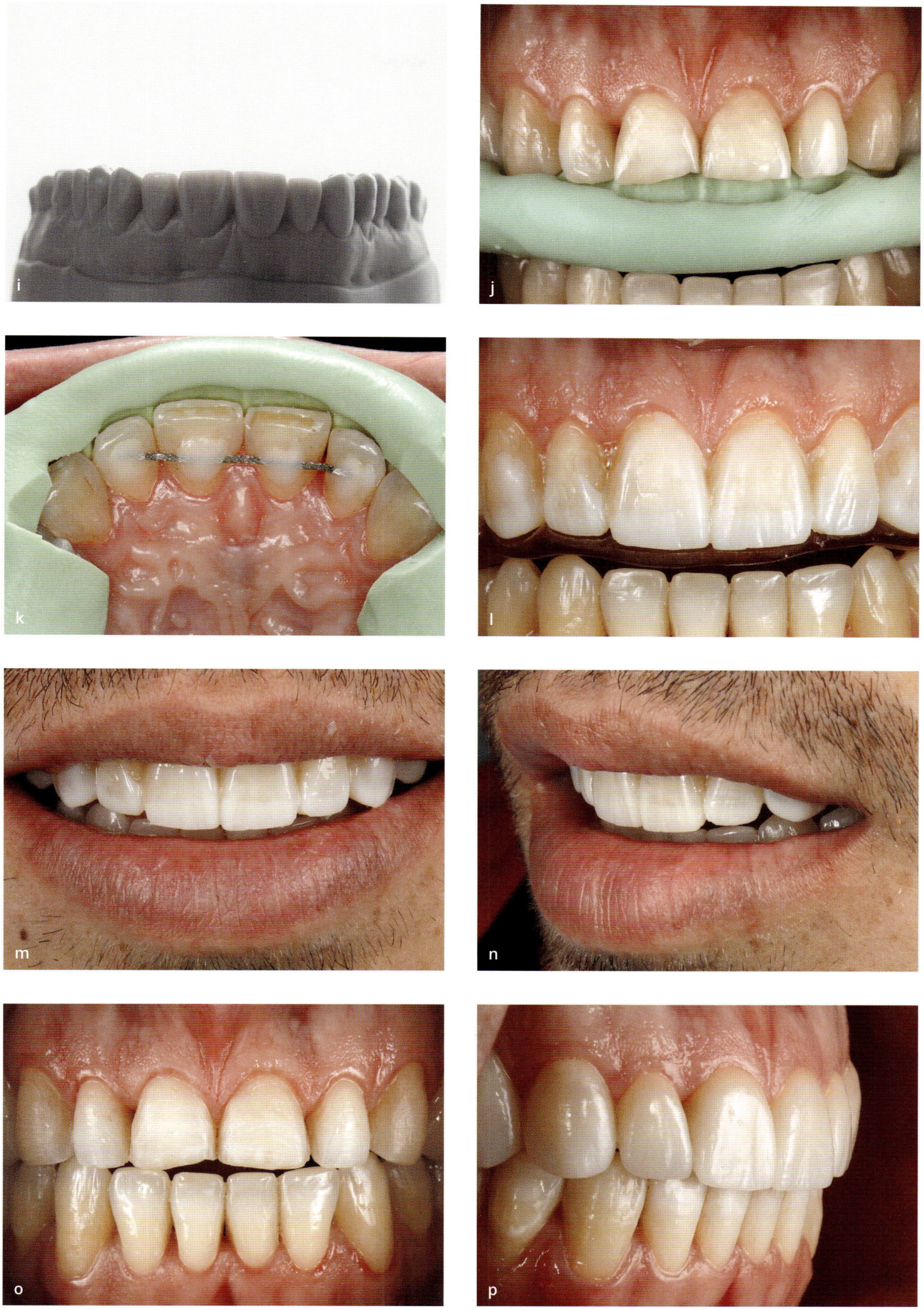

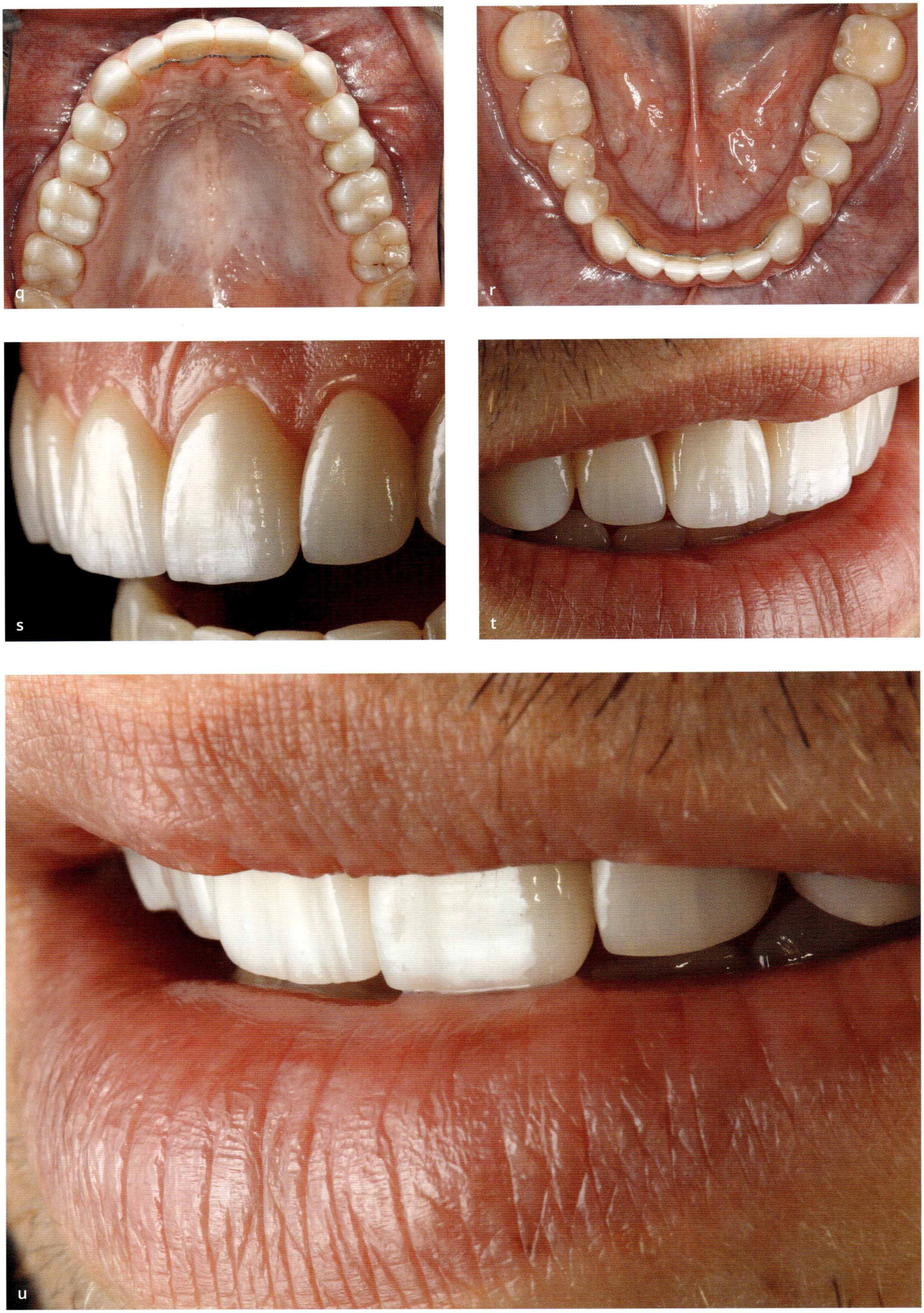
q
r
s
t
u

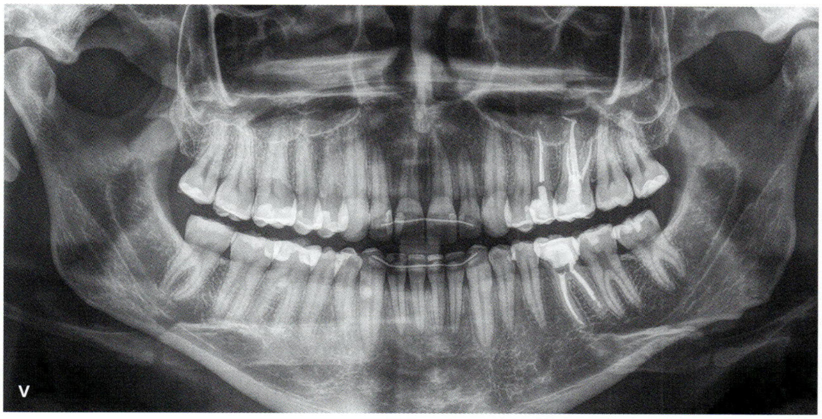


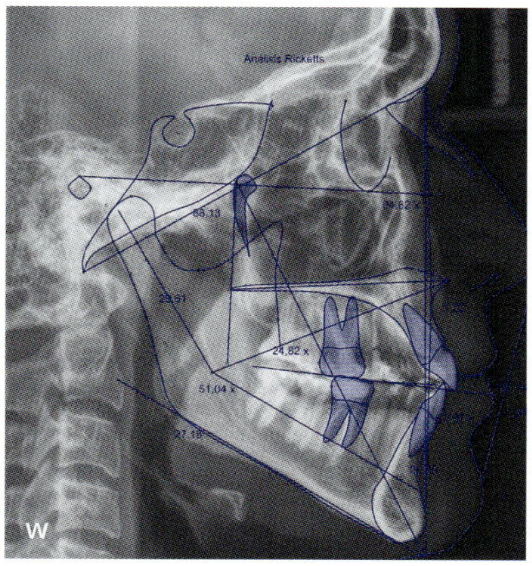


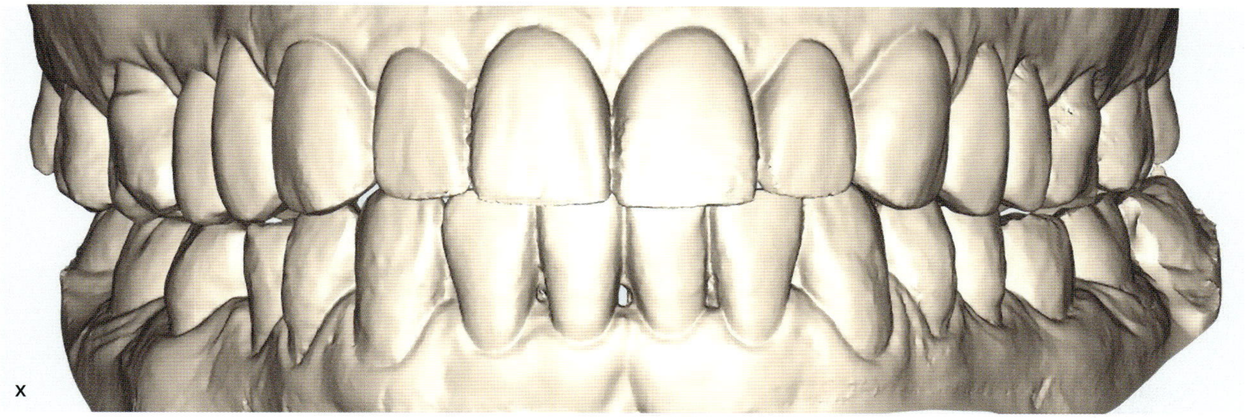


**Fig 8-12** *(continued)* The canine guidance is insufficient as a result of TW, and alternatively the restoration of the tips of the canin es can be done with freehand composite. This restoration can be retouched chairside any time wear is detected. Some patients have high esthetic demands, and the dentist might choose to combine direct composite and porcelain laminate veneers. In such a case, the esthetic evaluation and the reconstruction should be done first, followed by a functional dynamic evaluation in vivo along with the restoration of the tips of the canines to fulfill the canine guidance in the selected occlusal scheme (s to u). The final situation shows a more coherent occlusal curve and a better interincisal relationship as a result of the orthodontic and restorative combined treatments (v and w). The STL of the finished restoration is used for mouthguard fabrication and a prevention and monitoring program (x). Regular checkups and coaching are implemented in agreement with the patient as part of the TW follow-up (y). *(continued next page)*

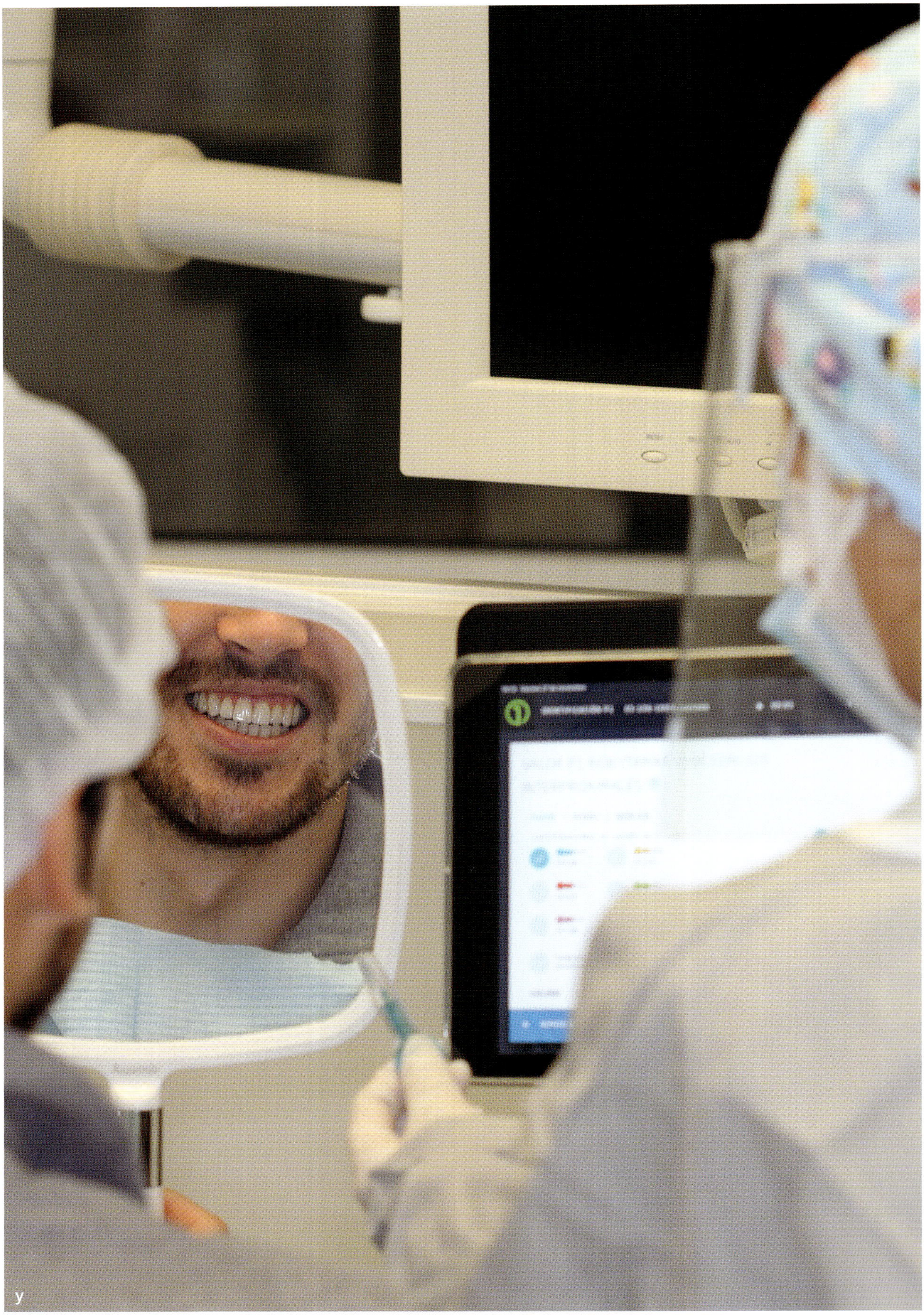
y

## 4. Communication: A Key Player in the Tooth Wear Outcome

Communication is the heart of medicine; it is indispensable. This refers to communication not only with our patients but also within our team. This is an important aspect in the delivery of high-quality health care. The orthodontist is one of the first dental professionals to see a patient and has traditionally developed certain abilities to communicate with the patient and educate them about their findings and the different possibilities available to address the orthodontic condition.

In fact, most complaints from patients are not related to clinical competency but to issues of communication that may break down trust in the doctor-patient relationship. However, many doctors tend to overestimate their ability to communicate even though they have not been trained in that field (Fig 8-13).

Furthermore, effective dentist-patient communication is indispensable in order to build the required mutual confidence that will best serve the patient's outcome and experience as well as the specialist's satisfaction. Dynamic bidirectional communication, described as "collaborative communication," will facilitate the patient's understanding.

On many occasions TW patients may not well understand the benefit of an orthodontic treatment prior to the restorative or the needed PPP (personalized preventive program) in order to minimize the risk of TW and erosion during orthodontics. The ability of the TW team to clearly communicate with patients will facilitate their understanding of the purpose of such care.

It has been proven that good communication inspires patients to feel respect for and confidence in the clinician, which will create a better treatment environment.[24] Interestingly, it has been proven that medical professionals who have better communication skills have a greater opportunity to provide less invasive treatments and also to intercept problems sooner while assuring stronger patient compliance.[25] In this sense, digital tools enable efficient transmission of data between several parties without the need for a synchronized connection between the members of the team involved. This allows modifications by multiple members, which may be a source of education and a better treatment outcome (Fig 8-14).

It is only logical that given the rising prevalence of TW in young patients it could well happen that the orthodontist is the first one to detect signs and symptoms of TW and/or a latent ED. Communication with the patient or patient's family is essential. In fact, several case studies have shown the precipitating role of fixed orthodontics in weight loss and the onset of EDs.[26] Moreover, patients with bulimia nervosa (BN) suffer from dental erosion that can be increased when fixed orthodontics appliances are started in a young population.[27] The orthodontist should suggest consultations with the general practitioner, family dentist, psychologists, and other relevant health care providers and be part of the monitoring and PPP for the TW patient, ideally being part of the TW team.

The term *self-esteem* is used to describe a person's overall sense of self-worth or personal value. There has been an increasing acceptance of the positive relationship between improvement in esthetics and an individual's psychologic profile.[24,28]

Orthodontically patients are classified following an anatomical, radiographic, mathematical, and metric analysis as Class I, Class II, Class III, and variations thereof. However, TW patients remain a true challenge, requiring discussions and agreements with the restorative team and the patient. The failure to anticipate the extent and type of restorations to be performed might condemn the prosthodontic-restorative team to sacrificing much more tooth structure than desired.[19]

Clinical experience shows that when the protocol described in this chapter is followed, tooth structure is saved, as a more additive approach will be easily implemented in the new occlusal arch upon finalization of orthodontic treatment. Implementing this protocol has been shown to minimize the number and extension of the restorative procedures, at least in some areas of the mouth, reducing the risk of failure and increasing the longevity of the teeth.

The orthodontist holds the most unique and influential position of any dental provider. Restorative teams with the vocation to treat TW patients would highly benefit from a close relationship with an orthodontic specialist, who can surely offer various paths. However, not every dental team has an orthodontist on hand. In such cases, the rapid communication tools available today should be used for the benefit of the patient and the TW team.[29]

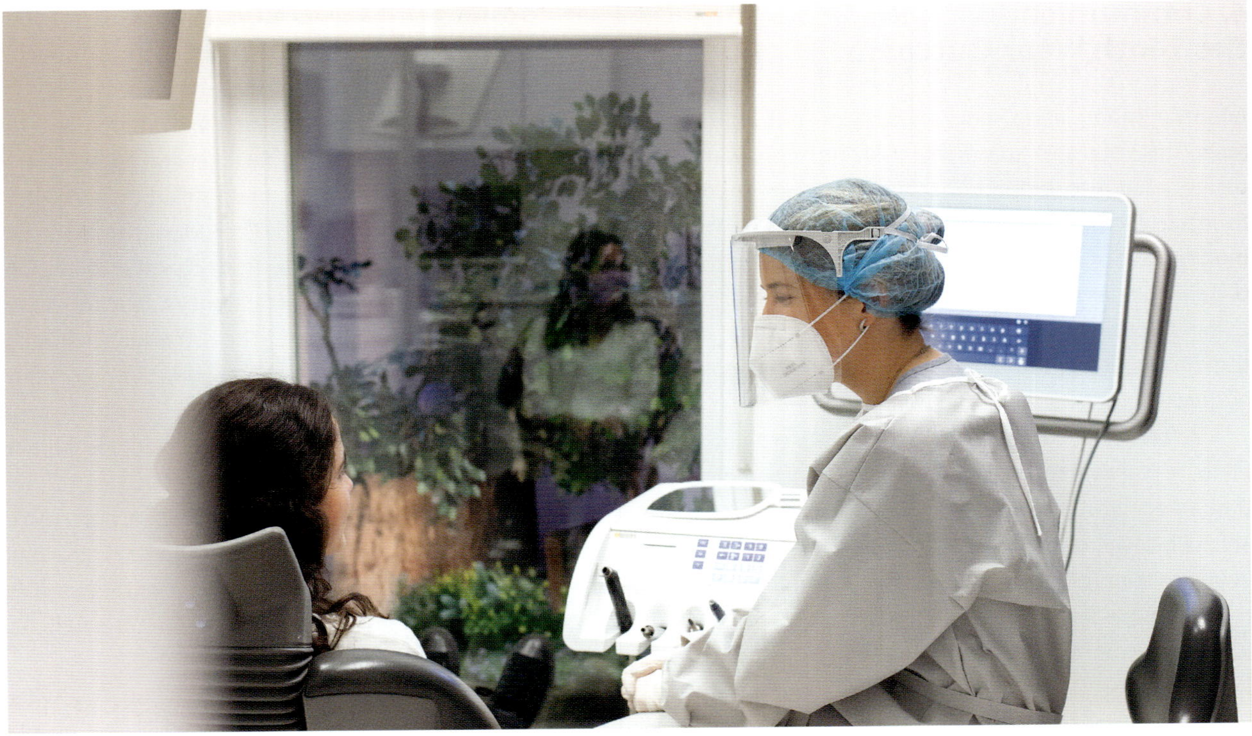

**Fig 8-13** Malocclusion often may be quite noticeable and therefore might lead to adverse social reactions and lowered self-esteem. Correction of malocclusion has been shown to improve not only dental but also facial features and body image. In addition, there are several key motives for seeking orthodontic treatment, such as social and psychologic effects. Oral health–related quality of life can be considered a useful supplementary measurement for orthodontic diagnosis and also treatment outcome. Similar to what happens after restoring a worn dentition, it should be presented to the patient as a means to improve not only oral but also general health.

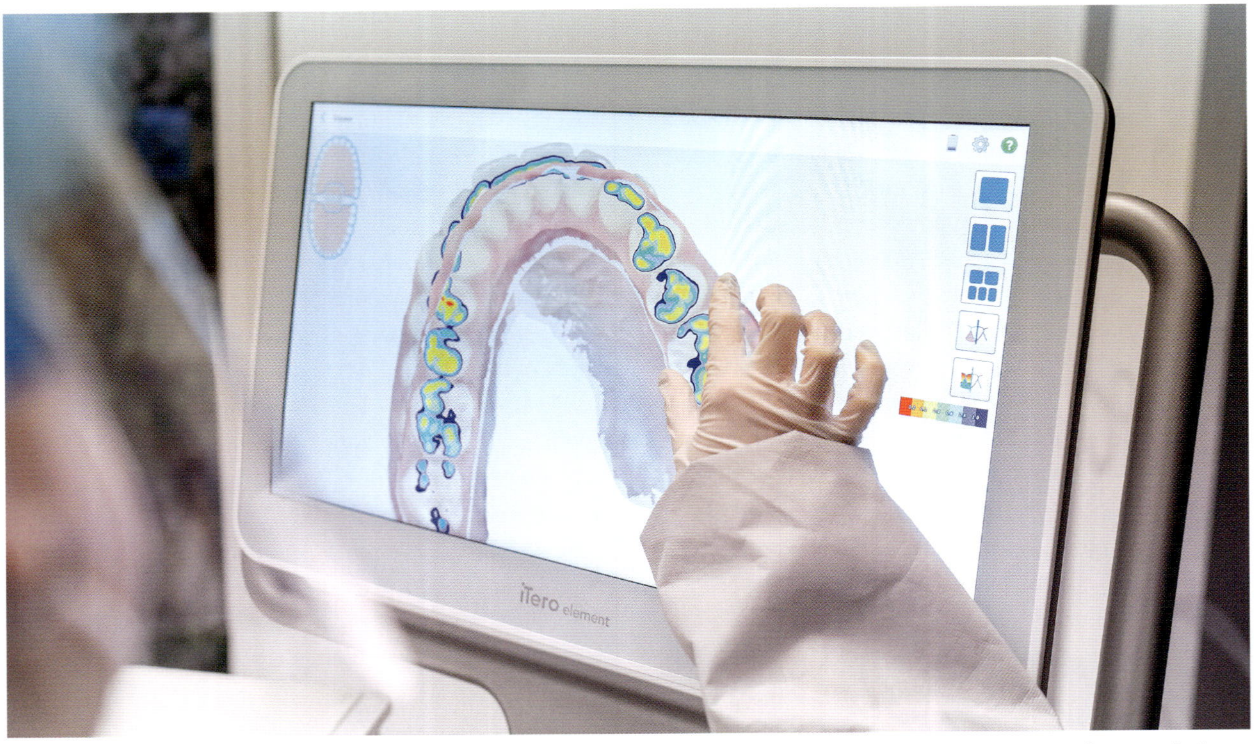


**Fig 8-14** Digitalization in orthodontics is a tool to help the patient visualize the three-dimensional changes often needed patients with TW. The compensatory eruption and adaptation mechanism to a changing anatomy in the TW patient may obscure some remarkable malocclusions. Enrolling the orthodontist in the comprehensive restorative treatment plan brings the opportunity to present the full treatment objectives to the patient.

## 5. Timing of Orthodontic and Restorative Interventions

All major malocclusions should be addressed before any restorative treatment is started. However, in some cases, the order can be altered, and restorations can be performed before the orthodontic treatment. This is the case in incipient TW, for which the restorative phase can be done before the orthodontic phase (see chapter 5).

In cases where the extent of the damage to the structure of the teeth dictates urgent reconstruction, if the priority is agreed to be tooth protection, the restoration of the teeth will take into consideration in the occlusal scheme to be achieved. Alternatively, this restoration can be addressed in a provisional/transitional manner. When the restorative phase is to be done after the orthodontic treatment, the orthodontist as a part of the TW team will decide whether the teeth should be aligned based on the gingival margins or the occlusal/incisal level, visualizing the permanent full anatomical restoration to be delivered at the final restorative phase.

## 6. Key Points: TW Treatment Planning: Considerations for the Orthodontic-Restorative Team

**Table 8-1** Considerations for the orthodontic-restorative team.

| |
|---|
| 1. Evaluate skeletal and dental class. Analyze tooth exposure and the patient's profile for esthetically driven orthodontics. |
| 2. Evaluate the anterior and canine guidance during function. |
| 3. Analyze the overbite and overjet. |
| 4. Does space need to be provided for restorations? |
| 5. Are the teeth going to be aligned based on the gingival architecture or the incisal plane? Align the teeth based on the gingival contour in the presence of incisal wear. |
| 6. Is the palatal aspect also worn? |
| 7. Consider options that minimize the need for more tooth reduction. Expand the arches and leave interocclusal space as planned with restorative team. |
| 8. Evaluate through cephalometric analysis the potential of adjusting tooth inclination. Would tooth angulation correction provide sufficient interocclusal space? |
| 9. Decide if the restorations will be performed before or after the orthodontic treatment. |
| 10. Does the patient have any TMJ complaints? If so, carry out TMJ therapy until the patient is asymptomatic before initiating the orthodontic-restorative treatment. |

## References


1. American Association of Orthodontists. Glossary of terms. https://www3.aaoinfo.org/blog/parent-s-guide-post/glossary-of-terms/. Accessed 30 Jan 2022.
2. Rasool G, Bashir S, Gul H, Afzal F, Nousheen A. Prevalence of tooth wear in different malocclusions of mixed dentition. Pak Oral Dent J 2014;34(2):309–312.
3. Marinelli A, Alarashi M, Defraia E, Antonini A, Tollaro I. Tooth wear in the mixed dentition: A comparative study between children born in the 1950s and the 1990s. Angle Orthod 2005;75(3):340–343.
4. Siluvai S, Kshetrimayum N, Reddy CV, Siddanna S, Manjunath M, Rudraswamy S. Malocclusion and related quality of life among 13- to 19-year-old students in Mysore City—A cross-sectional study. Oral Health Prev Dent 2015;13(2):135–141.
5. Janson G, Oltramari-Navarro PV, de Oliveira RB, Quaglio CL, Sales-Peres SH, Tompson B. Tooth-wear patterns in subjects with Class II division 1 malocclusion and normal occlusion. Am J Orthod Dentofacial Orthop 2010;137(1):14.e1–14.e7.
6. Kois DE, Kois JC. Comprehensive risk-based diagnostically driven treatment planning: Developing sequentially generated treatment Dent Clin North Am 2015;59:593–608.
7. Romano R. The future is here! CAD/CAM digital workflow in orthodontics: From planning to manufacturing predicted optimal smile. Clin Oral Implants Res 2018;29:26.
8. Gracis S. A simplified method to develop an interdisciplinary treatment plan: An esthetically and functionally driven approach in three steps. Int J Esthet Dent 2021;16(1):76–128.
9. Romano R, Bichacho N, Touati B. The Art of the Smile: Integrating Prosthodontics, Orthodontics, Periodontics, Dental Technology, and Plastic Surgery in Esthetic Dental Treatment. Chicago: Quintessence, 2005.
10. Romano R, Landsberg CJ. Reconstruction of function and aesthetics of the maxillary anterior region: A combined periodontal/orthodontic therapy. Pract Periodontics Aesthet Dent 1996;8:353–361.
11. Perakis N, Cocconi R. The decision-making process in interdisciplinary treatment: Digital versus conventional approach. A case presentation. Int J Esthet Dent 2019;14:212–224.
12. Cocconi R, Raffaini M, Fradeani M, van Doren E, Gori S, Rossi P. Team approach in esthetic dentistry. Int J Esthet Dent 2020;15:372–373.
13. Warreth A, Abuhijleh E, Almaghribi MA, Mahwal G, Ashawish A. Tooth surface loss: A review of literature. Saudi Dent J 2020;32(2):53–60.
14. Tollaro I, Defraia E, Marinelli A, Alarashi M. Tooth abrasion in unilateral posterior crossbite in the deciduous dentition. Angle Orthod, 2002;72:426–430.
15. Tamkin J. Impact of airway dysfunction on dental health. Bioinformation 2020;16(1):26–29.
16. Bachhav VC, Aras M. Altering occlusal vertical dimension in functional and esthetic rehabilitation of severely worn dentition. J Oral Health Res 2010;1(1):2–8.
17. Beyron H. Optimal occlusion. Dent Clin North Am 1969;13:537–554.
18. Patini R, Gallenzi P, Meuli S, Paoloni V, Cordaro M. Clear aligners' effects on aesthetics: Evaluation of facial wrinkles. J Clin Exp Dent 2018;10:e696–e701.
19. Magne P, Magne M, Belser UC. Adhesive restorations, centric relation, and the Dahl principle: Minimally invasive approaches to localized anterior tooth erosion. Eur J Esthet Dent 2007;2:260–273.
20. Poyser NJ, Porter RW, Briggs PF, Chana HS, Kelleher MG. The Dahl Concept: Past, present and future. Br Dent J 2005;198:669–676.
21. Dahl BL, Krogstad O, Karlsen K. An alternative treatment in cases with advanced localized attrition. J Oral Rehabil 1975;2(3):209–214.
22. Dahl BL, Krogstad O. The effect of a partial bite raising splint on the occlusal face height. An x-ray cephalometric study in human adults. Acta Odontol Scand 1982;40(1):17–24.
23. Mizrahi B. The Dahl principle: Creating space and improving the biomechanical prognosis of anterior crowns. Quintessence Int 2006;37:245–251.
24. Suarez-Almazor ME. Patient-physician communication. Curr Opin Rheumatol 2004;16(2):91–95.
25. Clack GB, Allen J, Cooper D, Head JO. Personality differences between doctors and their patients: Implications for the teaching of communication skills. Med Educ 2004;38(2):177–186.
26. Lee JY, Kim SW, Kim JM, Shin IS, Yoon JS. Two cases of eating disorders in adolescents with dental braces fitted prior to the onset of anorexia nervosa. Psychiatry Investig 2015;12:411–414.
27. Koukou M, Javed F, Michelogiannakis D. Is there an association between fixed orthodontic treatment and initiation of eating disorders? Quintessence Int 2021;52:565–566.
28. Johal A, Alyaqoobi I, Patel R, Cox S. The impact of orthodontic treatment on quality of life and self-esteem in adult patients. Eur J Orthod 2015;37:233–237.
29. Feudtner C. Collaborative communication in pediatric palliative care: A foundation for problem-solving and decision-making. Pediatr Clin North Am 2007;54:583–607.

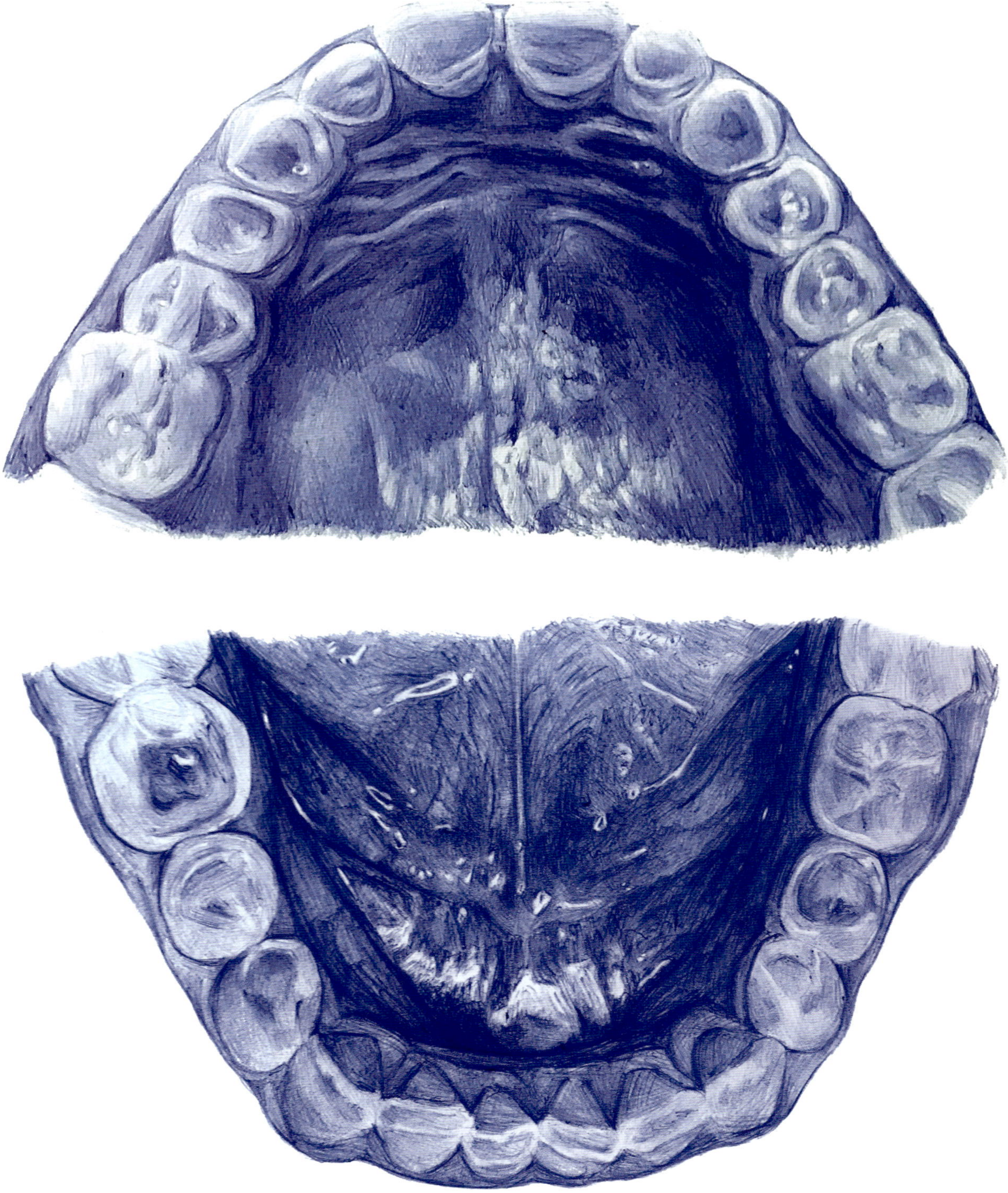

*The ability to find the answer is more important than the ability to know the answer.*

—Amit Kalantri, Indian illusionist

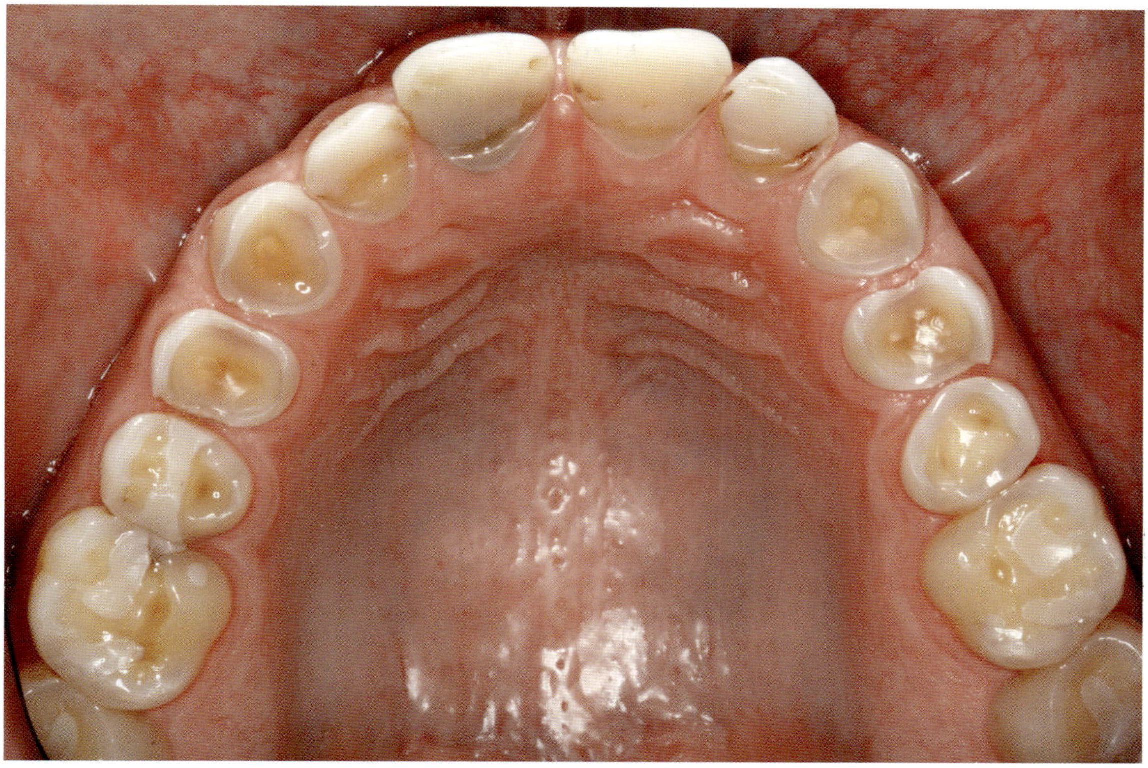

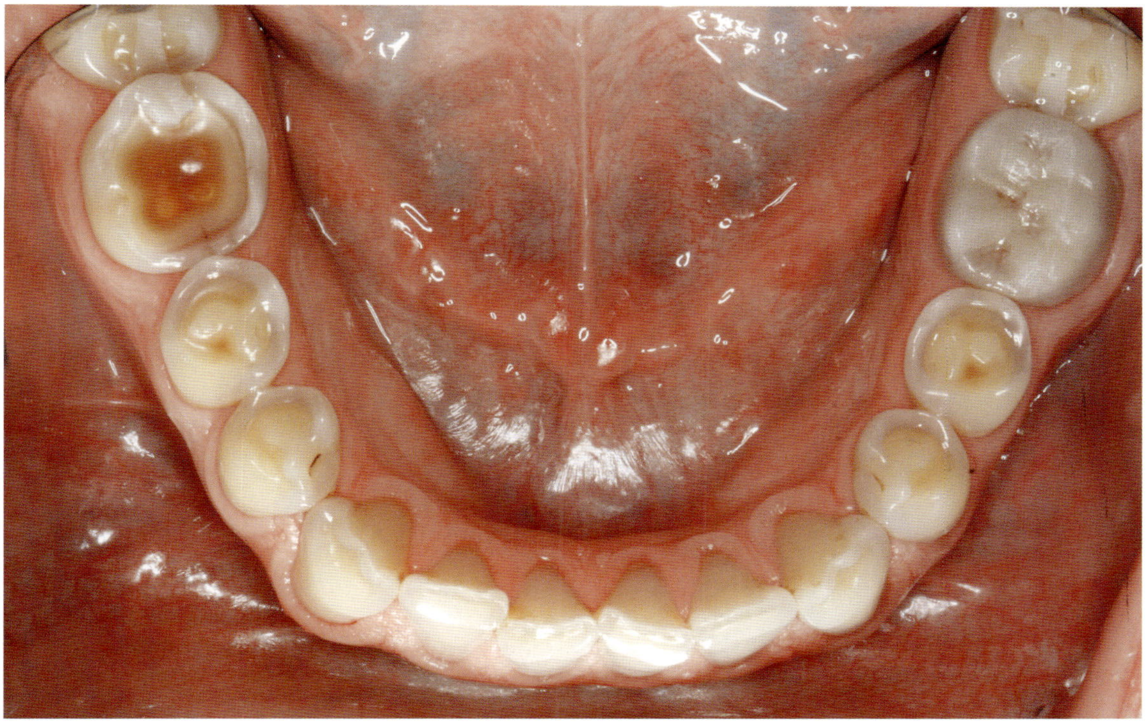

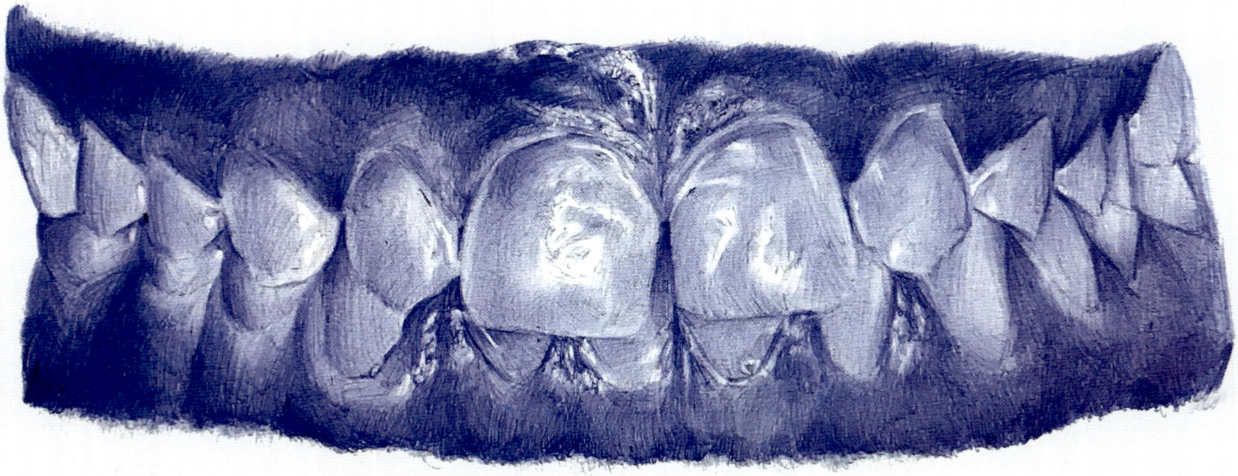

*Study nature, love nature, stay close to nature. It will never fail you.*

—Frank Lloyd Wright, American architect

CHAPTER 9

# IMPLANTS IN PATIENTS WITH TOOTH WEAR

The level of dental awareness and the prevalence of a preventive approach to dental care seem to be ever increasing in the general population. However, the increase in life expectancy, together with the omnipresent stress of daily life, mean that teeth are subject to wear and failure in a growing pattern due to reasons other than only caries and periodontal disease. When receiving an implant, patients sometimes take for granted that it should last for a lifetime. Clinicians are fully aware of the risk of bacterially originated diseases and are also experienced in dealing with mechanical complications. However, we tend to treat implant restorations very similarly to the way we treat teeth.

The functional and biodynamic properties of implants differ greatly to those of teeth or other kinds of prostheses. In this regard, clinicians should take the following aspects into consideration:

- The ankylotic nature of osseointegration
- The greatly reduced sensitivity of implants
- The restoration material, design, and mechanical properties
- Due to all of the above, the speed and pattern of wear of implant restorations

These characteristics make it necessary to revisit our rehabilitation and maintenance protocols in order to reduce the risk of not only peri-implant disease but also function-derived complications, especially in the patient with TW. It is also worth mentioning that there are no clear guidelines in the scientific literature as to which occlusal pattern and design should be used for each implant crown, bridge, or rehabilitation. This chapter aims to clarify some of the main aspects of implant dentistry in terms of occlusion, prosthetic design, and both mechanical and biologic failures related to oral functionality in the patient with TW.

## 1. Biologic and Mechanical Considerations

The concept of osseointegration has resulted in dramatic improvements in prosthodontics. Dental implants have allowed the rehabilitation of single teeth, multiple teeth, and full arches in a predictable manner.[1–8] The long-term success of dental implants is at least comparable to conventional fixed prosthodontics.[9] However, both the biomechanical behavior and the biologic interaction of an implant with the host bone are very different from that of a tooth.[10] There are two main considerations to bear in mind: first of all, the ankylosis-like union between the implant and the bone and, secondly, the fact that implant prostheses may have a different wear pattern and speed compared to a tooth.

This fundamental difference between teeth and implants means that the mechanical behavior of an implant is unique, and so is its functionality (Fig 9-1).

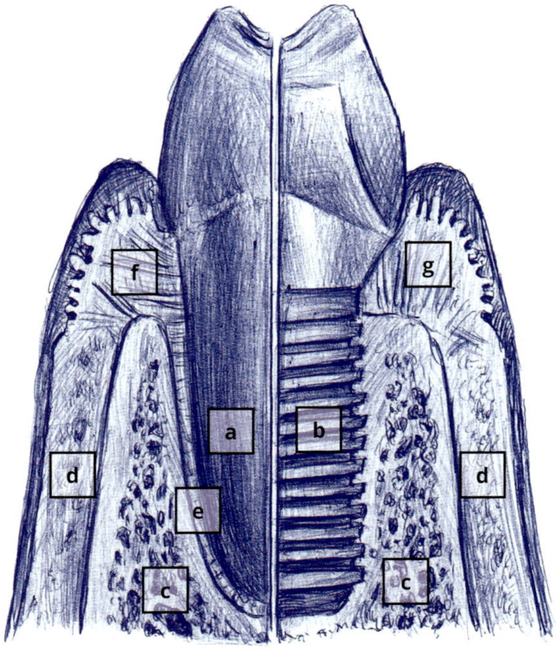


**Fig 9-1** Anatomical differences between tooth (a) and implant (b). Bone (c) and gjngival tissue (d) are common to both. The first clear difference is the lack of periodontal ligament around an implant (e). The second relevant difference between both entities is the disposition of the collagen fibers: around a tooth, collagen fibers are strongly attached to the root surface (f), whereas fibers around an implant run circularly without insertion to the surface (g). This confers to the implant reduced soft tissue protection against bacterial infections.

A healthy natural tooth will sink into the alveolar process under compression, mainly due to the resilience provided by the periodontal ligament. The movement that the osseointegrated implant will allow is considerably smaller.[10] This compressibility has the goal of minimizing stress to both tooth and bone at the time of chewing. In the absence of this physiologic movement, the tooth is submitted to greater stress and may be more prone to mechanical issues. For instance, ankylosed teeth are more prone to progressive replacement resorption, which leads to a higher risk of fracture.

Dental implants work on the basis of osseointegration. This means that there is a tight union between the metal fixture and the bone, and there is no periodontal ligament between them. In contrast, the periodontal ligament around a healthy tooth allows for a certain degree of motion upon compression. In the natural dentition, vertically, this movement is similar between anterior and posterior teeth, approximately 28 μm under light forces.[11] This displacement is accompanied by a horizontal component, which is much greater than the vertical, ranging from 56 to 108 μm, mostly depending on the site.[12] Additionally, once a larger amount of force is present, the viscoelasticity of the bone will allow for up to 40 μm further movement.[13] In contrast, implants only move approximately 2 to 3 μm in the vertical direction under light, initial forces.[14] This is likely due to the limited viscoelastic characteristics of the bone. However, if the implant is submitted to heavy loads, between 11 to 66 μm of movement can occur in the buccolingual direction[15] (Fig 9-2).

Furthermore, the reaction speed to occlusal forces is also considerably different between the entities. First of all, a tooth begins to move much sooner than an implant.[14] Thus, if an implant restoration is placed at the same level as the neighboring teeth, it will function for a longer period of time than a tooth on every chewing cycle. Secondly, the speed at which teeth and implants recover their initial position is also unequal; implants take around 1 millisecond to return after the load is finished, whereas teeth go back to their original place following a much slower viscoelastic movement. Once again, implants will function for a greater amount of time at each working cycle and will always be ready for the next biting movement.

The underlying bone is part of the structure that withstands occlusal forces. As a biologic entity, the amount of force that it can bear is also worth studying. The bones of the maxilla and mandible adapt their strength to the applied load; this continuous remodeling maintains the mechanical competence of the bone. This capacity also depends on the individual's bone characteristics.[16] These concepts were first developed in the field of orthopedics[17] and applied to dentistry by a group of orthodontists.[18] When moderate strain occurs (deformation induced by normal loading), the bone may experience three-dimensional growth. However, if a certain threshold is exceeded, micro- or macro-fractures may occur. Bone tolerates a microstrain of 0.0001% to 0.15% volume deformity.[19] In some cases, strains up to 0.3% can be counteracted as adaptation via reshaping and strengthening. More than 2.5% strain can induce whole bone fracture. If it is less than 0.0001%, functional atrophy may occur. It is important to point out that strain (flexing, deformation) is the issue and not the amount of force, which does not relate proportionally. Some publications have even pointed out that bone may grow after a long period of time supporting moderate biting forces.[18,20] It has also been proven that mechanically loaded implants are surrounded by more rigid bone[21,22] and a higher rate of bone-to-implant contact.[23]

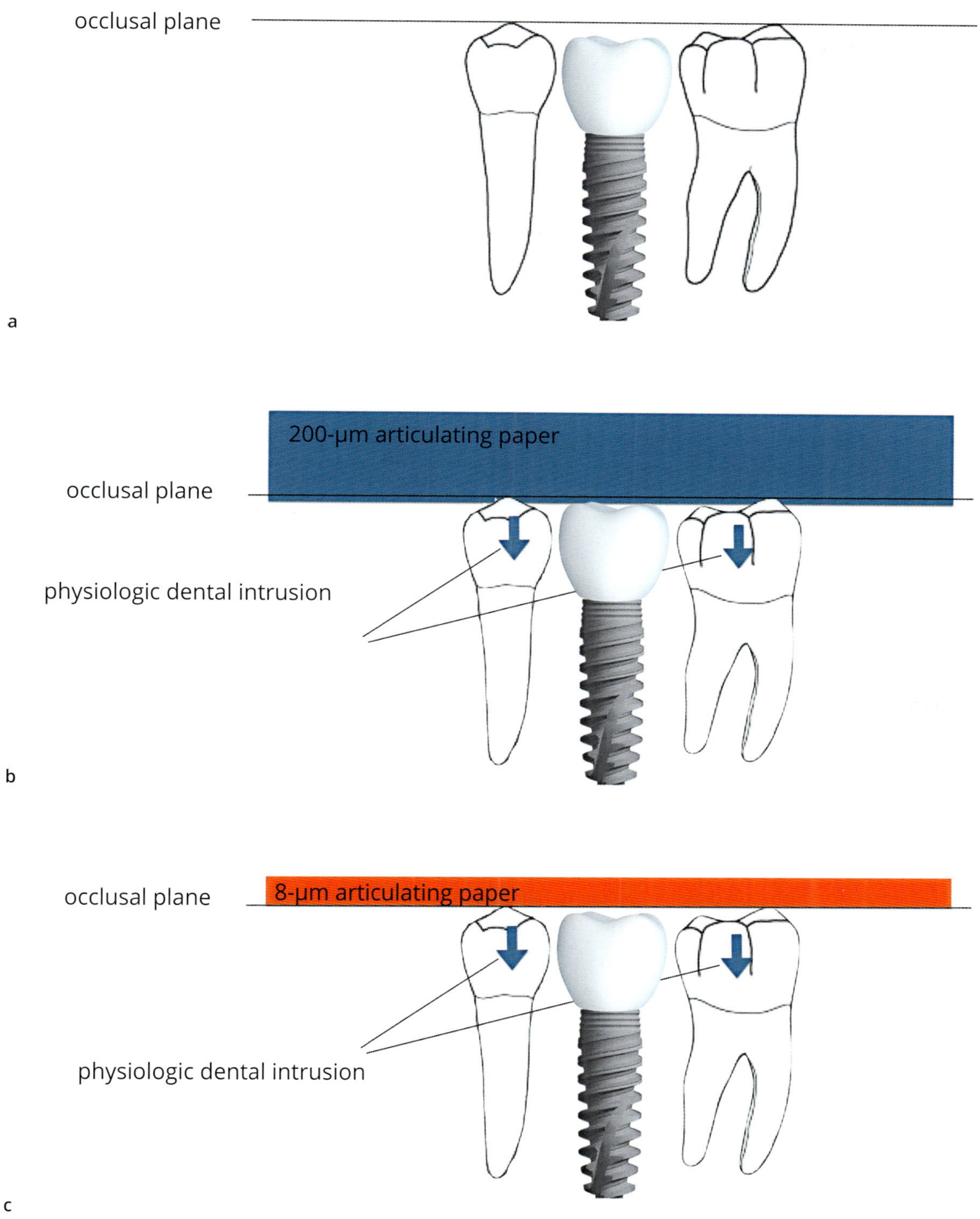


**Fig 9-2** Ideal occlusal function in a patient without TW. The slight infraocclusion of a single implant crown is based on the physiology of tooth movement (a). Upon chewing, the physiologic intrusion movement of the teeth allows for a 200-µm articulating paper to leave a trace both on the teeth and implant crown (b). The thicker articulating paper will first touch the teeth but will soon after be pierced by them, allowing for the implant restoration to be marked as well. In practical terms, this means that it is desirable that the first contact occurs on teeth, and once they start compressing, the implant crown will start to function. A thinner paper (8 to 40 µm) also leaves a trace on natural teeth upon chewing. However, this thinner paper should not be registered on the implant restoration; this is described as slight infraocclusion (c). In other words, the thinner paper should not be pierced to a degree that the implant crown is registered, as this would mean that the implant restoration would be vertically only a few microns away from the natural teeth. Bearing in mind that teeth compress approximately 150 µm, that trace would imply possibly excessive contact on the implant crown. In regard to the lateral component of occlusion (in the anterior sector), a similar criterion should be followed.

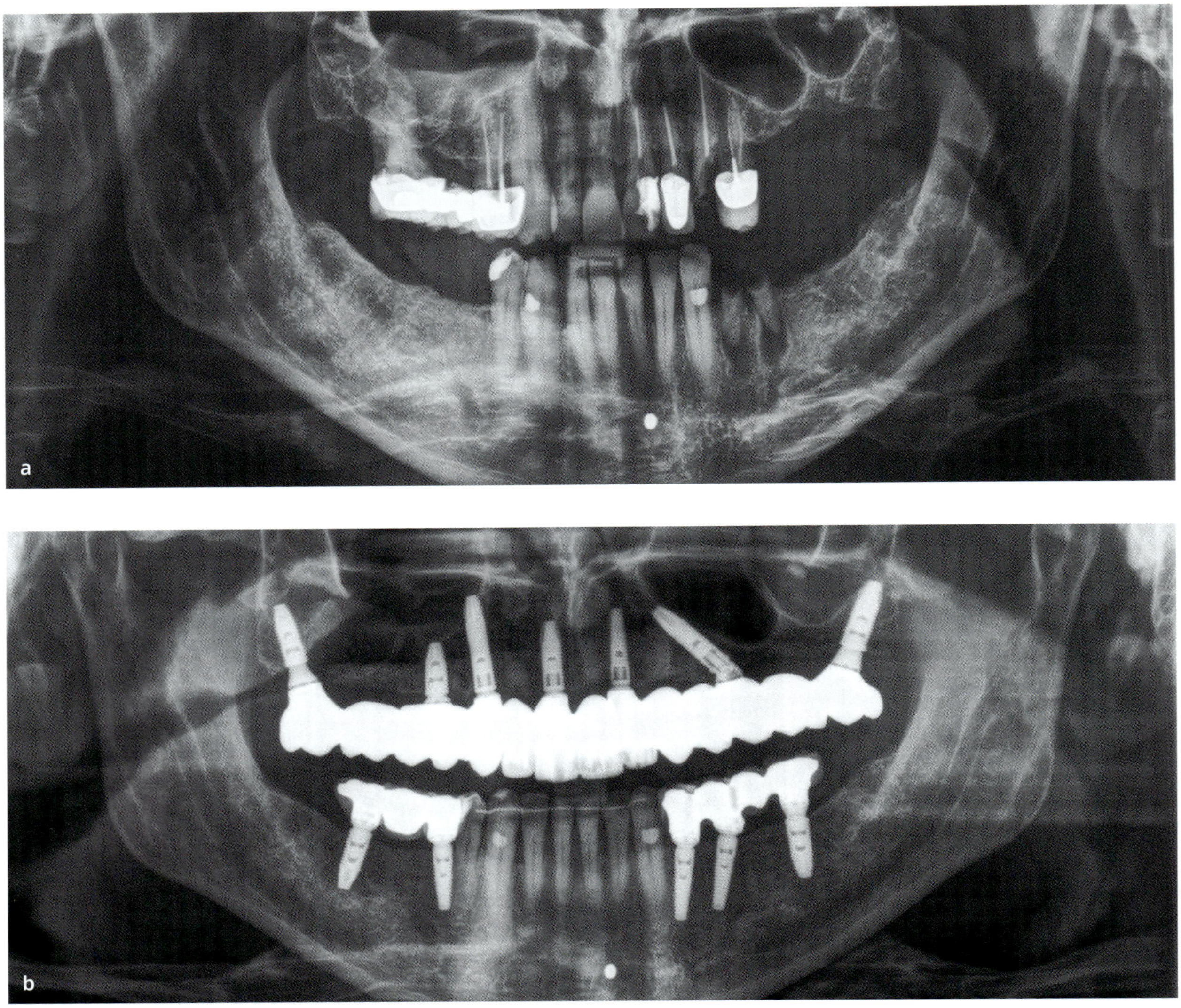

**Fig 9-3** Preoperative (a) and postoperative (b) panoramic radiographs of oral rehabilitation in a patient suffering from erosive TW since a young age. The patient claimed he used to go to bed with a two-liter soda bottle on his bedside table. The mandibular anterior teeth had been relatively spared thanks to the protection of the salivary flow and were orthodontically repositioned. In this case, preserving the natural mandibular dentition did not mean fewer implants; however, the preservation of the natural teeth along with their whole biologic complex allowed the patient to maintain a certain level of proprioception that may aid in the long-term survival of the reconstruction.

Another relevant characteristic of implant restorations is the reduced level of proprioception, with a tactile sensitivity up to 8.7 times lower on implants compared to teeth. In fact, whenever possible, the preservation of the natural proprioceptive capacity of natural teeth may prove beneficial and protective in the long term (Fig 9-3). This is particularly important in patients with bruxism. Excessive forces can lead to severe wear and other related complications. In these scenarios, some authors state that it may be reasonable to seek a unilaterally balanced or even bilaterally balanced occlusal scheme, should the initially chosen design be ineffective.[24]

## 2. Clinical Recommendations

Following the previously described concepts, certain parameters may be useful when restoring an implant. In spite of a lack of consensus in the literature, the guidelines described in this section should be considered in depth.

### Occlusal Table Surface Size

As a starting reference, a single implant crown for a molar replacement will be considered. The diameter of a

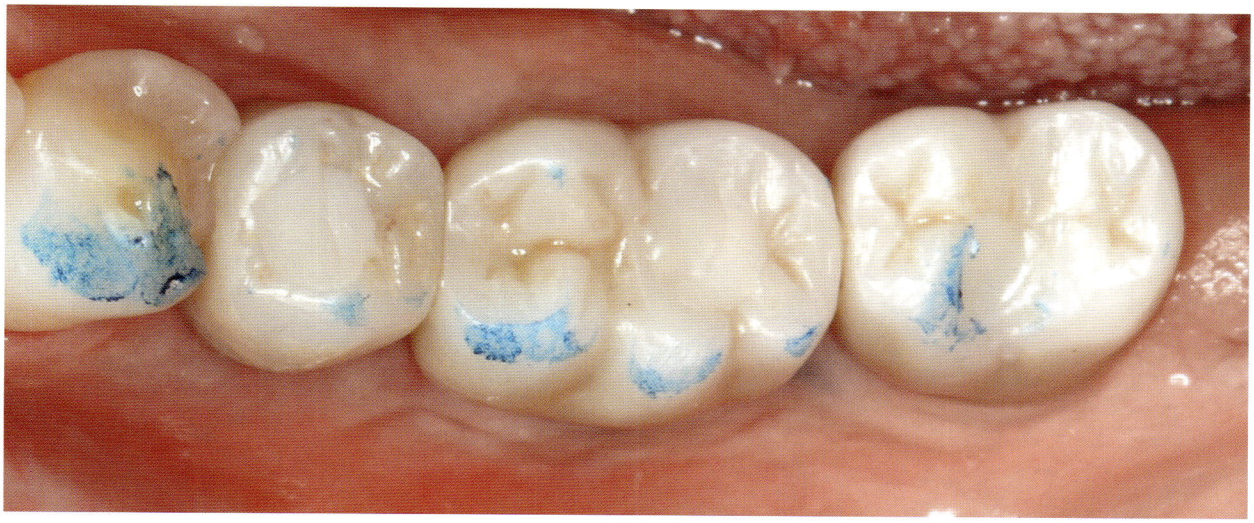

**Fig 9-4** In the case of a partial restoration, mechanical problems will most likely show at the occlusal surface of the restoration rather than at the implant-restorative interface, as the loads are shared among various implants, which helps counteract the nonaxial vectors. The narrow occlusal table design has been chosen in this posterior implant-supported partial denture in order to minimize dangerous, nonaxial forces. The buccolingual span of the molars is practically equal to that of the natural first premolar.

dental implant is usually considerably smaller than that of a tooth. For instance, the average width of a maxillary central incisor is 9.1 ± 0.62 mm,[25] and the most frequently used implants are between approximately 3.5 and 5 mm wide. This means that there is a large discrepancy between the occlusal surface of the tooth to be replaced and the implant width. Implants are most capable of resisting centric, axial (vertical) compressive loads.[26] This size difference between tooth and implant is even more pronounced in molars, where, additionally, occlusal forces are much greater. If these forces are applied on the perimeter of the occlusal surface, this will result in non-ideal shear forces.[27] These forces can lead to mechanical issues such as prosthetic screw loosening and crown surface damage (chipping), among others. The further the distance from the occlusal contact to the center of the implant in a horizontal dimension, ie, axial offset, the greater the torque induced on the whole implant-restoration complex.

One solution to this issue is to reduce the occlusal surface, at least in terms of buccolingual distance.[28,29] By designing a narrow contact area, the risk of undesirable forces is decreased (Fig 9-4). The clinician must nevertheless bear in mind that the restorations must provide adequate function; for instance, if a maxillary molar crown is reduced from buccal to palatal, an edge-to-edge bite may appear. This is not desirable, as it would provoke cheek biting.

## Cuspal Inclination

Premolars and molars are responsible for most of the work in chewing, as they provide a vertical stop for the jaws. As discussed in the previous section, nonaxial forces on an implant restoration should be avoided. Hypothetically then, a completely flat surface would be ideal, as cusps inherently generate a combination of vertical and lateral force vectors. However, a flat surface would be very inefficient for chewing.[30] Furthermore, the presence of vertical, pronounced cusps in posterior sectors makes it harder to avoid lateral interferences (Fig 9-5). Thus, some authors advocate for a reduction in cuspal inclination (ie, occlusal surfaces with relatively "shallow" fossae and low cusps).[27,28]

## Occlusal Contact Intensity

The degree of occlusal contact in implant restorations should also be addressed. As previously discussed, an implant prosthesis is not as prepared to cope with masticatory forces as teeth; the periodontal unit around a tooth acts as a spring that helps minimize the amount of force transmitted to the tooth and the bone. Thus, the amount of occlusal function borne by an implant restoration should be revisited. Due to the mechanical idiosyncrasy of osseointegrated prostheses, occlusal contact force should be adjusted depending on the situation, as described in the sections below.

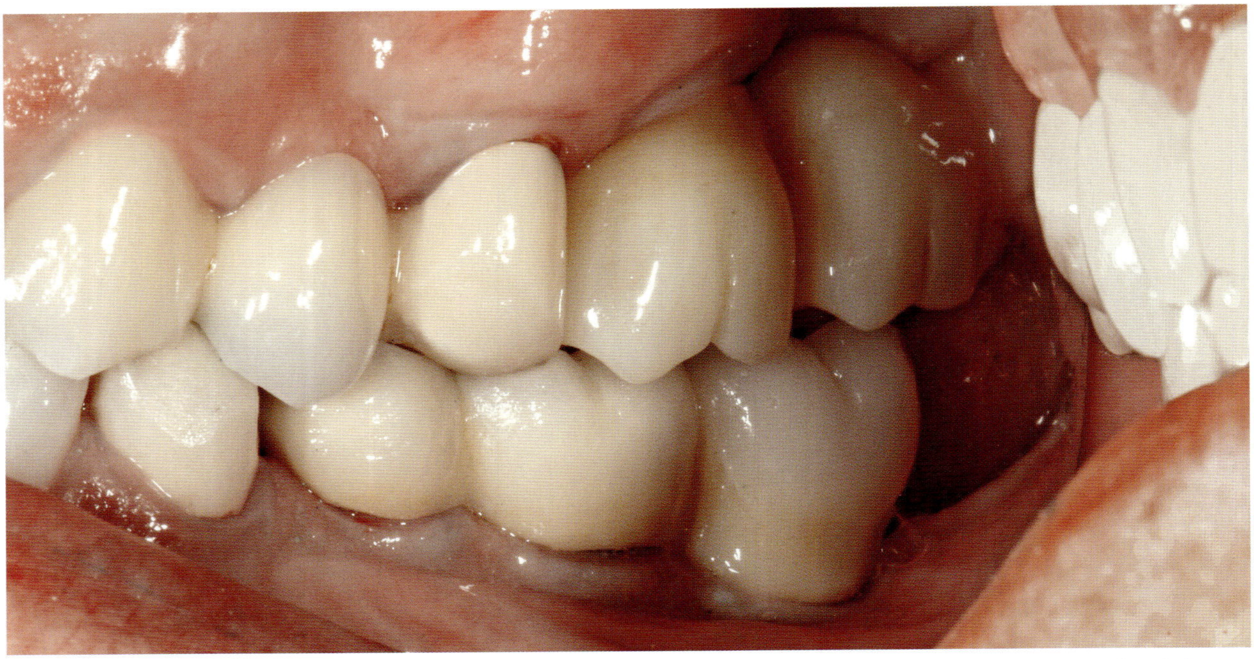

**Fig 9-5** Note the exaggerated buccal cusps on both molars in an implant-supported partial denture in the maxillary left quadrant. In order to avoid undesired contacts upon lateral movements, these pronounced buccal cusps were overtly separated from the antagonist surface. These cusps are not as relevant for masticatory efficiency and thus could have been designed more shallow and closer to the mandibular dentition.

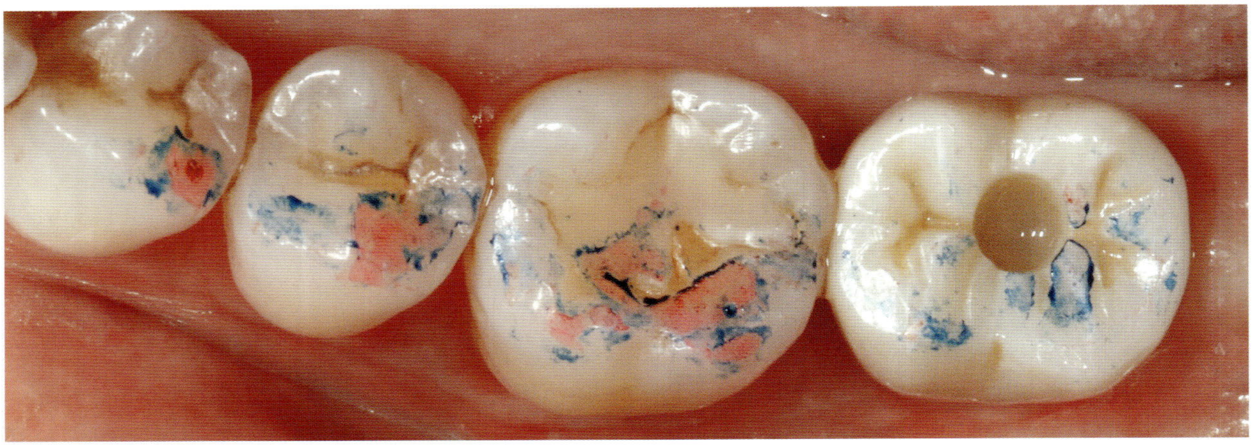

**Fig 9-6** Single implant crown on mandibular left second molar. Occlusal contacts are slightly less intense than on its natural tooth neighbors. Notice the absence of red marks (8-µm articulating paper) on the implant crown, as well as the narrower buccolingual dimension.

### Single implant crowns with adjacent natural teeth and an opposing natural dentition or fixed restoration

Once the occlusal contact is established, teeth will be depressed into the socket. If the implant crown is set at the same height as the teeth, once such depression takes place, the implant restoration will remain "emerged" and will bear more contact than the rest of the dentition (Fig 9-6). The opposing tooth or teeth will also suffer from overload in this scenario. In order to counteract this, a reduced occlusion has been recommended.[28] This means that initially only teeth will establish contact. Once the vertical compression takes place, the implant restoration will start to function.

If the occlusal scheme and anatomy were permanent, these guidelines would be easy to follow. Still, occlusal anatomy is subject to change. This is even more critical in the patient with TW, especially if erosion is present (Figs 9-7 to 9-9).

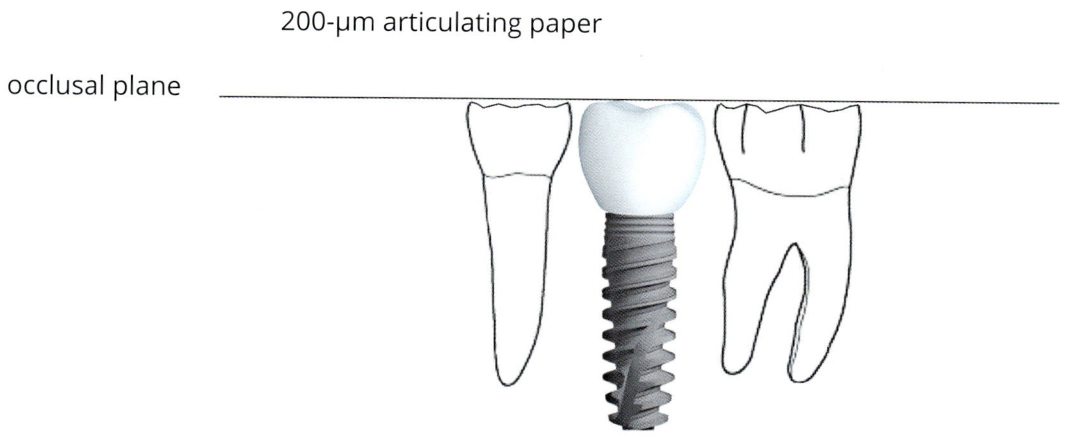


**Fig 9-7** Incipient-moderate TW. In general terms, in the patient with incipient to moderate TW, the eruptive compensation of the worn dentition may mislead us into thinking that the load is equally shared by implants and teeth. Nevertheless, the implant overload will depend on which is faster: compensatory eruption or wear on teeth. Usually, biting down on a regular 200-μm articulating paper will leave a trace both on teeth and the single implant crown. However, following the previously described concepts, the intrusion suffered by teeth upon chewing will be much greater than that suffered by the implant. Thus, a subclinical premature contact may induce an excessive load to this implant.

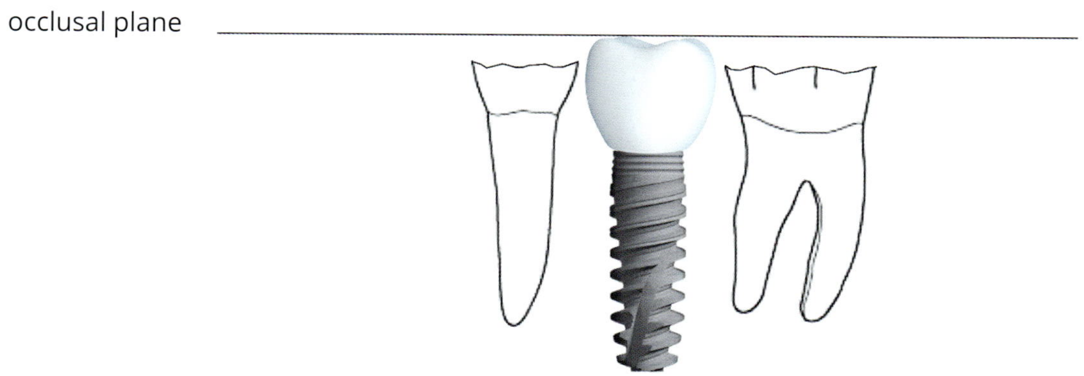


**Fig 9-8** Severe TW. In this scenario, premature contact on the implant crown may be clearly present at all times, especially in patients with acidic erosion, where the pace of tooth structure dissolution may be faster than compensatory eruption. A clear overload can even put osseointegration at risk. Moreover, in these cases, a reduced number of teeth due to extractions may multiply the risk.

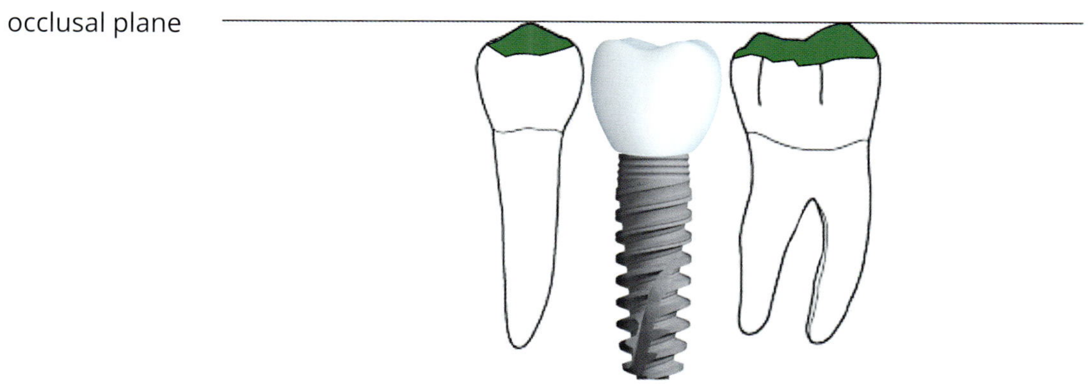


**Fig 9-9** Occlusal rehabilitation in the TW patient allowing for ideal occlusal anatomy is highly recommended and should be frequently monitored considering the chronic-phasic characteristics of TW. Because risk factors are not easy to control in the long term, periodic refurbishment or repetition of the restorations on the natural dentition have to be performed in order to keep the occlusal balance and safeguard the implant restorations, which will not wear at the same rate as teeth or tooth-borne restorations.

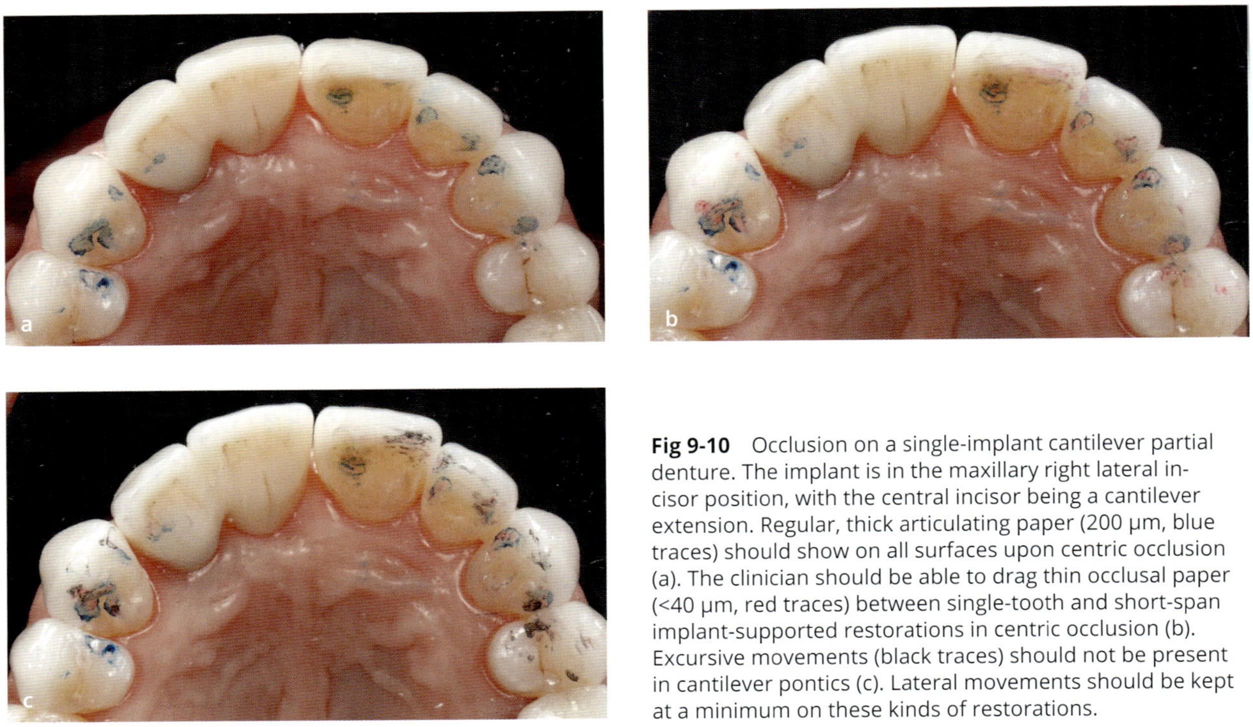


**Fig 9-10** Occlusion on a single-implant cantilever partial denture. The implant is in the maxillary right lateral incisor position, with the central incisor being a cantilever extension. Regular, thick articulating paper (200 µm, blue traces) should show on all surfaces upon centric occlusion (a). The clinician should be able to drag thin occlusal paper (<40 µm, red traces) between single-tooth and short-span implant-supported restorations in centric occlusion (b). Excursive movements (black traces) should not be present in cantilever pontics (c). Lateral movements should be kept at a minimum on these kinds of restorations.

### Small-span partial dentures

In terms of occlusal contact strength, these structures should be as similar as possible to single crowns as described previously, especially in terms of centric occlusion in the posterior sector (Fig 9-10).

### Large-span partial dentures

Large implant-supported partial dentures (four or more units) may represent a considerable part of an arch. If the partial denture only involves premolars and molars, the previously described criteria should apply to a certain extent, although it is also crucial to allow for a well-distributed occlusion. However, if the anterior sectors are involved, the implant-supported partial denture should be equally responsible for the function supported by the adjacent teeth. If the anterior sector is entirely restored via an implant-supported partial denture, the anterior function should be as close as possible to that of natural teeth, ensuring a mutually guided protection.

### Full-arch restorations

In these cases, where the whole arch behaves as a single piece, the centric occlusion should be designed and adjusted according to each individual scenario. This is dependent on the opposing arch and planned overall occlusal scheme. In case of an opposing natural dentition or fixed restorations, mutually protected guidance should be the goal. In case of a removable opposing prosthesis, a bilaterally balanced occlusion should be the aim in most cases.[31] In case of fixed prostheses, a large cantilever is directly related to the risk of mechanical complications but also to increased risk for peri-implant bone loss and implant failure.[32] It is also noteworthy that, even though distal implants on a cantilevered prosthesis seem to suffer from the highest forces, it is the mesial implants that show the highest rate of bone loss.[33]

Despite these considerations and guidelines, the clinician must always bear in mind the individual circumstances of the implant or implants, mouth, and patient; for instance, if an implant restoration is left in clear infraocclusion, the surrounding teeth will have to carry the functional load in that area. On the other hand, single implant crowns surrounded by heavily restored neighboring teeth or by teeth with more than physiologic mobility may be approached in a different manner; leaving the implant crown in slight infraocclusion may be beneficial for the implant as has been previously described, but those teeth may then be more susceptible to complications. In these scenarios, a frequent recall schedule for occlusal monitoring is recommended.

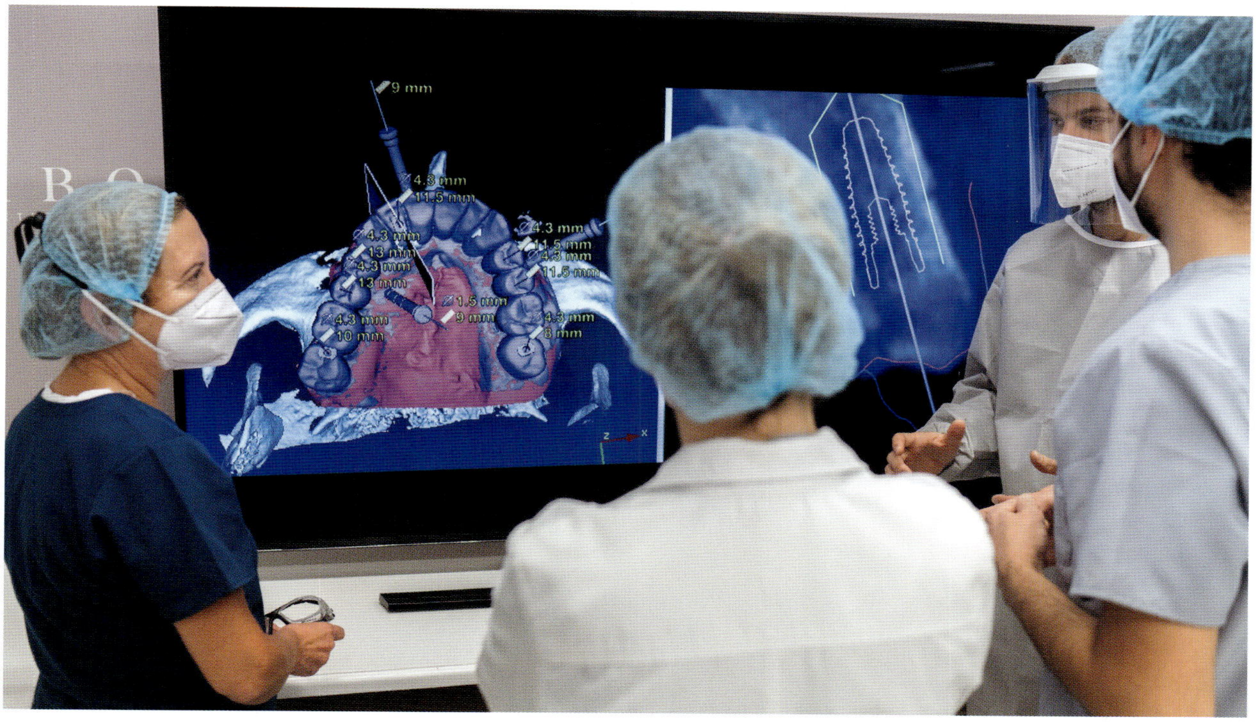


**Fig 9-11** Guided surgery should take into consideration the overall planning from the different specialties involved in the patient's treatment. Interaction between orthodontic, surgical, and restorative members of the team is beneficial to enhance the final outcome. The time schedule and provisionalization of the patient with TW is of great importance in the interdisciplinary approach.

## Surgical Considerations

Patients with challenging occlusal conditions, such as TW, may require an adaptation of regular implant dentistry protocols. Prevention of possible biomechanical issues, benefitting from the multidisciplinary intervention of other specialists to improve the overall oral health, leads to the reinforcement of the implant-restoration complex. Three different aspects must be taken into consideration, as outlined below.

### Implant choice

In light of a possibly higher risk of complications or even osseointegration failure, presurgical planning and implant choice should be adapted to the higher functional demands of patients with TW. Due to their increased resistance and reduced force transmission to surrounding bone, wide-diameter implants are indicated if conditions are appropriate.[34,35] On the other hand, the prosthetic space needed for a restoration must not be underestimated; if need be, the implant may be placed slightly deeper than usual.

### Implant number and distribution

A reduced number of implants, eg, an "all-on-four" protocol may not be indicated in patients with occlusal unstability such as TW patients. Even if no scientific literature supports the use of a high number of implants, in case of a single implant failure, the chances of prosthetic survival in a protocol with a reduced number of implants are lower than in, eg, an eight-implant solution. On the other hand, large distal cantilevers should be avoided. Splinted, multiple-unit prostheses should be considered whenever possible, as splinted implants show a lower rate of failure.[36]

### Planning and timing of the implant placement and rehabilitation

In severe TW, a general vertical and horizontal collapse can pose a limitation to the ideal time frame of the surgical intervention and the 3D positioning of the implant. A thorough integration of the implant planning into the overall treatment strategy is essential to avoid erroneous placement and provisionalization limitations in the patient with severe TW (Fig 9-11).

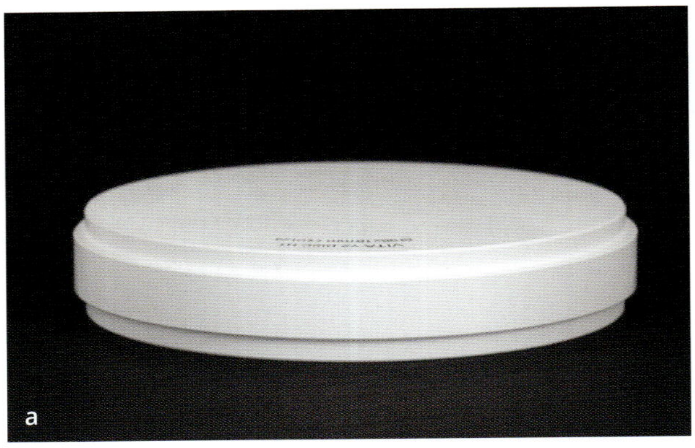


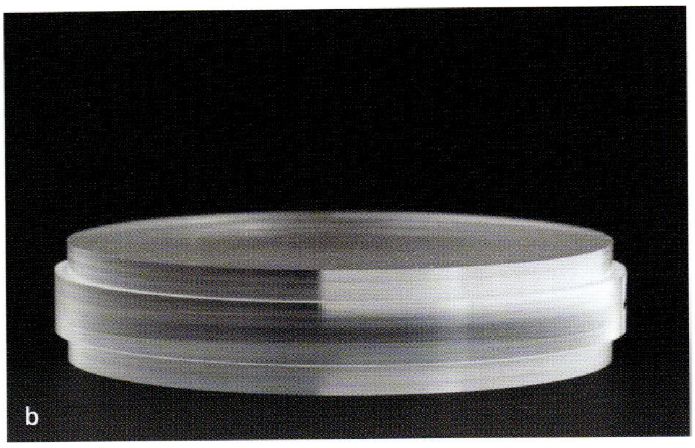


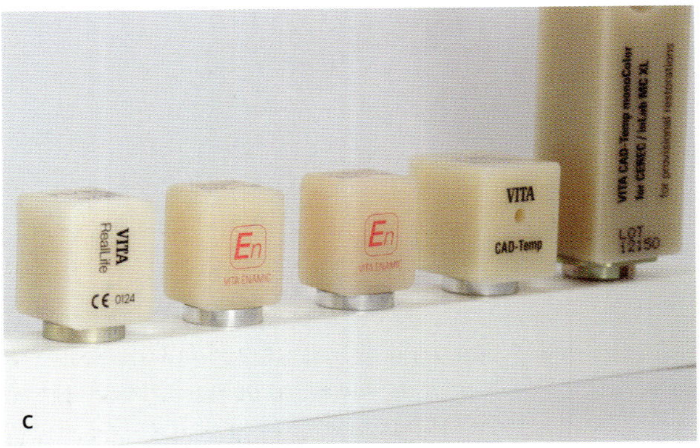


**Fig 9-12** Conventional, presintered zirconia block (VITA) (a). Highly translucent zirconia block (VITA) (b). Different CAD/CAM materials: feldspathic, polymer-infiltrated ceramic network, and resin-based (c).

## Material Selection for Implant Restorations in Patients with TW

The rate of wear may not be the same between a natural tooth and an implant restoration. The unique mechanical behavior, together with the materials used to restore an implant, make it very likely for teeth to wear faster than implant crowns. This means that a properly adjusted occlusal scheme will probably become unbalanced if left unattended for a long period of time. This fact renders material selection particularly relevant. Characteristics such as restoration wear rate, antagonist wear, and the modulus of elasticity of any given material are extremely important in implant prosthodontics.

The porcelain-fused-to-metal "gold standard" is considered as such due to its high level of long-term scientific support.[37] However, newer materials such as zirconia, lithium disilicate, and even hybrid ceramic-composite network restorations may pose an advantage in terms of resistance to oral functional demands. Furthermore, CAD/CAM protocols may improve the fit of implant restorations[38] (Fig 9-12).

In the case of zirconia, early-generation restorations showed comparable results to those of PFM.[39] Nevertheless, the rate of chipping on zirconia crowns was always higher than on their metal-ceramic counterparts.[40] Nowadays, monolithic zirconia is extremely popular over veneered zirconia as it foregoes the risk of ceramic chipping. This configuration makes sense especially for posterior implant crowns; its high modulus of elasticity confers great resistance to fracture to zirconia crowns.[41] Besides, and just as importantly, well-polished zirconia induces a very low rate of wear against the opposing dentition[42] as explained in chapter 7.

Lithium disilicate ($LiS_2$) has a lower flexural strength compared to zirconia (approximately 450 MPa for $LiS_2$ vs over 1000 MPa for zirconia).[43] In fact, it is closer to that of enamel (160 MPa).[44] This makes sense from the point of view of integration into the rest of the dentition.

New high-performance polymer (HPP) materials such as polymer-infiltrated ceramic network (PICN) and poly-ether-ether-ketone (PEEK) are relatively new in the implant restoration world, and thus, there is not enough long-term evidence to support their use. However, these solutions have the theoretical advantage of having a lower elasticity modulus, and this means they do not transmit the whole occlusal force to the bone-implant interface.[45] This could prove advantageous in patients with bruxism, as they might diminish harmful forces and reduce the risk of overload.

## 3. Overload and Implant Failure in Patients with Tooth Wear

A tooth suffering from occlusal trauma will generally provoke pain in the patient. Hyperemia and occlusal/thermal sensitivity will be present. In this situation, the patient will usually seek a professional solution. With more severe occlusal trauma, a tooth may become mobile. Overload is initially treated by reducing the amount of occlusion on the affected tooth, and the tooth will probably revert to its original degree of healthy mobility. In contrast, an overloaded implant may not develop associated symptoms but rather may end up with biologic complications such as microfractures of the surrounding bone and subsequent bone loss or mechanical complications such as porcelain chipping, screw loosening, etc. Moreover, and unlike a natural tooth, the traumatized, mobile implant most probably will not revert to its fixed status and will soon fail. In the presence of repeated trauma, a tooth may show wear facets, cervical abfraction, a widened periodontal ligament, sensitivity, and more. An implant will generally show trauma in form of a mechanical failure such as chipping of the restoration.

The topic of implant overloading is controversial in the scientific literature. Traditionally, orthopedic concepts of the capacity of bone to endure deformation or "strain" have been used to try to explain a non-plaque-related implant failure.[16,20] This has led to the general concept of "excessive load," which may induce such issues.[46] Nevertheless, even animal studies with remarkable forces have failed to establish a clear relationship between excessive load and osseointegration failure.[47]

If excessive forces are applied, an implant may lose its intimate contact with the bone, and this will be substituted by a fibrous union, which in turn is not able to withstand chewing. This may appear as a radiographic finding, although it is not always visible and is seldom detectable by probing, since the gap between the implant and the bone is usually very narrow (Figs 9-13 and 9-14). Besides the physical limits of the bone as a load-bearing entity, the osseointegration itself may be subject to challenges. Apart from the plaque-related diseases such as peri-implantitis, an implant may lose its capacity to function due to overloading (Fig 9-15).

Some authors state that even uniform premature contacts will not lead to osseointegration failure but will rather provoke an increase in bone density around the implant; however, this may lead to increased bone loss if combined with peri-implant disease.[48] However, other publications indicate that there is a clear connection between bruxism and implant failure.[49]

Patients suffering from severe TW are more prone to losing teeth.[50] As previously described, these patients will wear different materials in their mouth at a different rate. This is common to all patients, but it can be exacerbated in patients suffering from tooth wear. As an example, PFM crowns on natural healthy teeth will wear slower than the natural dentition. If left unattended, this wear differential will leave the PFM crown with a more intense occlusal function, which in turn can lead to occlusal trauma. This situation will likely lead to mechanical and/or biologic complications such as porcelain chipping, tooth fracture, loss of periodontal integrity, necrosis, or a combination of these.

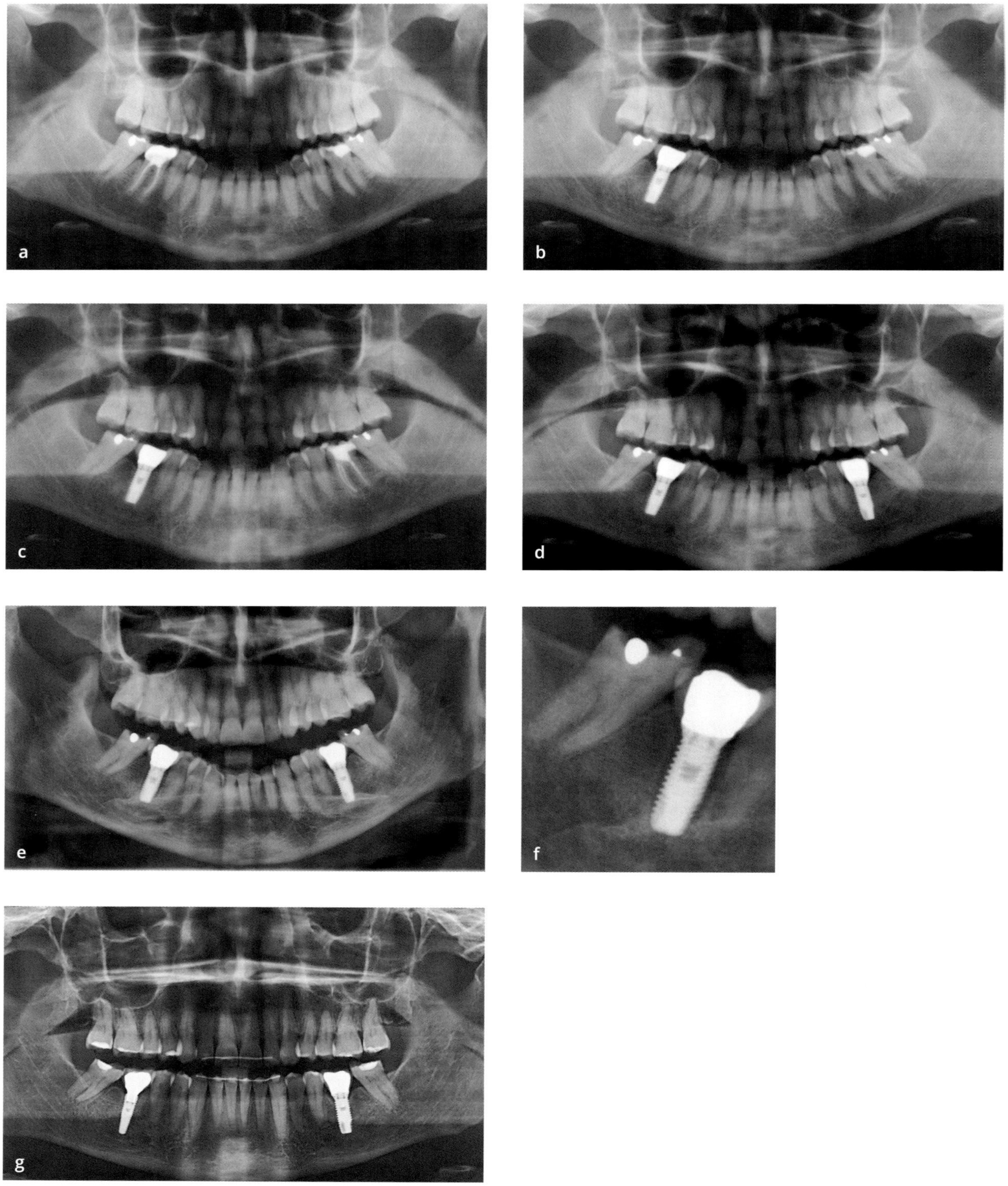


**Fig 9-13** Radiographic evolution of failure of mandibular first molars in a patient with stress-related bruxism and an erosive challenge. The rate of tooth wear on this patient was very high. In 2004, the patient received a root canal treatment on the mandibular right first molar due to pulp chamber exposure provoked by tooth wear (a). One year later, that tooth was extracted and replaced by an implant-supported prosthesis (b). Three years later, the contralateral molar underwent the same path; it was endodontically treated first (c) and some years later was replaced by an implant (d). Furthermore, the mandibular right implant developed a radiolucency, mobility, and mild pain upon chewing 4 years later (e). This implant had to be extracted and was replaced by a new one. In this case, the implant was extracted and the site was left to heal for 4 months. The newly placed implant was provisionally restored after 6 months for a 6-month period. Notice the severe wear and the difference in wear between the natural second molar and the implant restoration (f). This means that the implant probably suffered from traumatic loading that ultimately led to failure. An overall occlusal rehabilitation is mandatory in order to avoid future implant overloading and osseointegration failure (g).

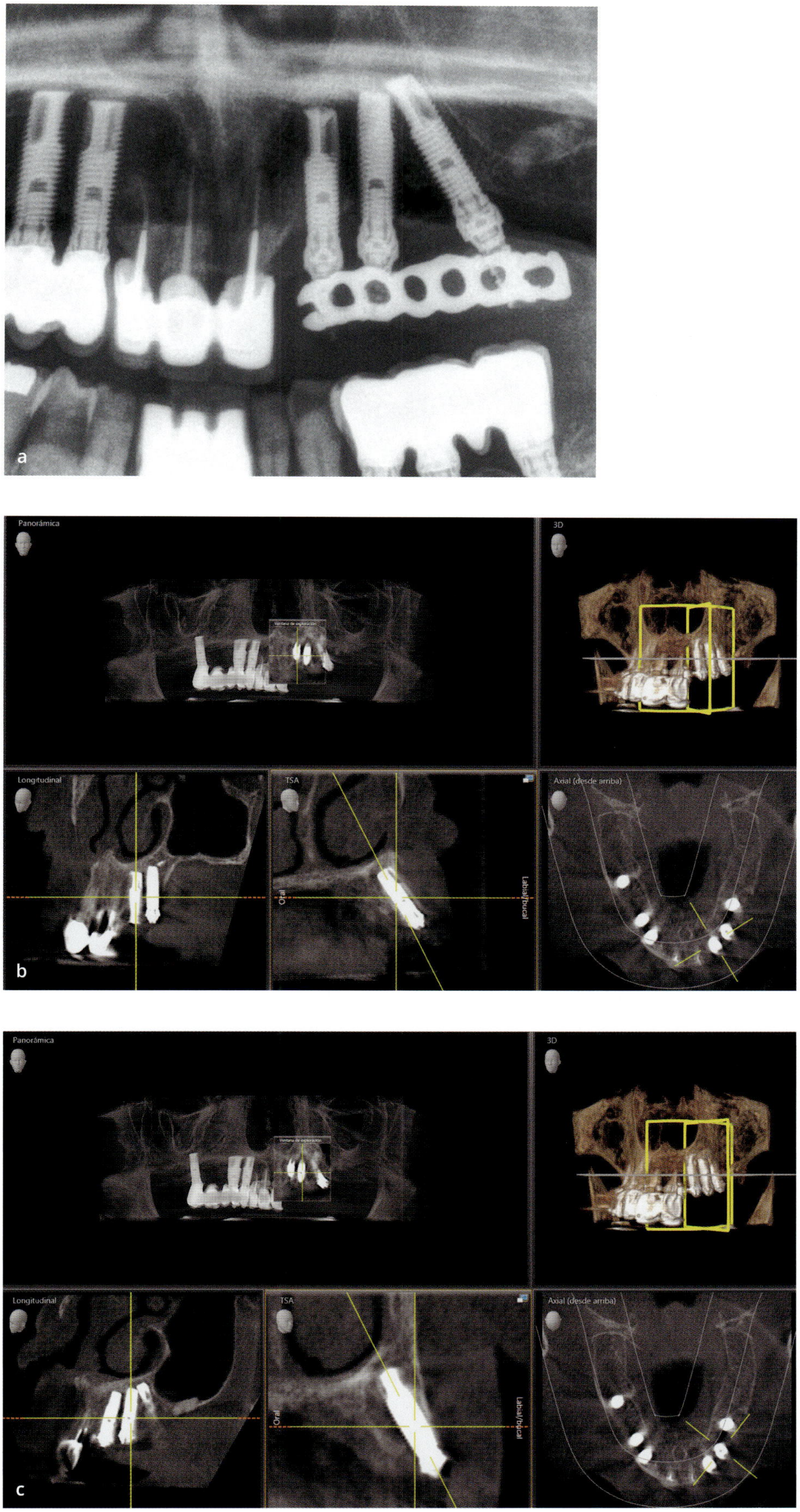


**Fig 9-14** This patient presented to our office complaining about her maxillary left implant-supported partial denture having "moved outwards" after years of service. A provisional partial denture had been adapted to the "new" position of her implants. No other symptoms were present other than very mild pain upon biting. Conventional, two-dimensional radiographic exploration showed no relevant findings except for the metal provisional framework (a). However, the CBCT scan showed that the mesial implant was buccally positioned, out of the alveolar process (b), and the central implant showed a radiolucent area around the whole implant (c).

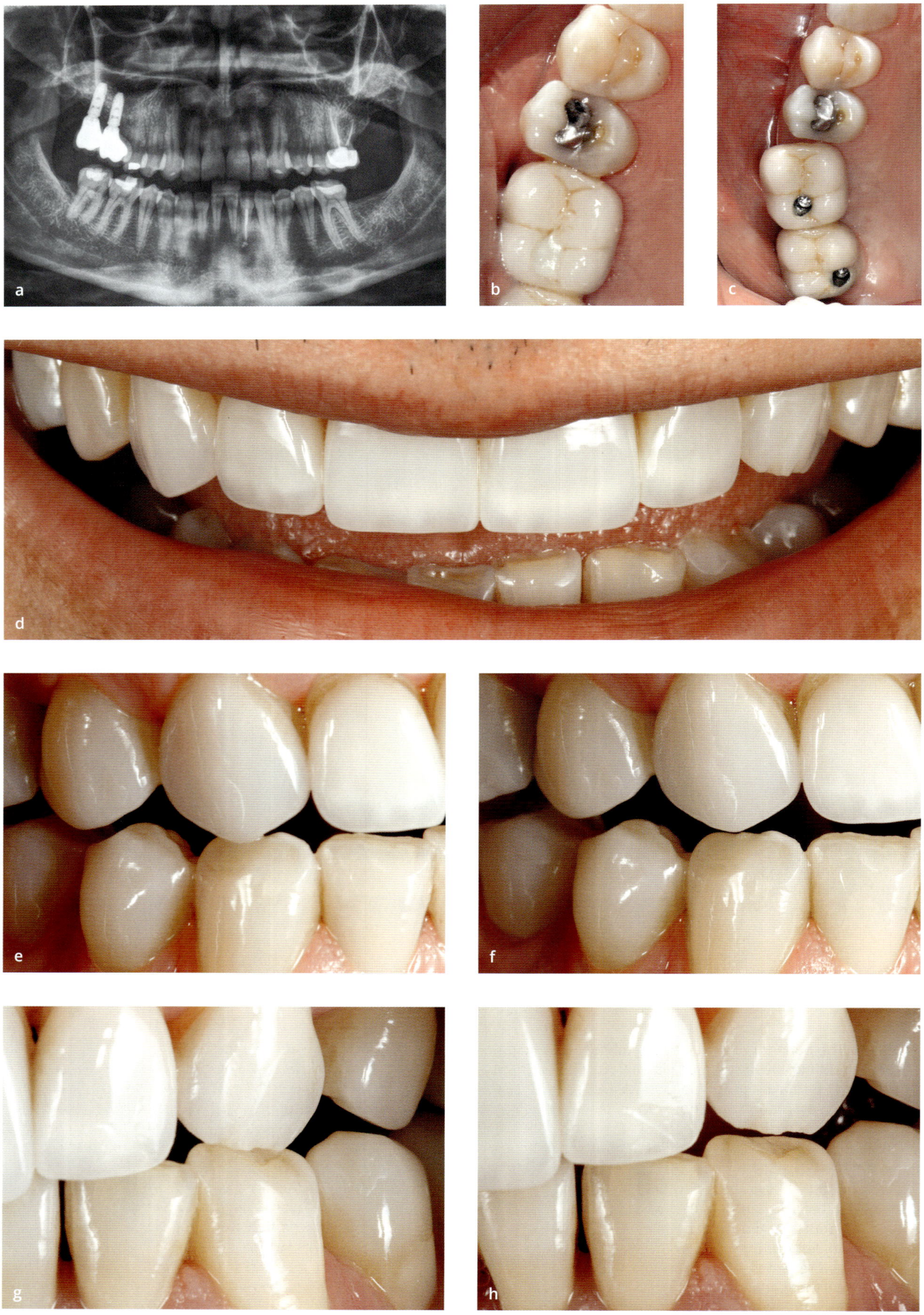
a
b
c
d
e
f
g
h

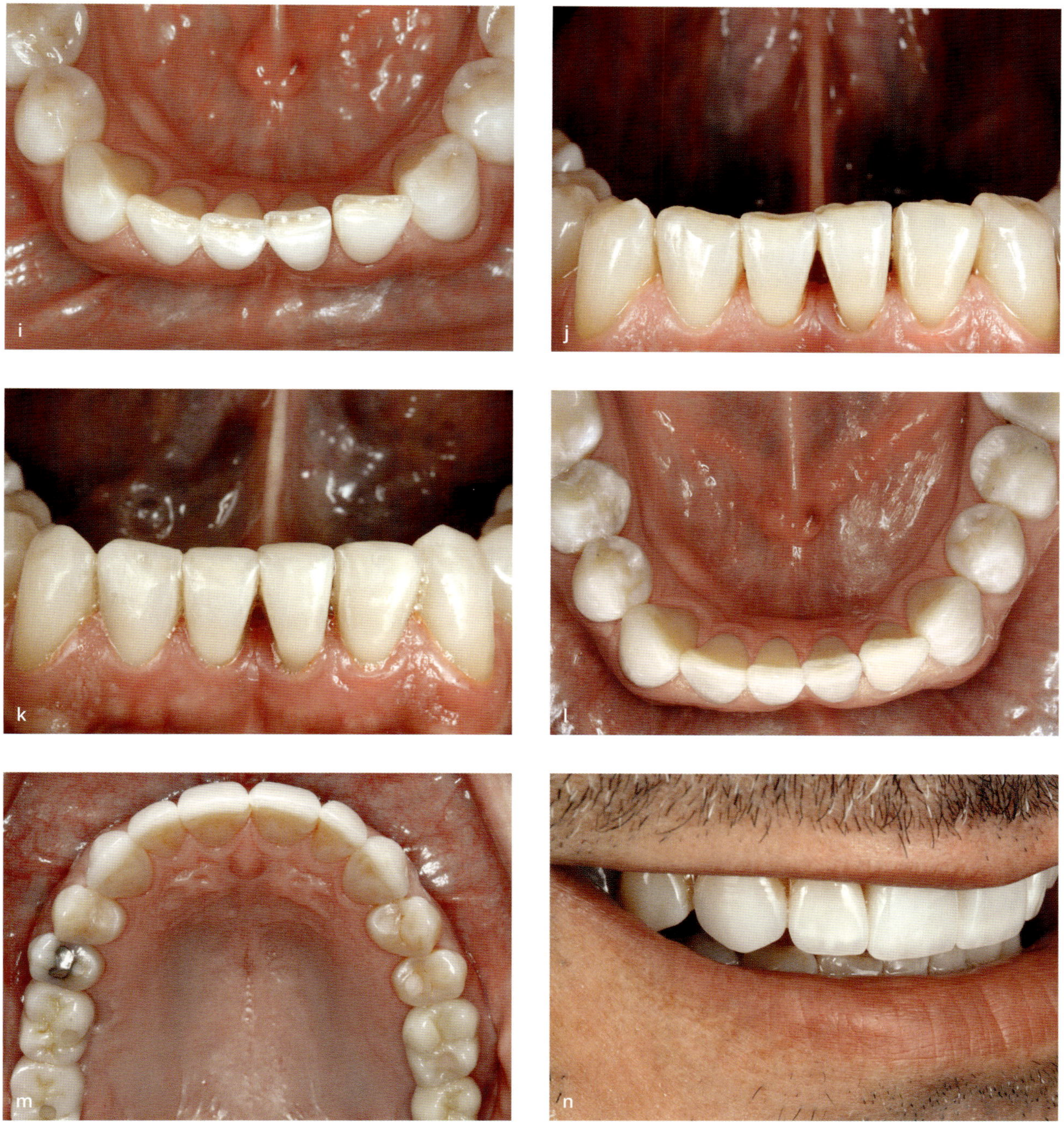

**Fig 9-15** The patient presented to the office with mild pain and reported implant restoration movement. The implants in the first quadrant had been restored via a two-implant-supported, two-unit partial denture approximately 1 year before (a and b). The two-unit partial denture appeared displaced, with a separation from the adjacent teeth (c). The diagnosis was failure of the implant restoration in the posterior sector. This semi-professional motorbike racer had a strong clenching/bruxism habit and TW that had been previously treated with porcelain laminate veneers to restore the anterior canine guidance (d). The worn mandibular teeth had not been restored and showed an impaired canine guidance and fracture of the maxillary left canine PLV (e to j). Upon clinical inspection, painful mobility of the implant restoration was apparent. After local anesthesia was administered, the partial denture was removed, and the implants came out attached to the partial denture with minimal force. After a 4-month healing period, three new implants were placed in order to compensate for the high biting forces (more implants than teeth to be restored, and one implant had a wide platform). In addition, two implants were placed in the maxillary left quadrant, on which two crowns were placed. To provide protection from parafunctional forces, mandibular TW lesions were restored by means of direct composite (k and l). The occlusal surfaces of the new implant-supported restorations follow the guidelines mentioned above (m). The canine guidance is improved in an easy-to-repair approach with direct composite on the mandibular teeth (n to p). *(continued next page)*

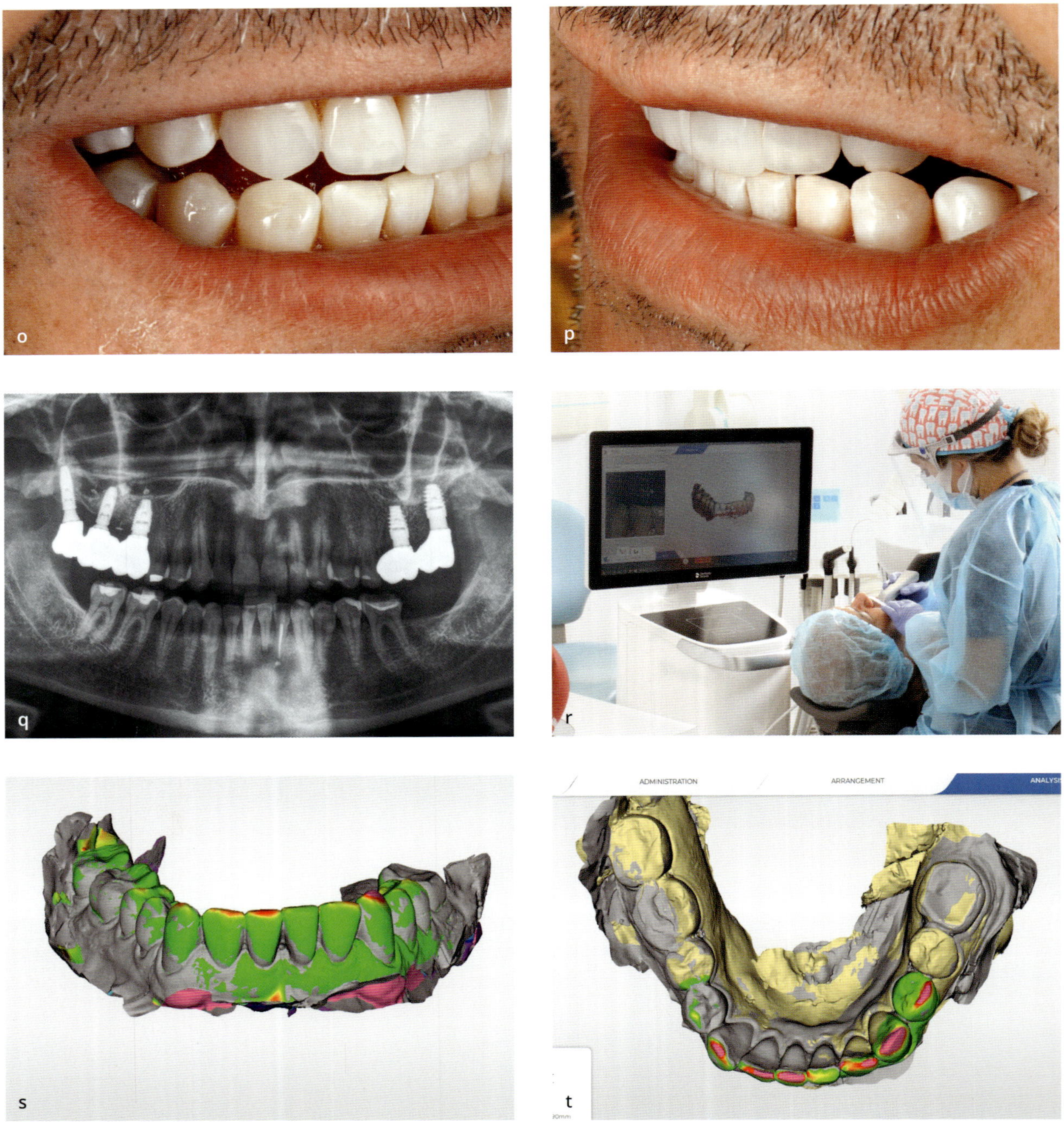


**Fig 9-15** *(continued)* The porcelain veneer on the maxillary left canine will be changed, and a new implant will be placed in the mandible after the race season (q and r). TW progression and restoration wear is to be digitally monitored with intraoral scans (OraCheck by Dentsply Sirona) (s and t). In addition to the regular Michigan-type nightguard (u), this patient has been instructed to wear a soft maxillary and mandibular Essix splint while participating in motorbike racing (v and w).

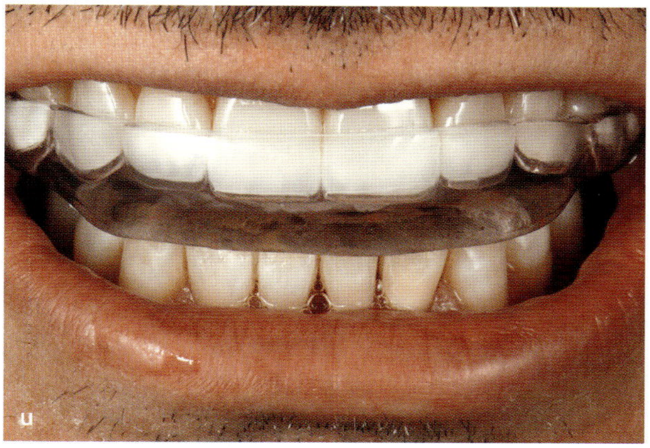
u

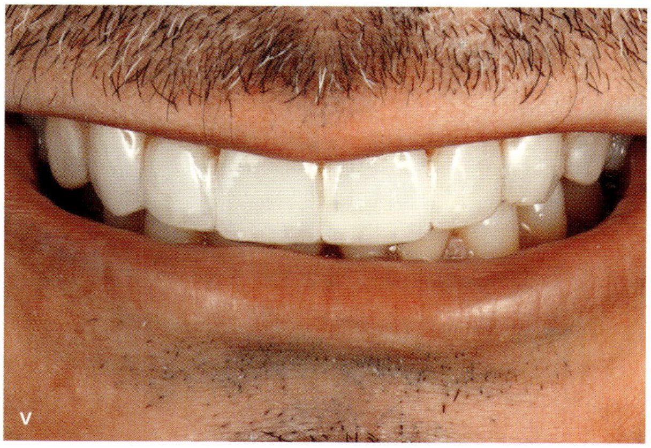
v

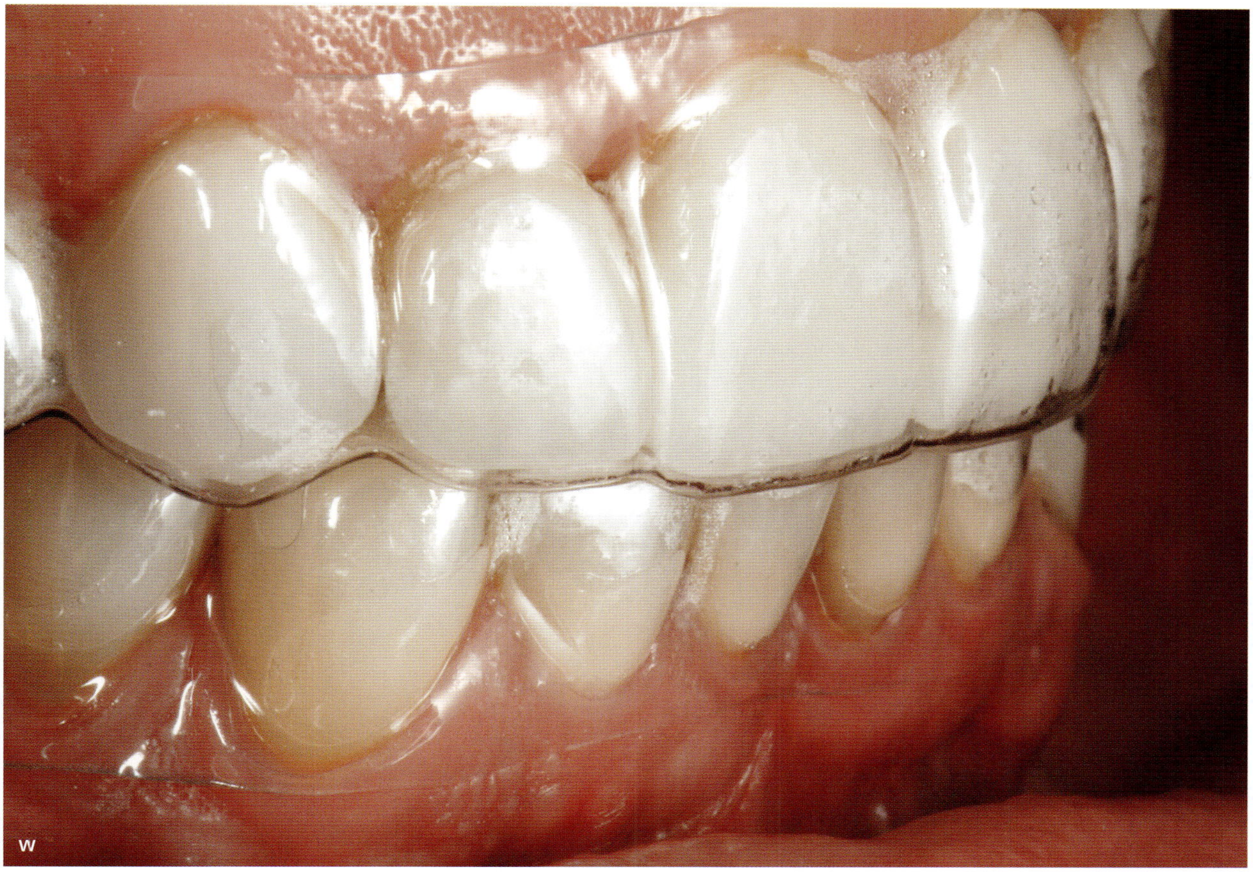
w

## 4. Implants and Occlusal Space in Patients with Severe TW: Management of Vertical Collapse

Several conditions or situations can lead to severe TW. For instance, eating disorders (EDs), prolonged stress, an unbalanced diet or abuse of acidic food and drinks, and gastric reflux (see chapter 3). The mechanism of tooth wear aggravation is both direct and indirect:

- Gastric acids severely erode enamel and dentin.
- Patients with ED usually suffer from malnutrition and hyposalivation—the quality and quantity of saliva is altered, and the protective mechanism provided by saliva is disrupted.
- Acidic food, stress, and a hyperconnected lifestyle all add erosive factors as well as tooth-to-tooth wear.
- Medication aggravates TW through impairment of saliva protection.

These patients are not only at high risk for rapid TW but are also prone to suffer from premature tooth loss and occlusal collapse. In fact, as explained earlier, they may also be more likely than the general population to lose osseointegrated implants. The reason behind this can be easily understood considering the higher rate of TW suffered by these patients, especially those with EDs, which can lead to premature occlusal contacts on implant restorations. This puts these restorations at risk of repeated trauma and overload. Additionally, factoring in the possible malnutrition suffered by these patients (and therefore poor bone metabolism and anti-inflammatory mechanisms), there is certainly a need for frequent occlusal checkups for these individuals. Furthermore, preventive or active treatment for TW is highly endorsed.

One critical consequence of the VDO collapse in severe TW is the diminished restorative space and the inherent difficulties for implant provisionalization. As in any case of TW, the restoration of the occlusal support should start with the mandibular teeth, then maxillary posterior teeth, and finally the anterior maxillary teeth together with the restoration of the anterior and canine guidance.

Scheduling the surgery at the correct time and with the correct VDO are key for a good surgical and prosthetic outcome, that is, once the posterior occlusal support that provides sufficient restorative space has been established. The lack of interocclusal space and the principle of preserving tooth structure pose a hidden difficulty. Provisionalization and immediate loading in severe TW can be highly advantageous.

A thorough case analysis is fundamental as a prompt surgical intervention without the appropriate occlusal scaffold will risk the overall outcome. Compensatory eruption in cases of severe TW in need of one or more implants has to be counteracted before addressing the tooth or teeth to be replaced, particularly if the challenge has had an erosive origin (Figs 9-16 to 9-35).

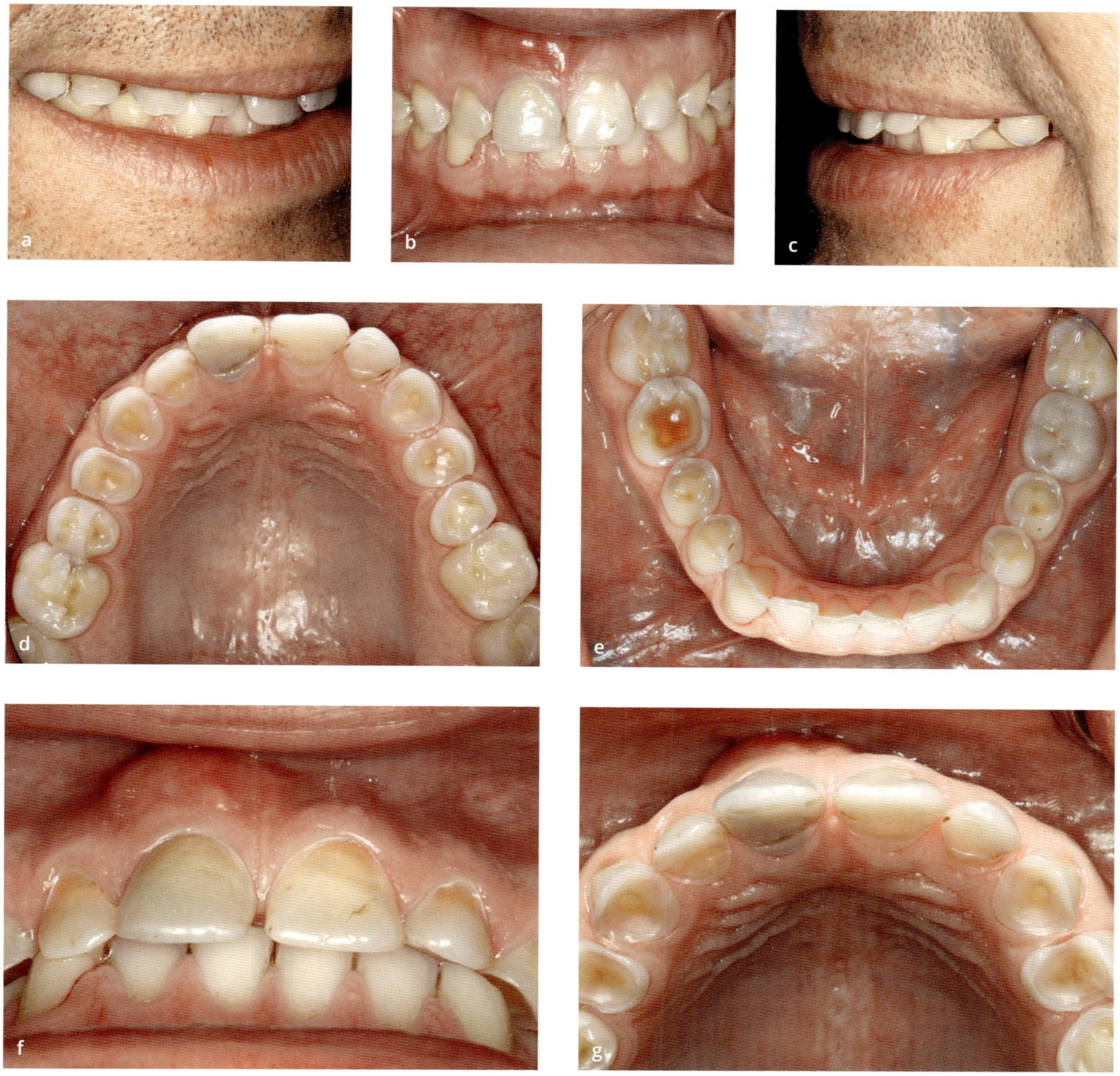


**Fig 9-16** Severe wear in a young male patient with non-relevant medical history except for a demanding, stressful professional life that had him connected 24/7. The patient's main concerns at his first visit were a desire to improve his smile and address a "lump" over his maxillary right central incisor, which remained after several endodontic treatment attempts in the past. The severe TW had already destroyed most of the tooth anatomy and negatively impacted the VDO (a to c). The erosive damage to the whole occlusal anatomy, including the palatal aspect of the maxillary anterior teeth, had been accompanied by compensatory eruption, leaving no interocclusal space for potential restorations (d to f). The patient had previously received localized, tooth-oriented treatments with poor results, and the abscess on the maxillary right central incisor had become a routine episode. Posterior sectors will have to be treated first in order to recover the VDO, as compensatory eruption has occupied the entire interocclusal space. The goal is to have an implant immediately placed at the time of extraction of the maxillary right central incisor, restored with an implant-retained crown (g).

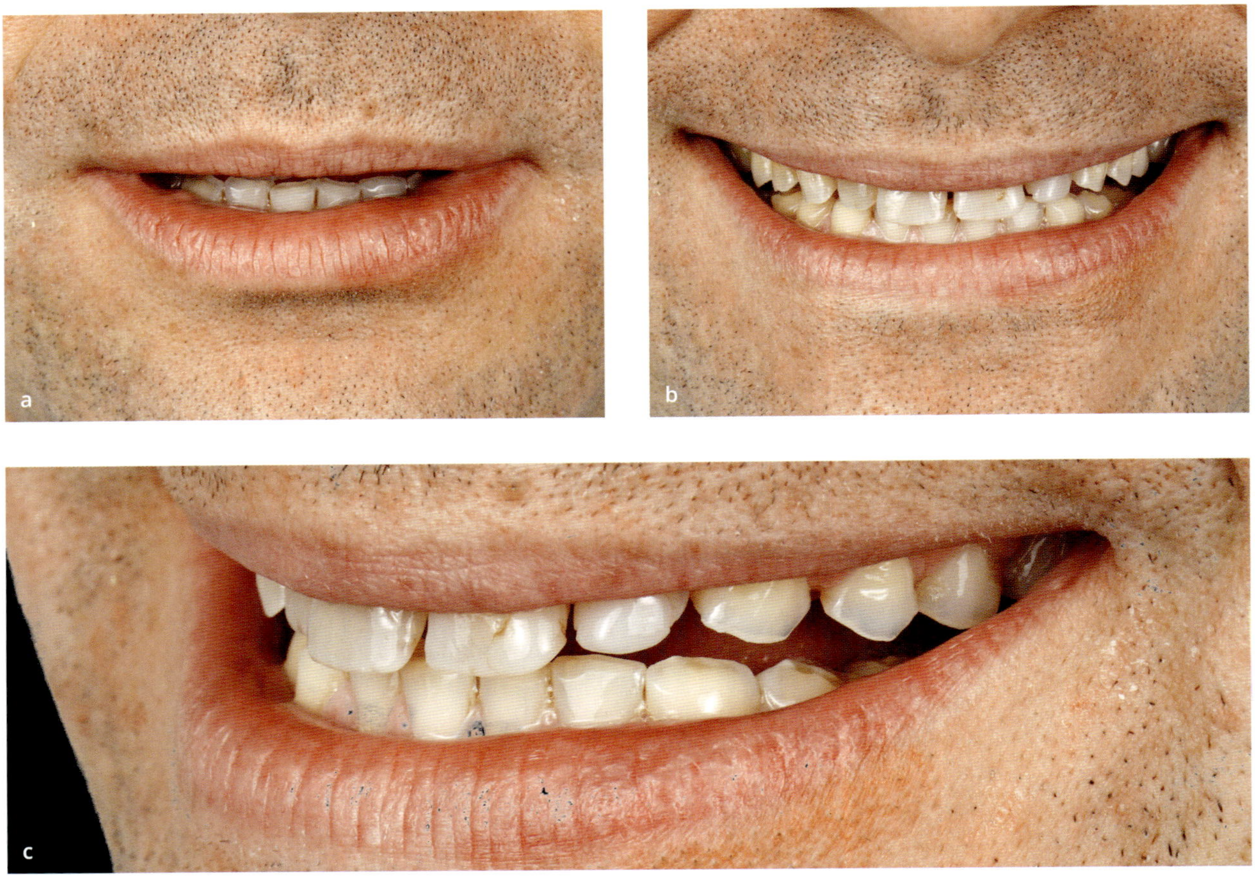

**Fig 9-17** The study of the smile reveals generalized, uniform damage to the overall esthetic appearance (a to c).

**Fig 9-18** *(right page)* Radiographic and CBCT examination (a and b) and intraoral scanning were performed (d to g). The CBCT shows an intraosseous lesion without history of trauma or caries. The CBCT as well as the intraoral and face scans are part of the digital data needed for diagnosis, planning, and treatment. The wear is probably partially responsible for the deterioration of the maxillary right central incisor, and after clinical and radiographical exploration, it is deemed to have a hopeless prognosis.

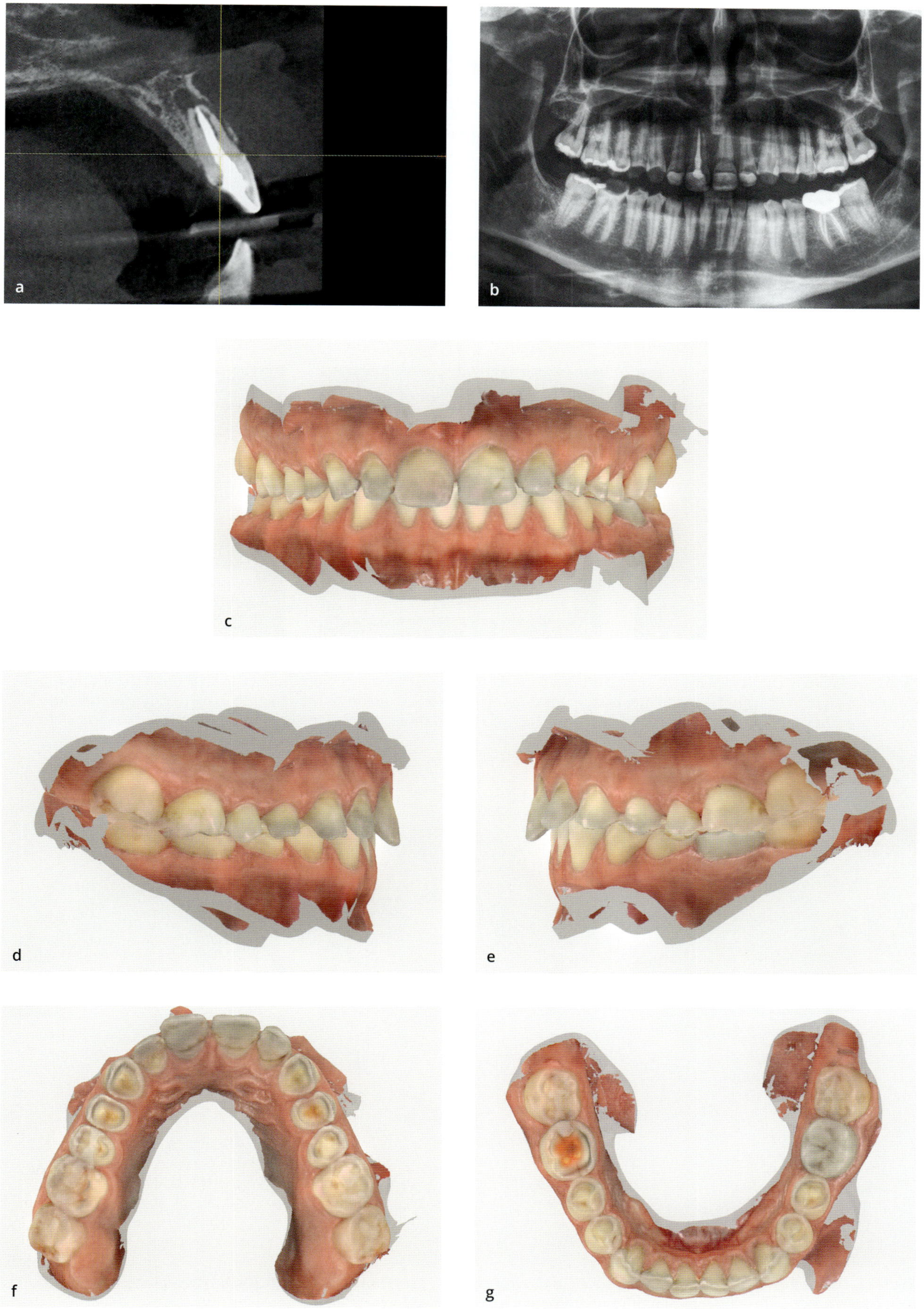
a
b
c
d
e
f
g

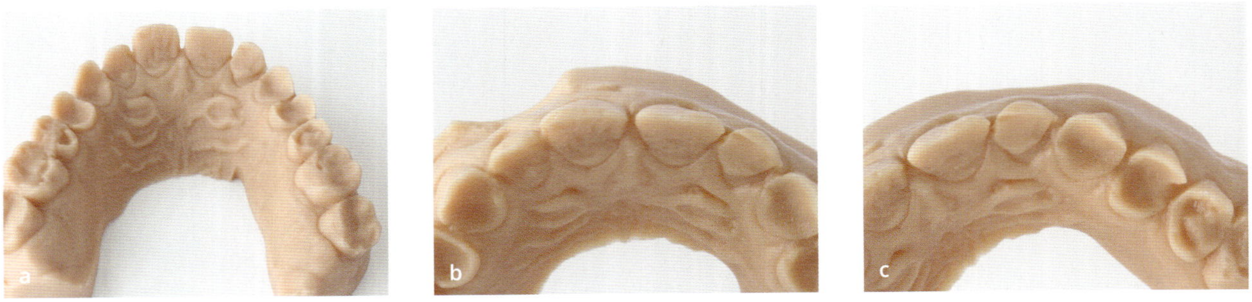


**Fig 9-19** Initial printed models. Note the saucer-like, severely eroded overall anatomy and sharp enamel edges (a to c). Once dentin is exposed to the oral cavity, erosive damage progresses more quickly than on enamel.

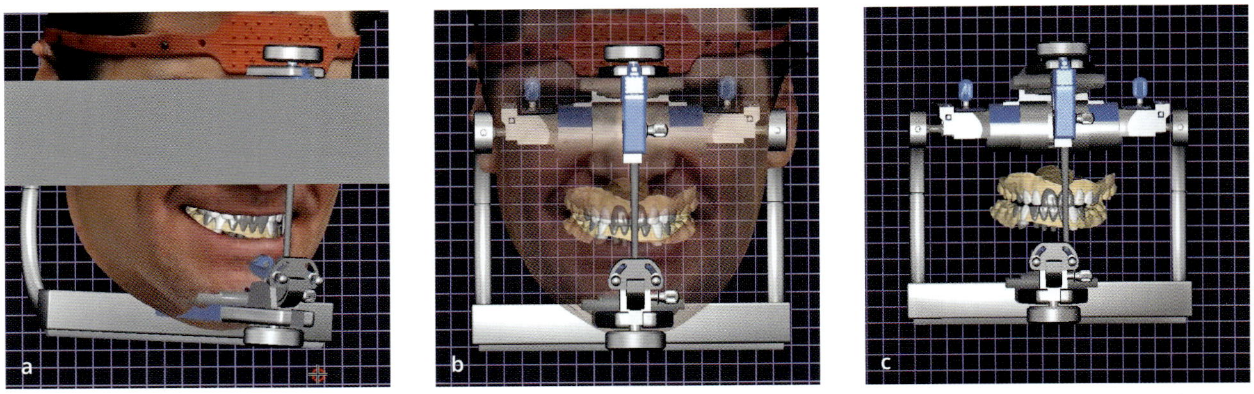


**Fig 9-20** The virtual setup is the frame in which the digital smile setup will be assessed first. The use of a virtual articulator helps the lab to accurately place the digital mock-up in the correct spatial dimensions (a to c). Even though the mock-up will only be applied in the anterior zone, the wax-up includes all teeth to be restored. The changes in arch width, overjet, and overbite as well as VDO are built into the digital wax-up and tested three-dimensionally by means of the virtual articulator.

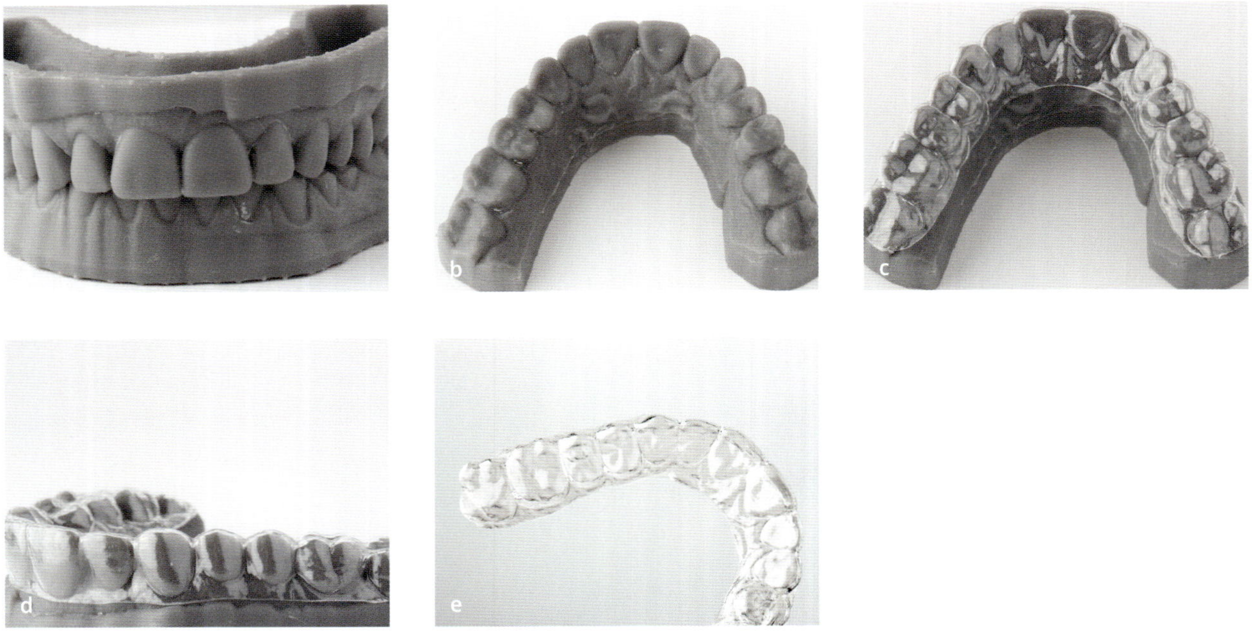


**Fig 9-21** Once the digital mock-up is approved, a model is printed (a and b) and a thin (0.20-mm) transparent Essix-like mock-up is vacuum-formed over the printed model (c to e).

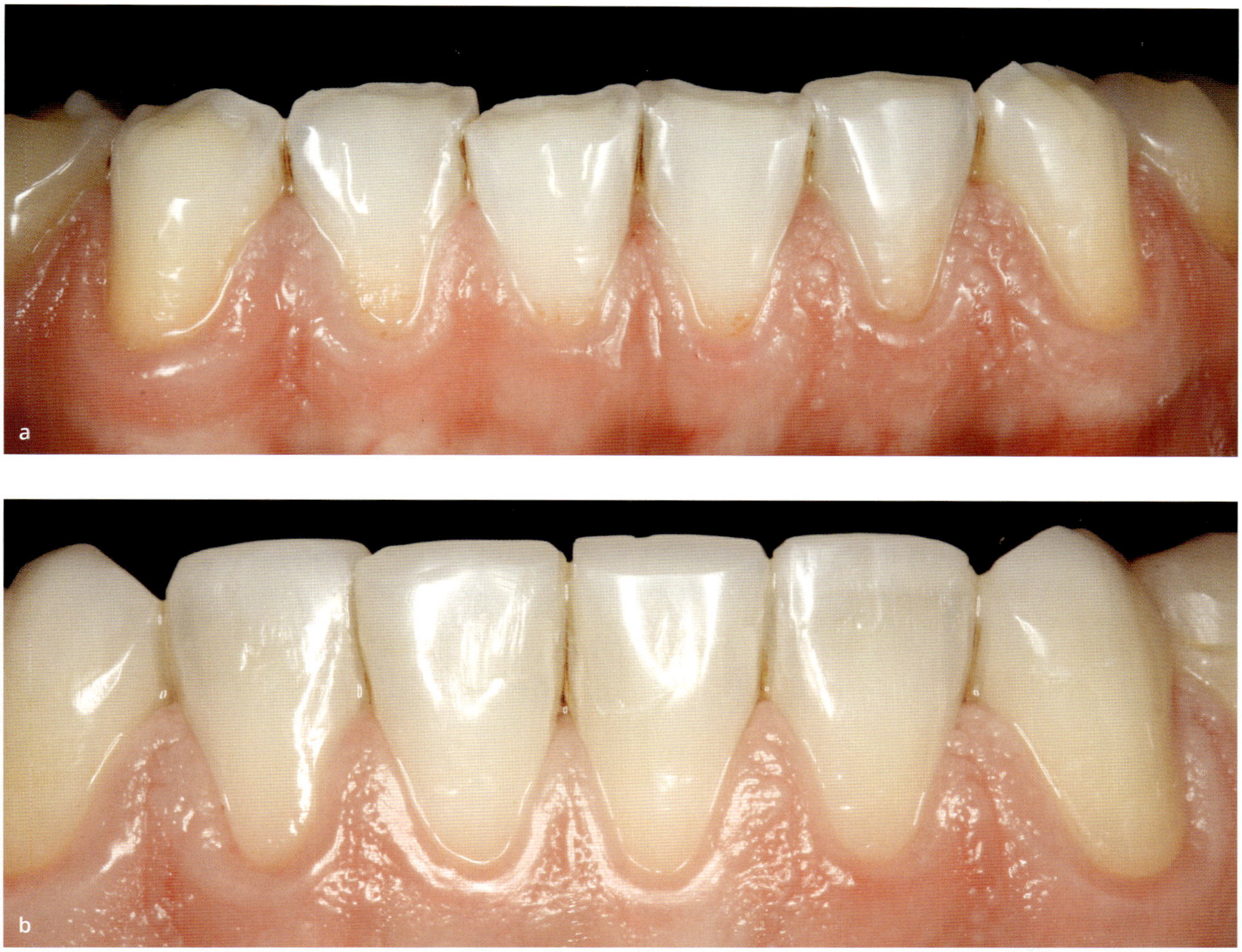


**Fig 9-22** Direct freehand composite is chosen for the mandibular anterior teeth (a and b), and indirect PICN (Enamic, VITA) overlays are selected for the posterior mandibular teeth at the planned VDO.

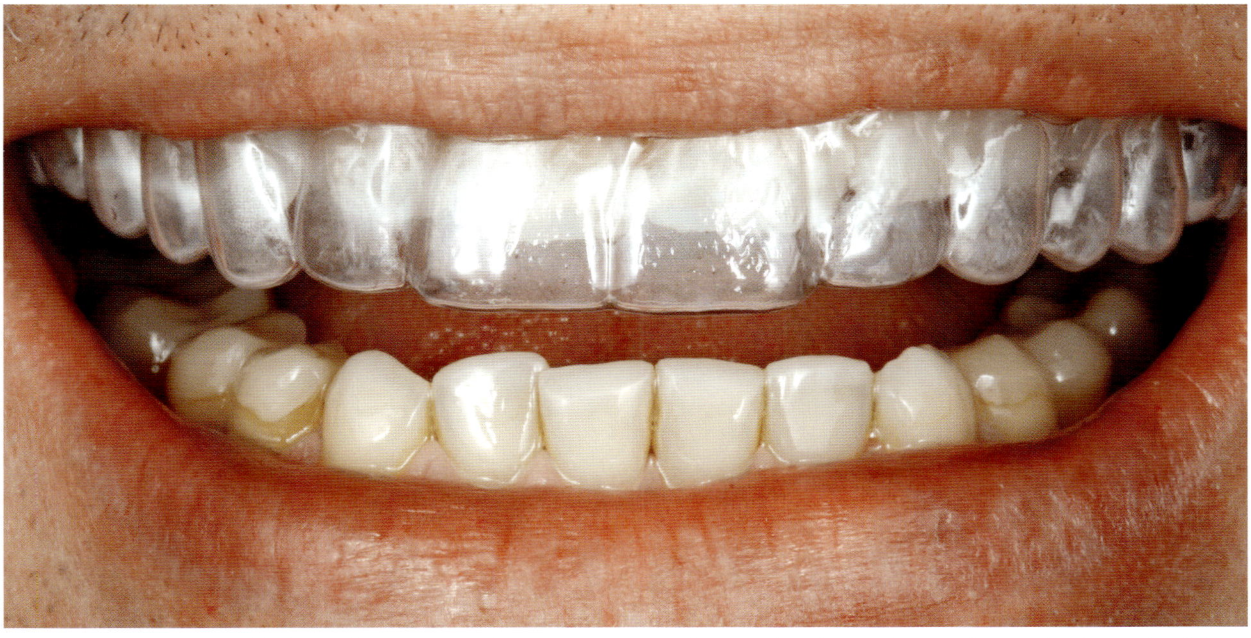

**Fig 9-23** Once the mandibular arch is restored, the transparent mock-up is placed over the maxillary arch. The try-in of the Essix-like mock-up shows the patient how much the maxillary teeth will be lengthened.

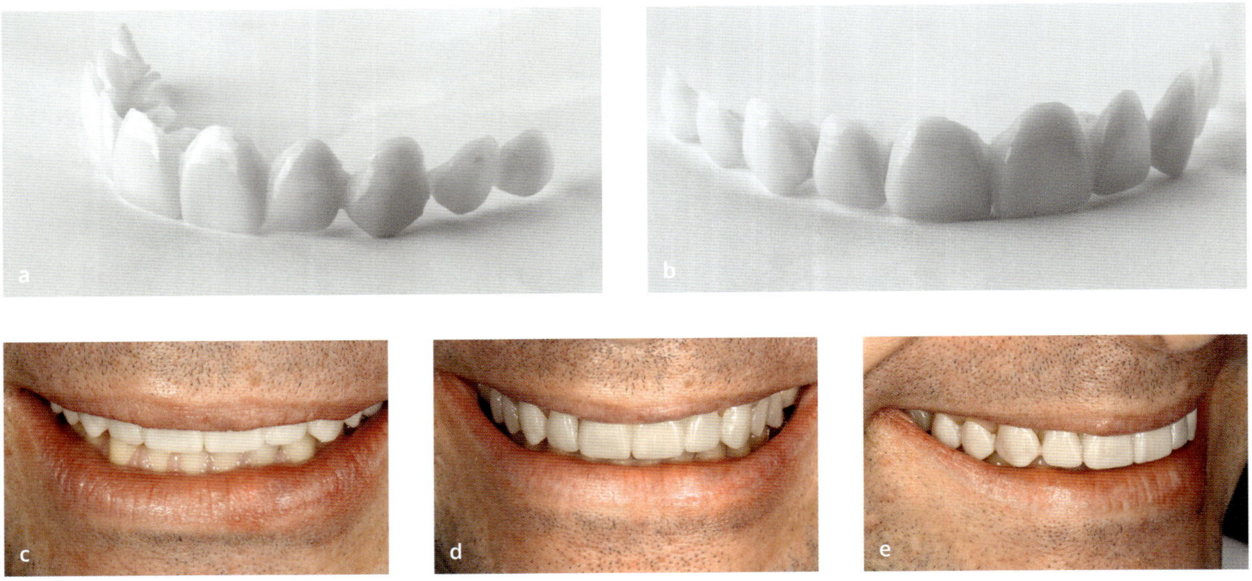

**Fig 9-24** In this case a cutback mock-up (a and b) is also tested intraorally, since the difference between the patient's anatomy and the previewed final restoration had to be fully understood and accepted by the patient. The initial digital wax-up and VDO serve as the blueprint throughout the whole process (c to e).

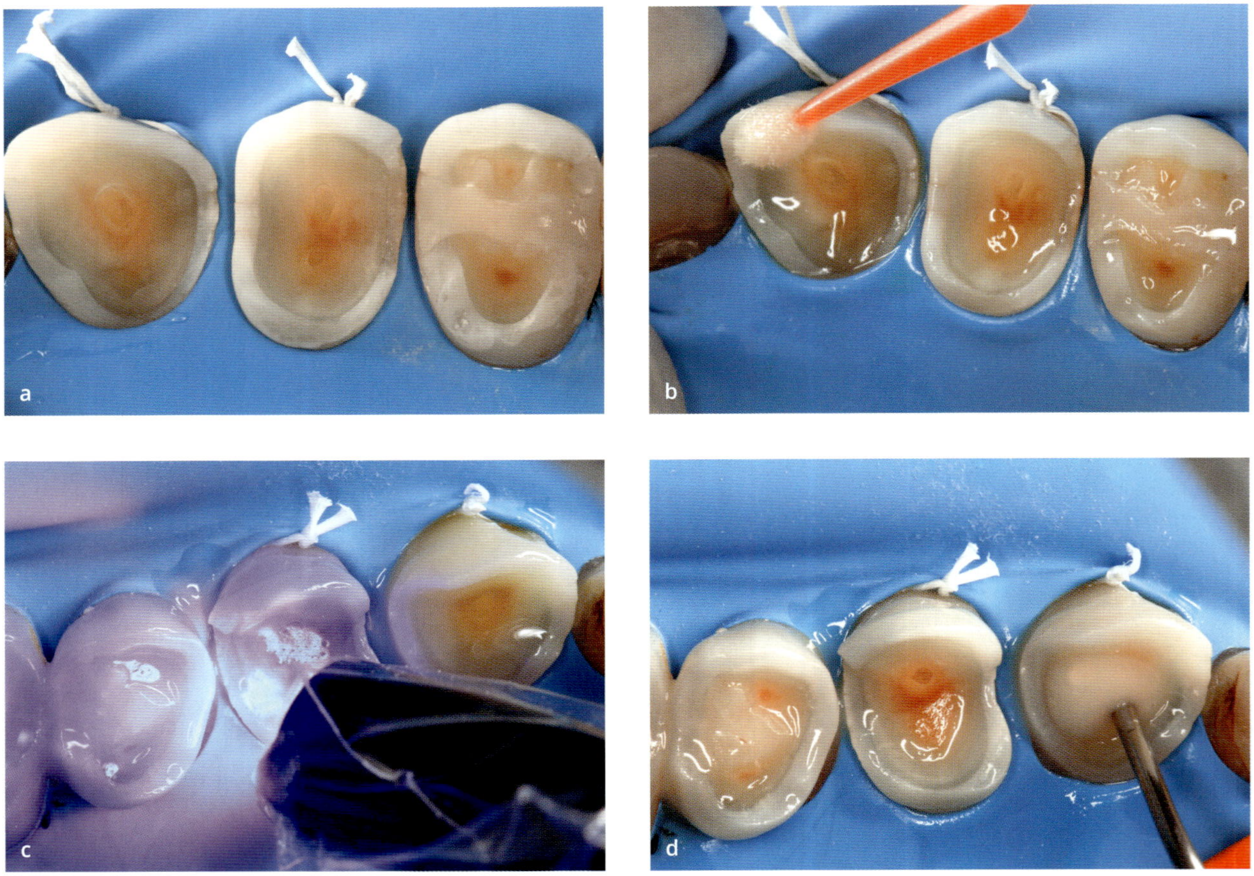

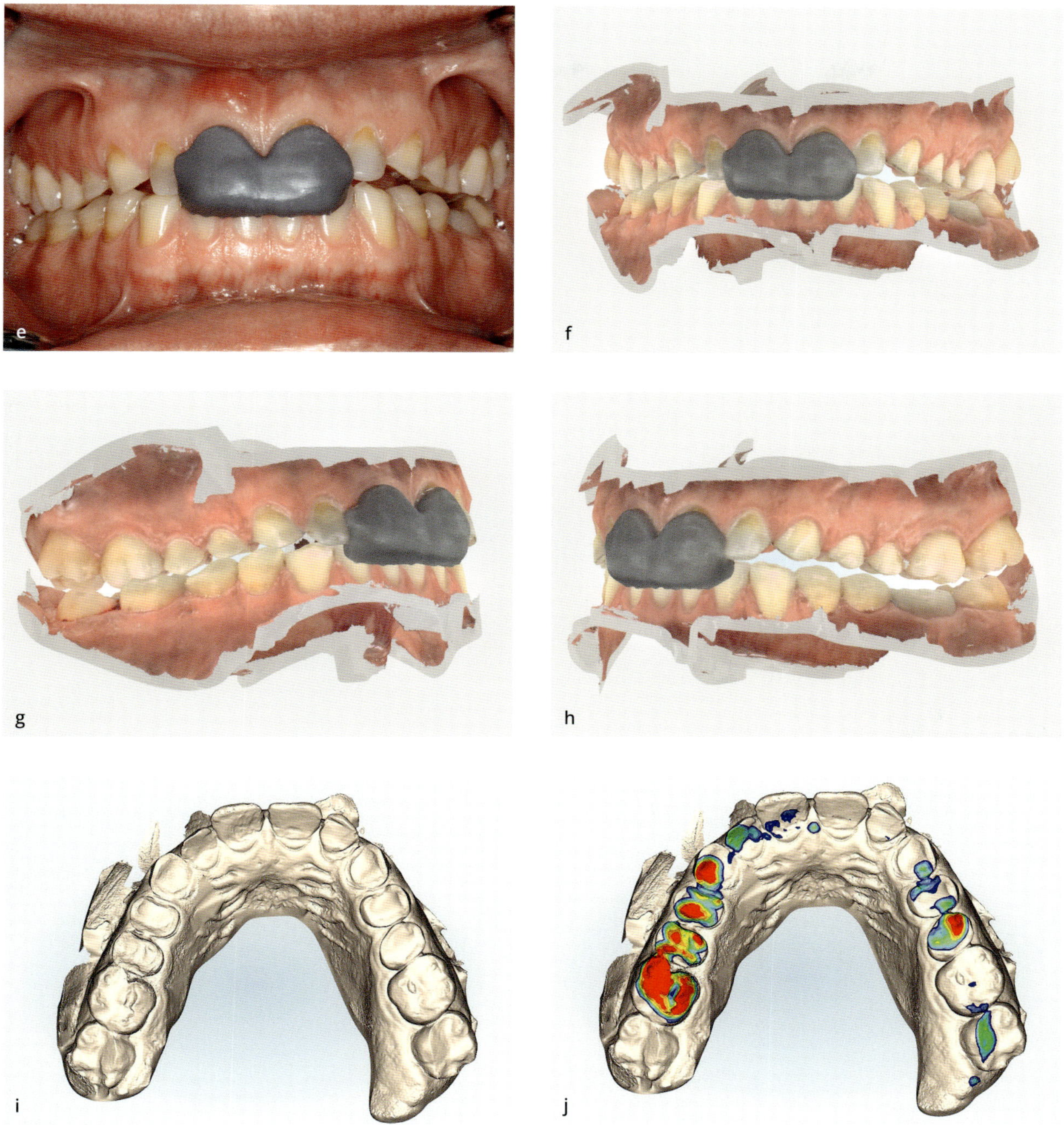


**Fig 9-25** One of the challenges of severe TW lies in the difficulties of stable provisionalization, as the overall vertical collapse imposes restrictions on the immediate temporalization of an implant. The principle of tooth structure preservation dictates avoiding the elimination of tooth structure as much as possible. In this case, as explained in previous chapters, the maxillary posterior teeth were restored after the mandibular arch had been completely restored at the chosen VDO. The severely damaged premolars and canines were evened out using flowable composite to avoid concave areas (a to d). Afterwards, this composite layer was gently roughened with a diamond bur as no preparation is needed or recommended, and an intraoral scanner was used to capture the prepared teeth. The superimposition and cross-mounting of the intraoral acquisitions saves time and procedures for the patient and the dentist. Alternatively, an analog work flow can be chosen. Once the VDO had been achieved, the extraction and implant surgery were performed. If it is preferred to do the surgery beforehand, these occlusal changes must be accounted for in the complete treatment. In order to stabilize the CR at the chosen VDO, a previously created printed jig was placed over the anterior teeth (e to h). The STL was processed at the lab; note the irregular occlusal contacts throughout the whole arch (i and j).

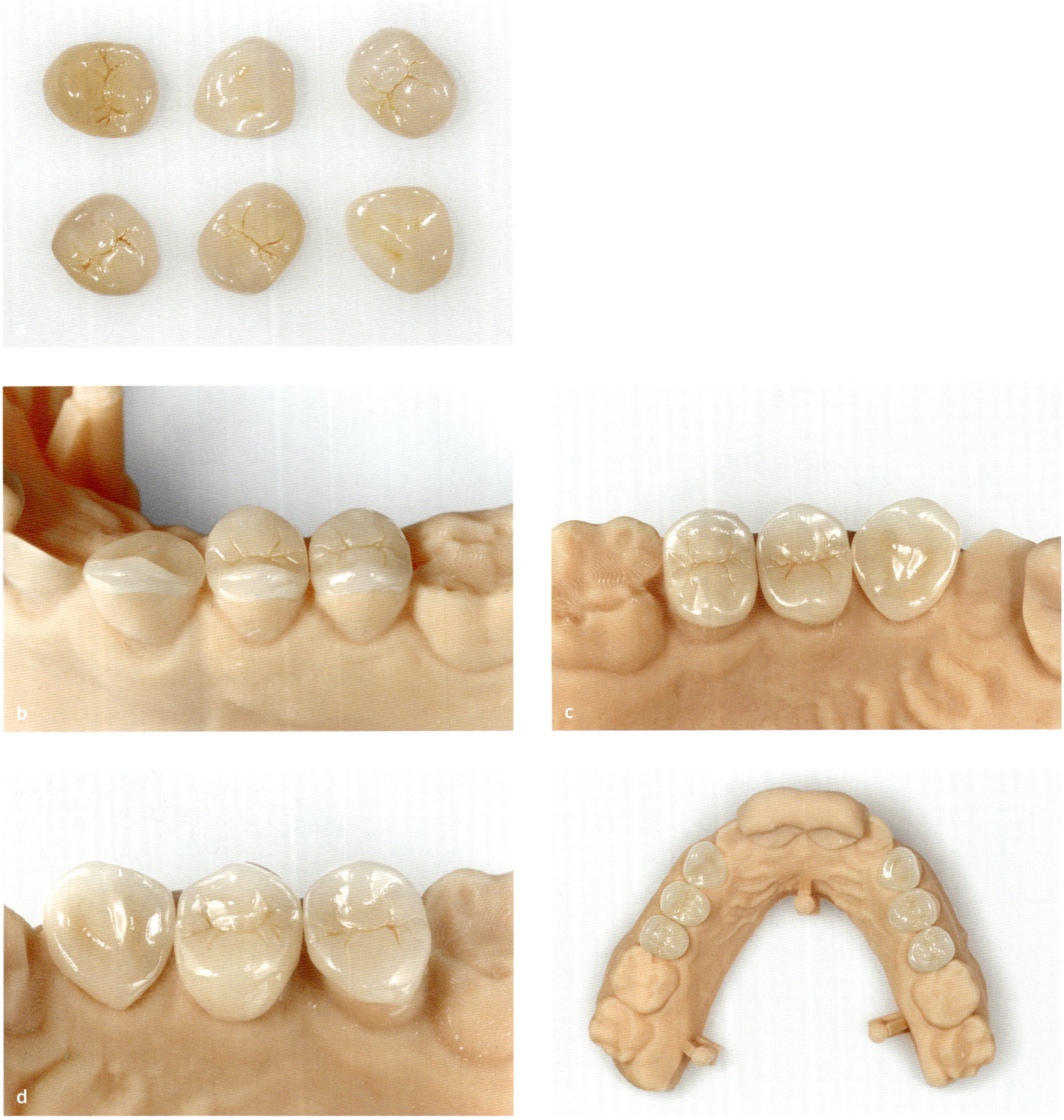

**Fig 9-26** The maxillary PICN overlays (Enamic), including for the palatal aspect of both canines, were milled at the chosen VDO and CR. The printed model reproduces the CR jig as the intraoral acquisition was done with it in place (a to e). The maxillary molars were planned to be directly restored with freehand composite as they had been relatively spared from the erosive attack in comparison with the rest of the maxillary teeth.

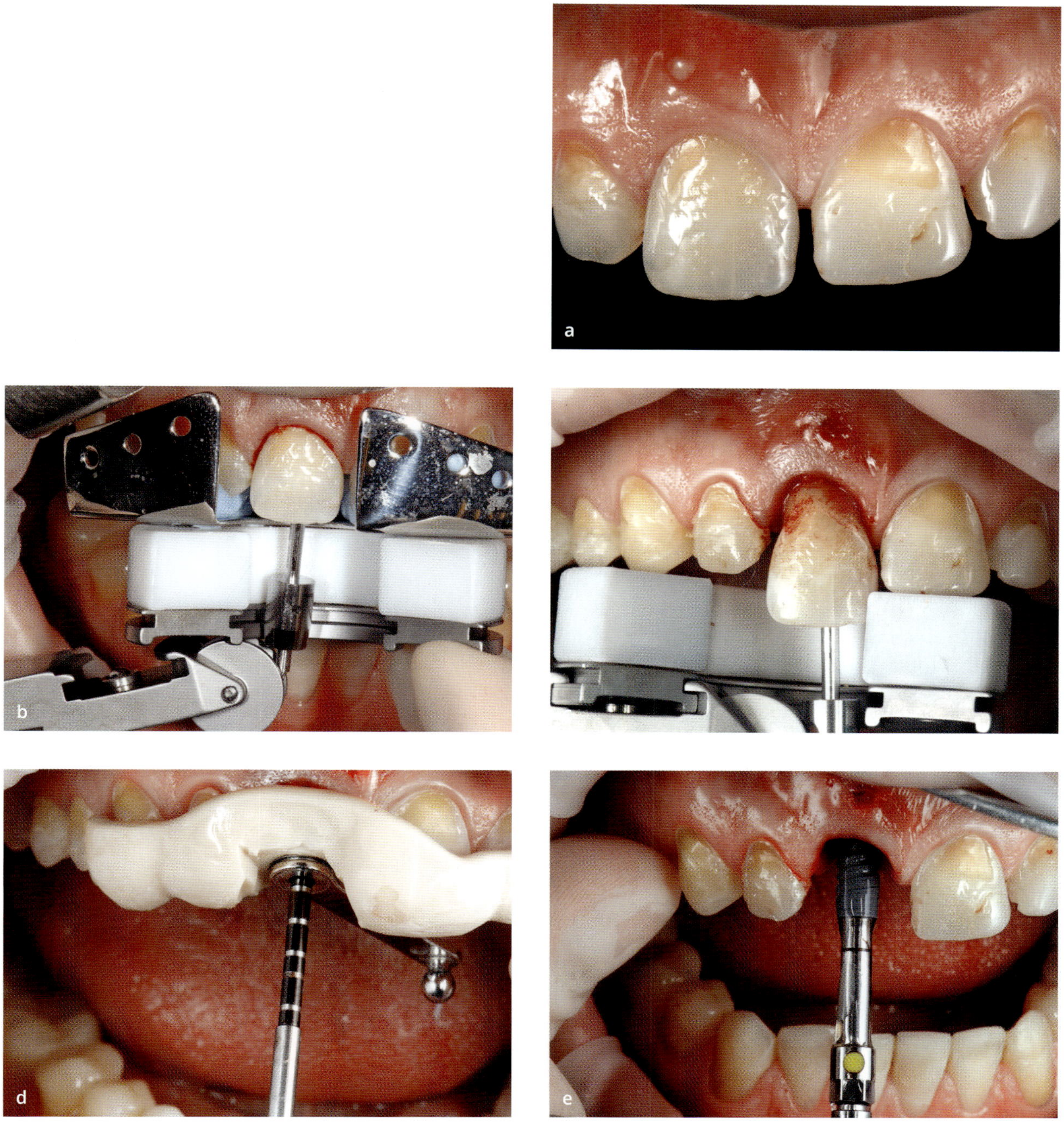


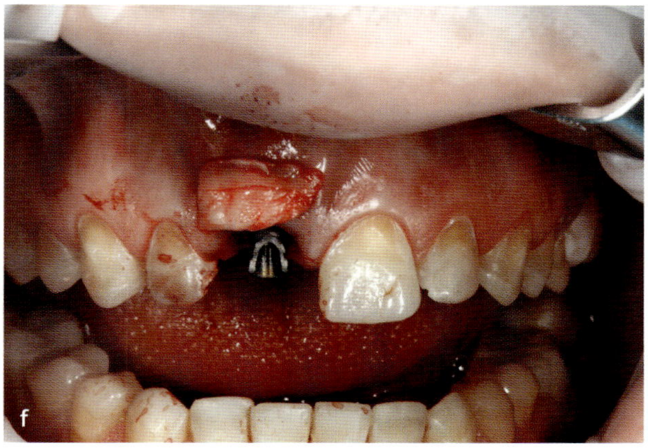


**Fig 9-27** At this stage, the VDO had been augmented with the posterior support provided by the restorations, and the surgery could be performed within a more convenient occlusal scenario (a). The extraction protocol was done without disrupting the overall gingival architecture. An immediate implant was placed with a surgical guide derived from the integration of the CBCT, face scan, and navigation software (DTX Studio, Envista) (b to f). A subepithelial connective tissue graft (CTG) as well as a particulate xenograft fill of the bone-to-implant gap were performed to try to counteract the expected volumetric resorption and thus improve the final esthetic outcome. The tuberosity was the donor site for the CTG in this case, since the highly fibrous characteristics of this area may provide long-term stability of the volumetric gain.

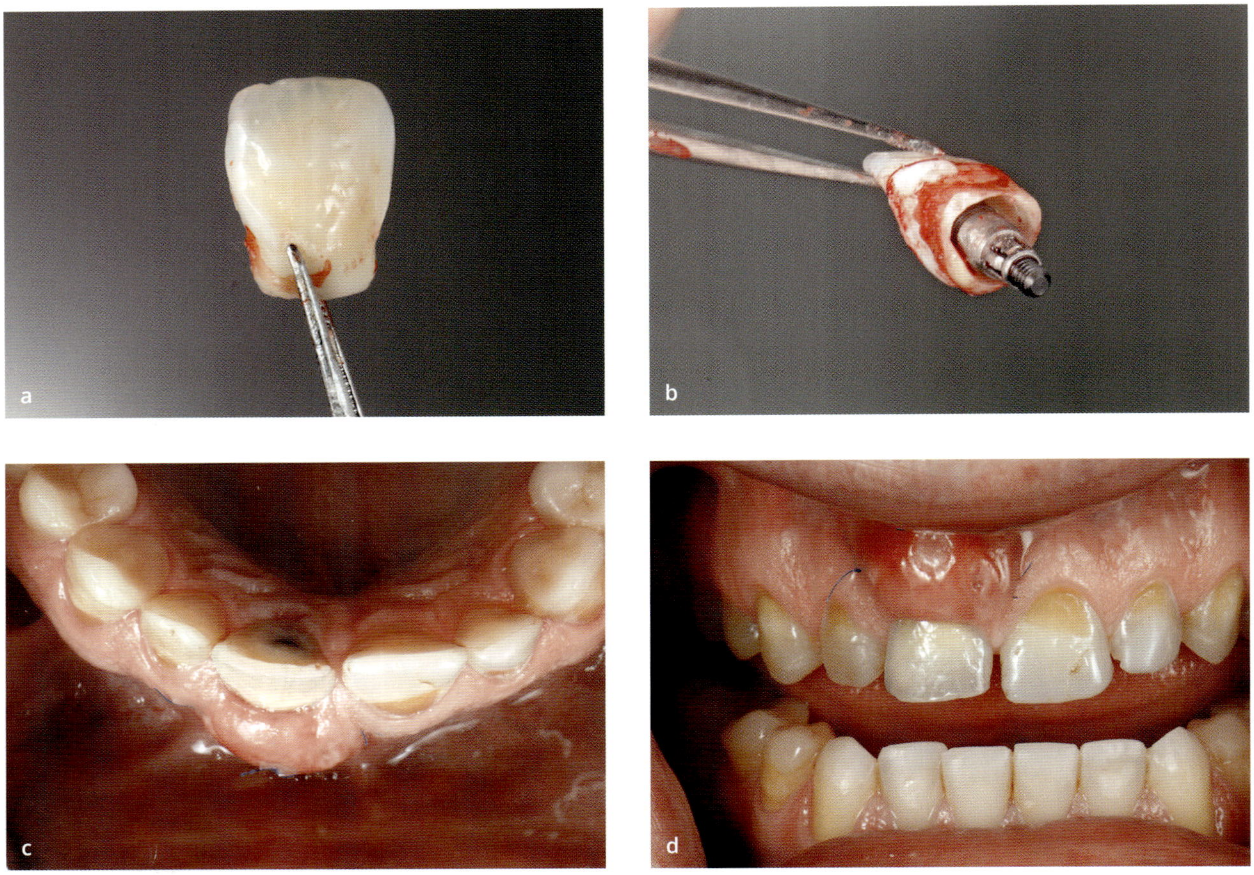

**Fig 9-28** A provisional restoration was fabricated using the patient's hollowed crown with a temporary titanium abutment in order to maintain the natural emergence profile of the tooth (a to d).

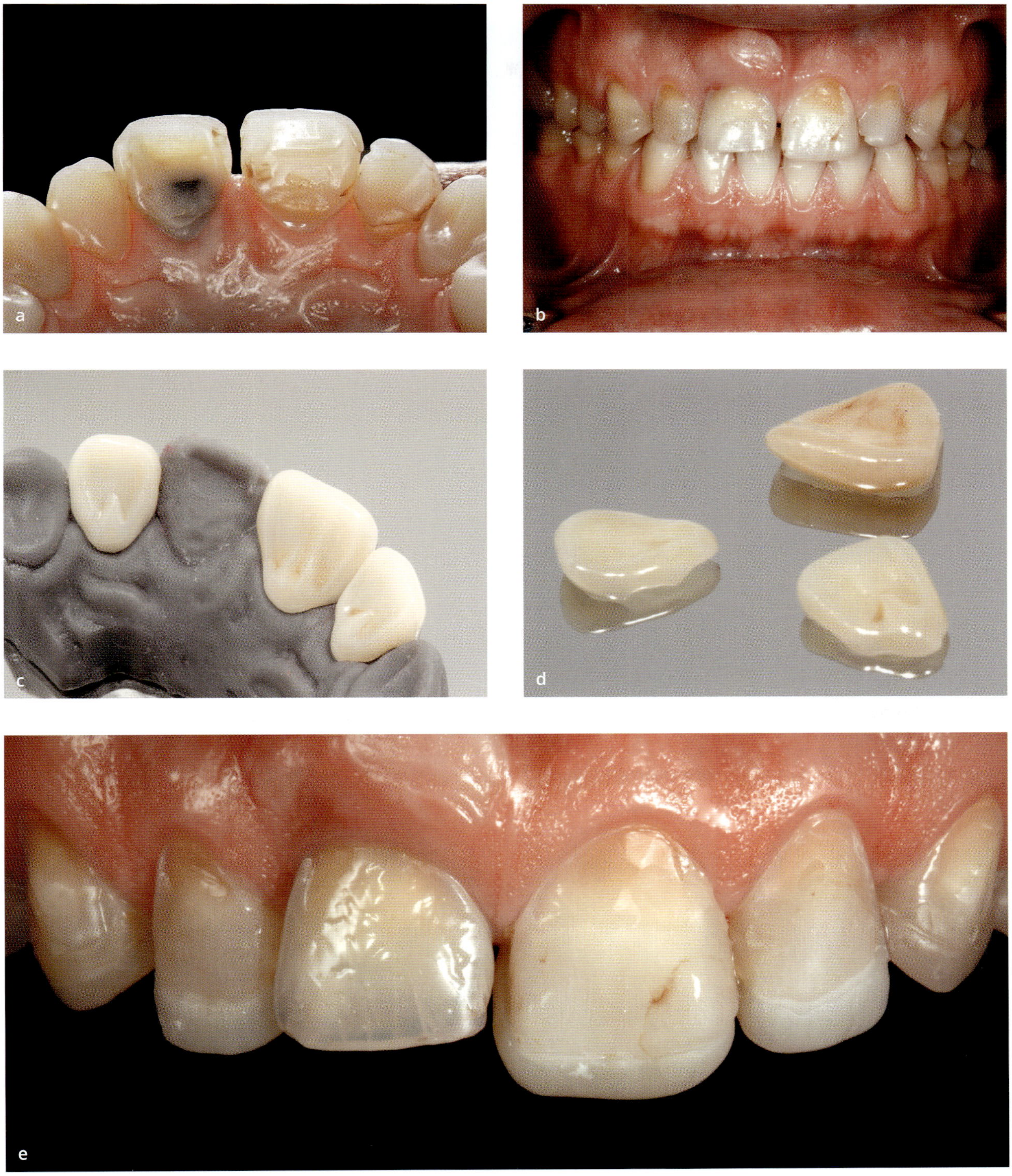

**Fig 9-29** The palatal aspect of the three anterior incisors was planned to be restored with palatal onlays (a to e); the canines had already been restored with onlays at the same time as the premolars (see Fig 9-26). The new length of the anterior teeth was built into the palatal onlays. The implant provisional crown was still the original patient's hollowed tooth with the natural anatomy and length. A shallow preparation was done before a silicone impression was taken and sent to the lab. Note the translucent halos of the three palatal onlays that were visible at the incisal margins until the buccal indirect PLVs were delivered to nine maxillary teeth. In this case, a handmade (analog) flow was chosen for the feldspathic PLVs and the final implant-retained crown. Some authors recommend letting the patient experience the new VDO for some weeks before proceeding with further phases of treatment. If the patient declares discomfort or difficulties, VDO is adjusted until approved before anterior and canine guidance are addressed. In this case, the patient was pleased from the first moment as he was conscious of the considerable collapse his muscles and facial anatomy had suffered as a result of the severe destruction. However, unless the anterior sector is restored directly or the restorations are done on the same day, in any case 1 or 2 weeks will pass before cementation, allowing time for minor adjustments on the posterior restorations.

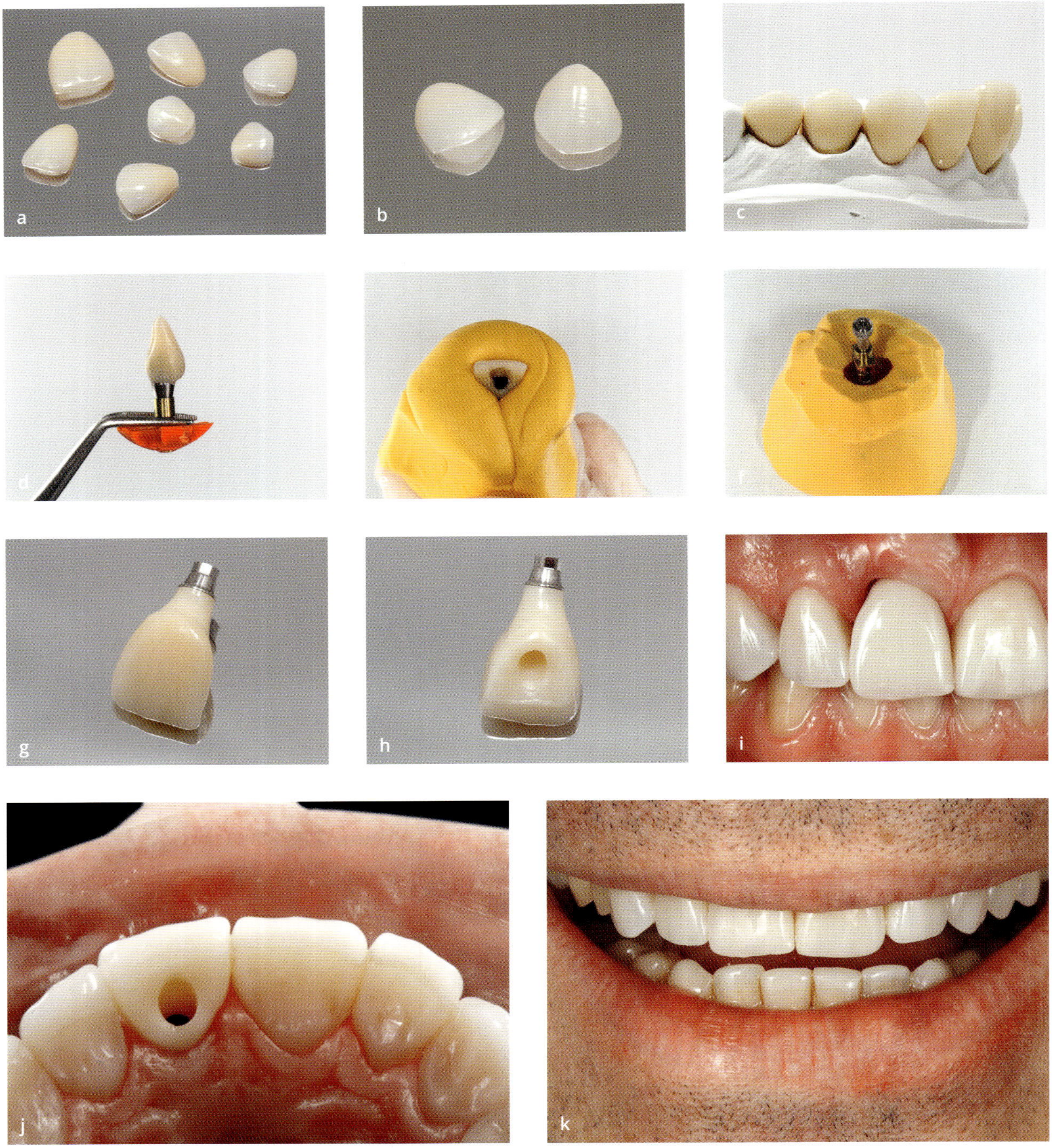

**Fig 9-30** Nine feldspathic PLVs were delivered to the patient in order to minimize the need for tooth reduction and, at the same time, reinforce the severely damaged tooth structure (a to c), and a new provisional crown was placed on the maxillary right central incisor. A traditional work flow was chosen as the porcelain veneers were to be done by the lab technician by hand to help in the integration of the different restorations. In order to replicate the emergence profile of the provisional restoration, a customized impression coping was fabricated; if the clinician were to place a conventional, cylindrical impression coping, the soft tissue anatomy would quickly collapse. After the 4-month healing period, the provisional restoration was removed and screwed onto the implant analog (d). Notice the analog tip was surrounded by resin in an irregular shape in order to reduce its rotation during the process. This was embedded into silicone at a depth that allows the anatomy of the provisional crown to be replicated up to its equator (e). Once the silicone was set, the provisional was removed, an open-tray impression coping was placed, and the emergence profile anatomy was filled with resin (f). This can be placed directly onto the implant, allowing for the best possible anatomy replication (g to k). Note the initial extra space that was created in order for the distal papilla of the central incisor to be able to creep in over the following weeks (i); this had been communicated to the lab technician.

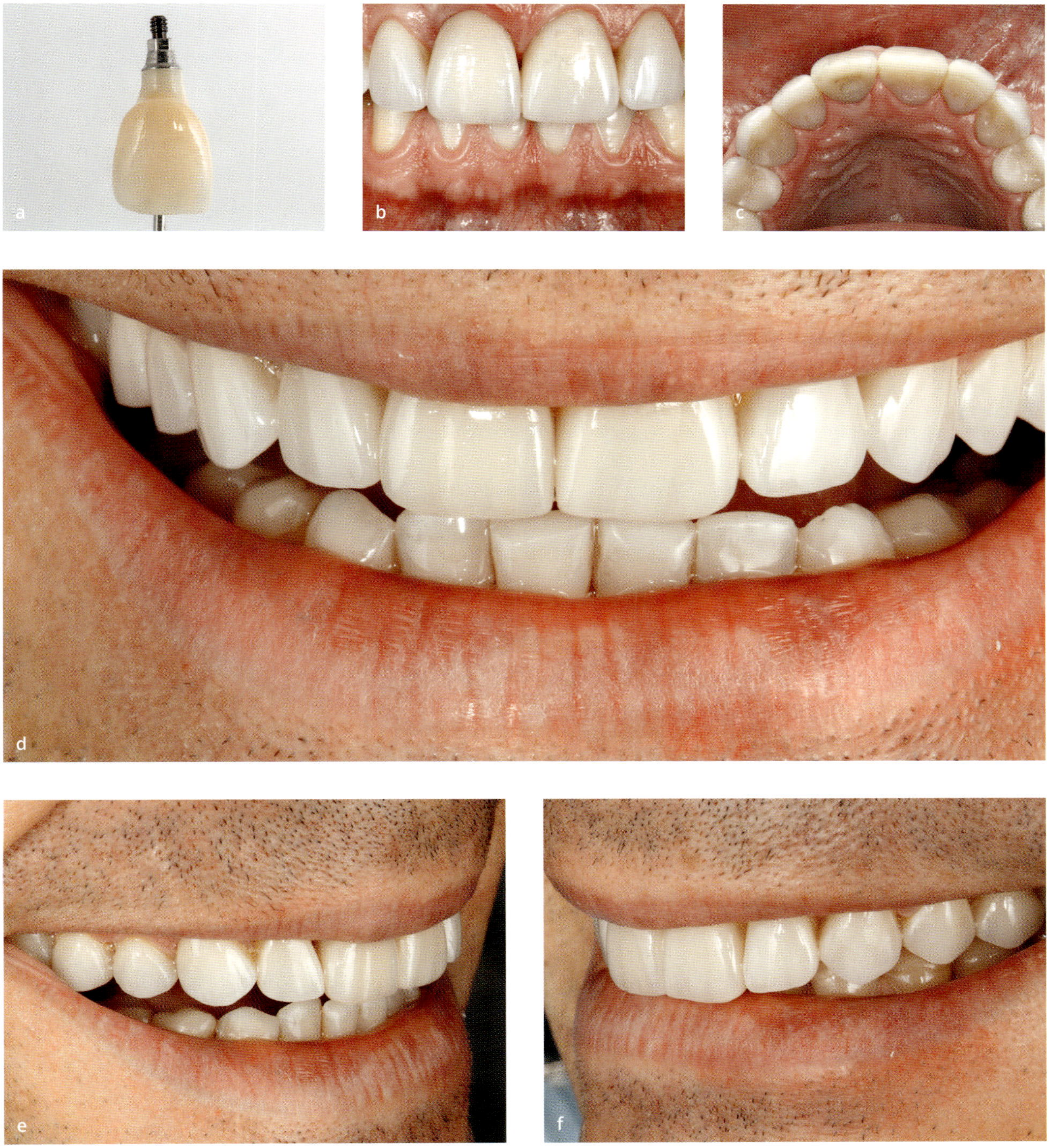


**Fig 9-31** The implant-supported crown in place (a and b). The occlusal view shows the implant crown and palatal and occlusal onlays on the neighboring teeth (c). The integration of the implant crown might improve in time thanks to creeping of soft tissue in the papillary region. The feldspathic vestibular layering of the implant-supported crown allows for optimal matching with the feldspathic veneers (d to f).

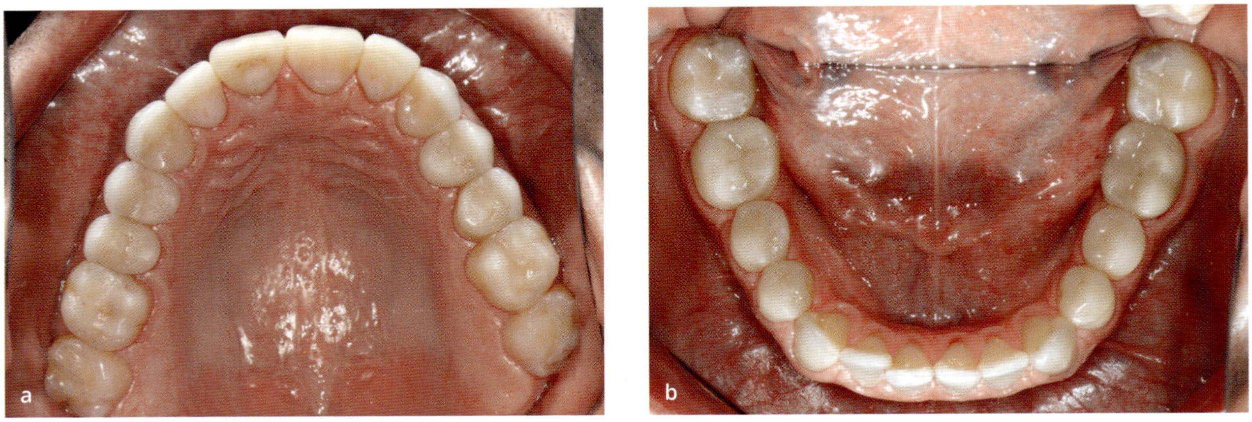

**Fig 9-32** As previously mentioned, by the time the final implant crown is in service, the overall occlusal rehabilitation needs to be finalized in order to provide the adequate VDO that assures long-term survival. At this point neither the patient nor the TW team should forget the risk factors that have caused oral collapse in such a young patient. A personalized preventive program (PPP, see chapter 10) including regular checkups must be implemented (a and b).

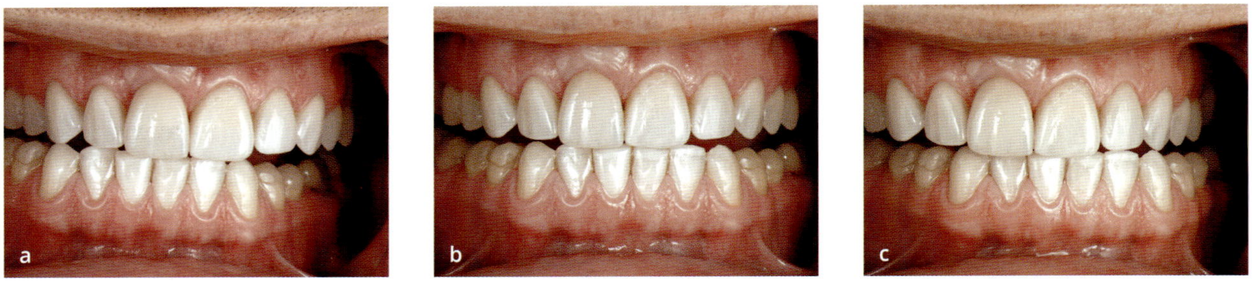

**Fig 9-33** Functional analysis shows competent anterior and canine guidance (a to c).

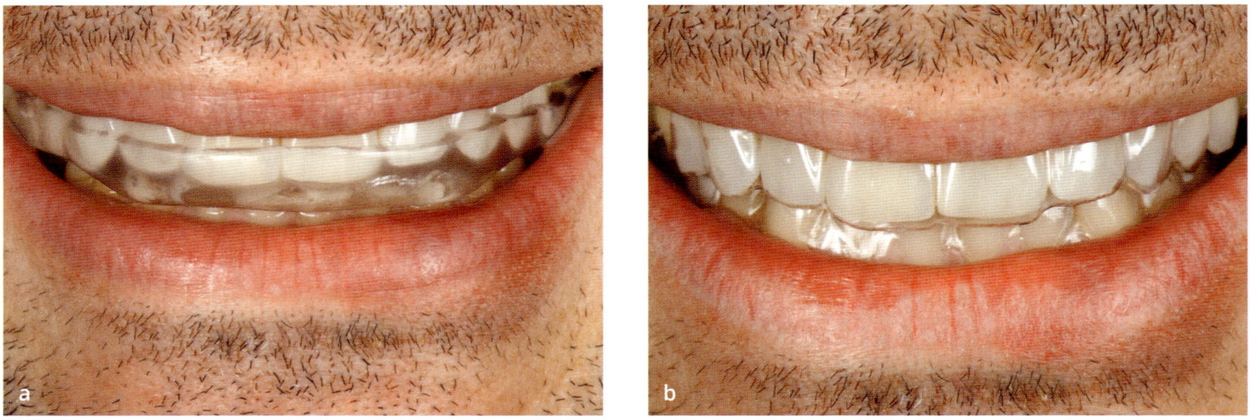

**Fig 9-34** The PPP for this young patient affected by severe TW recommends changes in lifestyle, and, if and when possible, also the use of protective guards. A Michigan guard (a) is to be used during the night, while soft Essix guards (b) are to be worn during stressful working hours and very frequent transoceanic flights.

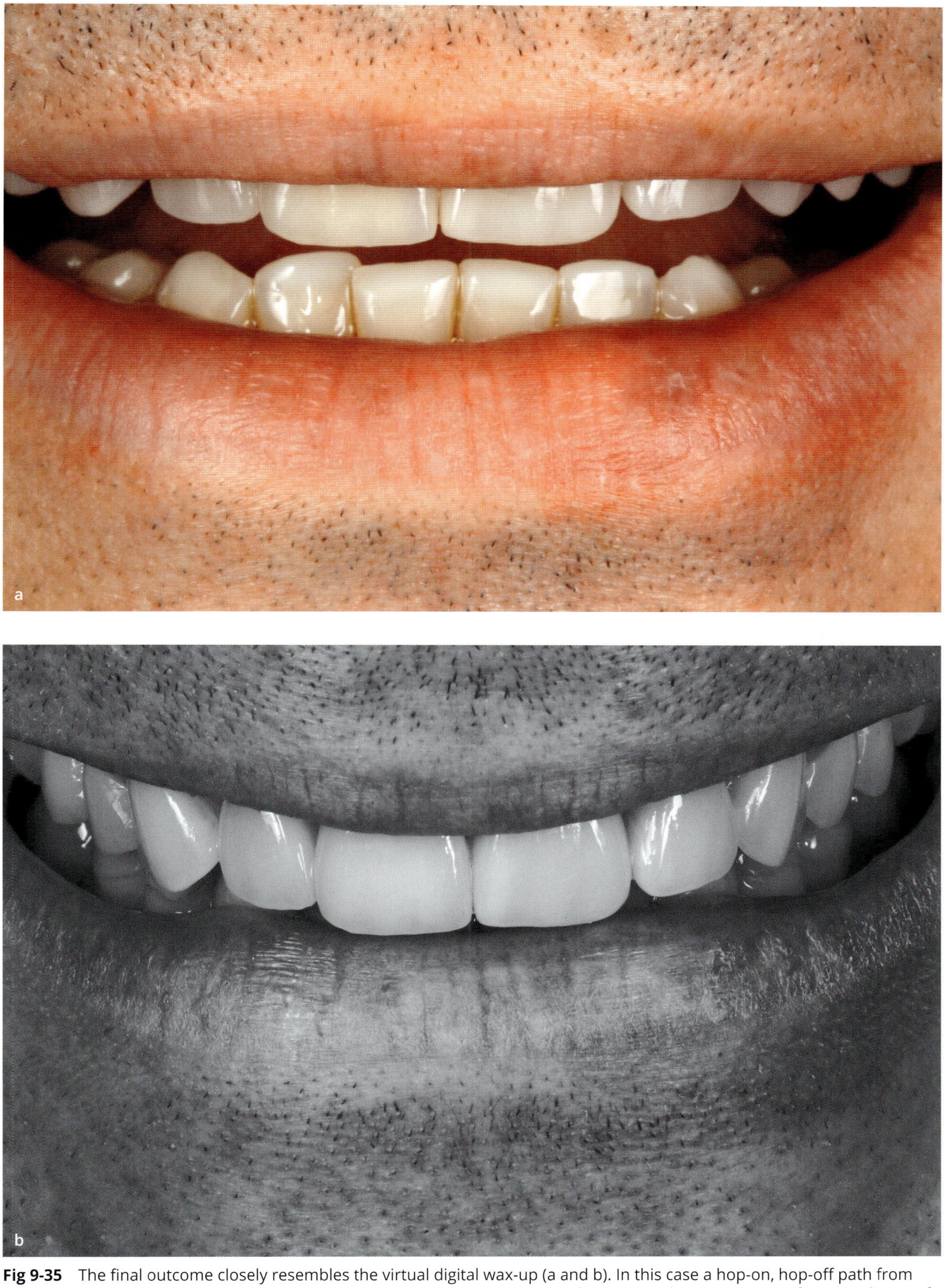

**Fig 9-35** The final outcome closely resembles the virtual digital wax-up (a and b). In this case a hop-on, hop-off path from digital to analog work flows allows the initial 3D planning to be integrated in the handmade restorations. After completion of treatment, the patient was digitally registered and checked at regular intervals. Future STL files will be compared to the post-treatment ones by the software to monitor for TW progression.

## 5. Digital Cross-Mounting and Advantages of Digital Protocols in TW Treatment

Digital protocols are highly useful in patients with TW. For didactic purposes, we will focus on a single implant crown. If the crown were to suffer from chipping, fracture or wear, the dental technician can easily refabricate the crown as it was initially placed. Moreover, if the clinician recorded the final anatomy of the crown after delivery and occlusal/interproximal adjustment, there should be virtually no changes needed to the new crown's anatomy, except for possible minor occlusal surface modifications. A new digital impression can be performed, and the initial design can be fused with the present situation in order to create a new restoration. This is just another advantage of monolithic restorations: They do not need the technician's handcrafting in the same manner as conventional PFMs do, and therefore a high degree of reproducibility can be expected.

As mentioned in previous chapters, intraoral scanners allow for precise and early monitoring of deterioration of hard surfaces (eg, iTero TimeLapse, Align Technology and Primescan OraCheck, Dentsply Sirona). In case of rapid abrasion, interceptive or corrective treatments can be applied. When applied to full-arch implant rehabilitations, these systems can vastly accelerate the restoration protocols. After a certain period of time in function, a prosthesis may be subject to repair or complete refurbishment. Such is the classic case of reparation of a worn-down or damaged full-arch prosthesis after years in function. An analog protocol would normally imply centric relation and vertical dimension registration, try-in of a tooth setup, and finally refurbished prosthesis delivery. If the mounted casts had been properly stored, it should not present any major technical difficulty, as the clinician only needs to reposition the casts in the articulator. However, if the available casts are not mounted on the articulator, the reparation will take several appointments and is a technically difficult and time-consuming procedure. Digital protocols allow for the "matching" of different models and their comparison. This means that the technician is able to superimpose different models and, if need be, refabricate a certain part of the prosthesis, with particular efficiency in the case of monolithic structures and a probable reduction of the number of appointments and the amount of chair time.

Sometimes it is not easy to understand the reasons behind overall oral failure in such patients. Even though there may not be any clear signs of TW, this does not mean that it is not present. For instance, premature tooth loss and full-contour restorations in the remaining teeth can hide TW signs. This is the reason why thorough anamnesis is key to coming to a TW diagnosis in such patients with this level of deterioration.

When addressing a patient with TW and multiple implants, it is even more critical to keep in mind that the risk factors that caused the severe TW should not be forgotten. Such risk factors and environmental changes in the oral cavity may play a negative role in the long term. A digital work flow may be of help in future reparations and/or retreatments (Figs 9-36 to 9-47).

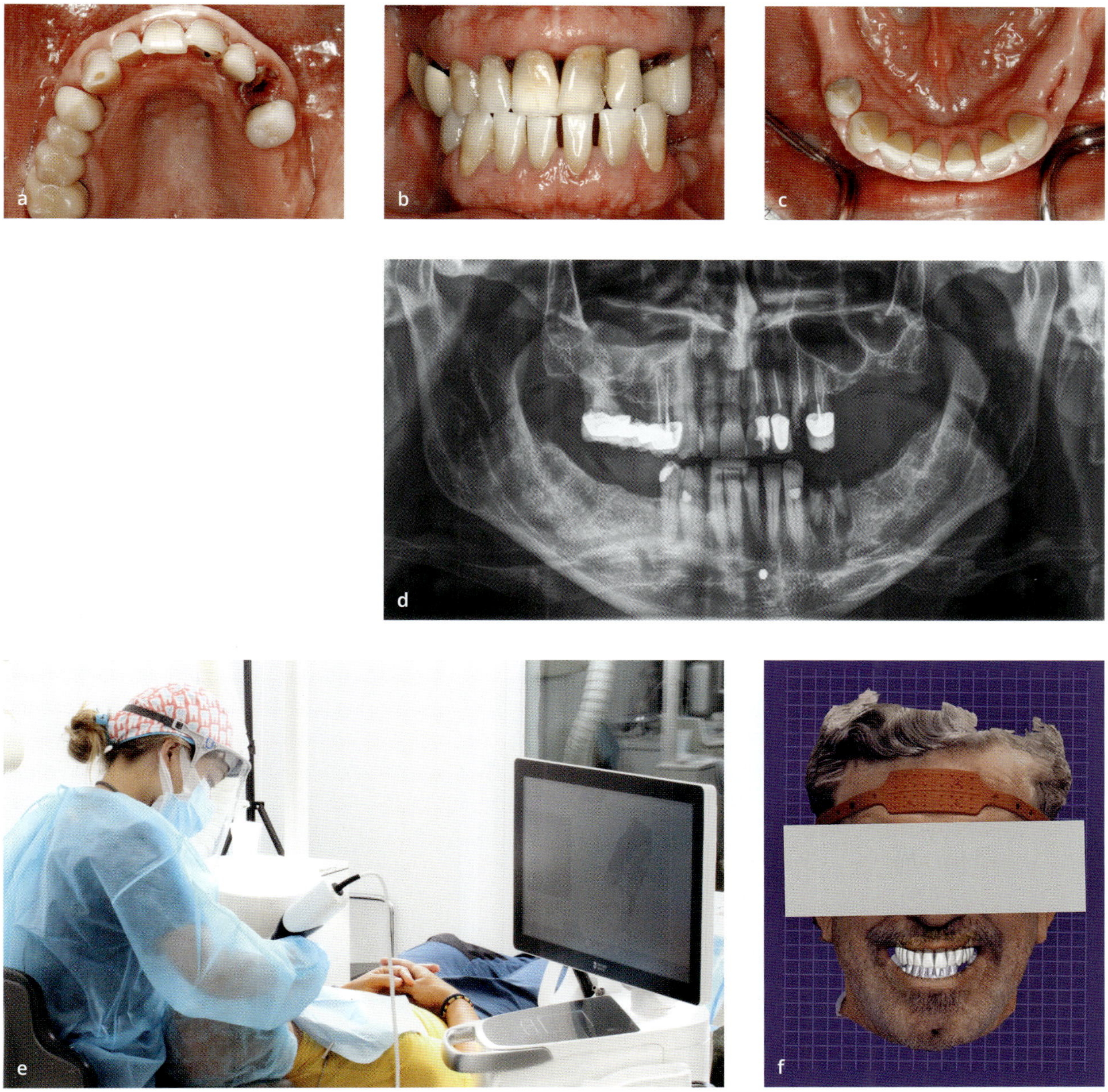

**Fig 9-36** This patient's history of intense soda drinking caused severe damage to the dentition and numerous visits to the dentist. The erosive TW trace could easily have been lost due to the premature loss of teeth and extended restorative treatments that obscure or impede the detection of erosive signs. The patient also has rampant caries associated with the highly erosive cariogenic diet (a to d). The rampant caries had progressed subgingivally in several of the maxillary teeth. It is also relevant to note that the patient had a history of sinusitis that contraindicated sinus grafting for implant placement in the posterior sectors. A diagnosis of severe TW with multiple tooth failure is shared with the patient. It is agreed to extract all maxillary teeth and infected mandibular premolars and keep the six mandibular anterior teeth. In the maxilla, a fixed complete dental prosthesis (FCDP) supported by seven implants is planned. A combined orthodontic-restorative approach will be taken to rehabilitate the mandibular anterior dentition. As explained, the proprioceptive advantage of keeping natural teeth may help lessen the fracture and overload risk of patients with TW. The patient's oral and facial anatomy is digitalized (e). An esthetically driven full-mouth rehabilitation is planned; digital impressions, photos, and a facial scan are sent to the lab in order to create a virtual prototype of the patient's smile. This is created considering the esthetic characteristics of the patient's face (f).

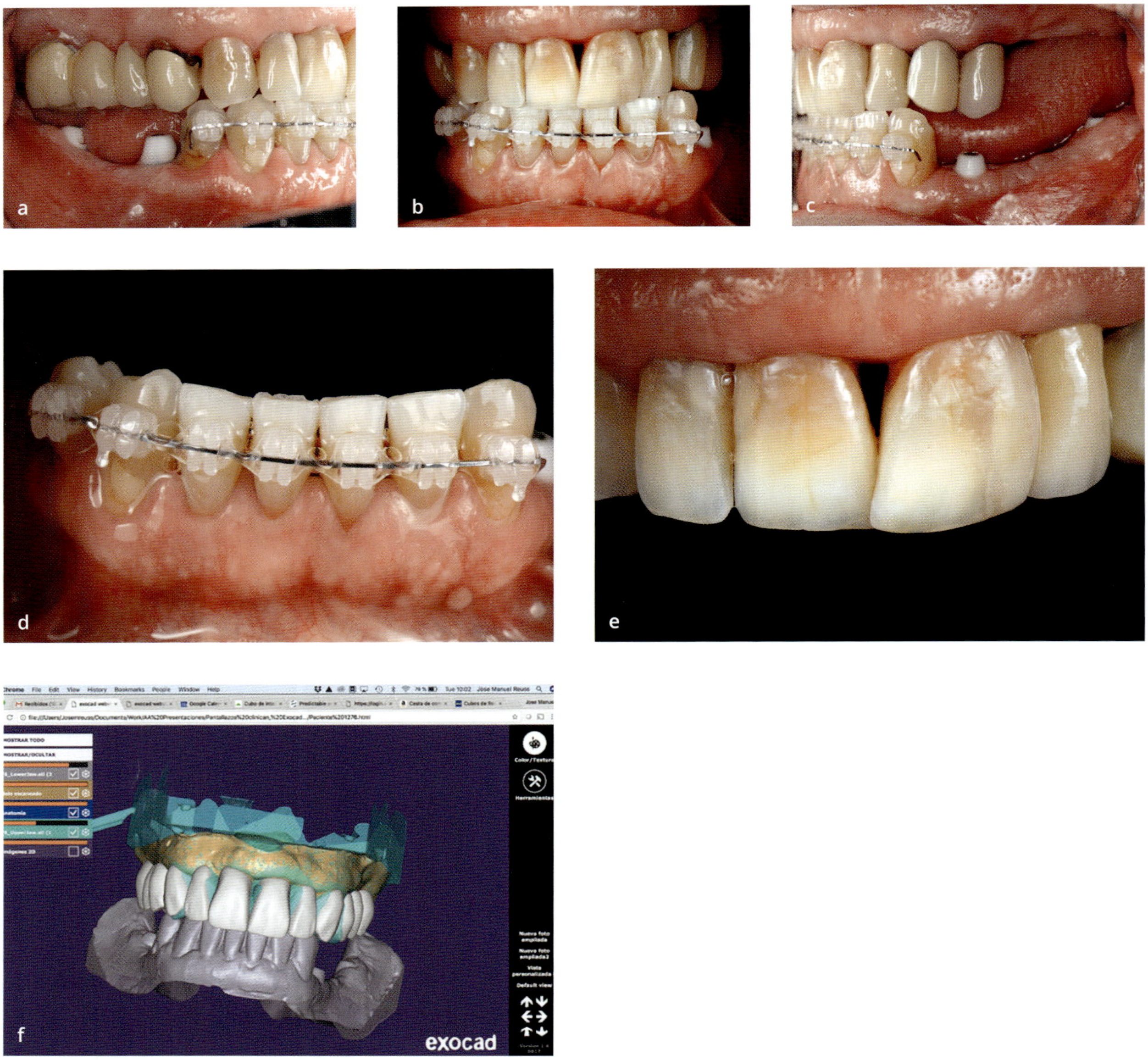


**Fig 9-37** Mandibular posterior implants are placed during the first weeks of treatment, prior to maxillary extractions, in order to provide posterior occlusal support as soon as possible for the full-arch maxillary restoration (a to c). Since the lab technician has a comprehensive set of information, the virtual prototype is very close to the ideal smile. This will be used as a guide for the implant rehabilitation in the maxilla as well as for the orthodontic treatment in the mandible (d). The maxillary teeth have been provisionally restored in order to avoid a removable phase (based on the patient's wishes) and improve the patient's esthetics (e). Meanwhile, the minor realignment of the mandibular teeth is executed with sectional orthodontics after nonsurgical periodontal treatment. A fixed orthodontic appliance is placed in the mandibular anterior dentition in order to meet the demands of the virtual smile prototype, including retrusion and alignment of these teeth (f).

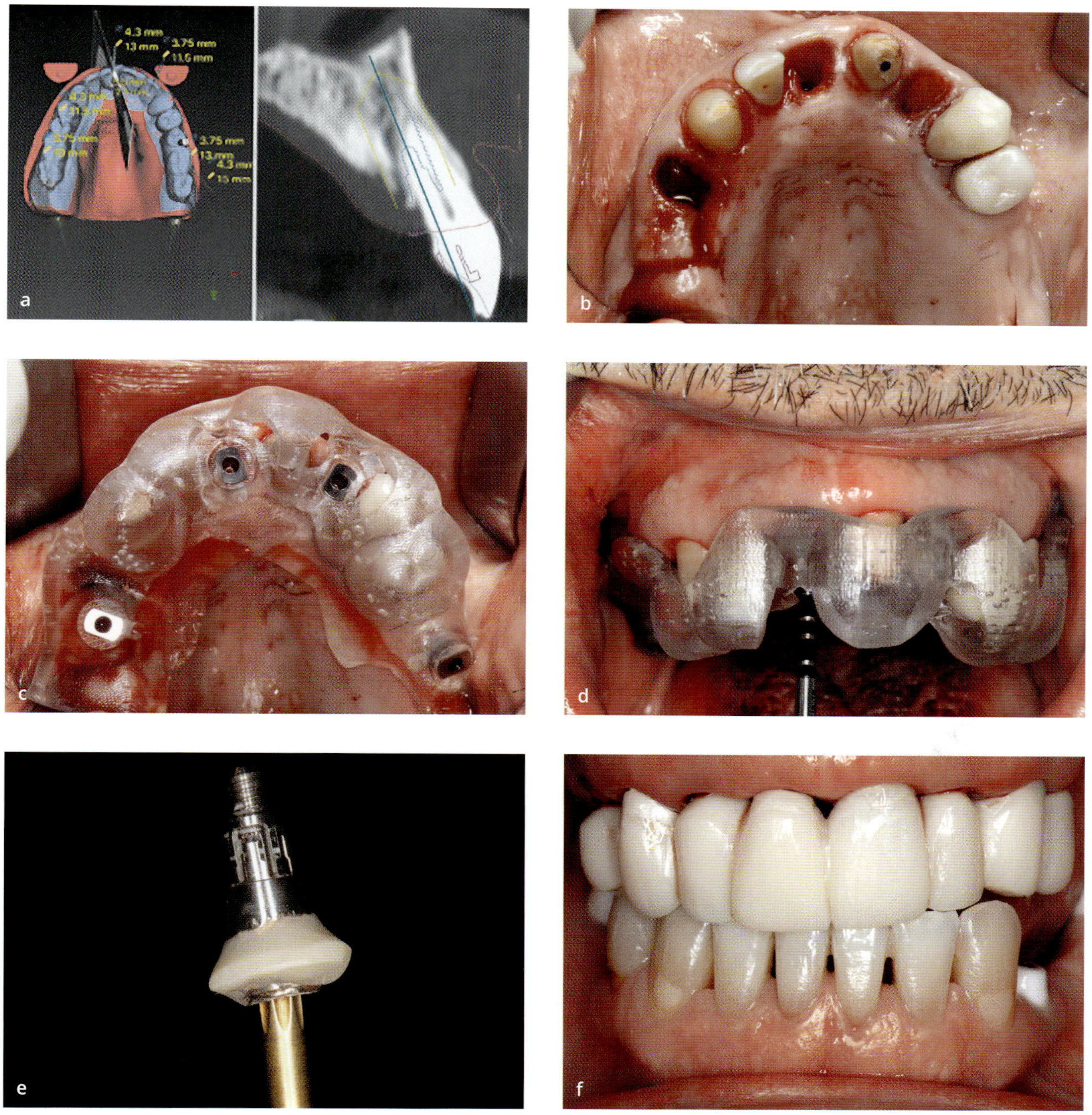


**Fig 9-38** The maxillary dentition is going to be extracted in two stages. During the first maxillary implant surgery, five teeth will be kept as transitional abutments for a fixed restoration, while five implants are to be placed following the guided surgery plan (a). The failing distal teeth in the right quadrant are removed. Strategic teeth are used as abutments for a provisional fixed acrylic shell-type restoration (b). A surgical template using a guided surgery system is used for the placement of the maxillary implants (c and d). A customized healing abutment is delivered on the implants in the right central and left lateral incisor sites to preserve the emergence profile (e). Orthodontic movement of mandibular teeth is finished at this point; brackets are removed, and a fixed lingual retainer is cemented. A maxillary provisional acrylic fixed partial denture is cemented to the strategic natural tooth abutments (f).

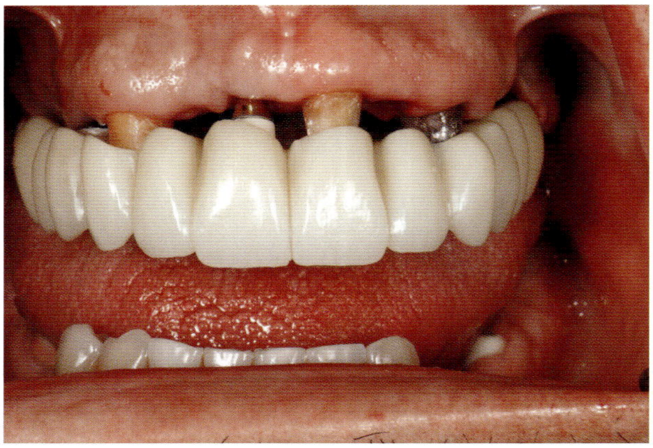

**Fig 9-39** After the osseointegration healing period for the first five implants, an implant-supported partial denture is created. This is ready for the day of the extraction of the remaining teeth, with hollow pontics in the areas of these teeth for esthetic try-in. After extraction, those voids were relined chairside.

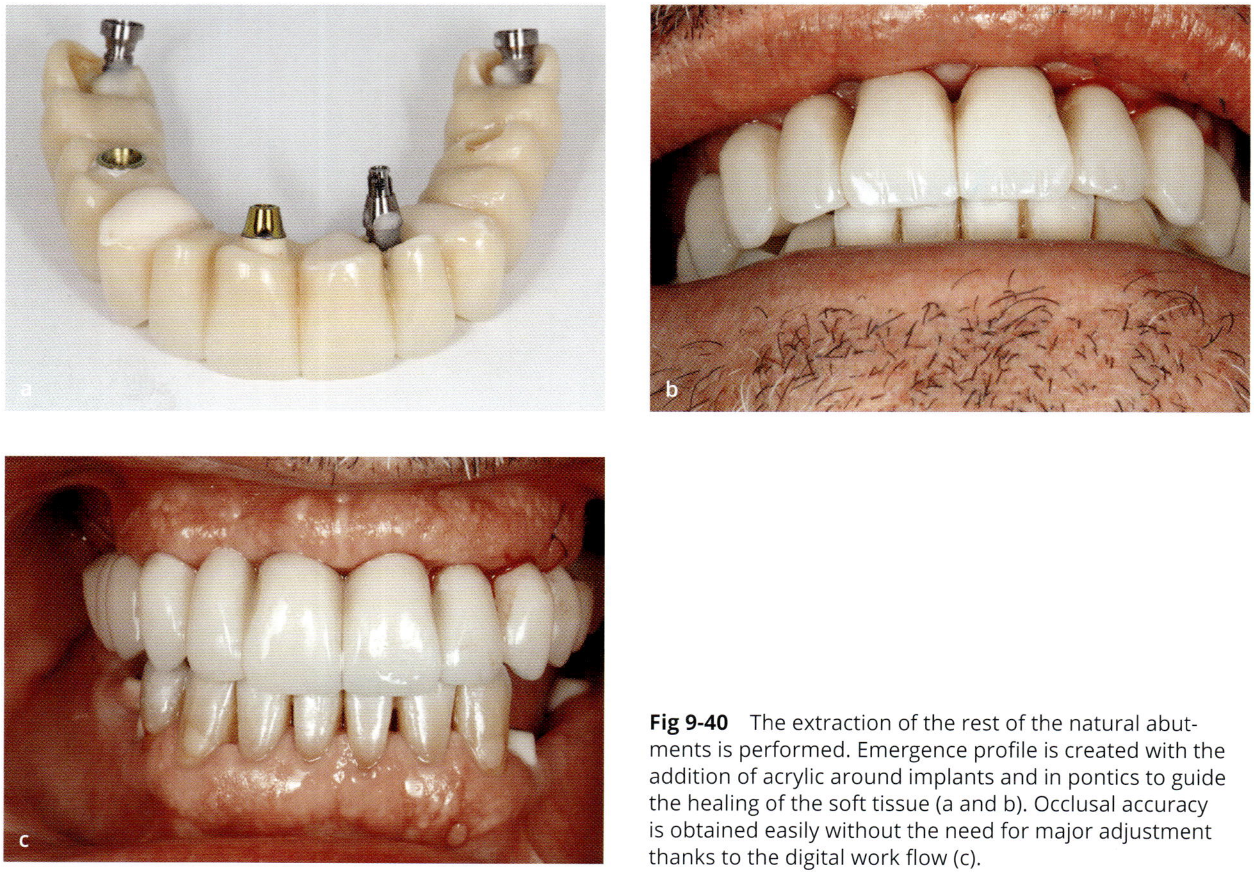

**Fig 9-40** The extraction of the rest of the natural abutments is performed. Emergence profile is created with the addition of acrylic around implants and in pontics to guide the healing of the soft tissue (a and b). Occlusal accuracy is obtained easily without the need for major adjustment thanks to the digital work flow (c).

**Fig 9-41** *(right page)* Four sets of information are used for the final prosthesis fabrication. First, the stone implant cast is digitalized. Second, right after prosthesis removal, a digital intraoral impression is taken without the prosthesis, with only two intraoral scan bodies; the goal of this impression is to quickly capture the soft tissue anatomy before it flattens out after prosthesis removal (in comparison to the traditional silicone impression, an optic scan is much faster). Due to the superior reliability of silicone impressions, this digital impression only captures these two implants in order to be able to "match" this impression with the conventional impression. Third, an intraoral impression of the slightly modified printed prototype is done to transmit the information of such changes and the behavior of the soft tissues to those modifications. Finally, the initial digital wax-up is superimposed onto these three digital models (a to f). A printed prototype is tried in, following the initial face scan protocol (g). The digital wax-up is the blueprint throughout the whole process. The try-in prototype follows and guides the soft tissue architecture (h). Most of the preservation and scalloping work should be done prior to the final prosthesis delivery.

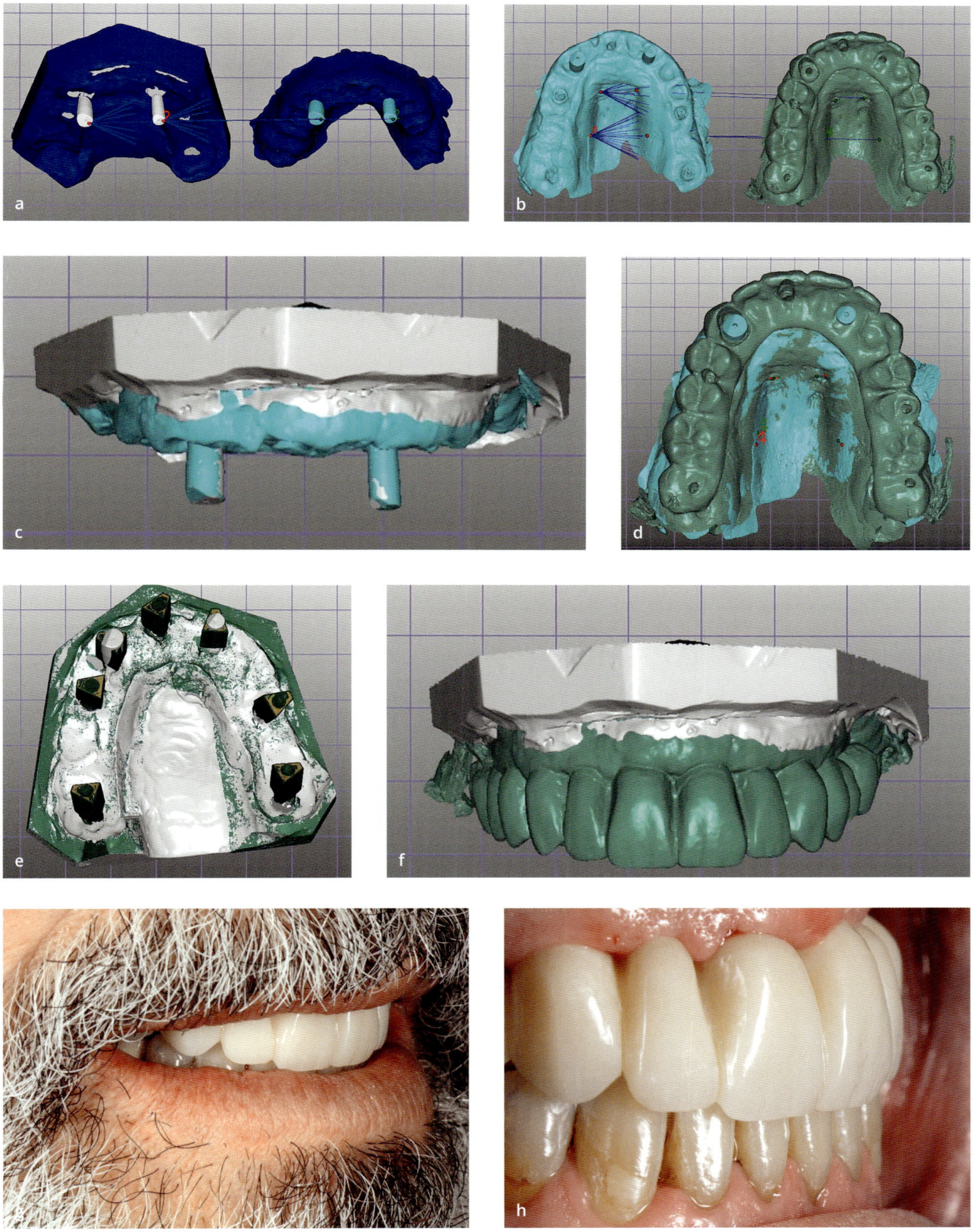
a
b
c
d
e
f
h

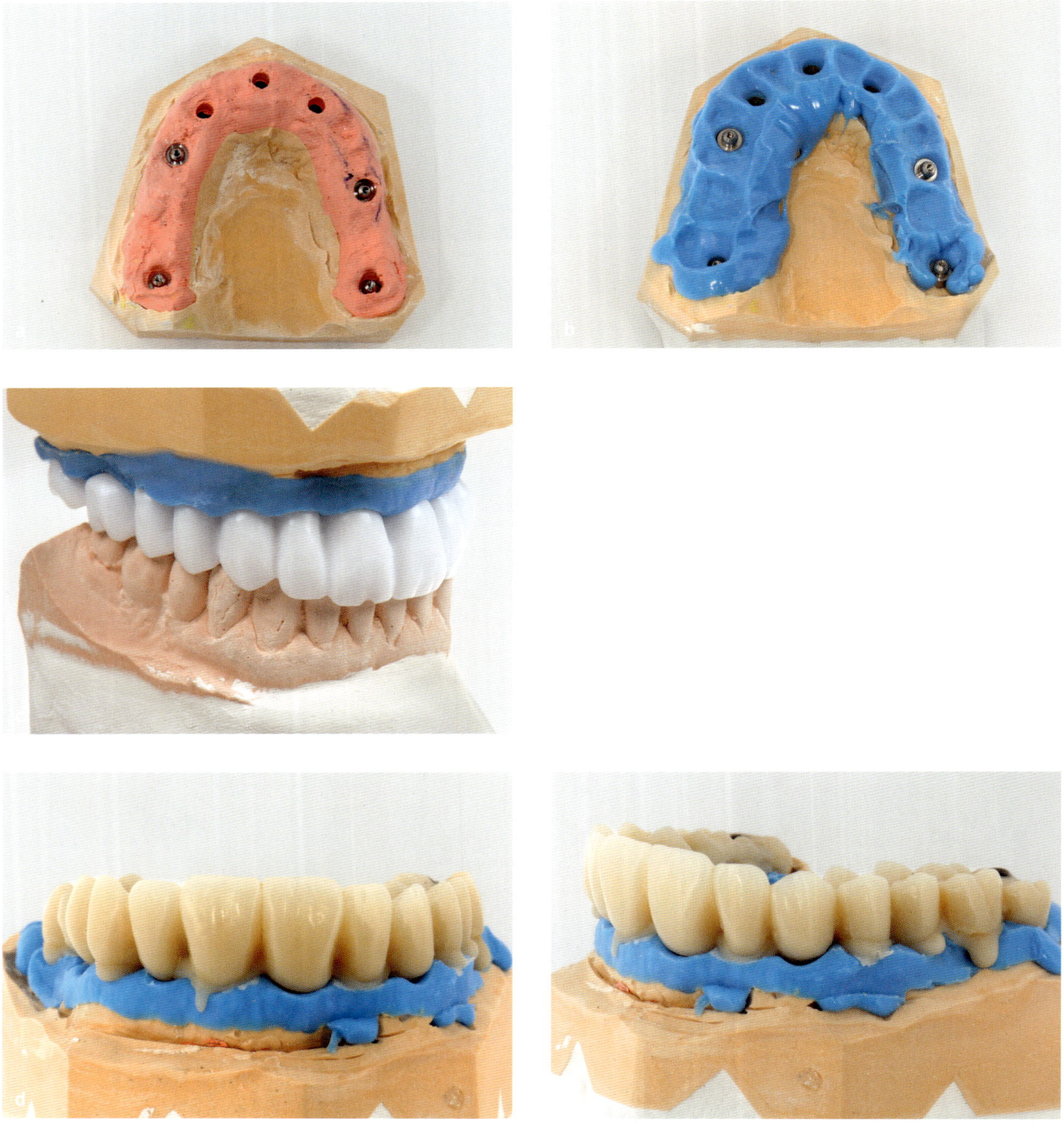

**Fig 9-42** Comparison between final impression and modified gingival architecture thanks to the fusion of the previously mentioned digital files (a and b). The "modified" model allows the creation of a new prototype with subtle esthetic improvements compared to the provisional prosthesis (c). After an intraoral try-in, the implant-supported provisional restoration is mounted on the model and modified, adding resin where the printed prototype had shown the need for improvement (d and e).

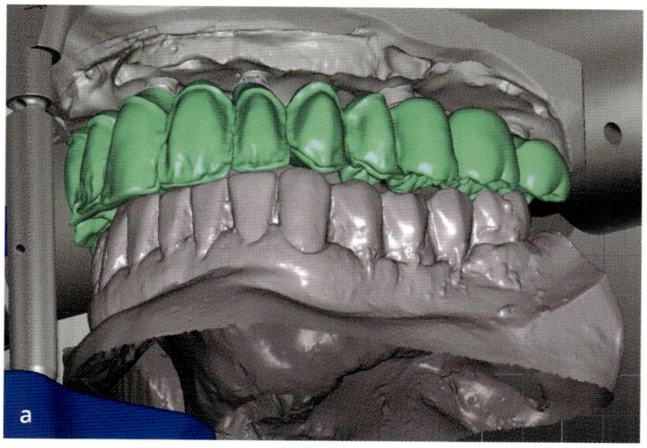

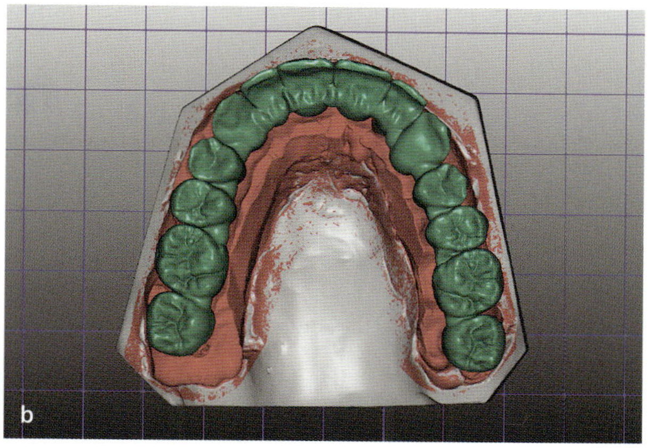

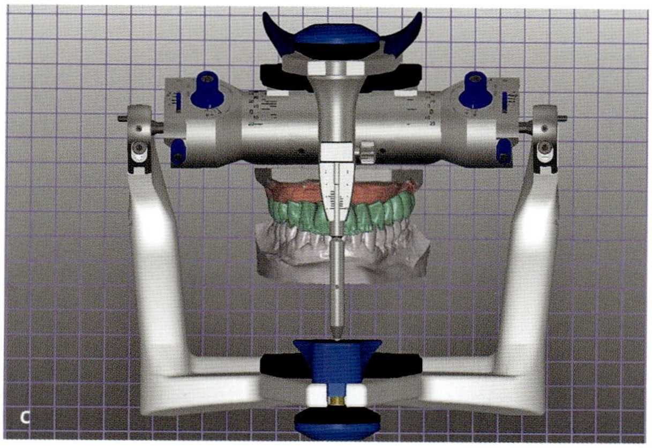

**Fig 9-43** Final wax-up in the digital articulator. Note the cutback on the maxillary anterior teeth for porcelain veneering (a to c).

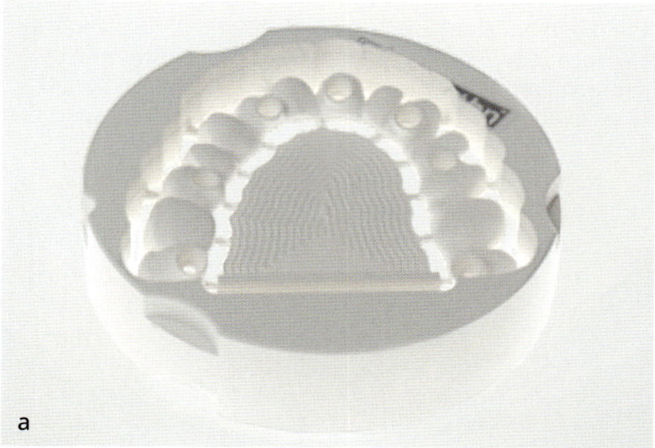

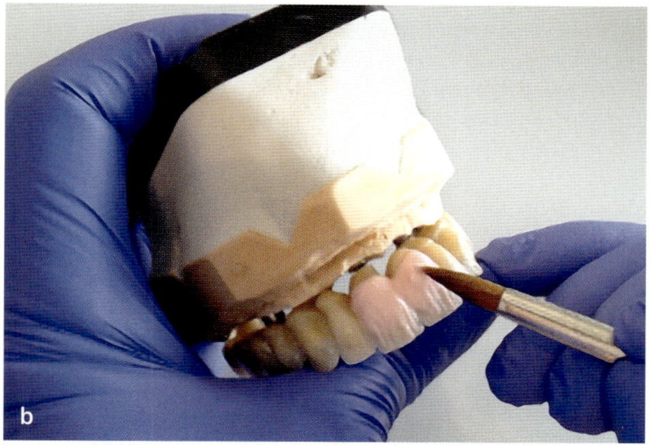

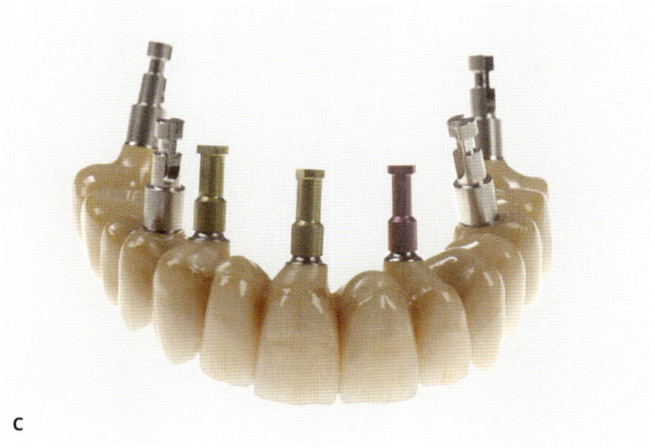

**Fig 9-44** The work of the lab technician is key to the esthetic outcome. The zirconia prosthesis is milled (a), and the buccal surfaces of the 10 anterior teeth are veneered with porcelain (b). The layering of the porcelain is a paradigmatic step in providing a natural, attractive appearance (c).

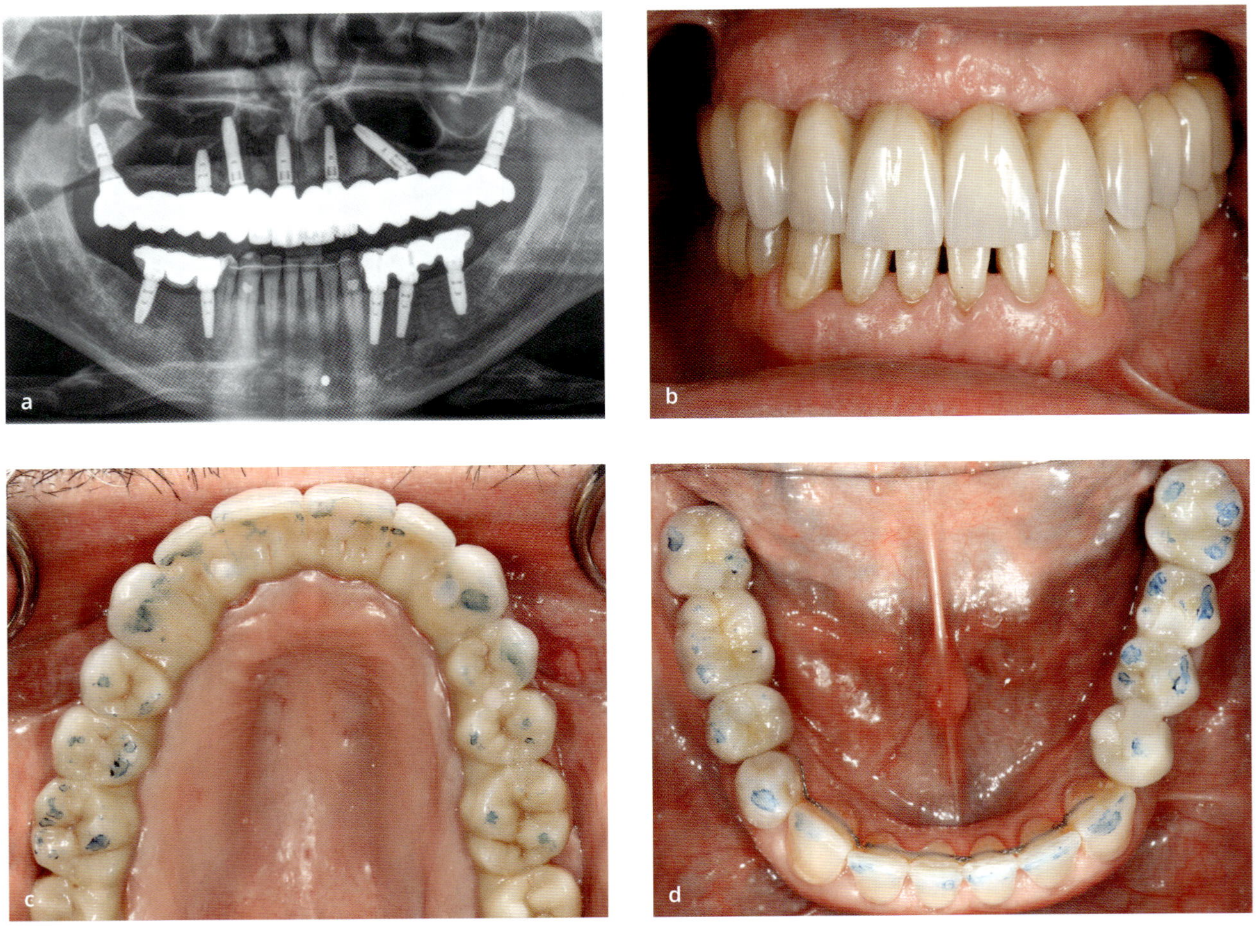


**Fig 9-45** Final restoration. Note the restored natural dentition in the mandibular anterior arch. A direct freehand composite approach was chosen to restore the worn incisal edges, lost canine cusp, and NCCLs (a and b). Occlusion right after prosthesis placement reveals a balanced distribution of contacts, following the occlusion that was adjusted in the try-in prototype (c and d). The posterior sectors are full-contour zirconia for the sake of avoidance of wear and chipping. The buccal aspects of the eight anterior teeth are veneered with porcelain.

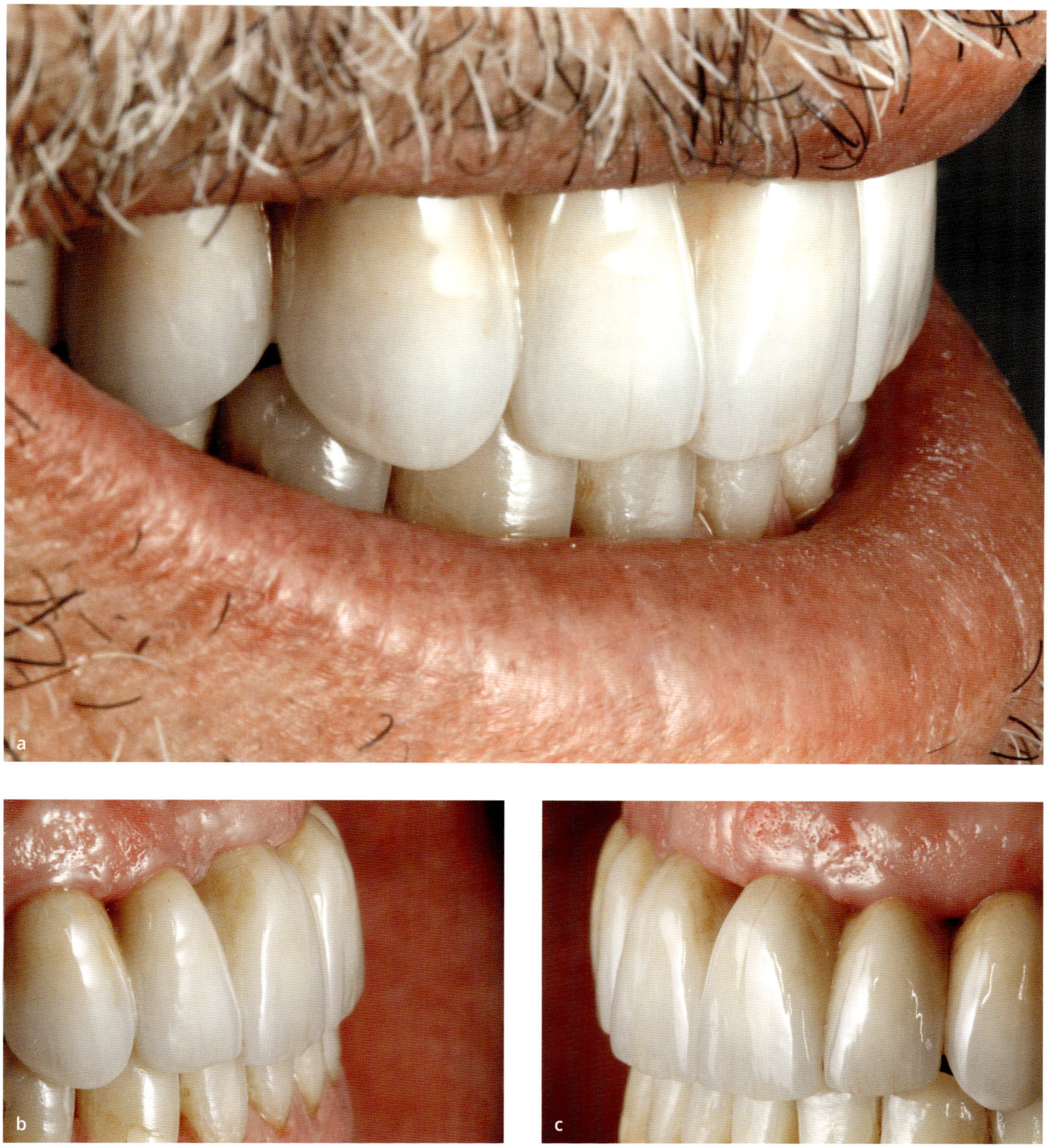


**Fig 9-46** Detailed profile views of the gingival embrasures show soft tissue embracing the highly biocompatible zirconia-based prosthesis (a to c).

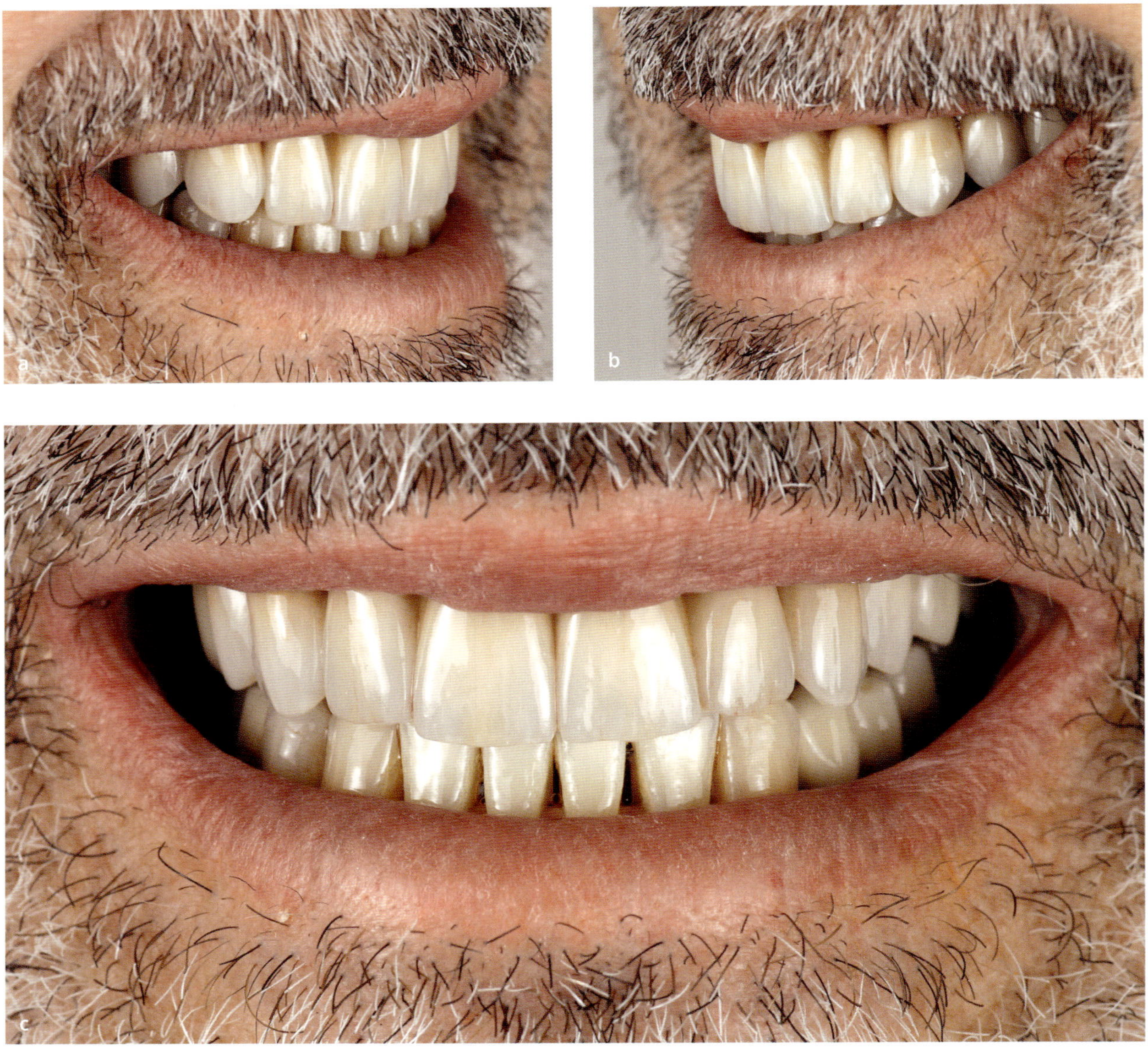


**Fig 9-47** The final outcome resembles the initial digital planning, even though a hop-on, hop-off (digital-analog) protocol was chosen (a to h).

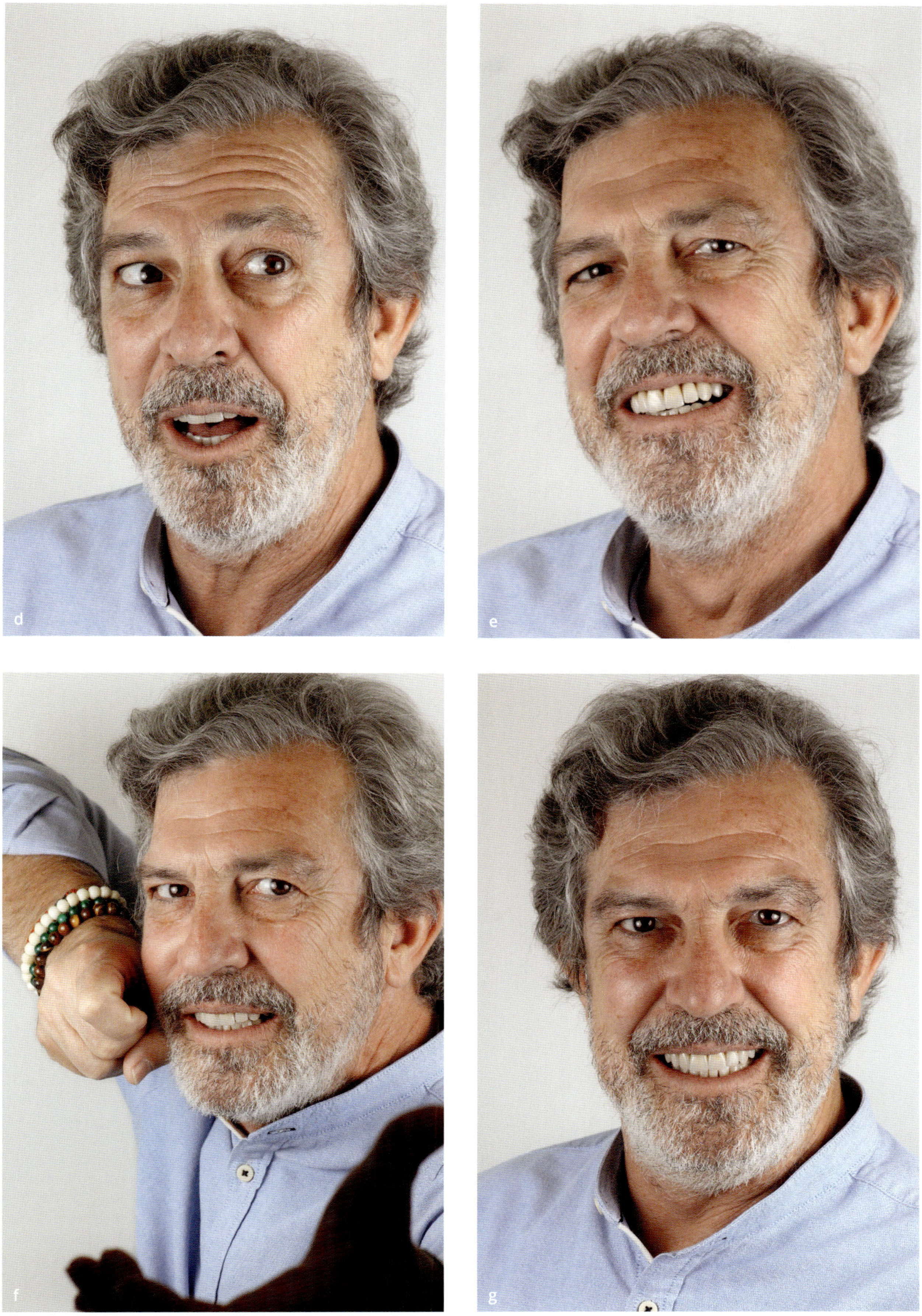
d
e
f
g

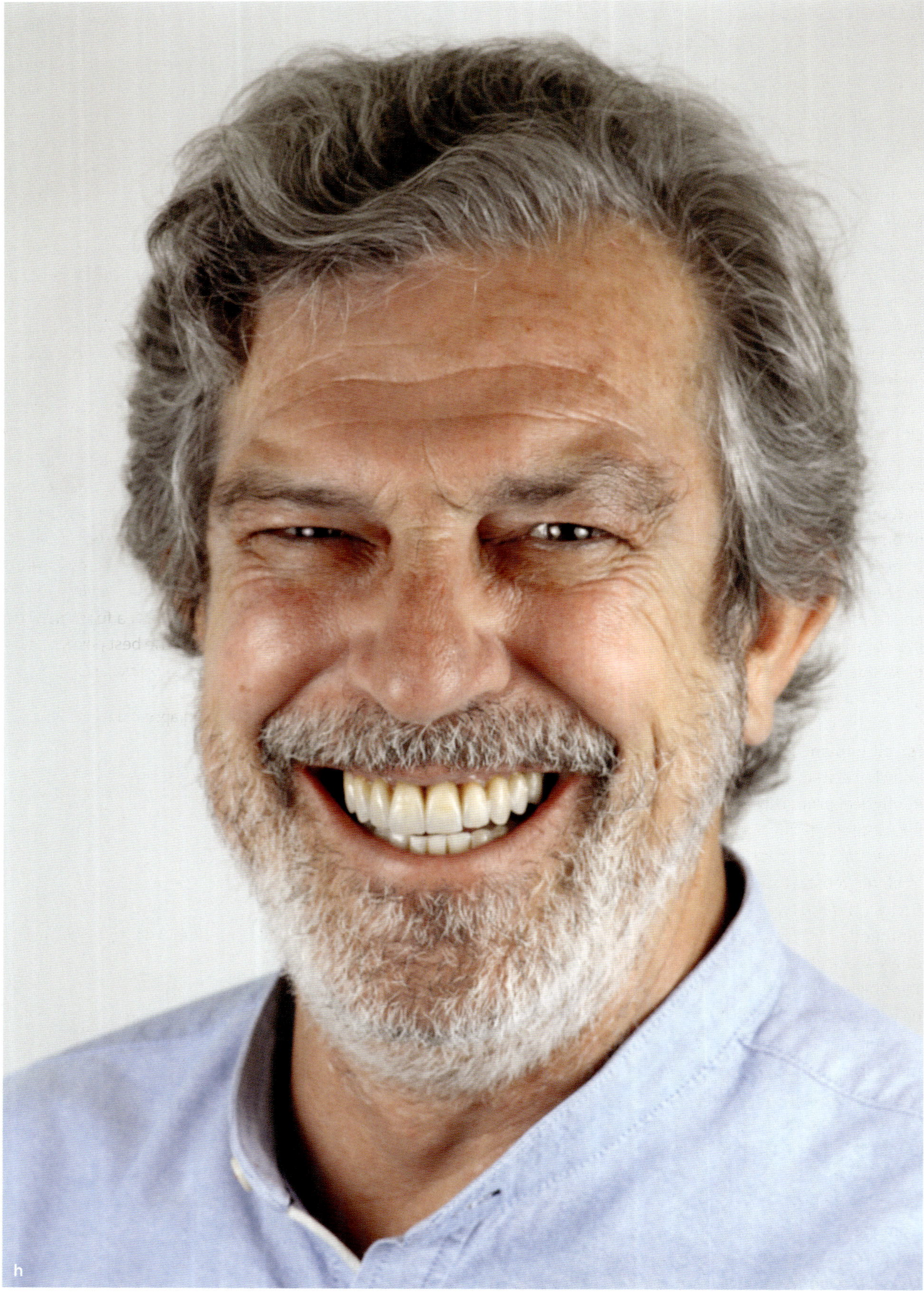


**Fig 9-47** *(continued)*

## 6. Maintenance Protocols in Patients with TW and Implants

Xerostomia and/or hyposalivation is usually associated with severe TW. The absence of proper salivary function is an indication for dental implants versus a removable prosthesis, as a mucosa-supported prosthesis may be unbearable in the absence of proper lubrication.[44,45] Nevertheless, this dryness may come at the cost of a higher risk of peri-implant disease due to the very same reasons[46,47]; xerostomia can lead to delayed healing, early osseointegration failure, and peri-implantitis. Once more, patients with severe TW and implants should be recalled at short intervals to assess their capacity to maintain peri-implant health. While peri-implantitis is a totally different condition than implant overload, these conditions are often mistaken. However, the one characteristic that they do share is the possible fatal ending of an implant. Peri-implantitis can be defined as the inflammation of the mucosa surrounding an osseointegrated implant with accompanying destruction of supporting bone.[51,52] The etiology is bacterial-inflammatory, and it is a highly prevalent disease. This entity is clearly different from TW and overload-related issues, although as previously mentioned, bone loss can be worsened in the presence of overload. Monitoring for peri-implant hygiene and health is vital.

A strict follow-up protocol should be established for all implant patients. The maintenance protocol is heavily related to the previously described difference in physical properties and wear characteristics between implant restorations and teeth or other entities present in the mouth. Traditionally, checkups for patients with implants mostly focus on peri-implant health, while the occlusion is not always closely monitored. It is highly recommended in the patient with TW to perform a thorough occlusal analysis and, if need be, an adjustment. Tooth wear patients, those with an unstable occlusion or with a history of fractures, or those suffering from parafunctional habits should be monitored closely, with more frequent visits. Protective mouthguards, be it a Michigan hard acrylic splint or a soft Essix-like splint, will also help over the long term.

Risk factors associated with lifestyle habits such as unbalanced diets, stress, sleep disturbances, polymedication, and others should be addressed with the patient from the start of the treatment. Modification of lifestyle is not an easy task; therefore, close monitoring is essential for such patients. An oral care regimen ensuring saliva stimulation is desirable in many cases.

## 7. Key Points: Implants in TW

Implant dentistry has come a long way since its beginnings many decades ago. The advent of minimally invasive protocols, use of highly biocompatible materials, and enhanced prosthetic designs have mainly brought biologic advantages to this form of treatment. However, occlusal concepts and maintenance are of utmost importance when it comes to TW patients. Monitoring wear, establishing prevention protocols, and providing interceptive treatments are perhaps the best strategies to increase the longevity of implant restorations, biologic and risk factors aside. This is especially relevant in patients with TW and a bruxism habit.

Due to the biomechanical nature of an implant restoration, special considerations must made. In general terms, occlusal design on implant restorations should adhere to the principles of optimization of load bearing: minimizing the size of the occlusal table, avoiding undesired interferences, and, when possible, slightly reducing the intensity of occlusion on the implant. In regard to material selection, special attention must be given to the opposing arch and the patient's individual occlusal characteristics. We must then choose which complications we are willing to deal with, in order to provide the patient with a functional and biocompatible implant solution with the best possible long-term outcomes. In summary, the key points are:

1. Diagnosis: Identify TW, VDO collapse, hopeless teeth, and risk factors.
2. Integrate the whole team into an esthetically driven treatment work flow. Do not perform isolated restorative, orthodontic, or implant treatments in the patient with TW.
3. Analyze restorative space. Take an orthodontic and/or restorative path to increase VDO if needed.
4. Choose an occlusal design/scheme depending on the kind of implant restoration and the individual patient's characteristics. The patient with TW should never be addressed using a "tooth-oriented approach"; a comprehensive occlusal rehabilitation is essential.
5. Implant biomechanics are conceptually different than that of other kinds of restorations or teeth. Namely, there is much-reduced mobility upon function. Interferences are to be avoided, and the intensity of occlusal contacts should be reduced.
6. Prosthetic design should preferably reduce the occlusal table in the patient with TW.
7. Timing: definitive implant restorations usually come last! If the remaining dentition is worn, restore it prior to delivery of implant prostheses.
8. Maintenance protocols: A personalized preventive program should be implemented. Monitor gingival/peri-implant health, TW risk factors, and occlusion.

## References

1. Peršić S, Čelebić A. Influence of different prosthodontic rehabilitation options on oral health-related quality of life, orofacial esthetics and chewing function based on patient-reported outcomes. Qual Life Res 2015;24:919–926.
2. Moraschini V, Poubel LA, Ferreira VF, Barboza Edos S. Evaluation of survival and success rates of dental implants reported in longitudinal studies with a follow-up period of at least 10 years: A systematic review. Int J Oral Maxillofac Surg 2015;44:377–388.
3. Rohlin M, Nilner K, Davidson T, et al. Treatment of adult patients with edentulous arches: A systematic review. Int J Prosthodont 2012;25:553–567.
4. Graetz C, El-Sayed KF, Geiken A, et al. Effect of periodontitis history on implant success: A long-term evaluation during supportive periodontal therapy in a university setting. Clin Oral Investig 2018;22:235–244.
5. Gil A, Müller P, Hämmerle C, Jung R. Team approach in esthetic dentistry. Int J Esthet Dent 2021;16:142–143.
6. Bichacho N, Feraru M. Replacing hopeless maxillary incisors with adjacent implants via an integrative biologically oriented approach. Compend Contin Educ Dent 2019;40:434–443.
7. Mankoo T, Frost L. Rehabilitation of esthetics in advanced periodontal cases using orthodontics for vertical hard and soft tissue regeneration prior to implants—A report of 2 challenging cases treated with an interdisciplinary approach. Eur J Esthet Dent 2011;6:376–404.
8. Schoenbaum TR, Moy PK, Aghaloo T, Elashoff D. Risk factors for dental implant failure in private practice: A multicenter survival analysis. Int J Oral Maxillofac Implants 2021;36:388–394.
9. Roccuzzo M, Bonino F, Aglietta M, Dalmasso P. Ten-year results of a three arms prospective cohort study on implants in periodontally compromised patients. Part 2: Clinical results. Clin Oral Implants Res 2012;23:389–395.
10. Misch CE. Dental Implant Prosthetics, ed 2. St. Louis: Elsevier Mosby, 2015.
11. Parfitt GJ. Measurement of the physiological mobility of individual teeth in an axial direction. J Dent Res 1960;39:608–618.
12. Rudd KD, O'Leary TJ, Stumpf AJ Jr. Horizontal tooth mobility in carefully screened subjects. Techn Docum Rep Sam-Tdr-64-12. Tech Doc Rep U S Air Force Syst Command Electron Syst Div 1964;94:1–6.
13. Mühlemann HR. Tooth mobility: A review of clinical aspects and research findings. J Periodontol 1967;38(6 Suppl):686–713.
14. van Steenberghe D (ed). Tissue Integration in Oral Maxillofacial Reconstruction: Proceedings of an International Congress, May 1985, Brussels, no. 29, Current Clinical Practice Series. Amsterdam: Excerpta Medica, 1986.
15. Albrektsson T, Zarb GA, Brånemark PI. The Brånemark Osseointegrated Implant. Chicago: Quintessence, 1989.
16. Isidor F. Influence of forces on peri-implant bone. Clin Oral Implants Res, 2006;17(Suppl 2):8–-18.
17. Wolff J. The Law of Bone Remodeling. Maquet P, Furlong R (trans). Berlin: Springer-Verlag, 1986.
18. Frost HM. Wolff's law and bone's structural adaptations to mechanical usage: An overview for clinicians. Angle Orthod 1994;64(3):175–188.
19. Frost HM. Perspectives: Bone's mechanical usage windows. Bone Miner 1992;19:257–271.
20. Frost HM. A 2003 update of bone physiology and Wolff's law for clinicians. Angle Orthod 2004;74(1):3–15.
21. Piattelli A, Ruggeri A, Franchi M, Romasco N, Trisi P. An histologic and histomorphometric study of bone reactions to unloaded and loaded non-submerged single implants in monkeys: A pilot study. J Oral Implantol 1993;19:314–320.
22. Piattelli A, Corigliano M, Scarano A, Quaranta M. Bone reactions to early occlusal loading of two-stage titanium plasma-sprayed implants: A pilot study in monkeys. Int J Periodontics Restorative Dent 1997;17(2):162–169.
23. Berglundh T, Abrahamsson I, Lindhe J. Bone reactions to longstanding functional load at implants: An experimental study in dogs. J Clin Periodontol 2005;32:925–932.
24. Hämmerle CH, Wagner D, Brägger U, et al. Threshold of tactile sensitivity perceived with dental endosseous implants and natural teeth. Clin Oral Implants Res 1995;6(2):83–90.
25. Magne P, Gallucci GO, Belser UC. Anatomic crown width/length ratios of unworn and worn maxillary teeth in white subjects. J Prosthet Dent 2003;89:453–461.
26. Misch CE. Implant design considerations for the posterior regions of the mouth. Implant Dent 1999;8:376–386.
27. Weinberg LA, Kruger B. A comparison of implant/prosthesis loading with four clinical variables. Int J Prosthodont 1995;8:421–433.
28. Lundgren D, Laurell L. Biomechanical aspects of fixed bridgework supported by natural teeth and endosseous implants. Periodontol 2000 1994;4:23–40.
29. Klineberg IJ, Trulsson M, Murray GM. Occlusion on implants—Is there a problem? J Oral Rehabil 2012;39:522–537.
30. Prinz JF. Abrasives in foods and their effect on intra-oral processing: A two-colour chewing gum study. J Oral Rehabil 2004;31:968–971.
31. Strub JR, Kern M, Türp J, et al. Curriculum Prothetik III. Kombinierte und abnehmbare Prothetik Implantologie Nachsorge Psychologie, 4. Berlin: Quintessence, 2011.
32. Kim Y, Oh TJ, Misch CE, Wang HL. Occlusal considerations in implant therapy: Clinical guidelines with biomechanical rationale. Clin Oral Implants Res 2005;16(1):26–35.
33. Lindquist LW, Rockler B, Carlsson GE. Bone resorption around fixtures in edentulous patients treated with mandibular fixed tissue-integrated prostheses. J Prosthet Dent 1988;59(1):59–63.
34. Termeie D, Klokkevold PR, Caputo AA. Effect of implant diameter and ridge dimension on stress distribution in mandibular first molar sites—A photoelastic study. J Oral Implantol 2015;41(5):e165–e173.
35. Lü J, Liu C, Lan J, Gao X. Three-dimensional finite element analysis of the effect of the location and diameter of implants on the stress distribution in three-unit implant-supported posterior cantilever fixed partial dentures under dynamic loads [in Chinese]. Hua Xi Kou Qiang Yi Xue Za Zhi 2013;31:552–556.
36. de Souza Batista VE, Verri FR, Lemos CAA, et al. Should the restoration of adjacent implants be splinted or nonsplinted? A systematic review and meta-analysis. J Prosthet Dent 2019;121(1):41–51.
37. Heintze SD, Rousson V. Survival of zirconia- and metal-supported fixed dental prostheses: A systematic review. Int J Prosthodont 2010;23:493–502.
38. Pelekanos S, Pozidi G, Kourtis S. Restoration of divergent implants with a 2-piece screw-retained fixed, complete dental implant prostheses. J Prosthet Dent 2016;115:389–392.
39. Sailer I, Gottnerb J, Kanelb S, Hammerle CH. Randomized controlled clinical trial of zirconia-ceramic and metal-ceramic posterior fixed dental prostheses: A 3-year follow-up. Int J Prosthodont 2009;22:553–560.
40. Cantarella J, Pitta J, Mojon P, Hicklin SP, Fehmer V, Sailer I. Mechanical stability of restorations supported by titanium base, zirconia, and polyetherketoneketone abutments on one- and two-piece zirconia implants. Int J Oral Maxillofac Implants 2021;36:313–321.
41. de Kok P, Kleverlaan CJ, de Jager N, Kuijs R, Feilzer AJ. Mechanical performance of implant-supported posterior crowns. J Prosthet Dent 2015;114(1):59–66.
42. Gou M, Chen H, Kang J, Wang H. Antagonist enamel wear of tooth-supported monolithic zirconia posterior crowns in vivo: A systematic review. J Prosthet Dent 2019;121: 598–603.
43. Kwon SJ, Lawson NC, McLaren EE, Nejat AH, Burgess JO. Comparison of the mechanical properties of translucent zirconia and lithium disilicate. J Prosthet Dent 2018;120(1):132–137.
44. Arola DD, Reprogel RK. Tubule orientation and the fatigue strength of human dentin. Biomaterials 2006;27:2131–2140.
45. Huang ZL, Shi JY, Zhang X, Gu YX, Lai HC. The influence of the shock-absorbing restorative materials on the stress distributions of short dental implant rehabilitations. Eur Rev Med Pharmacol Sci 2021;25(1):24–34.
46. Quirynen M, Naert I, van Steenberghe D. Fixture design and overload influence marginal bone loss and fixture success in the Branemark system. Clin Oral Implants Res 1992;3(3):104–111.
47. Chambrone L, Chambrone LA, Lima LA. Effects of occlusal overload on peri-implant tissue health: a systematic review of animal-model studies. J Periodontol 2010;81:1367–1378.
48. Naert I, Duyck J, Vandamme K. Occlusal overload and bone/implant loss. Clin Oral Implants Res 2012;23(Suppl 6):95–107.
49. Chrcanovic BR, Kisch J, Albrektsson T, Wennerberg A. Bruxism and dental implant failures: A multilevel mixed effects parametric survival analysis approach. J Oral Rehabil 2016;43:813–823.
50. Mengatto CM, Coelho-de-Souza FH, de Souza Junior OB. Sleep bruxism: Challenges and restorative solutions. Clin Cosmet Investig Dent 2016;8:71–77.
51. Sicilia A, Gallego L, Sicilia P, Mallo C, Cuesta S, Sanz M. Crestal bone loss associated with different implant surfaces in the posterior mandible in patients with a history of periodontitis. A retrospective study. Clin Oral Implants Res 2021;32:88–99.
52. Fickl S, Kebschull M, Calvo-Guirado JL, Hürzeler M, Zuhr O. Experimental peri-implantitis around different types of implants—A clinical and radiographic study in dogs. Clin Implant Dent Relat Res 2015;17(Suppl 2):e661– e669.

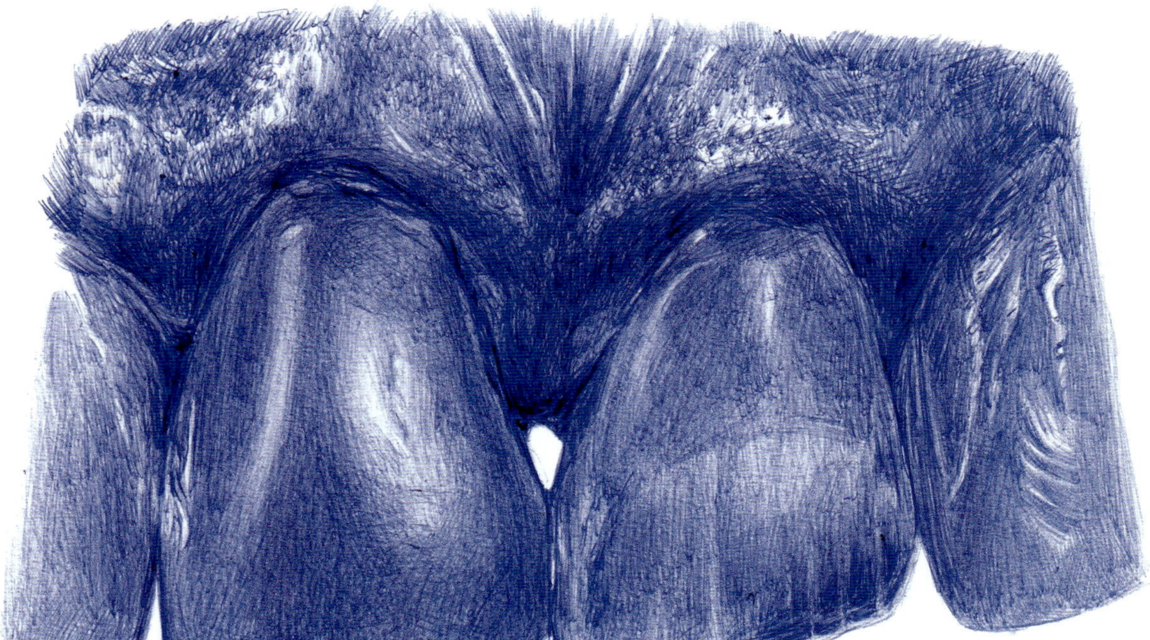

*Here comes the sun, and I say, 'It's all right.'*

—The Beatles, rock band, born in Liverpool

# SECTION III
# PREVENTION AND LONG-TERM MAINTENANCE IN TOOTH WEAR TREATMENT

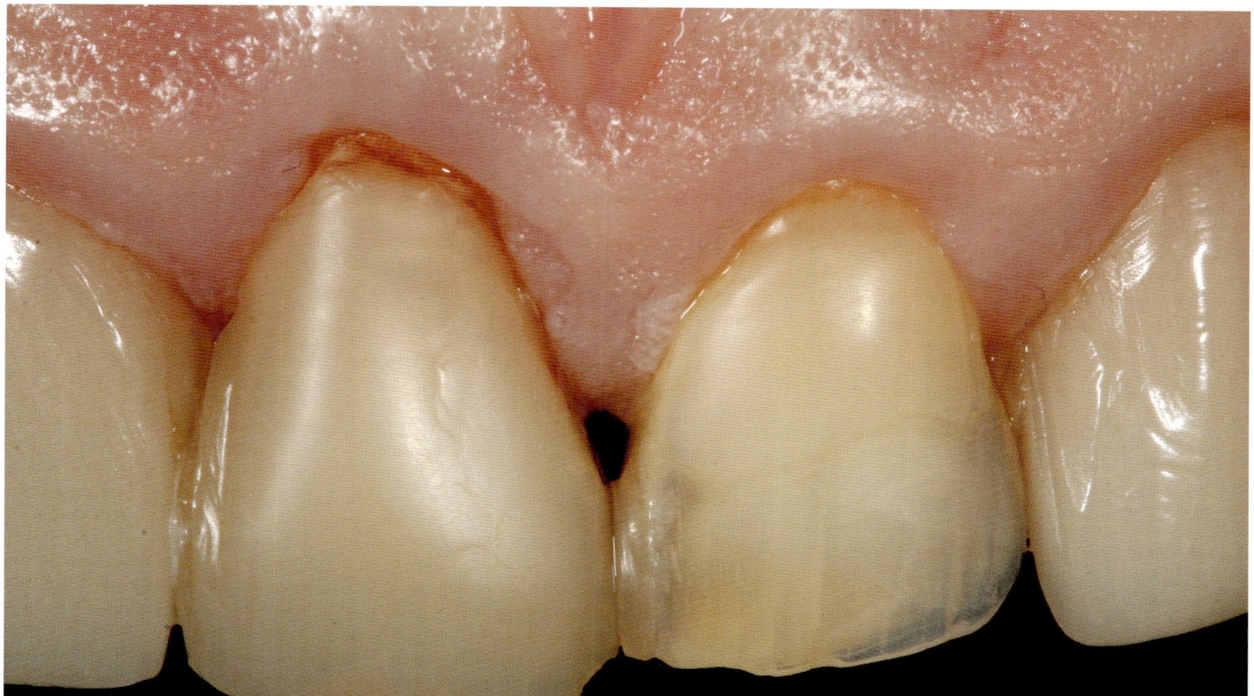

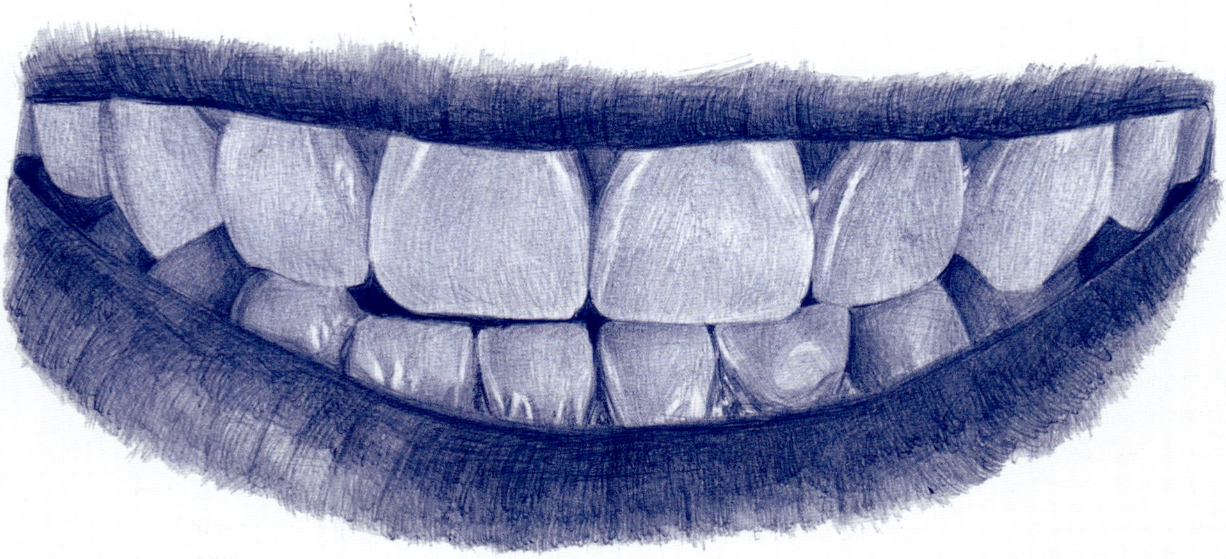

*It is health that is real wealth and not pieces of gold and silver.*

—Mahatma Gandhi, father of the independence of India

CHAPTER 10

# ARE WE IN TIME TO FLATTEN THE TOOTH WEAR CURVE?

Medicine in the 21st century aims to become preventive rather than curative. This may be possible only because of the ongoing identification and understanding of risk factors that lie behind disease. The exhaustive study of risk factors in the cardiovascular field has enabled cardiovascular management to shift to preventive cardiology; lifestyle reeducation and minor cardiovascular interventions intercepting future damage as well as removing the damaged tissue in the initial stages have changed the game.

Yet, cardiovascular disease is the leading cause of death in developed countries today because of the so-called behavioral risk factors. Patient education powered by the passion and motivation of health professionals is making a significant change in this field of modern medicine. Dentistry as a medical discipline has the duty to move forward in this direction in order to facilitate the prevention of disease.

However, the road ahead is long and winding. It requires being able to educate the patient into commitment through the understanding of the benefits of preventive measures, even if this involves a change of lifestyle. Furthermore, it also requires training of the dental team in the philosophy of health promotion and in communication skills.

## 1. 30 Years of Treating Tooth Wear: What Have We Learned?

Just as seismic scientists are able to determine which areas of the Earth are more susceptible to earthquakes, dentists and other dental professionals should be able to determine which patients are at higher risk of developing TW. Specialists who predict earthquakes study movement and the personality of tectonic plates, while dentists should get their information from a comprehensive medical history, without underestimating the effect of the patient's personality. Medical history can be enriched with a self-assessed Lifestyle and Health TW Questionnaire (see appendix 1) to facilitate the gathering of information. The analysis of such a questionnaire will help to detect TW before it manifests its clinical and anatomical consequences, and chances are that, by the modification of a coexisting condition or lifestyle habit, prevention of TW may be achieved in a timely manner. Dentist-patient communication should be fluid in order to succeed in this task (Figs 10-1 and 10-2).

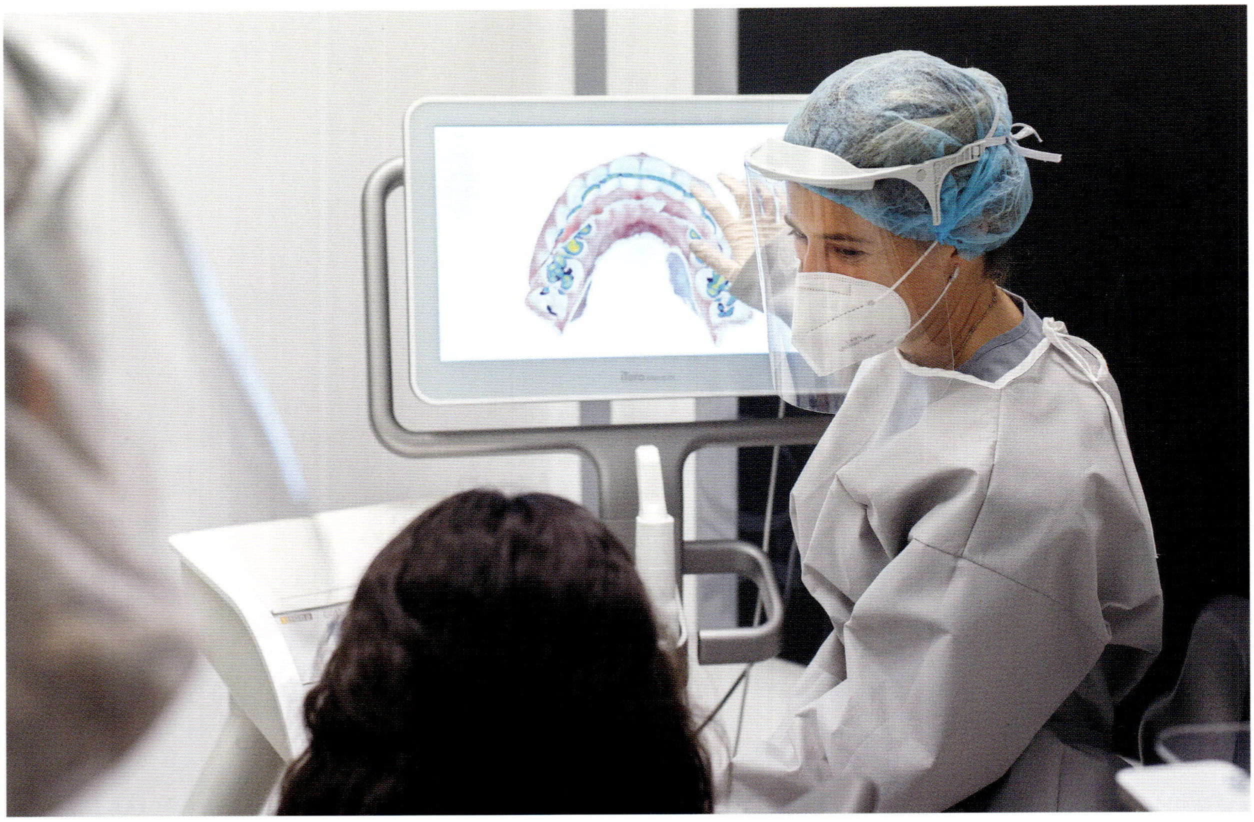

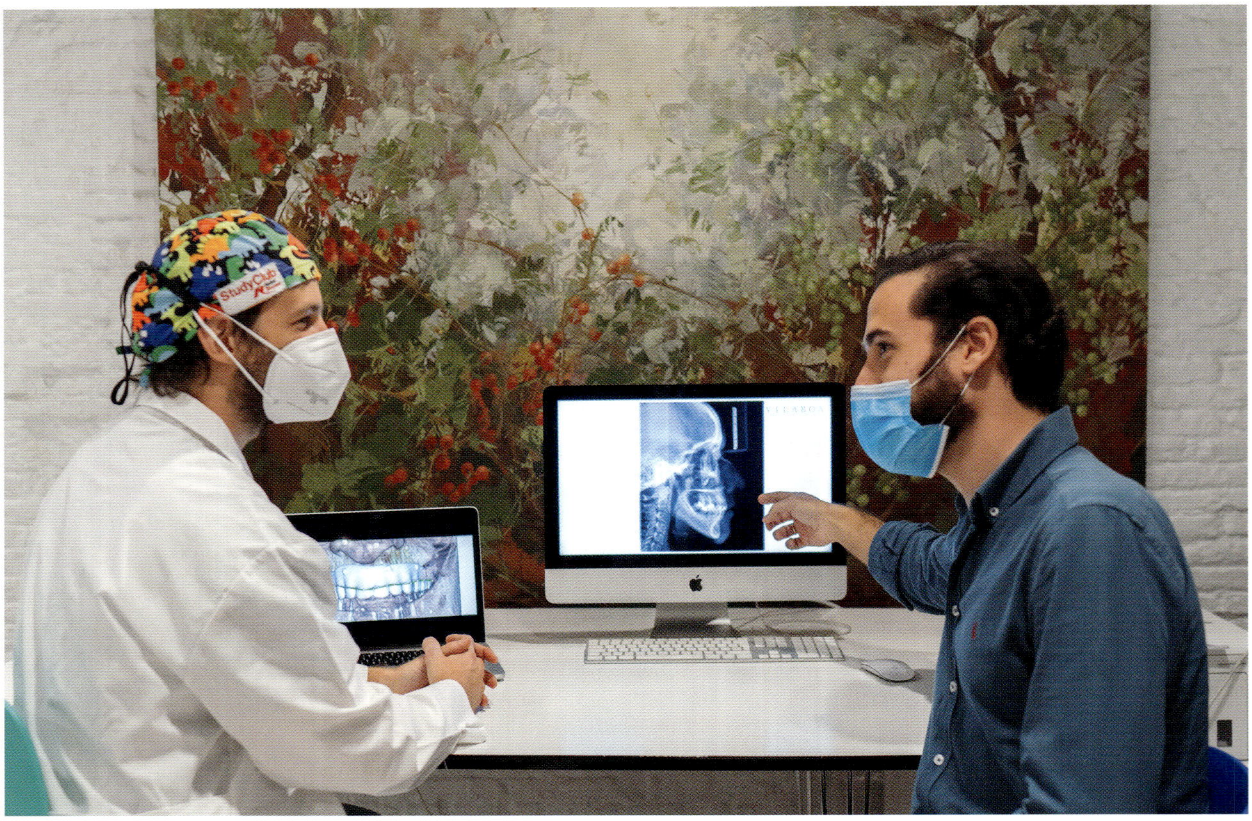

**Figs 10-1 and 10-2** The end of the paternalistic era in medicine, predominant up until the 20th century, must necessarily be followed by a new method of care whereby thoughtful shared decision making will yield better treatment outcomes. Active listening to the patient will lead to a mutual improvement in understanding that, in its turn, will reinforce the decision-making process when treating TW.

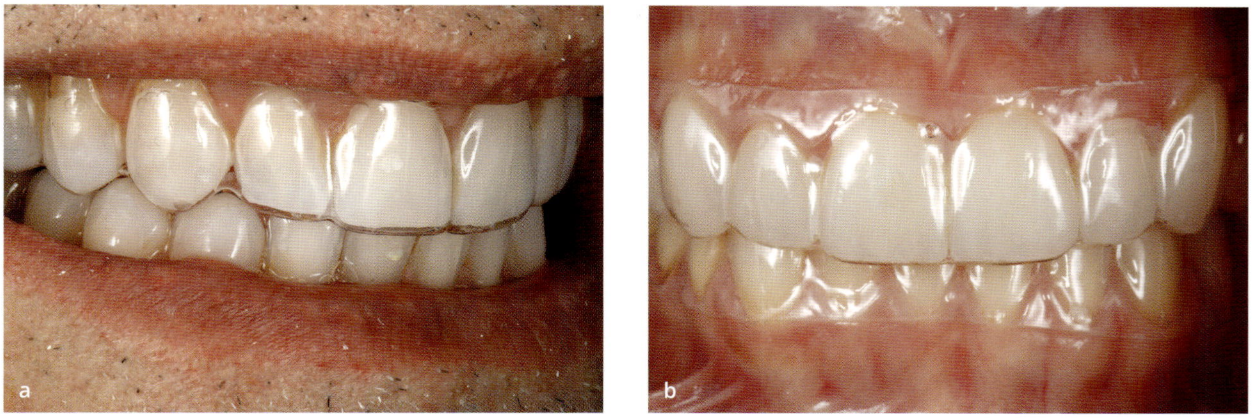


**Fig 10-3** Soft full-arch protective splints are meant to protect both restorations and, most importantly, teeth from erosive TW. They are to be worn mostly during the night and sometimes during the day. They are well accepted by patients, are cost-effective, and have shown good patient compliance while providing protection for restorations in the patients with TW. Individualizing the type of mouthguard protection depending on the type of TW origin helps in the patient's compliance. The classical Michigan-type mouthguard is only meant to be used during sleep except for episodes of acute TMJ crisis for mechanically induced occlusal alterations. Soft protective guards serve as orthodontic retainers and for protection of composite restorations in Fig 10-3a, while they protect porcelain laminate veneers in the patient shown in Fig 10-3b.

In the same manner as the European Federation of Periodontology's (EFP) recent EFP Manifesto encourages medical and dental teams to proactively work toward the identification of periodontal disease,[1] over recent years European expert consensus management guidelines have outlined the path to raise awareness of the importance of early detection of TW in order to minimize its impact on oral health and general well-being.[2]

It is increasingly evident that TW risk factors and clinical parameters should be taken into consideration when evaluating the oral health of a patient, alongside the clinical recording of caries, periodontal disease, and oral pathology.[3] As explained in previous chapters, an easy-to-use clinical TW index would be an effective tool to help dental teams (dentists and hygienists) in the detection of early signs of TW. The already detailed and increasingly used Basic Erosive Wear Examination (BEWE) is still mainly applied in the domain of the academic world for research and publication purposes.[4–6] A Wear Easy Clinical Classification (WECC) is proposed in this book for its use in the everyday practice, as well as a Wear Aggravation Severity Scale (WASS) to help in the detection of those cases where a more rapid and severe evolution is expected (see chapter 4).

In the same way as risk assessment protocols for digestive health have encouraged health professionals to prescribe histamine H2-receptor antagonists not only in cases of duodenal or gastric ulcers, stress gastritis, and gastroesophageal reflux disease, among others, but also whenever a challenge to the digestive mucosa is suspected (intake of any gastro-erosive drug, for example), after a proactive identification of TW risk factors it would be desirable to activate special recommendations that may, in some cases, be enough for the primary prevention of TW.

Being able to determine in a given patient the major cause of TW, even if combined with other causes, is vital to the implementation of specific measures to control or counteract the predisposing factors. Erosion is regarded as the main cause of TW in Europe, while attrition is more relevant in other localizations.[7,8]

Although no scientific evidence seems to exist in regard to whether the use of a hard acrylic occlusal splint is effective in the prevention of the consequences of sleep bruxism (SB),[9] the general clinical consensus regarding these cases has favored the use of such occlusal appliances. If the TW is mainly erosive, this type of stabilizing occlusal splint will not prevent teeth from dissolving in an acidic environment. Nevertheless, long-term maintenance of the restorations provided will result from the regular use of protective Essix-like guards, which are more suitable in cases of erosive damage. Hence precision targeting is essential in order to obtain reliable results in TW prevention (Fig 10-3).

## 2. Modern Lifestyle: Change What Is Possible

From an epidemiologic point of view, most of the approaches for reducing TW involve modern lifestyle modifications, a complicated task indeed if we take into consideration, for example, how difficult the prevention of cardiovascular disease, diabetes, and other diseases is, even after decades of national and worldwide campaigns. Preschool children are already confronted with healthy or unhealthy lifestyle choices. Prevention of the universe of diseases linked to lifestyle behaviors should start early enough to be able to mold the way we live.[10–12] As an example, the well-known television show *Sesame Street,* first aired in 1968, has devoted great effort toward the promotion of healthy habits inspired by breakthrough innovations in cardiovascular and general health. Titanic educational efforts would be futile without the help of the media.[13] Furthermore, educating the young into adopting healthy habits is happening today through new technologies such as digital games that, even if in contradiction with their sedentary use, help promote the value of physical activity in their games[14] (Fig 10-4).

However, while society gets acquainted with the emerging TW data and receives education about how to prevent it, the role of the dentist and the dental team is of paramount importance in implementing a Personalized Preventive Program (PPP) for the patient with TW. It may well happen that no signs of TW are visible yet, but TW risk behaviors or conditions are declared by the patient. This would be the ideal moment to implement a TW PPP.

As explained in previous chapters, the wide variety of TW predisposing factors and the fact that TW is often multifactorial may make this task seem unattainable. However, promoting specific countermeasures as soon as possible is decisive in the prognosis of the case and the patient's commitment and trust. This is certainly a time-consuming mission; therefore, the involvement of other members of the dental team would make it more feasible and sustainable. Communication skills are mandatory to succeed. Educating in parameters such as pH, buffer capacity, titratable acidity amongst other factors related to tooth structure dissolution is very important (Fig 10-5).

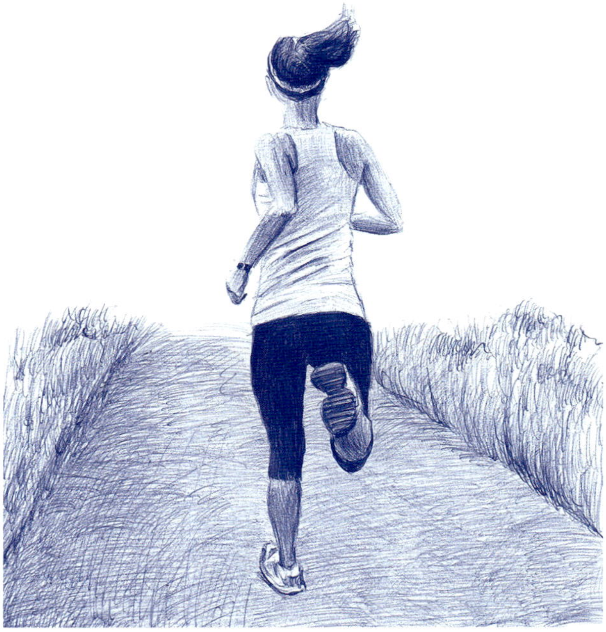

**Fig 10-4** Lifestyle coaching has been proven to be effective in helping overweight children and adults reach a healthier lifestyle in in countries such as the Netherlands and appears to be a tool that is exportable to TW prevention. Topics such as nutritional and dietary re-education, reinforcement of the values of sustainable physical activity, and teaching good sleep hygiene and stress management are addressed by the lifestyle coach, a new profession that will offer great value also in TW prevention and maintenance.

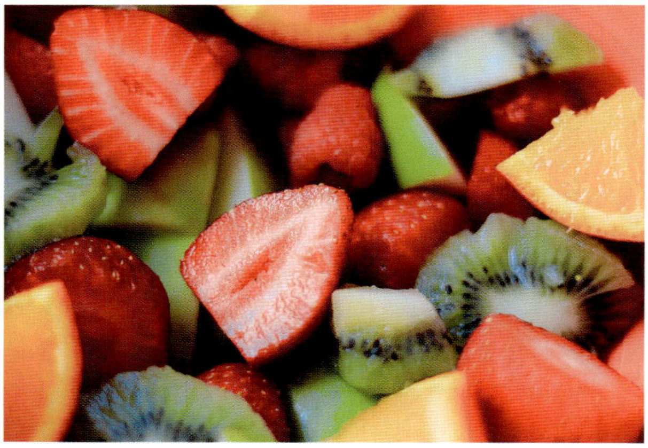

**Fig 10-5** Consumption of acidic fruits or beverages, when in excess, especially in vulnerable patients, can produce devastating erosive damage in the dentition. Dietary habits, dietary fashions, and acidic fizzy drinks are behind the rising figures of erosive TW.

### Activation of Preventive Measures to Minimize the Impact of TW Risk Factors

The moment TW risk factors have been identified, with or without detection of TW signs or symptoms, a prompt activation of individualized countermeasures should be considered and discussed with the patient. As per evidence that has been gathered, the preventive countermeasures outlined in Tables 10-1 and 10-2 are proposed for adults and children.[15–56]

**Table 10-1** Tooth wear risk factors and preventive countermeasures in adults.

| | Risk Factors | Countermeasures |
|---|---|---|
| Dietary Risk Factors | ▪ Soft drinks<br>▪ Fruit juices<br>▪ Sport drinks | Restrict acidic drinks to main meals. Reduce intake.<br>Substitute with milk, water, or yogurt whenever possible.<br>Use a straw. Control and modify manner, frequency, and duration of contact time with acidic food.<br>Sport drinks should not be consumed after intense performance that leads to dehydration and potentiation of erosive damage. |
| | ▪ Acidic fruits<br>▪ Vinegar<br>▪ Lemon<br>▪ Salad dressings | Chewing fruits is preferable to fruit juices as it allows saliva production. Use other options such as olive oil and soy sauce. Reduce acid intake. Combine yogurt or olive oil with acidic fruits. |
| | Caffeine | Reduce intake, especially close to bedtime. |
| | Alcohol | Reduce intake. Do not "hold" in the mouth. |
| | Red/white wine | Do not "hold" in the mouth. Drink in combination with cheese or olives. |
| Lifestyle | Practice of intense sports | Avoid dehydration. Avoid sports drinks. Use protective mouthguards. |
| | ▪ Presence of stress<br>▪ Hyperconnected life | Promotion of healthy lifestyle and relaxation. Educate patients so that they understand anxiety can produce low salivary flow and TW. |
| | ▪ Vegetarian diet<br>▪ Fruitarian diet | Balanced diet. Mediterranean diet. Dietary intake should include protein, carbohydrates and lipids, preferably coming from olive oil. Fiber and vitamins from vegetables and fruits must not be overlooked. |
| | ▪ Low or vocational educational level | Associated with unbalanced diet. Promote nutritional education and coaching. |
| | ▪ Swimming in chlorinated water<br>▪ Wine tasters | Seen in professionals. Explain risks.<br>For nonprofessionals, combine with cheese or olives. |
| Oral Hygiene Habits | Use of a hard-bristle manual toothbrush | Switch to medium-soft bristles. |
| | Use of high-speed electric toothbrush | Reduce force/speed. Switch to manual toothbrush (medium-soft). |
| | Use of abrasive toothpaste | Choose toothpaste with low or nonabrasive RDA value. |
| | Use of acidic oral care product in patients with xerostomia | Choose saliva-stimulating oral care line with neutral pH. |
| | Tooth brushing immediately after consuming acidic food or beverages | Wait preferably 30 minutes before tooth brushing. Use regular application of fluoride. |
| Parafunctional Habits | Nail biting<br>Lip biting<br>Cheek biting<br>Pen biting | Stop the habit. Use full-arch soft Essix-like guards at night to deprogram the habit. |

**Table 10-1** *(continued)* Tooth wear risk factors and preventive countermeasures in adults.

| | Risk Factors | Countermeasures |
|---|---|---|
| Malocclusion | | Eliminate prematurities and/or interferences when existing. Orthodontic treatment. |
| Sleep Disorders | Sleep bruxism or clenching<br>Day clenching | Nighttime hard acrylic bite splints. Oral hygiene regimen to stimulate saliva and serve as lubricant.<br>Use of lubricants. |
| Sleep Disorders | Snoring | Reduce tobacco and alcohol use and lose weight (if applicable). Stimulate salivary flow. |
| Sleep Disorders | Sleep apnea | Mandibular advancement device (MAD), CPAP, salivary moisturizers. |
| Medical Conditions | Gastritis or heartburn<br>Hiatal hernia<br>GERD<br><br>Easy or frequent vomiting, eating disorders (BN/AN)<br>Food intolerance | Consult physician.<br>Stop caffeine, tobacco, and alcohol use, especially close to bedtime. Avoid fatty food. Choose small and frequent meals over big meals. Consult physician about use of proton pump inhibitors. Lose weight. Use erosion-protective oral hygiene regimen. Earlier dinnertime and take a walk before bed when possible.<br>Consult physician, counselor, psychiatrist, and/or psychologist. Use manual toothbrush and erosion-protective oral hygiene regimen. Stimulate salivary flow.<br>Consult physician and/or nutritionist. |
| Medical Conditions | Intake of medication | Consult physician. If possible, switch to less xerostomic drugs. If possible, change medication dosage and/or number of medications. Change formulation and type of medication. Tooth damage may be caused by xerostomic or acidic effects of medication. Stimulate salivary flow. |
| Medical Conditions | Chewing vitamin C, aspirin with vitamin C, or iron tablets | Swallow tablets instead. |
| Medical Conditions | Oncological condition (based on type and use of chemo- and/or radiotherapy) | Use erosion-protective oral hygiene regimen. Stimulate salivary flow. |
| Medical Conditions | Dry mouth / xerostomia | Check the cause. Reduce acid in diet. Use erosion-protective oral hygiene regimen. Stimulate salivary flow. Educate patient in erosion-protective diet. Restore missing dentition to facilitate chewing and salivary stimulation. |
| Medical Conditions | Stress<br>Anxiety<br>Depression | Consult physician, counselor, psychiatrist, and/or psychologist. Educate patients so that they understand stress will produce low salivary flow and TW. Promote stress-reduction techniques. Avoid xerostomic drugs such as tricyclic antidepressants if possible (new-generation antidepressants are less xerostomic). |
| Medical Conditions | Any other major medical condition | Consult physician. Stimulate salivary flow. |

**Table 10-2** Tooth wear risk factors and preventive countermeasures in children.

| | Risk Factors | Countermeasures |
|---|---|---|
| Dietary Risk Factors | ▪ Soft drinks<br>▪ Fruit juices<br>▪ Candies<br>▪ Sweets<br>▪ Popsicles, slushies, and shakes | ▪ Substitute with milk, water, or yogurt. Reduce intake. Use a straw. Control and modify manner, frequency, and duration of erosive food consumption. Combine with yogurt or cheese.<br>▪ Educate in erosion-protective diet. Avoid providing bottles with acidic drinks to babies and toddlers at night. |
| Oral Hygiene Habits | Use of a hard-bristle manual toothbrush | Switch to medium-soft bristles. |
| | Use of high-speed electric toothbrush | Reduce force/speed. Switch to manual toothbrush (medium-soft). |
| | Use of abrasive toothpaste | Choose toothpaste with low or nonabrasive RDA value. |
| | Use of acidic oral care product in patients with xerostomia | Choose saliva-stimulating oral care line with neutral pH. |
| | Tooth brushing immediately after consuming acidic food or beverages | Wait preferably 30 minutes before tooth brushing. Use regular application of fluoride. |
| Parafunctional Habits | Nail biting<br>Lip biting<br>Cheek biting<br>Pen or toy biting | Stop the habit. Use soft Essix-like guards during the day to deprogram the habit. |
| Malocclusion | | Eliminate prematurities and/or interferences when existing. Orthodontic treatment. |
| Sleep Disorders | ▪ Snoring<br>▪ Insomnia | Orthodontics to intercept upper respiratory tract constriction. Consult physician. |
| Medical Conditions | Easy or frequent vomiting, eating disorders (BN/AN)<br>Food intolerance | Consult physician, counselor, psychiatrist, and/or psychologist. Look for bullying (including cyber-bullying). Use erosion-protective oral hygiene regimen to stimulate salivary flow. Consult nutritionist and/or provide dietary coaching. |
| | ▪ Stress<br>▪ Difficulty sleeping<br>▪ ADHD | Consult physician, counselor, psychiatrist, and/or psychologist. Check salivary flow and use oral hygiene regimen to stimulate saliva. |
| | Bullying (including cyber-bullying) | Consult counselor, psychiatrist, and/or psychologist. Children subjected to long-term bullying may develop eating and sleeping disorders. Check salivary flow and use oral hygiene regimen to stimulate saliva. |
| | Intake of medication | Consult physician. If possible, switch to less xerostomic drugs. Stimulate salivary flow. If possible, change medication dosage and/or number of medications. Change formulation and type of medication. Tooth damage may be caused by xerostomic or acidic effects of medication. |
| | ▪ Allergies<br>▪ Asthma<br>▪ Use of aerosols for allergies and/or asthma | May induce both xerostomia and erosive damage. Stimulate salivary flow via oral care and chewing (choose solid foods over liquids). Use erosion-protective oral hygiene regimen. |
| | Oncological condition (based on type and use of chemo- and/or radiotherapy) | Stimulate salivary flow via oral care regimen. Use erosion-protective oral hygiene regimen. Educate patient and/or parents in erosion-protective dietary habits. |

## 3. Targeting Nutritional Risk Factors: The Benefits of Erosion-Protective Foods

Teaching children to reduce the amount and frequency of their intake of soft drinks and citrus fruit juices and modifying the manner of intake, even if it involves nutritional education campaigns, may prove a cost-effective measure in preventing or reducing TW incidence in the younger population. Substitution with water, milk shakes, or yogurt-drinks is safe and will ensure better oral status over the longer life expectancy of future generations (Figs 10-6 and 10-7). Keeping a comprehensive diet diary will provide a lot of information regarding the patient's nutritional habits.[57]

Citric acid is frequently part of the composition of such drinks, and therefore several approaches, including supplementation with minerals, are currently under analysis to determine whether this strategy offers a protective effect.[58–61] The erosive potential of citric beverages is mainly due to the chelation of calcium complexes and does not depend exclusively on the minerals but also on pH, amount of titratable acidic content, and buffering capacity, among others. Research shows controversial results of adding minerals to citric acid–containing beverages.[58–62] Further studies are required in order to clarify strategies for this approach.

Regarding erosion-protective food, it has been documented that yogurt does not induce erosion, even when it contains fruit and acidic flavors[63] (Fig 10-8). Dairy products such as cheese produce an immediate rise in pH, driving dental plaque to a neutral pH scenario. Casein also helps reduce enamel solubility. The rapid pH rise after the intake of cheese or dairy products appears to be linked to stimulation of the salivary flow and its inherent beneficial effects. Taking this into consideration, dairy products should be included in diet counseling.[64] Cleverly, traditions of serving cheese with wine in Mediterranean countries offers a natural protection from wine's erosive damage (Fig 10-9).

There is a growing body of opinion that the Mediterranean diet is compatible with general good health.[65–67] The main components of this diet are fiber, fruits, vegetables, fish, and fats coming mostly from olive oil (Figs 10-10 to 10-12).

Special attention should be given to apparently innocent healthy habits. Chewing vitamin C tablets (rich in ascorbic acid), aspirin with vitamin C, or iron tablets on a long-standing basis can cause erosive tooth damage.[68,69] Swallowing instead of chewing is a good alternative.

Erosive signs have also shown prevalence in certain professions, such as wine tasters, who unfortunately cannot benefit from simultaneous erosion-protective foods as they may alter their taste[70] (Fig 10-13). Wine's high acid content and the drinking manner, savoring and holding the wine in the mouth, pose a challenge to dental structure. In Mediterranean countries, traditionally wine is served accompanied by cheese and/or olives that may naturally counteract the erosive potential of wine. Alternatively fish, preserved or smoked, can serve this purpose.

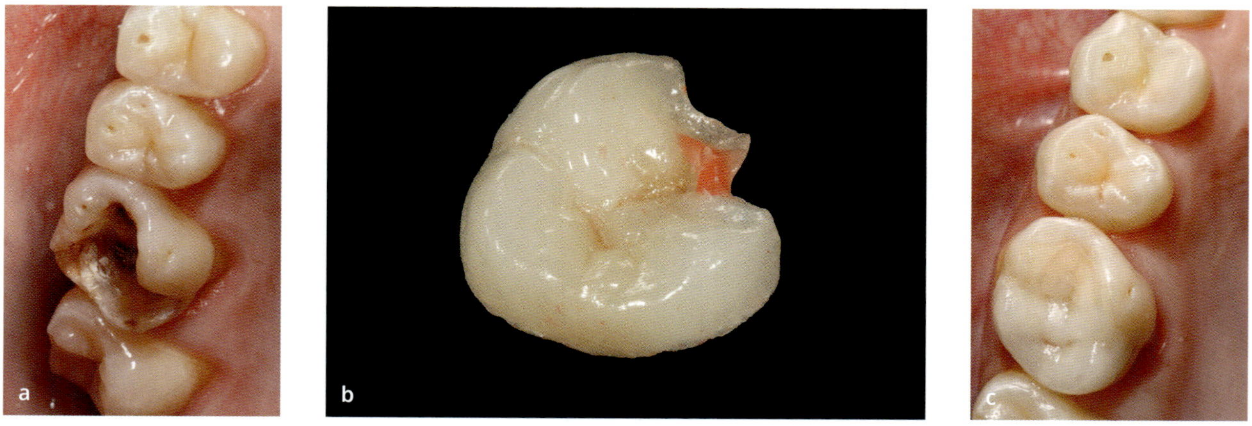


**Fig 10-6** Signs of incipient erosion or so-called biocorrosion should not be understimated in initial visits and/or regular checkups. Incipient erosive lesions have been overlooked, especially when the patient is in need of other treatments (a to c). At that point, a conversation with the patient with the aim to discover, if possible, etiologic risk factors is desirable. Consumption of soft drinks, sodas, and acidic fruit juices is a predisposing factor for dental erosion. Note the incipient minor erosive lesions in the tip of the cusps of this woman in her early 20s.

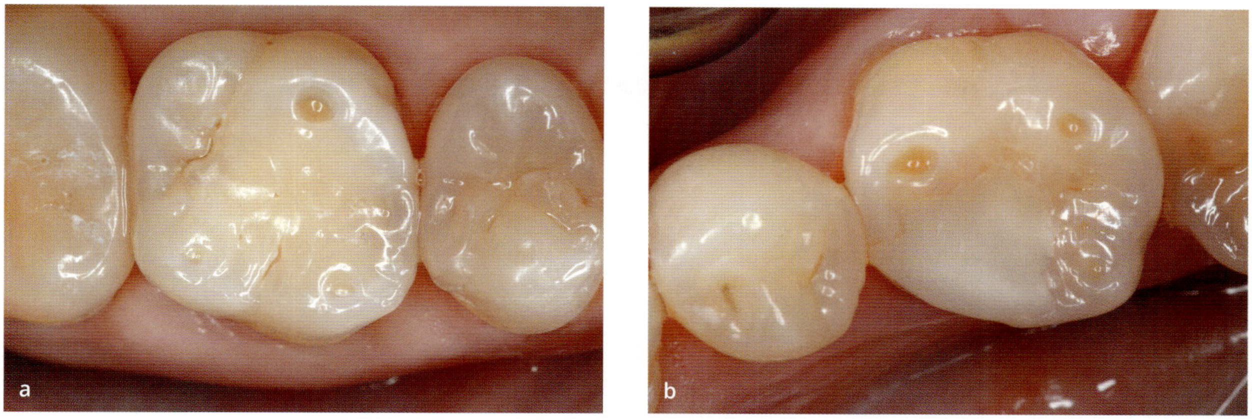


**Fig 10-7** Evident signs of gingival inflammation may obscure the diagnosis of incipient well-like erosion lesions on the tips of the cusps in this patient (a and b). Soft tissue disorders, such as gingival or papillae inflammation, have been linked to erosive challenges.

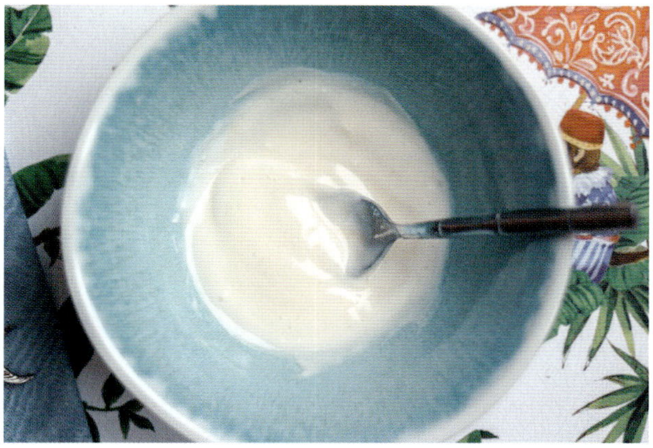

**Fig 10-8** Although yogurt and milk have a pH close to 4.5, their high content of calcium and phosphate, among other characteristics, render them nonerosive food and beverage choices.

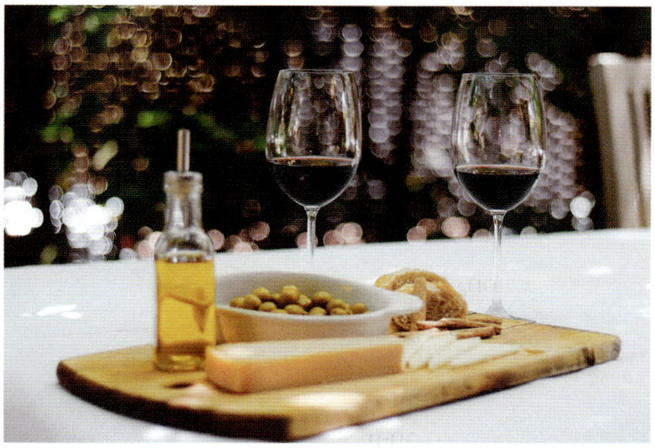

**Fig 10-9** Abundant content of phenolic acids and polyphenols seem to stand behind the highly regarded reputation of daily moderate wine consumption among the general population.

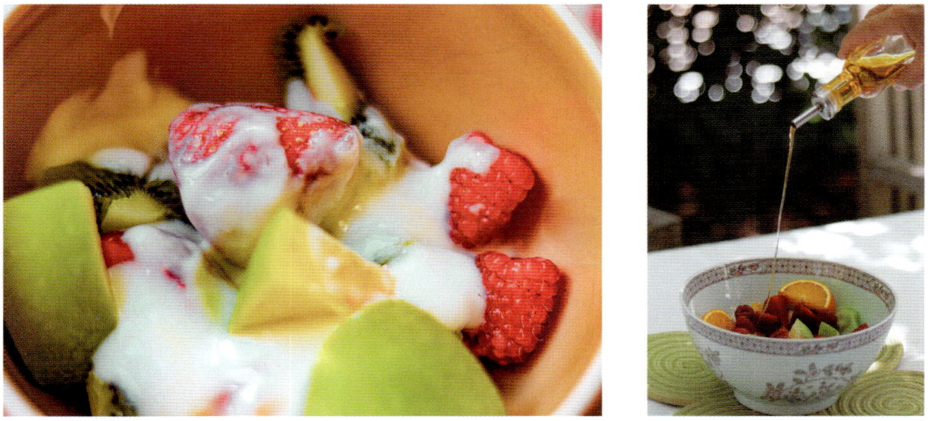

**Figs 10-10 and 10-11** The health benefits of fruit are unquestionable. In patients with erosion risk, its intake in the form of fruit salads with dressings such as yogurt or extra-virgin olive oil might be an interesting approach to reducing the acidic challenge.

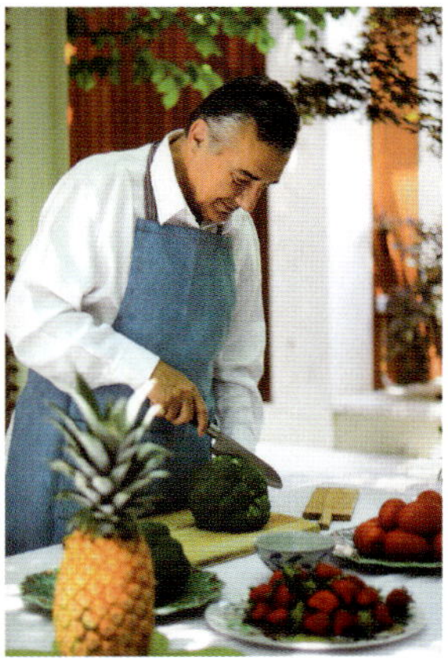

**Fig 10-12** Educating families in nutritional and cooking strategies offers a better window of opportunity for patients at high risk of erosion to avoid TW.

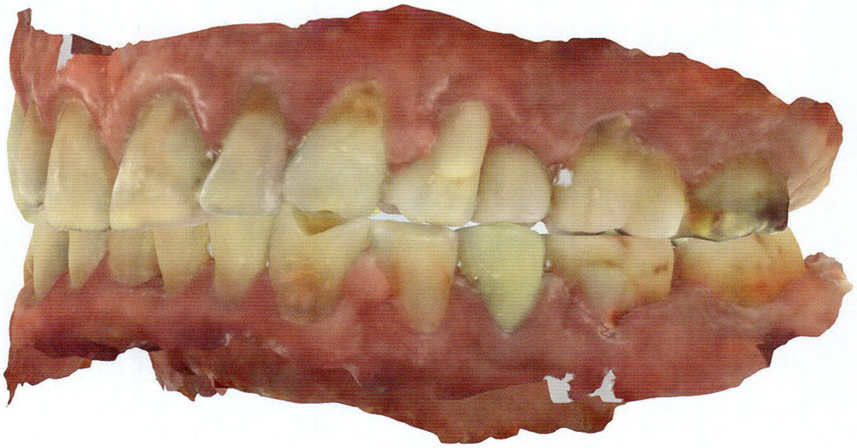

a

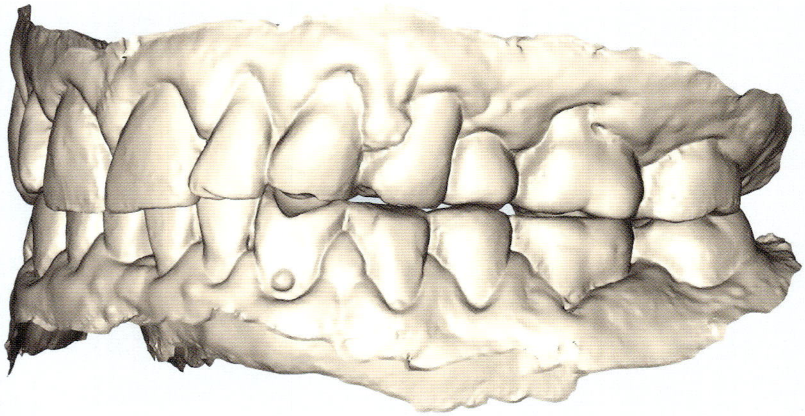

b

**Fig 10-13** The clinical evidence on erosion/biocorrosion lesions in professional enologists and viticulturists supports the recommendation to ask about drinking habits. Note the erosive damage and flattening of the occlusal plane revealed by intraoral scanning in a professional wine taster (a and b).

## 4. Parafunctional Habit Control and Ideal Occlusal Scheme: Keys to Long-Term Maintenance

Diagnosis and treatment of malocclusions are not only tools to treat the TW patient but also therapeutic tools to prevent and intercept the onset of TW. Premature contacts and interferences should be identified. The patient should be occlusally equilibrated to meet the dentist's preferred occlusal scheme. Exploration in maximal intercuspation and in centric relation should always be part of the initial visits and, if needed, follow the guidelines of the fathers of occlusion to provide an appropriate occlusal scenario and the required space to restore the dentition.[71-74] If TW is already present, alternative measures to remove tooth structure by occlusal adjustment should be considered. Additive therapies are more suitable in general than subtracting from the worn dentition (Figs 10-14 and 10-15).

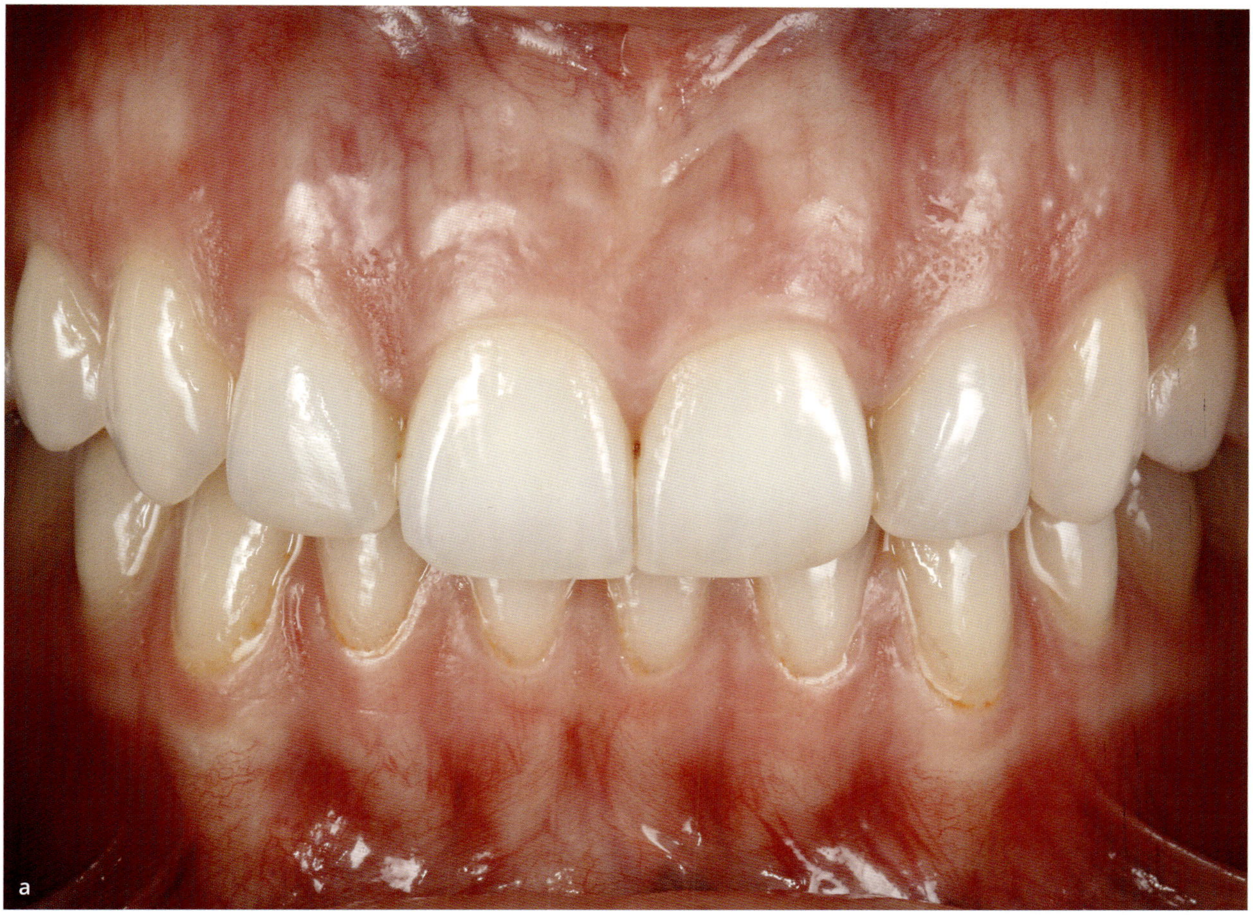


**Fig 10-14** Performance of occlusal equilibration as a general method to provide an optimal functional scenario should always be kept in mind. An additive approach to occlusal equilibration in the patient with TW will save tooth structure and in many cases provide a safe occlusal scheme appreciated in TW management. Routine monitoring to evaluate if composite-restored anterior/canine guidance is still in good function in a young female patient is shown here (a).

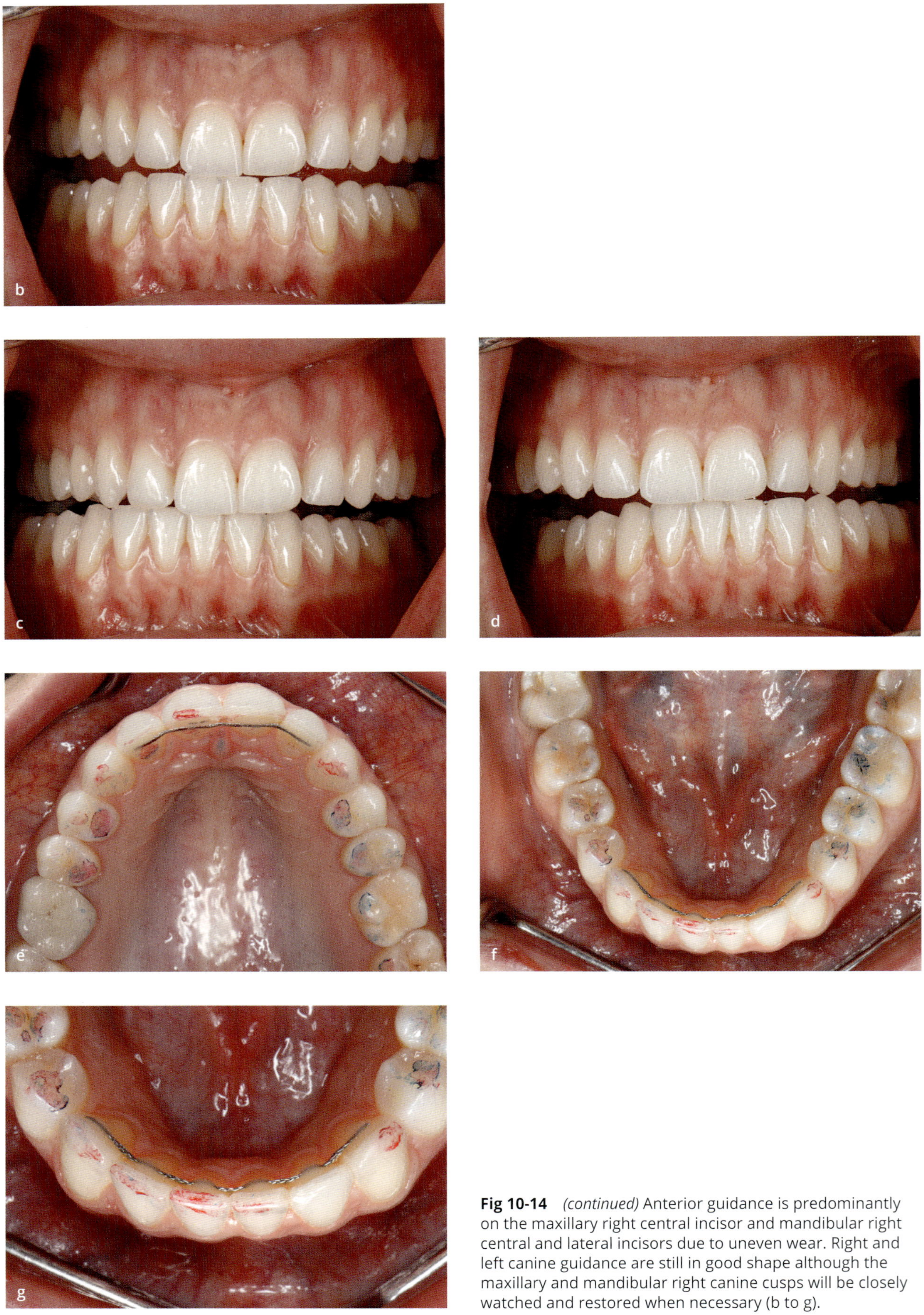


**Fig 10-14** *(continued)* Anterior guidance is predominantly on the maxillary right central incisor and mandibular right central and lateral incisors due to uneven wear. Right and left canine guidance are still in good shape although the maxillary and mandibular right canine cusps will be closely watched and restored when necessary (b to g).

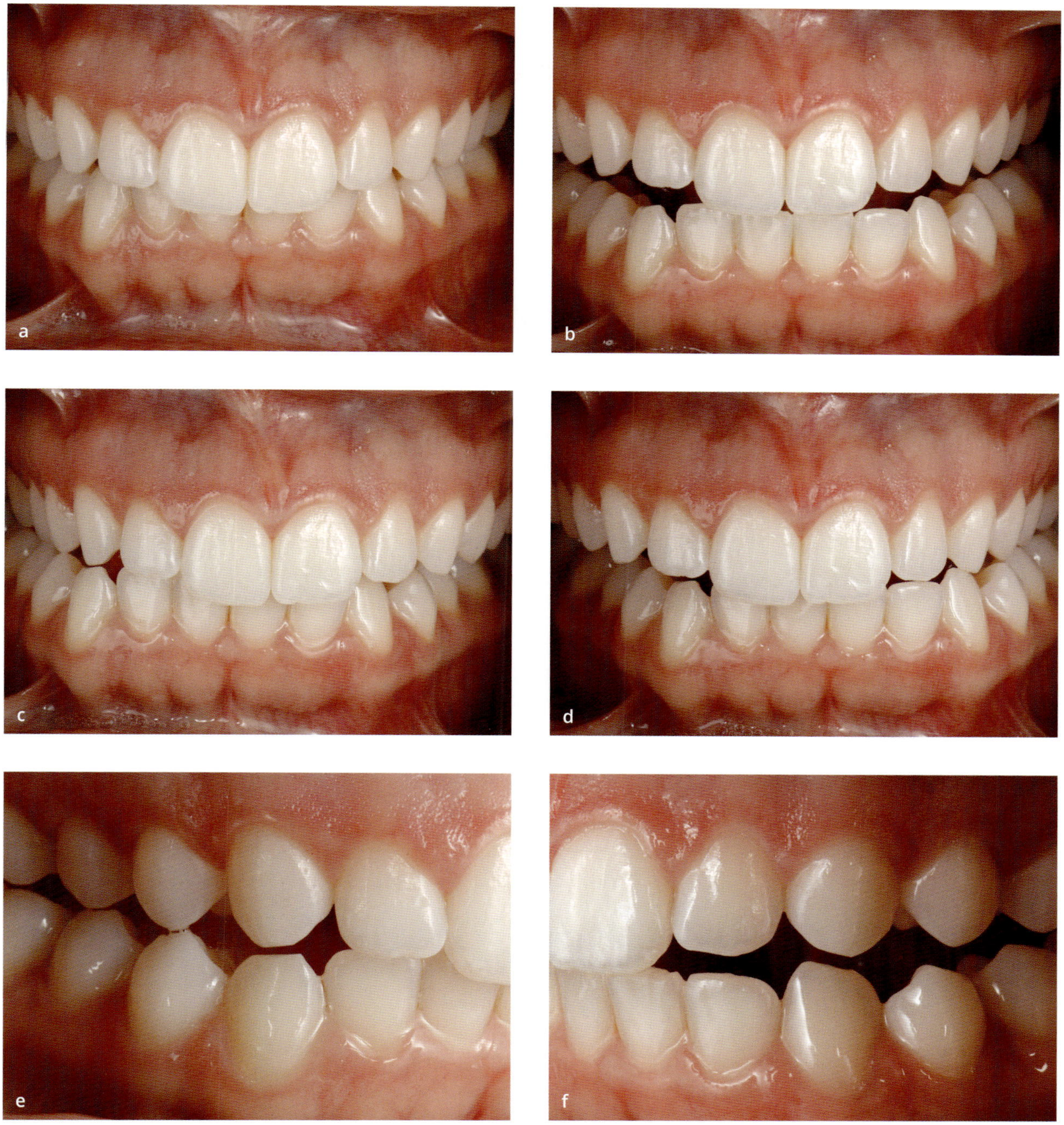

**Fig 10-15** When confronting young patients with overall excellent oral condition, the dilemma to treat or not to treat is always present and should be discussed with the patient and/or the patient's family. If the patient decides not to be treated, frequent recalls must be implemented. The young female patient in this figure is the sister of the patient shown in Fig 5-15 in chapter 5. Interestingly, both sisters show the same premature tooth-to-tooth wear. Group function appeared as a consequence and adaptation to premature wear in the tips of the canines (a to f). *(continued next page)*

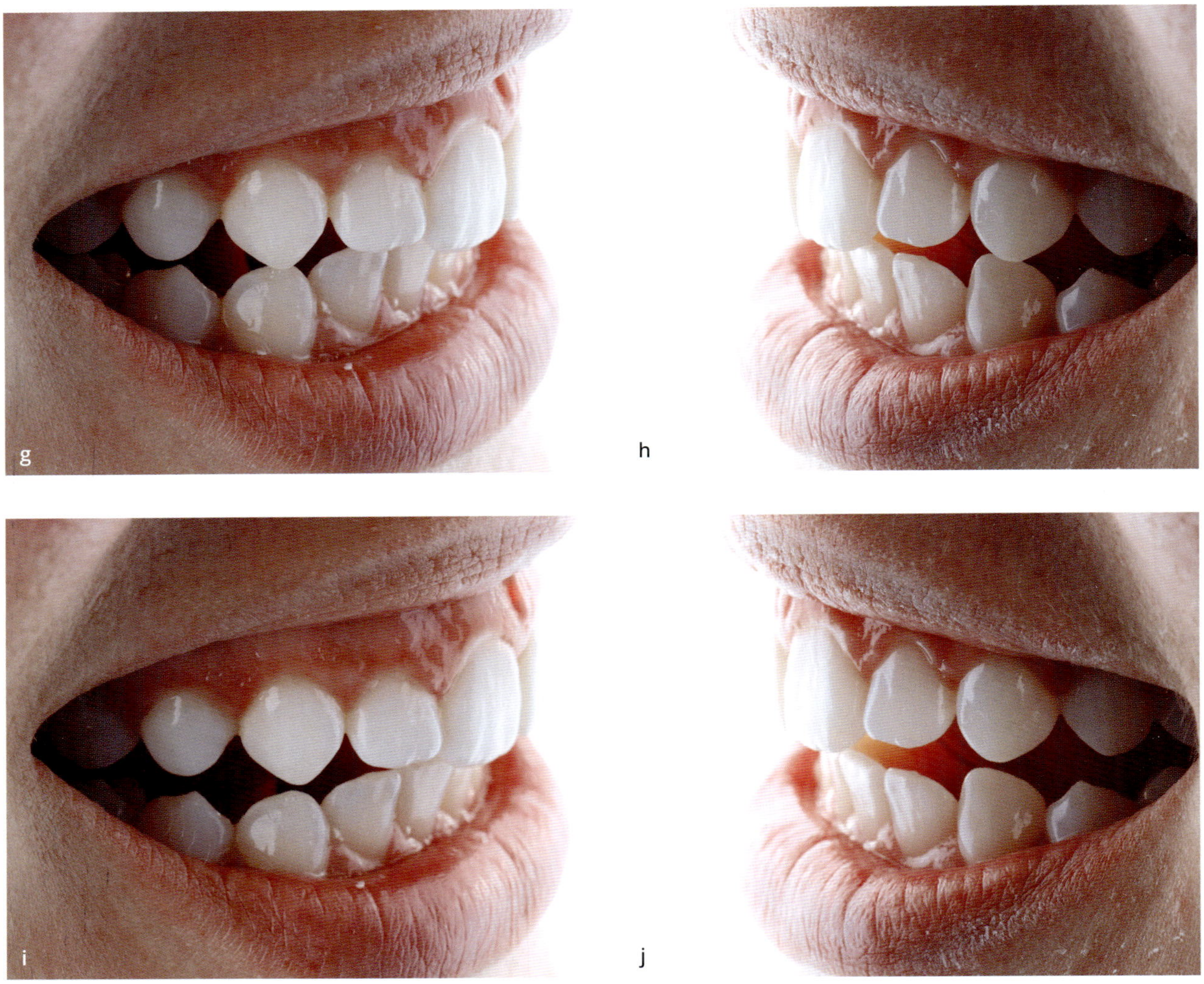

**Fig 10-15** *(continued)* Restoring the four canines at this early stage will prevent further wear in this healthy patient in her early 20s (g to j).

# 5. Oral Hygiene and Tooth Wear

## TW, Tooth Brushing, and Toothpaste Abrasiveness

Oral hygiene is essential for oral health. In view of data from the literature, oral hygiene could be regarded as a TW risk factor; however, its benefits exceed the risks.[75]

The array of oral care products on the market can make it difficult for patients to choose. The choice is also difficult for the dental professional. Patient-dependent factors such as the intensity, frequency, and timing of tooth brushing in relation to eating or drinking have a key influence on oral health and may have an impact on TW.

Tooth brushing has traditionally been linked to abrasion, to some extent considered as physiologic by many authors. Abrasion related to tooth brushing is induced both by the characteristics of the toothpaste and/or toothbrush and by patient-dependent modus operandi, such as the aforementioned frequency and timing[75] (Fig 10-16).

Tooth brushing has also been connected to the removal of the demineralized eroded enamel and or dentin and the appearance, and/or aggravation of erosive damage. Studies evaluating abrasion from tooth brushing on eroded dentin and enamel have shown that dentin and enamel loss increase relative to the increasing abrasiveness of the toothpaste slurry. Tooth loss is also influenced by the stiffness from toothbrushes filaments[76,77] (Fig 10-17). There is general agreement that a toothpaste with a low abrasive index is determinant in preventing erosion.

A long-term in vitro study compared four types of toothbrushes (rotating-oscillating, sonic, and two types of manual toothbrushes) with the same brushing force on eroded dentin lesions. Results from the study showed that manual toothbrushes were significantly less abrasive compared to power toothbrushes.[78] Furthermore, when gingival erosion is to be considered, a controlled brushing force, controlled toothbrush stiffness, and controlled toothpaste abrasiveness are essential to minimizing not only the hard tissue damage but also the erosive consequences on soft tissue in an overall acidic scenario.

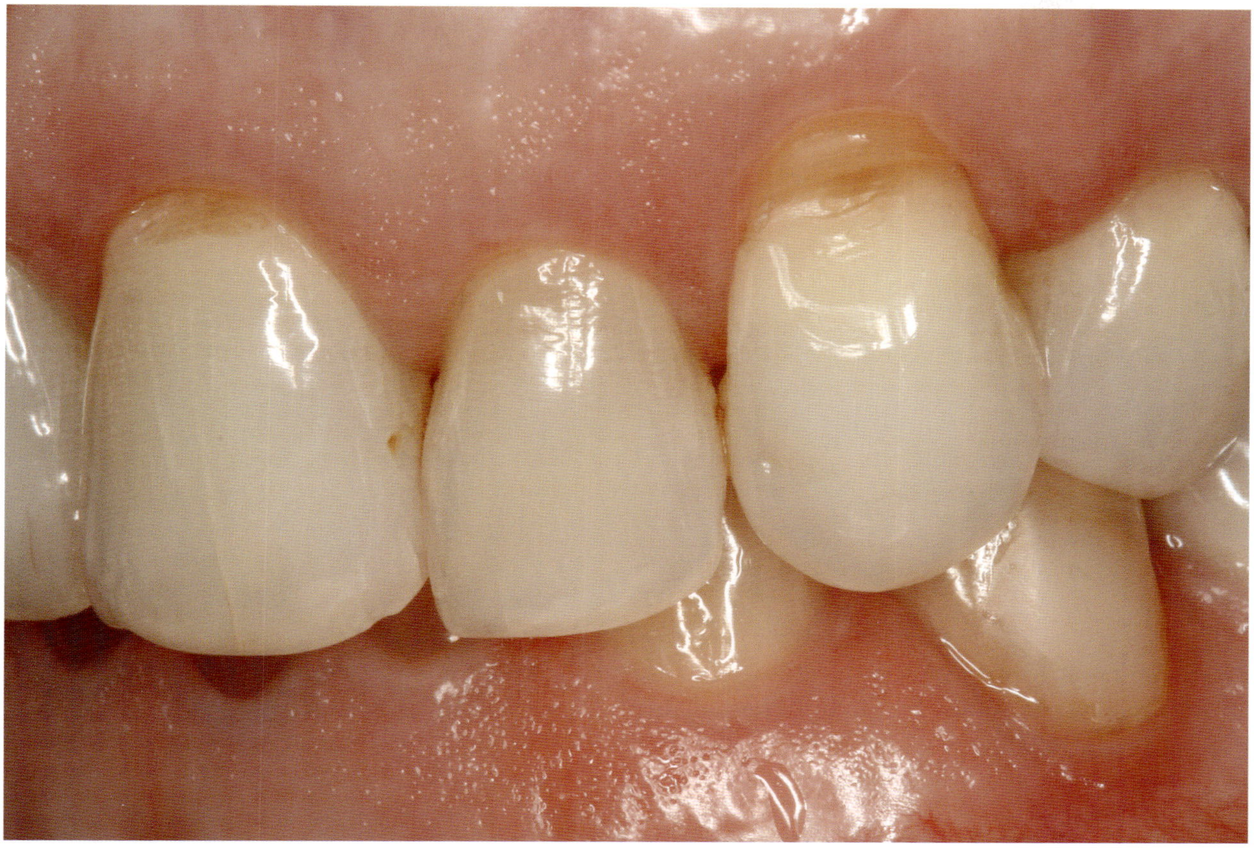

**Fig 10-16** Abrasion risk related to tooth brushing should be controlled in patients with high TW risk. Malocclusion-related overloading might also be influencing the abrasion found in this patient, producing a so-called abfraction pattern.

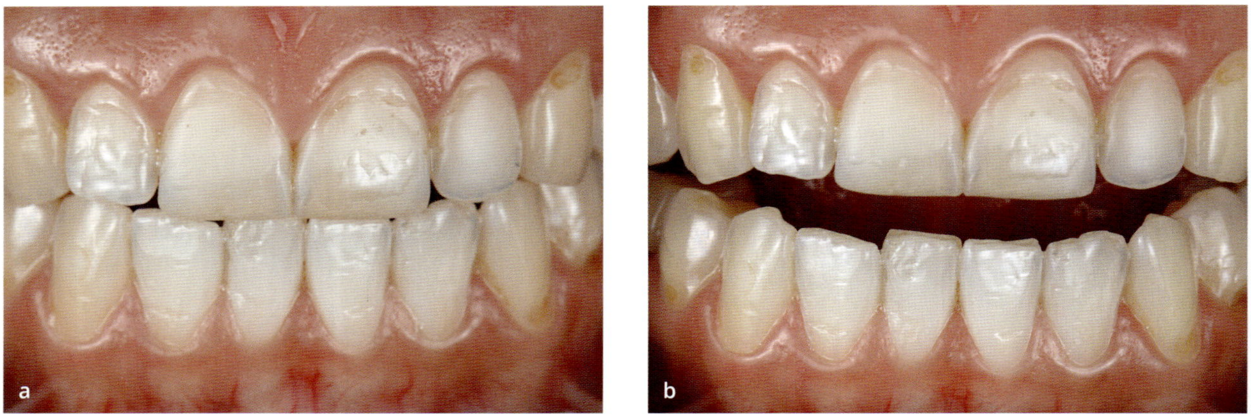

**Fig 10-17** The detrimental role of inadequate tooth brushing mode and/or tools can be critical in those patients suffering from moderate or severe erosion. Preexisting impaired enamel microhardness and dentin exposure in this type of patient offers very poor resistance to tooth brushing mechanical forces (a and b).

Another study comparing manual and sonic toothbrushes found that the average brushing force of manual toothbrushes was significantly higher than sonic ones. The conclusion of the study stated that patients with no wear or with wear lesions limited to enamel will have a better outcome using manual toothbrushes, while patients suffering from severe wear and exposed/eroded dentin will benefit more from sonic toothbrushes.[79]

Notwithstanding the existing discrepancies in terms of the type of toothbrush, there seems to be a consensus regarding the relevance of the brushing mode and force.

## Gingival Erosion in Erosive TW

More than 30 years of treating patients with TW opens the eyes to unexplained common findings, such as the gingival macroscopic changes associated mostly with the erosive type of TW. Niemi et al described how stiffness of toothbrush filaments and abrasiveness of dentifrices influence the degree of what they described as gingival erosion,[80] utilizing the same term as applied to hard tissue.

The impact from the erosive acidic environment and the overall microbiome modification conditioned by the major environmental pH shift in erosive TW is to be further analyzed. This acidic atmosphere is changing the habitat of the oral cavity, and soft tissues have to adapt to this new environment. In fact, recent research coming from Japan has shown the significant prevalence of oral soft tissue disorders that accompany acidic challenges such as the one presented in GERD. The relevance is such that oral soft tissue disorders appeared to be as frequent as tooth erosion in this type of patient.[81] A new concept of tooth and gingival erosion is already occupying researchers at the same time as we are asking ourselves why. Pushing this group of patients to excel in hygiene measures without addressing the erosive condition might not offer the expected benefit.

## Remineralization, Fluoride, and TW

TW and especially erosion require preventive measures that combine several strategies, such as nutritional reeducation, industrial modification of acid-containing drinks, specifically targeted oral hygiene with compounds that might prove effective in erosion prevention, and the use of oral hygiene products that have been shown to be effective in stimulating salivary flow.

The remineralization process described for caries requires the existence of sound enamel, under which the subsurface offers an adequate matrix for crystal growth. This is only possible if there is a supersaturation of minerals in saliva in relation to the tooth. Therefore, correct salivary quantity and quality are sine qua non conditions for remineralization to take place. When erosion is the issue, the enamel surface is affected in such a way that there is no matrix for crystal regrowth, and mineral deposition is impeded, even if the existing saliva is supersaturated with the required minerals. This is the reason behind the statement that describes erosion as irreversible[82] (Fig 10-18).

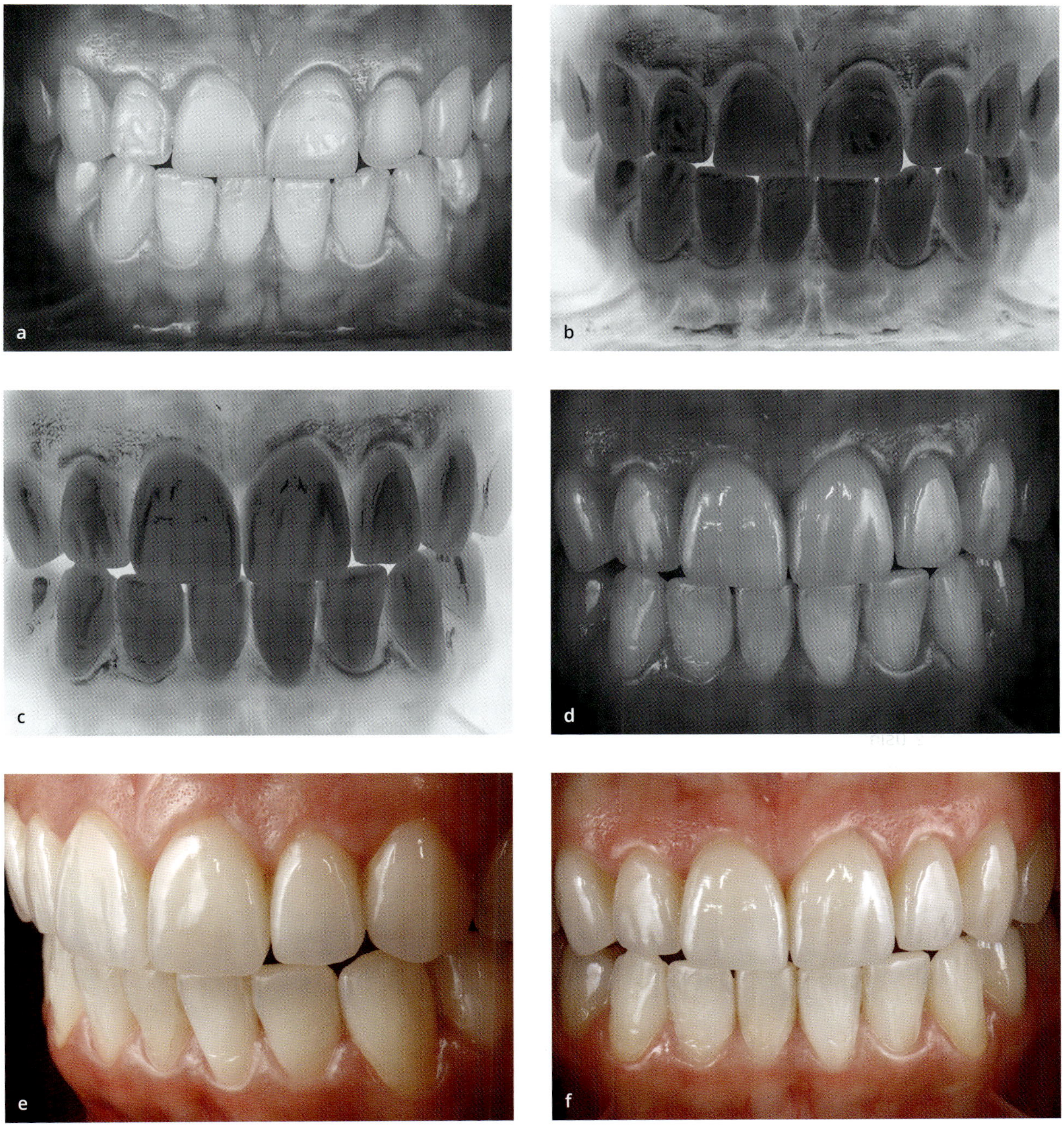

**Fig 10-18** Collection of unstimulated salivary flow can be performed chairside in a simple and easy way. Hyposalivation has been classically diagnosed when unstimulated salivary flow is <0.1 mL/min. However, minimal reductions of salivary flow can render the teeth unprotected against a TW challenge or a health hazard such as a common virus influenza infection. Note enamel dissolution, probably in relation to hyposalivation, in a 30-year-old female patient who has undergone previous treatments, which were mere attempts to fill the multifactorial lesions in a timid and insufficient mode (a). TW is usually detected in the occlusal, incisal, cervical, or palatal aspects of teeth. However, the overall volume of the tooth is reduced. The black-and-white images reveal a matte, flattened surface anatomy that shows the incremental comparative volume before and after the additive porcelain laminate veneers in the maxillary teeth and the direct freehand composite in the mandible (b to d). A very shallow preparation enables recuperation and correct integration in many cases of TW as the challenge—erosive or mechanical or both—has already reduced the teeth. Note that the partial direct approach in the mandible does not intend to cover the teeth but restore what is worn (e and f). The maxillary indirect feldspathic porcelain partial coverage helps endure the required hygiene routine.

The anticariogenic effect from fluorides does not perform equally when protecting from erosion as the $CaF_2$ precipitates that are formed on the enamel surface are soluble in acids. Therefore, erosion cannot be inhibited or prevented totally with fluorides in daily recommended doses.[82] Metal-containing fluorides such as tin-containing fluorides seem to provide anti-erosive protection. However, the secondary effects such as discoloration of the teeth and the dryness sensation, together with its extremely low pH, does not permit safe self-application and makes it necessary to pursue further research.[83-87]

Moreover, the acidic pH at which fluoride compounds have proven anti-erosive efficacy poses a dilemma in relation to patients suffering from hyposalivation with both low saliva quantity and poor buffering capacity.[42,56] Conclusions from the World Workshop on Oral Medicine on the protective effect of saliva advocate for saliva natural stimulation[88] (Fig 10-19).

Remineralization requires synergistic action from fluoride, calcium, and phosphate. Innovative approaches in order to boost mineral gain in challenging situations such as erosion are under study not only in regard to fluoride but also other minerals. In this sense, studies proclaim the benefits of using calcium-phosphate systems.[89] The combination of fluoride, calcium, and phosphate is essential for effective remineralization.[90] The added value of the proven saliva stimulation provided by a composition comprising olive oil, betaine and xylitol (Saliactive) is not to be underestimated[40] (Fig 10-20a). Other innovative approaches have been presented with what seem to be good results[91,92] (Fig 10-20b). Traditional fluoride-containing toothpastes have had a revival, with high concentrations of this ingredient to be used for short periods of time (Fig 10-20c). In fact, a published study coming from the university of Zurich proved that conventional toothpastes are not as effective at preventing extrinsic and/or intrinsic erosion when compared to anti-erosive toothpastes or those with a high concentration of fluoride.[93]

Although remineralization in severe TW today is still a chimera, in cases of incipient TW all efforts should be made in order to gain enamel resistance. It is in these cases, where the softened enamel has not yet caused noticeable TSL, that all available means should be used for remineralization and the prevention of further erosive damage. In this sense it is worth mentioning an innovative new strategy to stimulate remineralization that promotes bleaching as a pretreatment prior to the remineralization protocol.[94] Interestingly, research published in the *Journal of Clinical Pediatric Dentistry* shows an increase of enamel microhardness after the use of a bleaching system that combines carbamide peroxide, xylitol, and fluoride[95] (Fig 10-21).

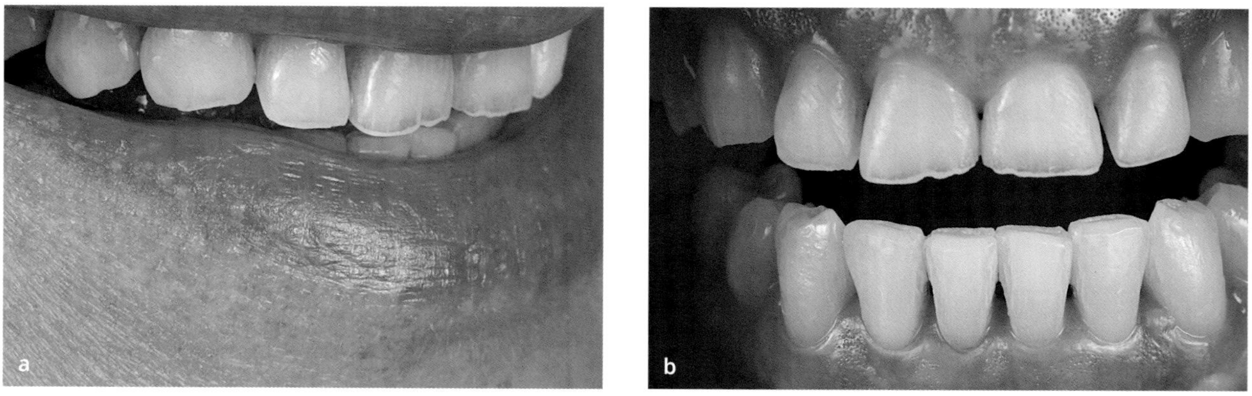


**Fig 10-19** Chewing is the major stimulus for salivation. Impaired anatomy in patients with TW impede masticatory function and therefore optimal saliva production. While an esthetic issue affecting the anterior sector of the mouth might be the patient's major concern, rehabilitating the posterior anatomy is essential in patients with TW. Essix-like guards in this case will serve both as orthodontic retainer and as protection for restorations (a to h).

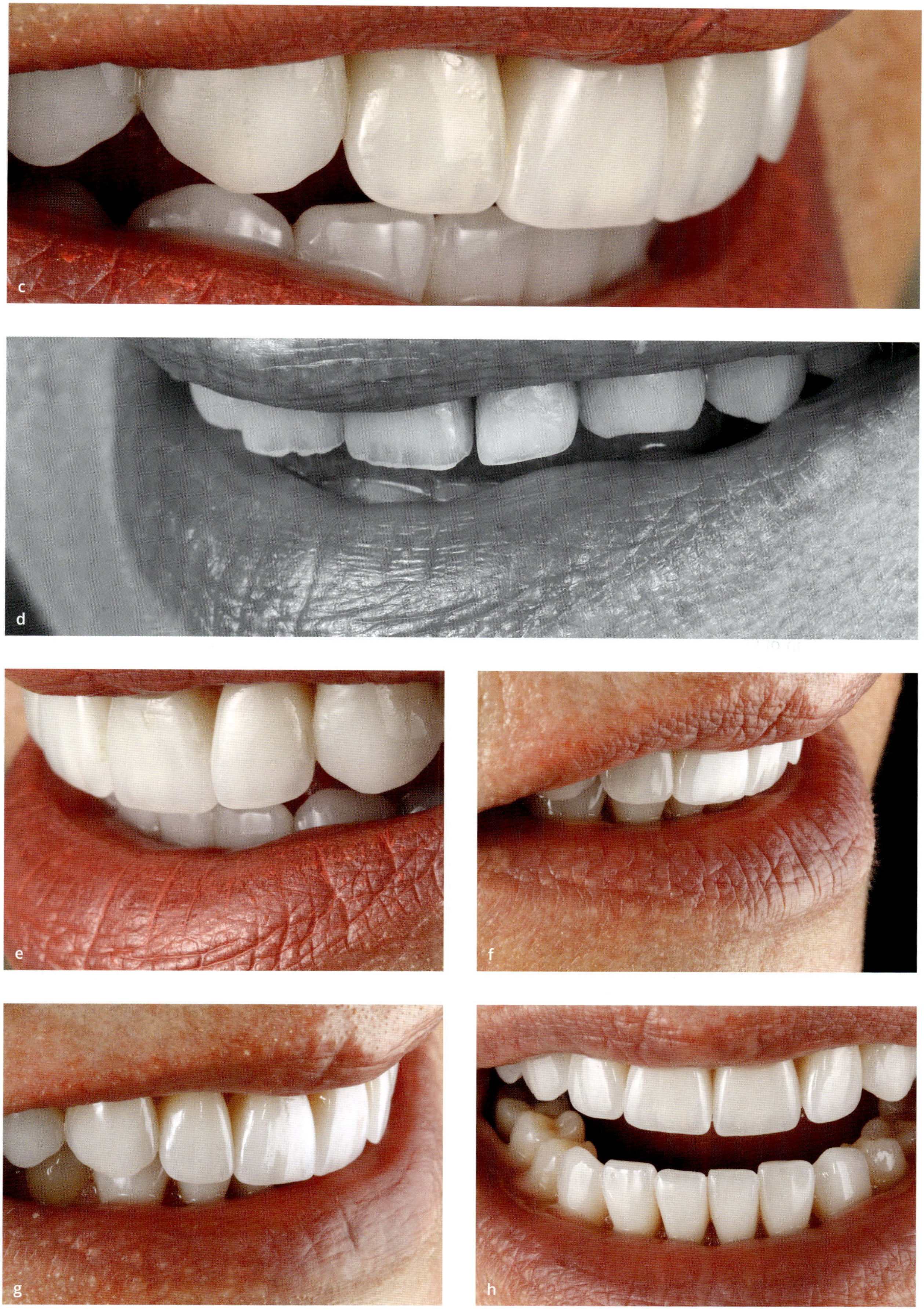
c
d
e
f
g
h

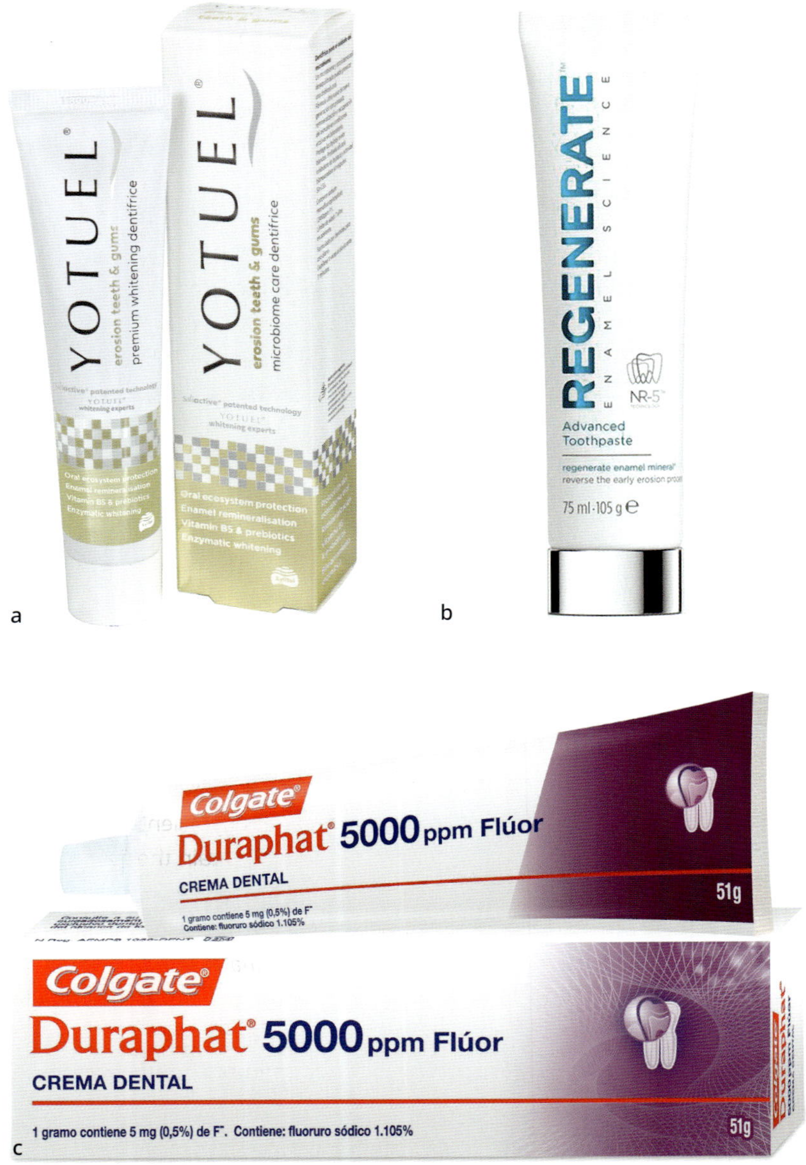


**Fig 10-20** The industry is making a substantial effort to meet the needs of contemporary TW. Erosion toothpastes are current pioneers in the field of oral hygiene. The combination of a remineralization and anti-erosive, non-abrasive buffer formula with the benefits of saliva stimulation is an innovative approach in this hygiene product, indicated in erosion and attrition. (a). This product supplies minerals with the aim of replicating enamel's hydroxyapatite (b). High concentrations of fluoride may be indicated in specific situations, such as before radiotherapy or critical hyposalivation (c).

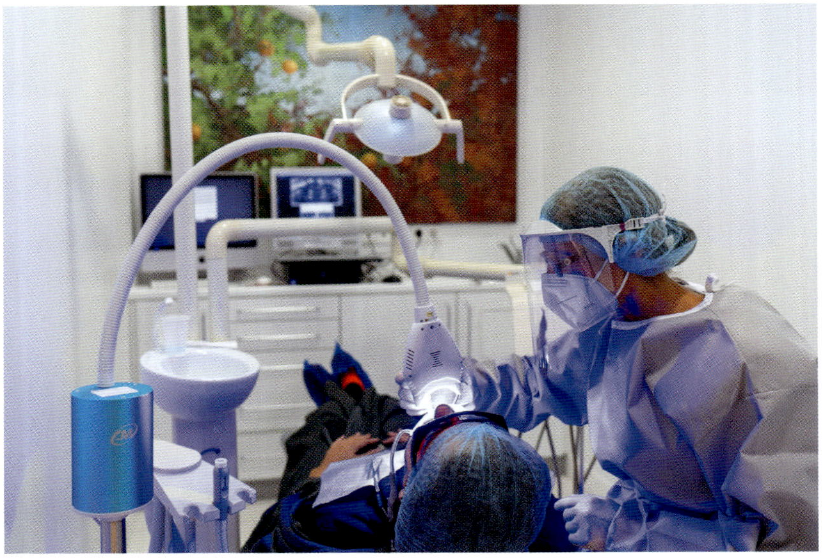

**Fig 10-21** Incipient TW should be faced with a proactive attitude in order to enhance enamel protection. A strategy of including a bleaching protocol prior to a remineralization protocol has shown beneficial effects in promoting mineral gain in white lesions (inactive caries). The image depicts in-office bleaching combining carbamide peroxide, xylitol, and fluoride.

## 6. New Strategies in TW Prevention: Enhancing Healthy Saliva, the Day and Night Bodyguard

Bearing the previously described considerations in mind, there is a palpable need to discover new approaches in oral hygiene formulations in order to obtain protection from acid attack while ideally producing salivary flow stimulation. Saliva is to be regarded as an asset providing value to both the digestive and respiratory systems.

Several groups have reported that some lipids, namely olive oil, could act as a diffusive barrier, creating a defensive coating and restricting the dispersion of acids and minerals.[96,97]. As aforementioned, a proof of principle study[56] has shown that a solution of olive oil combined with other compounds offers a protective effect against enamel and, surprisingly, dentin erosion even under severely erosive conditions. Another previously mentioned study has shown olive oil can be used as a lubricant for patients suffering from bruxism in view of lack of compliance from some patients in using nightguards. A positive effect of reducing attrition lesions with the use of olive oil as a lubricant has been demonstrated.[35]

Recent research proved the efficacy for salivary stimulation of a 1% malic acid sialagogue spray,[98] although it is not indicated for patients under erosive challenge as malic acid can potentially induce erosion.[88] Another study showed unclear results on a mucin-containing spray for erosion prevention.[99]

A mucoadhesive lipid-based bioerodible tablet applied to the palate has also been investigated.[100] Taking into consideration that TW challenges may remain active throughout a patient's life, the ideal approach for the patient should be safe, effective, and easy to implement in their everyday routine. Otherwise, the patient's compliance will be seriously compromised. Whenever possible, a balanced savory diet, preferably with olive oil as a lipid source and natural salivary stimulants, should be encouraged. The physical value of chewing in salivary stimulation should never be underestimated; therefore, rehabilitating the masticatory surfaces to provide posterior support is key for these patients.

Each approach has its limitations, and some do have relevant secondary effects that hinder continuation of the therapy. Side effects of cholinergic agonists are usually the result of generalized parasympathomimetic stimulation such as vasodilatation, headaches, urinary frequency, sweating, bronchoconstriction, bradycardia, hypotension, and others. Experts share the conclusion that nonpharmacologic stimulants should be the first choice before contemplating systemic pharmacologic approaches due to their collateral effects (Figs 10-22 to 10-25).

The mouth is directly connected to both the digestive and the respiratory apparatus. Saliva secreted by multiple salivary glands scattered throughout the oral cavity is known to have valuable properties in terms of protecting oral tissues, favoring digestive functions, and even preventing or mitigating the severity of respiratory infections[101] (Fig 10-26).

The saliva stimulation mechanism is switched on by taste, food, and mastication. Taking into consideration that humans spend one-third of their lifetime sleeping, the protective capabilities from saliva should also be in place throughout the night. However, during the night, saliva lacks the masticatory stimulation. During sleep, oral motor activities such as muscle movements may well be providing the stimuli in order to obtain the fundamental lubrication for the oral cavity in the absence of mastication. Dryness may well be the triggering factor to initiate muscle activity in order to stimulate saliva production[102] (see chapter 2).

A decrease in saliva quantity or impaired saliva quality has been related to augmented tooth damage by erosion, attrition, and abrasion. Moreover, the existence of the so-called salivary highways in the oral geography create zones of higher protection, demonstrating that the presence or lack of saliva is a crucial factor in the oral defense[103–105] (Figs 10-27 to 10-29).

Saliva wets not only the oral territory but also the digestive and respiratory mucosa, facilitating health-promoting conditions. Saliva acts as a defensive barrier that, far from being passive, has been shown to exert a unique and sophisticated effect.

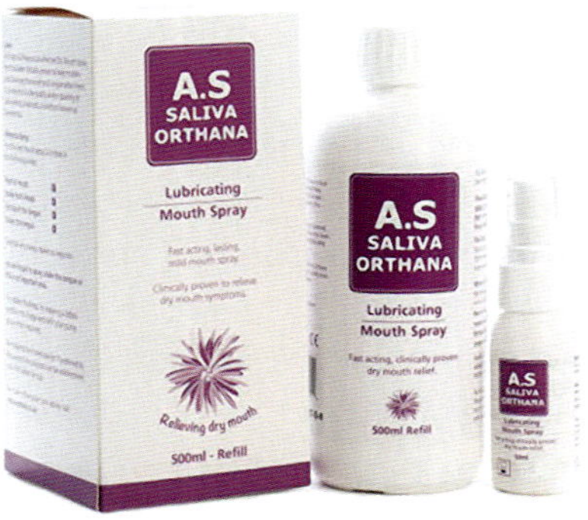


Fig 10-22 Malic acid–containing products have shown promising results in saliva stimulation and in improving the patient's quality of life. However, attention should be paid to the pH of the solution, as an acid challenge could be a concern in patients suffering from erosion.

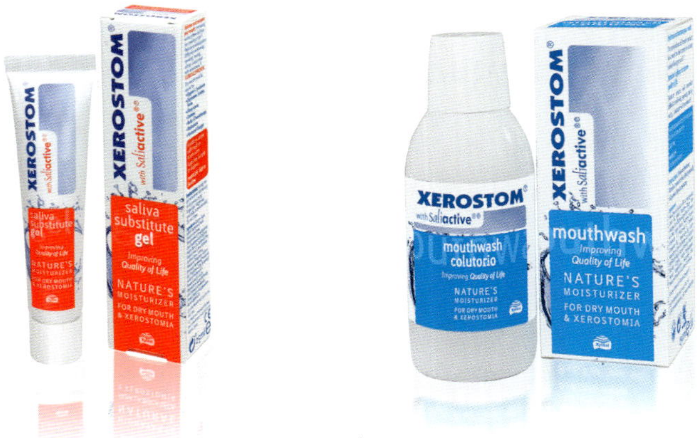


a b

Fig 10-23 An over-the-counter oral care regimen with a composition of olive oil, betaine, and xylitol has shown an increase in unstimulated salivary flow and positive impact on quality of life in polymedicated and vulnerable patients, such as patients with cancer. In comparison with cholinergic agonists, no side effects have been found, thus enabling good patient compliance (a and b).

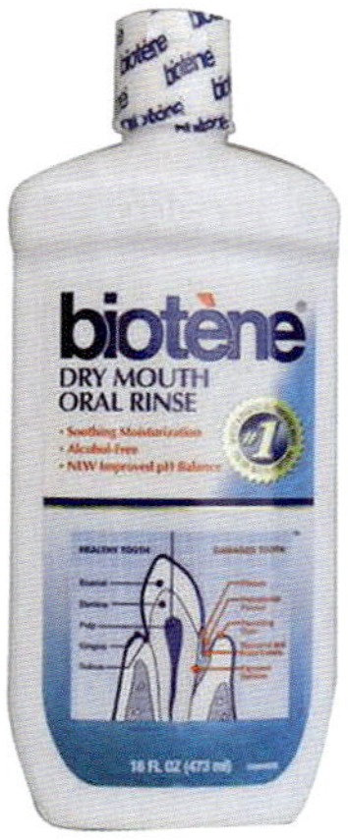


Fig 10-24 Usually the dentist is the first specialist encountering the patient with dry mouth. Furthermore, in the vast majority of the cases, the dentist establishes a diagnosis of dry mouth without the patient having been aware of the ongoing condition. Over-the-counter oral care products provide better quality of life for patients with dry mouth.

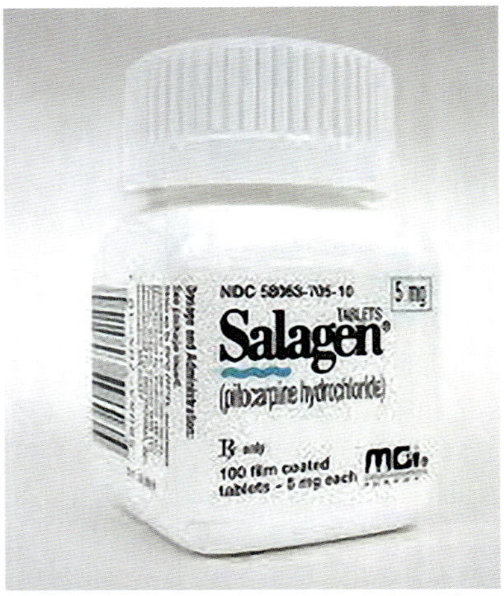


Fig 10-25 Cholinergic systemic therapies should be used with caution in patients with cardiovascular and pulmonary diseases.

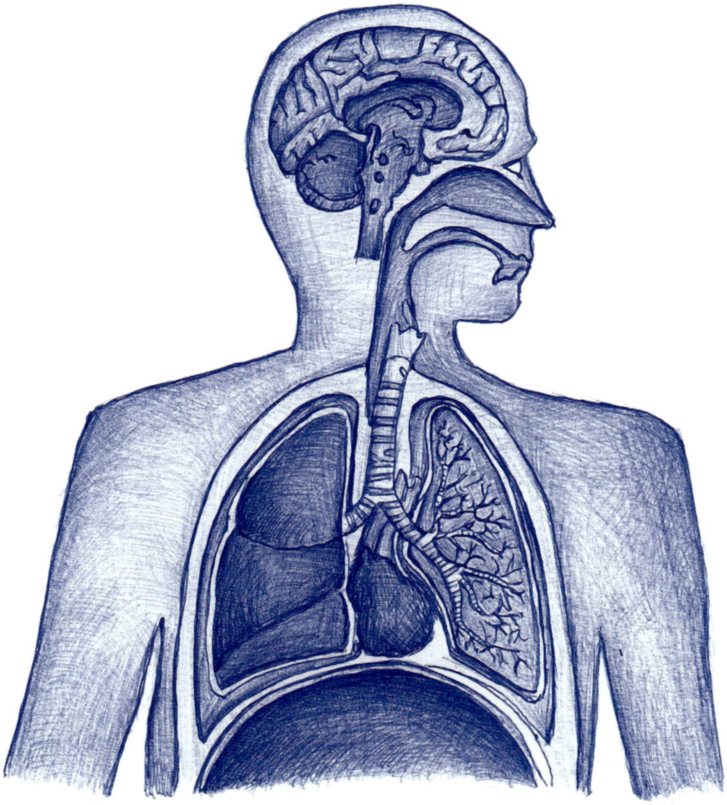

**Fig 10-26** The oral cavity is the entry to the body, belonging at the same time to the digestive and respiratory apparatuses. It is full of scattered salivary glands that excrete saliva, the principal secretion of the oral cavity, regarded today as indispensable for oral and general health.

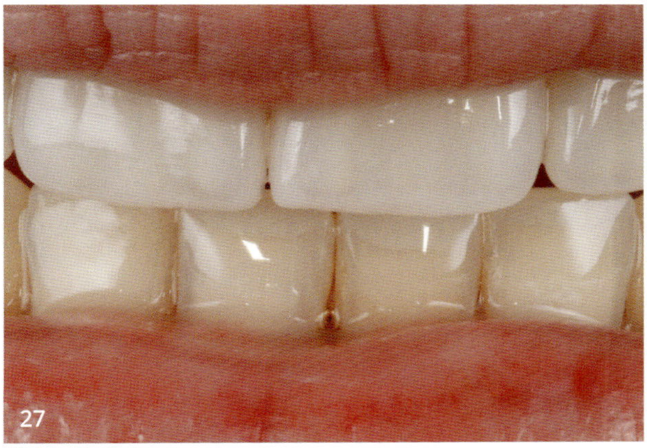

27

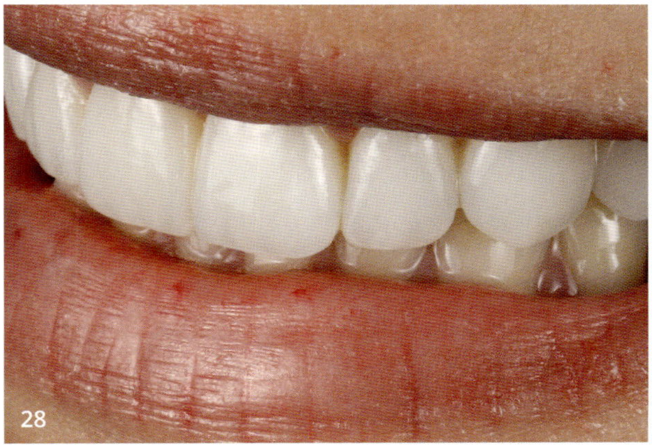

28

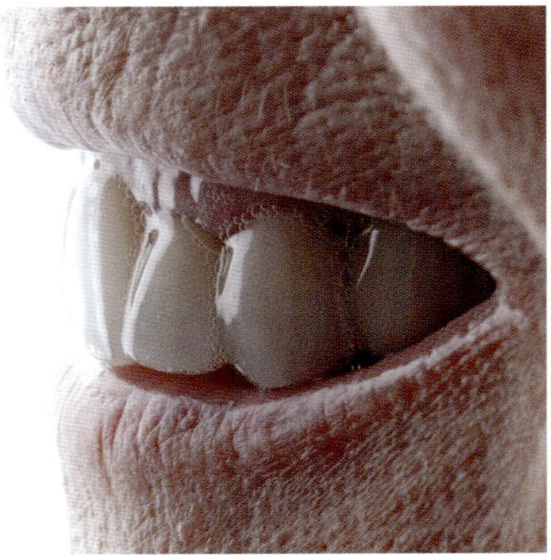

29

**Figs 10-27 to 10-29** Note the saliva bathing the mandibular teeth once tooth structure is restored and chewing capacity is at its optimal level thanks to the restoration of proper chewing support in this patient (Fig 10-27). Saliva-promoting oral care regimens are not to be forgotten in patients with TW. Benefits provided by saliva will definitely play a role in the overall prognosis of this patient with TW who has undergone restoration (Fig 10-28). The use of soft protective guards together with lubrication from saliva help in the long-term maintenance of restorations and the natural dentition. Hard acrylic night splints may be of help in patients suffering from bruxism. The thin acrylic guard has a capillary effect, helping saliva spread over the teeth (Fig 10-29).

## 7. Long-Term Maintenance of the Patient with TW

The literature describes TW as a progressive, sometimes phasic, irreversible, multifactorial, and chronic condition that challenges tooth integrity as well as oral and general health. A long-term maintenance protocol is desirable to prevent further wear and to maintain restorations in order to avoid more invasive strategies.

Each patient requires a specific personalized preventive program (PPP) depending on the origin of TW. In many cases, lifestyle coaching is mandatory. Nutritional reeducation is a highly recommended approach to reducing TW risk. Trying to determine if TW-originating factors are still active is very useful when a PPP is implemented.

The PPP should always include periodic checkups at which digital or analog measurement should be implemented to detect signs of TW progression. In order to assure stability, the efficient performance of anterior and canine guidance must be monitored. Prompt detection of wear, decementation, or fracture of TW restorations is ideal. Salivary stimulation through safe and effective methods should be implemented.

For years, nightguards seemed to be the gold standard for preventing TW from evolving into more severe dental wear. However, today we know that the complexity of TW requires individualized approaches on many occasions.

Research has shown that keeping the same physician can reduce the need for emergency hospitalizations.[106] Another study showed how being under the supervision of the same physician can even extend the patient's life.[107] In the same manner, checkups with the same dentist may offer advantages to improve the prognosis as a comprehensive overview of the timeline of the TW condition is highly desirable in this chronic condition. Several factors play an important role in the evolution of TW in a given patient. General maintenance guidelines described in section 9 of this chapter tend to help, whether patients have treated or untreated TW. Figures 10-30 to 10-40 illustrate these guidelines.

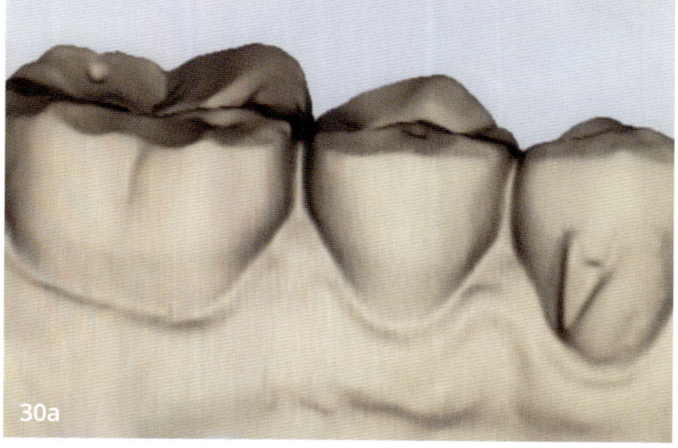
30a

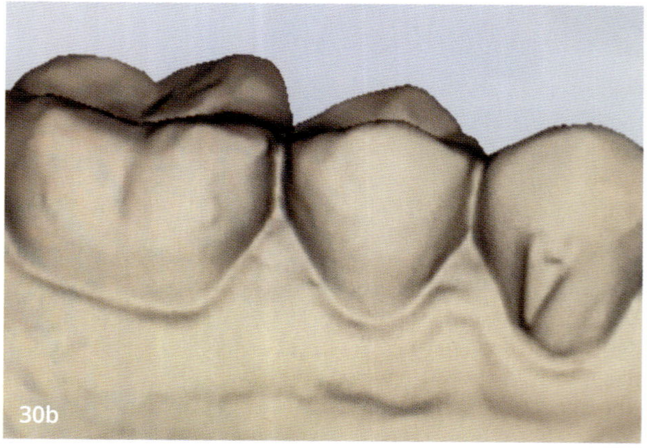
30b

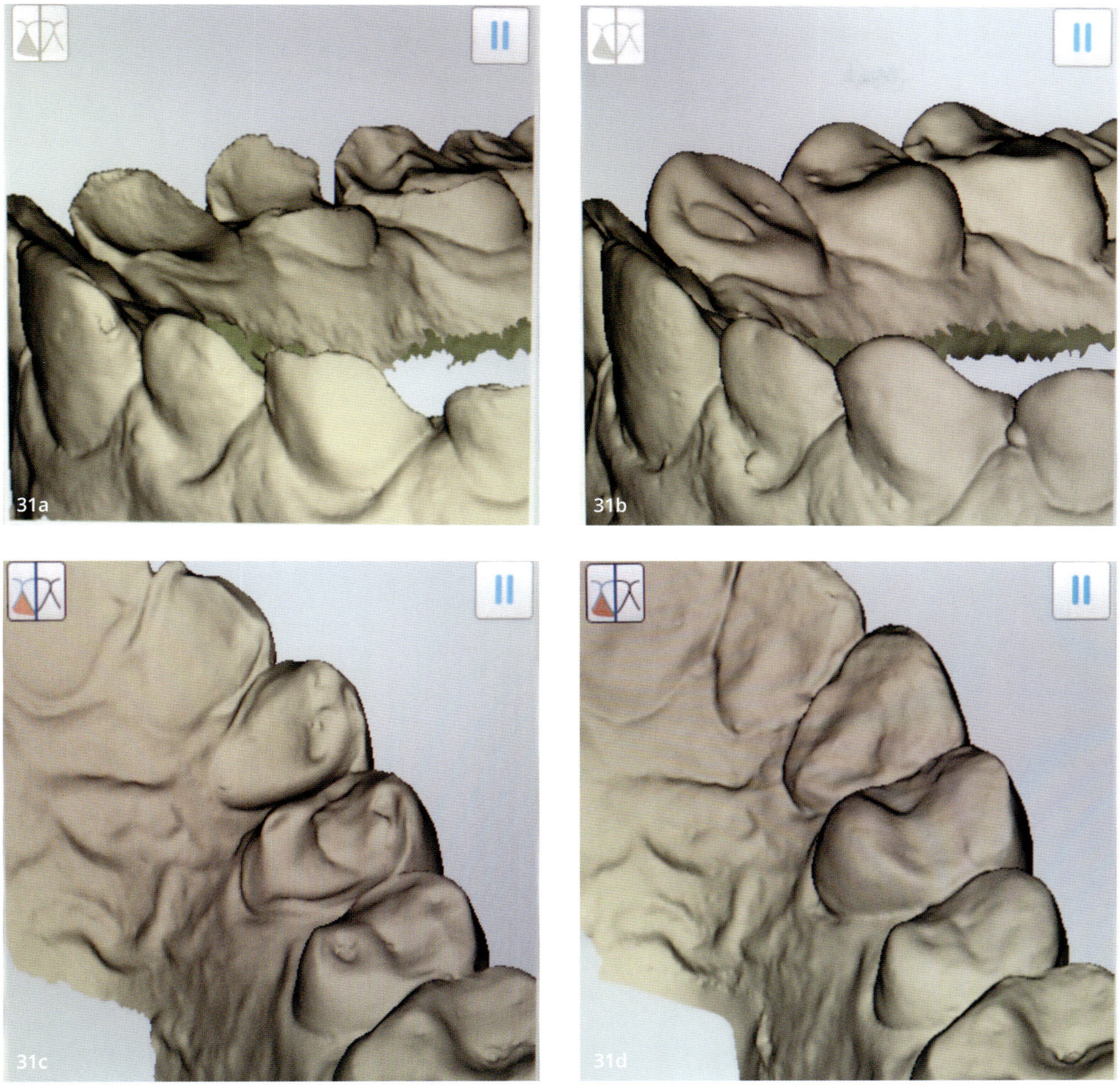


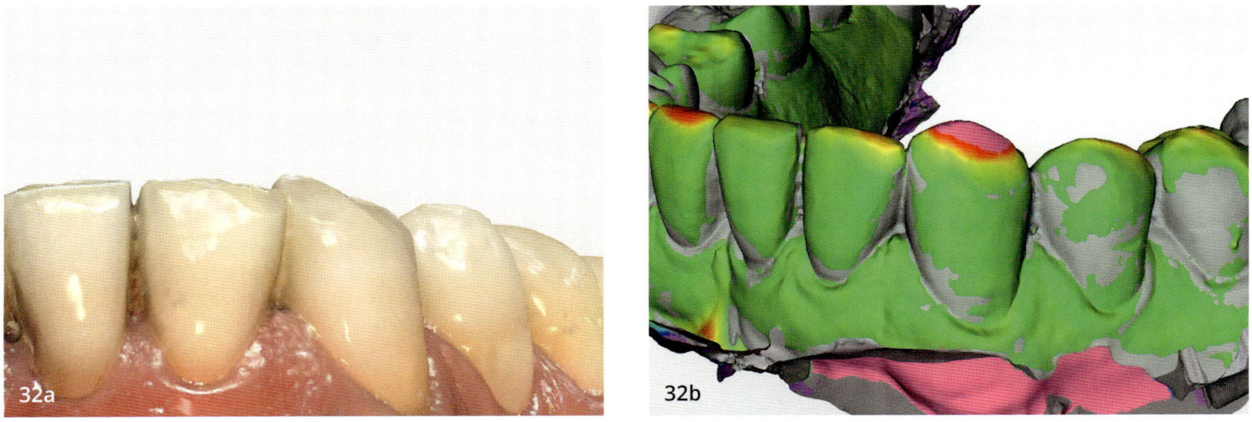


**Figs 10-30 to 10-32** Monitoring TW evolution will help the clinician determine the pace at which TW is advancing and discuss this information with the patient. Digital programs associated with intraoral scanners (eg, iTero TimeLapse,(Align Technology) that are able to compare anatomy over the passing of time can be used both to monitor the behavior of the previously worn and restored dentition and also to monitor the evolution of TW in untreated patients.

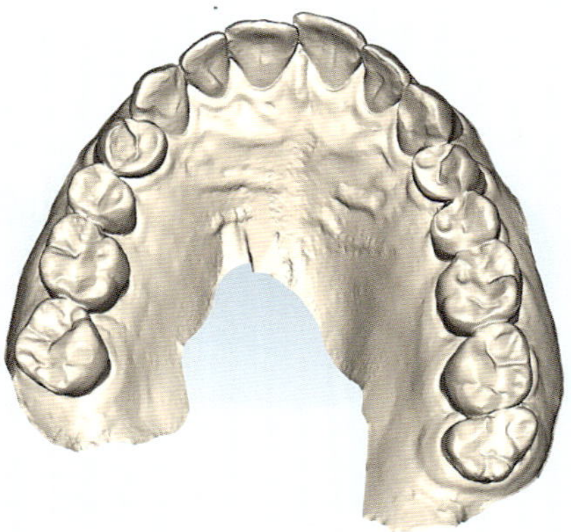

a

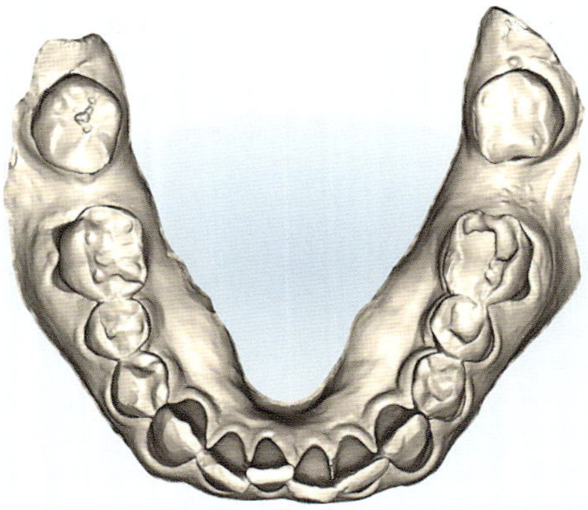

b

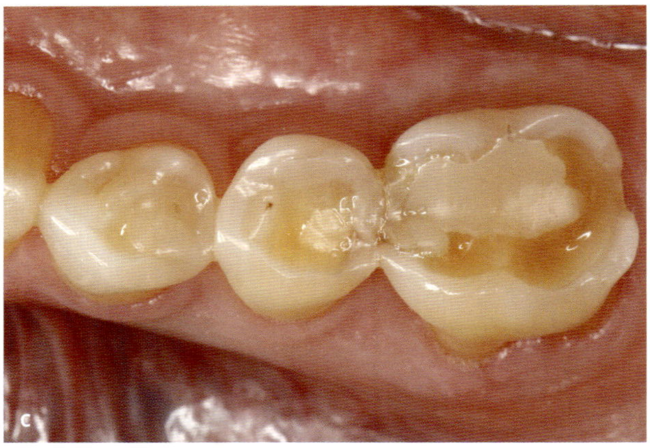

**Fig 10-33** Intraoral digital scanning provides accurate information that facilitates TW diagnosis, treatment planning, treatment, and long-term maintenance. This tool also has a forensic utility as it can superimpose images, offering a quantification of lost or deteriorated dentition and/or restorations. When the patient is reluctant to undergo treatment, it may be practical to capture the situation in order to help in the control measures. Note the severe TW in the mandible, mainly the mandibular left first molar and second premolar that so far have received only one treatment with poor results (a to c).

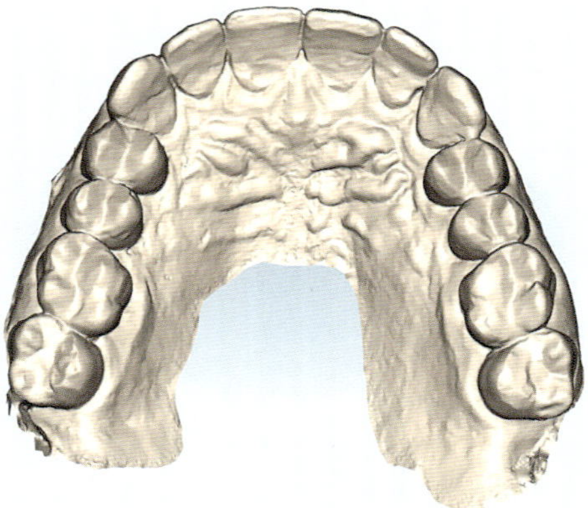

a

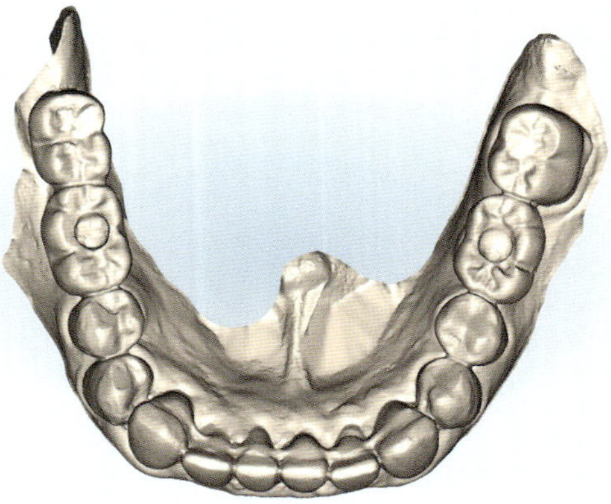

b

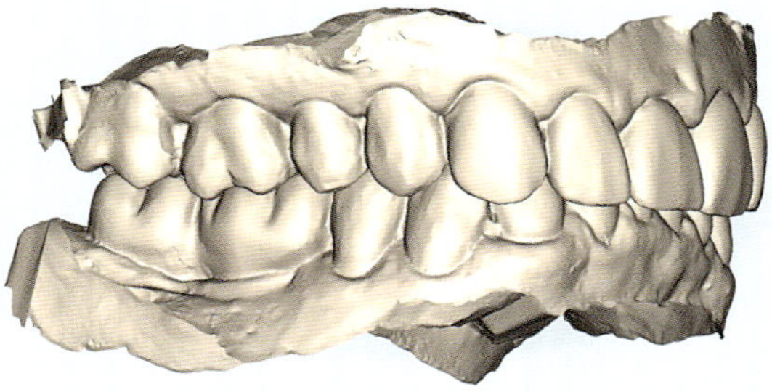

c

**Fig 10-34** Regular checkups in the TW patient should include extra records, such as intraoral digital scans, in order to monitor evolution. A comprehensive rehabilitation was performed in this patient with TW, including a variety of treatment modalities such as direct composite restorations, laminate veneers, and tooth- and implant-supported crowns. Note how wear of the palatal direct composite restorations is detected in the intraoral digital scans during a regular checkup, and thus refurbishment of the aforementioned will be scheduled (a to c).

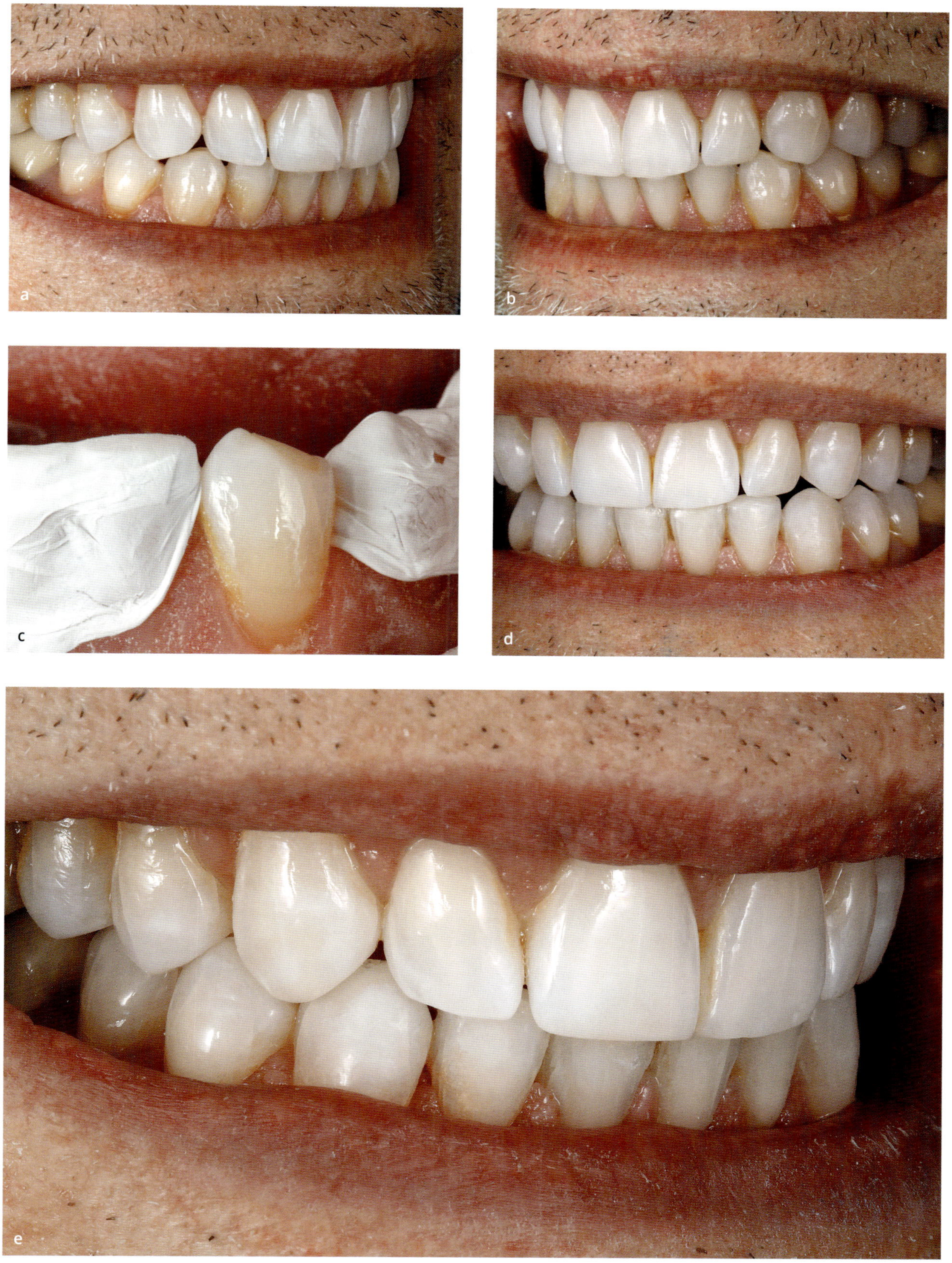

**Fig 10-35** Prompt canine cusp rehabilitation provides effective interception of further wear and should be considered a TW prevention procedure. The use of a nightguard and saliva stimulation through a topical oral care regimen are key to long-term maintenance. Periodic monitoring to check that restorations are in good shape and providing anterior and canine guidance protection are to be included in the PPP (a to e). *(continued next page)*

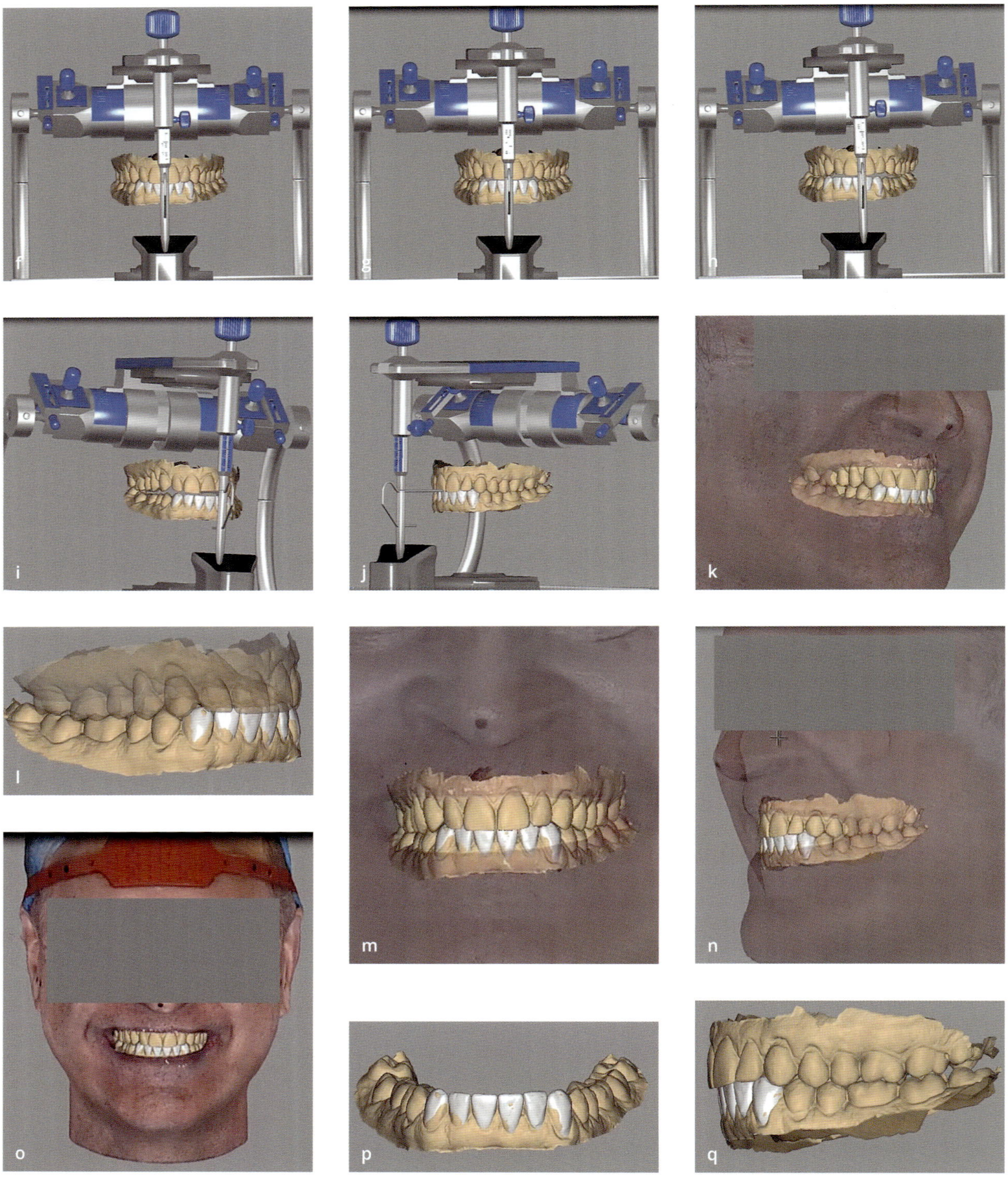


**Fig 10-35** *(continued)* The use of a face scan and virtual articulator is a noninvasive, non–time consuming, low-cost procedure that helps in the functional analysis and is performed at the initial analysis of the case and at the periodic patient check-ups in the dental office (f to q). It is likely that in the future, the patient will be able to have the face scan application on their mobile phone, and the recording of the images will be controlled remotely at the dental office. In this way, the patient can be called in when necessary. This distant monitoring is already a reality today in cardiology.

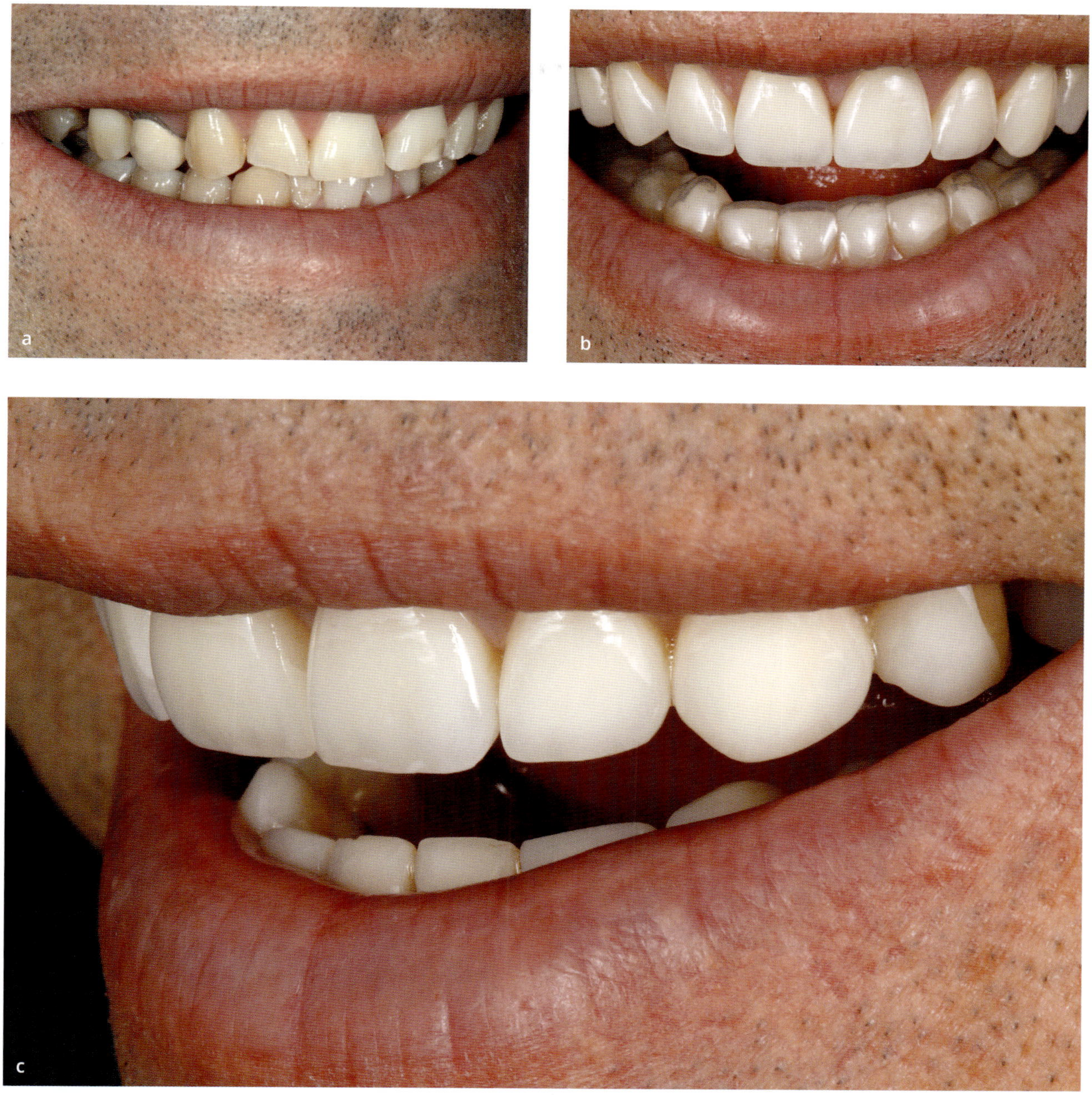

**Fig 10-36** The chronic and cyclic personality of TW requires sustained compromise from the patient and the TW team. Anticipation of fractures, debonding, or aging of restorations should be shared with the patient at the beginning of the treatment. Maxillary and mandibular soft Essix-like guards are provided to the patient. It may be ideal for the patient to wear both simultaneously, but they may feel more comfortable using one at a time. Patient commitment is mandatory. A restoration fracture has been detected in the regular check-up of the patient (a to c).

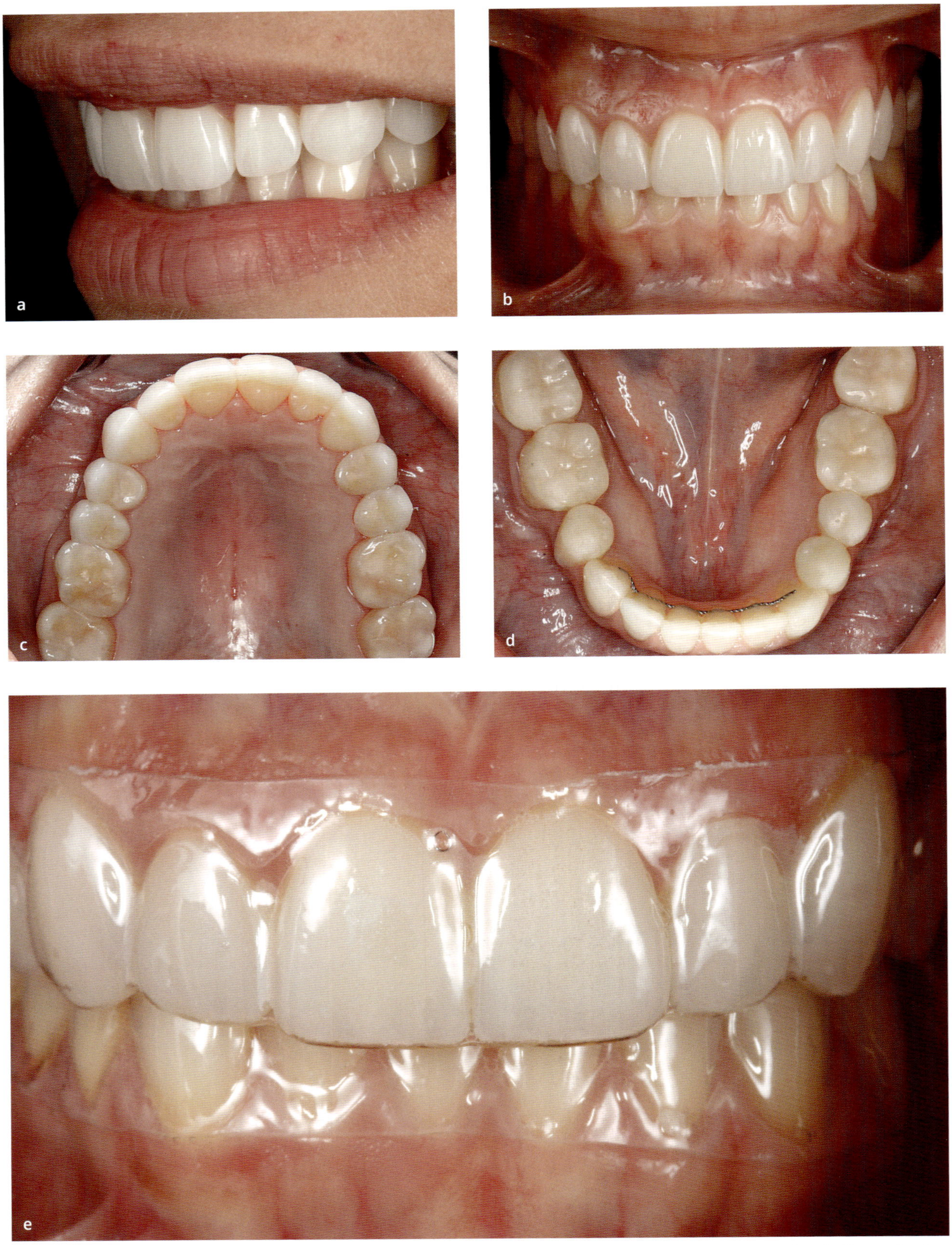

Fig 10-37 Occlusal wear on canines frequently leads to group function in patients with TW, a condition that facilitates further TW. In this case, restoration of the maxillary anterior teeth with indirect porcelain veneers enables reestablishment of anterior and canine guidance (a and b). Monitoring of this patient has detected slight wear in the maxillary right posterior composite restorations, requiring a refurbishment (c and d). The use of soft Essix-like guards is normally well tolerated by the patient (e).

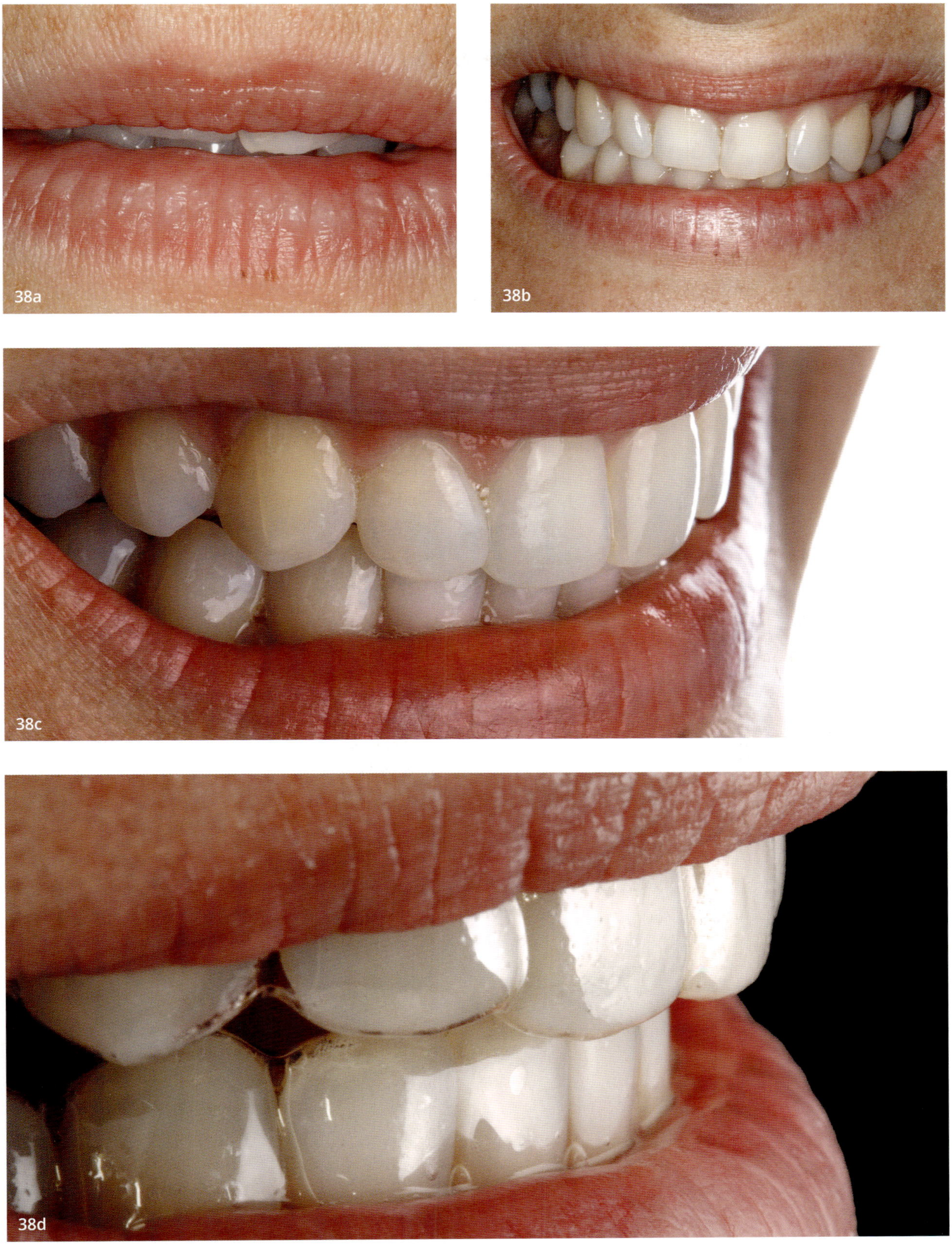


**Figs 10-38 to 10-40** Volume is the counterpart of narrow spaces. Capillary action is the process of a liquid flowing in narrow spaces without the influence of any force. When volume is restored in a worn dentition, saliva exerts its capillary action in the interproximal areas, at the labial aspects of teeth in intimate contact with the lips, and at the lingual aspects of teeth in touch with the tongue. The close contact between the thin splints and teeth also causes saliva to move around and over the teeth, exerting its protection. *(continued next page)*

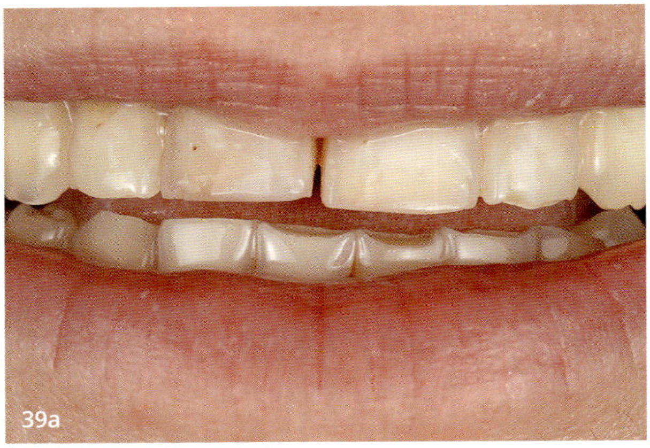


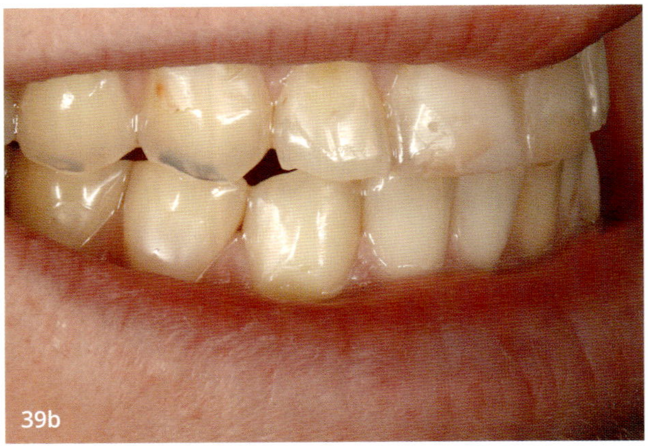


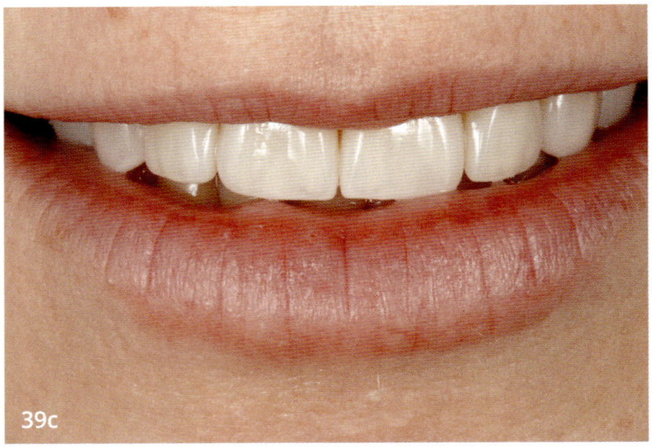


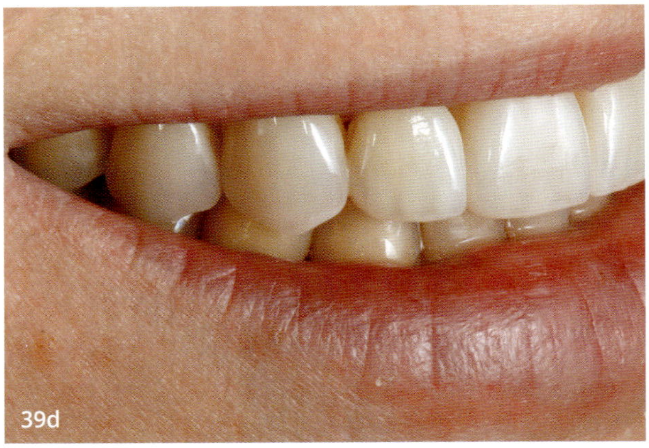


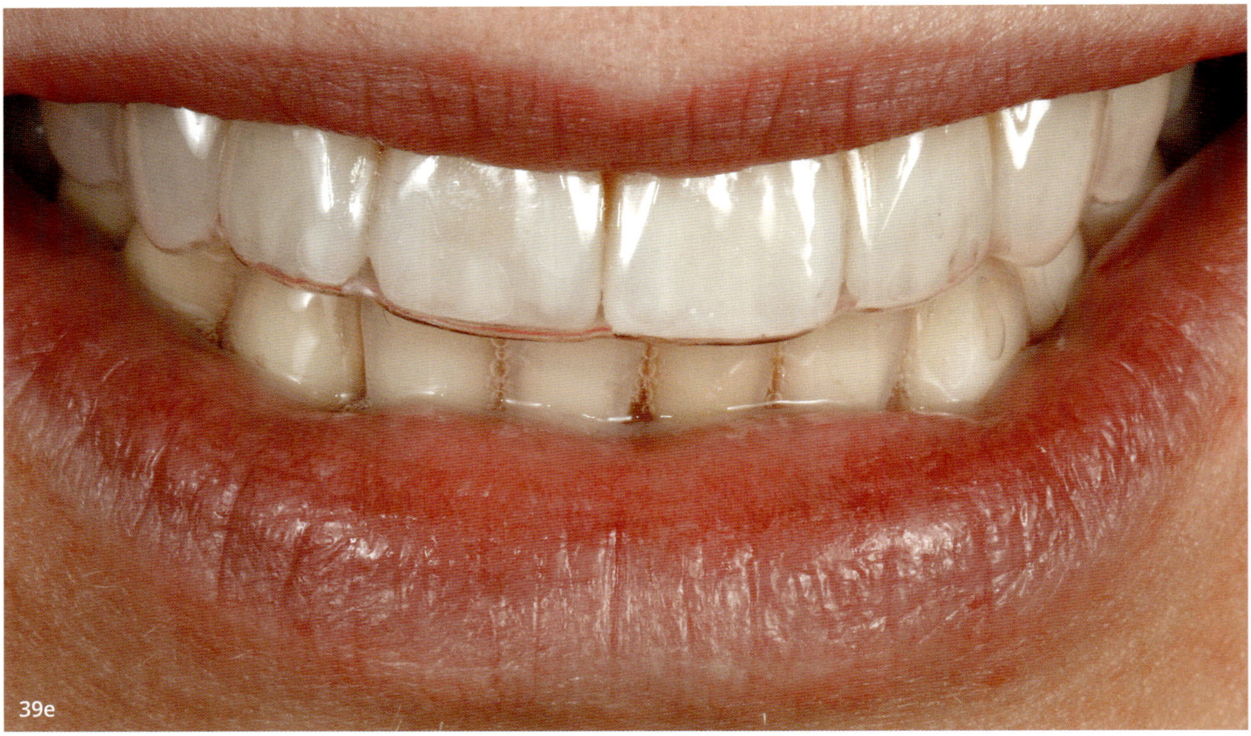


**Figs 10-38 to 10-40** *(continued)*

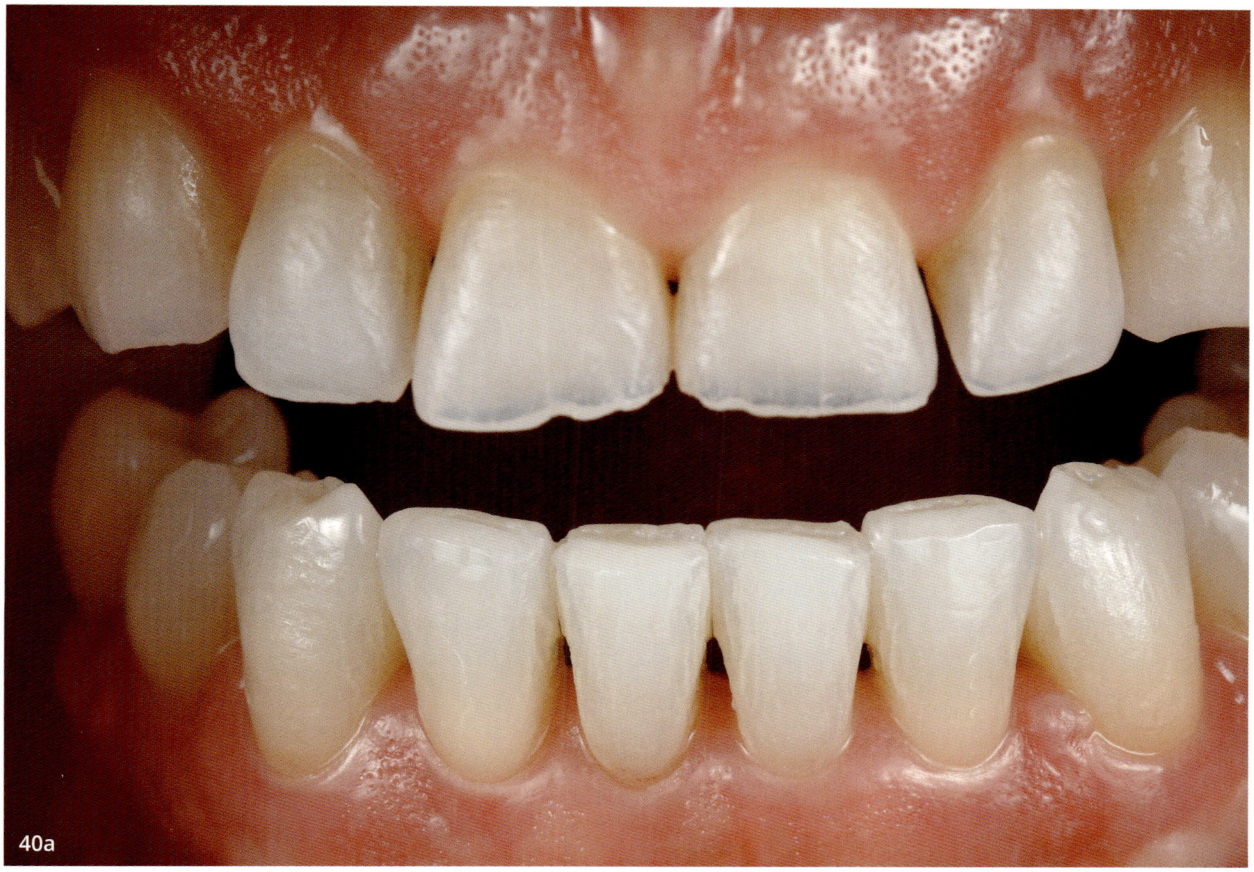

40a

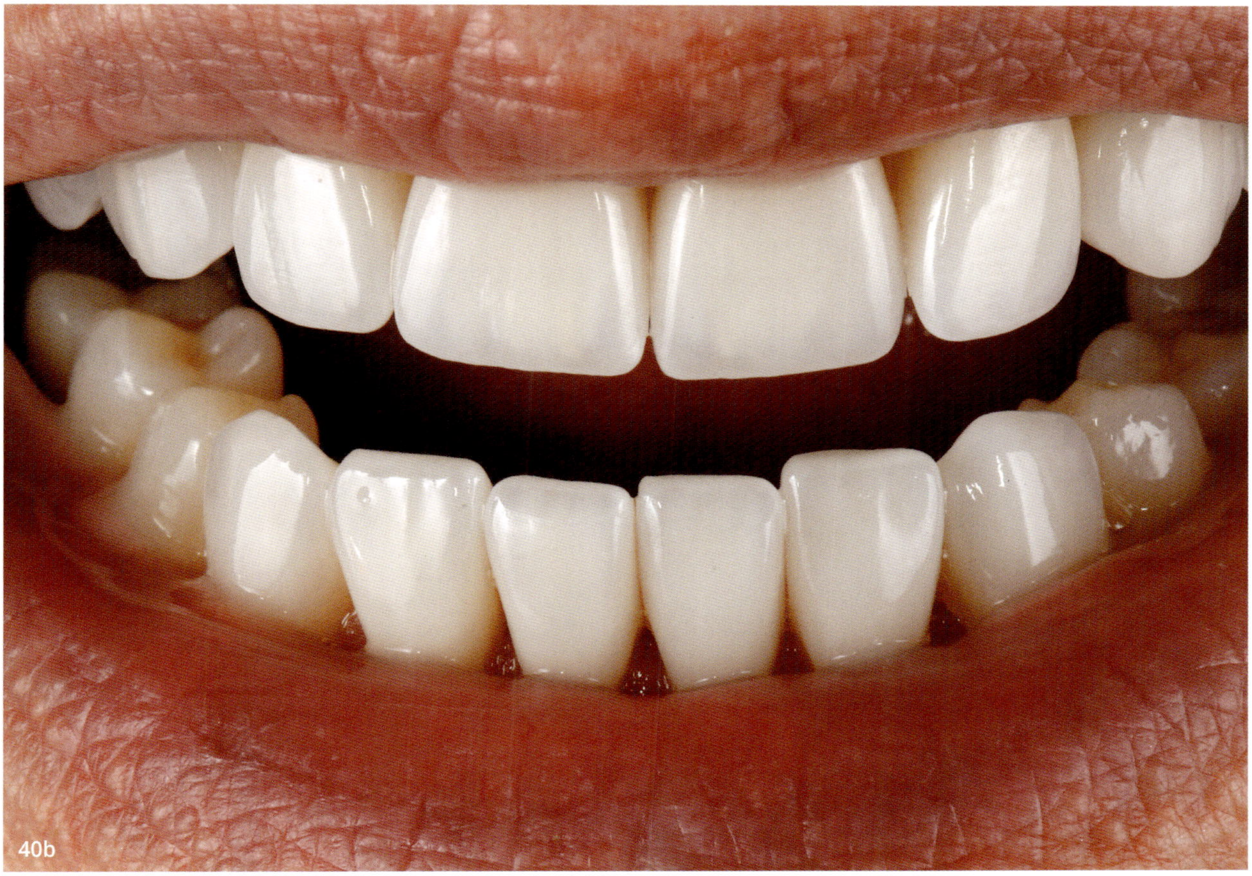

40b

## 8. Patient-Centered Long-Term Management of TW: Quality of Life, PREMS, and PROMS

The term *quality of life* was first used by Wolfgang Zapf in the architectural domain.[108] The WHO describes quality of life as "an individual's perception of their position in life in the context of the culture and value systems in which they live."[109–111] Oral health–related quality of life takes this same concept and relates it specifically to oral health.[112–114] The need to measure and quantify the manner in which a specific health issue impacts quality of life has enabled the development of measuring instruments[110,111] such as the Oral Health Impact Profile-14 or the Oral Health Impact Profile-49.[115–118]

The value of the aforementioned questionnaires consists in the self-reported evaluation of quality of life from the patient before and after treatment. Patient-reported quality of life should always be taken into consideration when treating the patient with TW.

Quality of life measured by PROMS and PREMS is another approach to quantifying a patient's perception and experience. PROMS (patient-reported outcome measures) quantify the patient perception of the result of a procedure. PREMS (patient-reported experience measures), quantify the patient perception of the accessibility of the treatment. PROMS and PREMS questionnaires have gained significant respect from clinicians and researchers after the European Medicines Agency (EMA) and the US Food and Drug Administration (FDA) indicated in 2005 and 2009 that both efficacy and improvement of qualify of life could be considered co-primary endpoints in the evaluation of a medicament.[119]

Furthermore, the unequivocal evolution of the health care provider model has been seen, from the very paternalistic model where the doctor knew what was best for the patient, to the informed consent model in which information was provided to the patient who was still not openly invited to the decision-making process, to the most recent shared decision-making model in which negotiation and agreement is to be expected between the parties. TW management, which involves lifestyle modifications, will have better chances to succeed when the patient is given an active role in the process of deciding what to change in their everyday routines and how and when treatment will be carried out.[120] A doctoral thesis reviewing the different outcomes in quality of life between treated and untreated patients with TW offered a confirmation of the benefits of treatment.[121]

Patient commitment and a trained team are essential for a long-term positive outcome in the patient with TW. Patient-centered care is likely to play a major role in the welfare and medical care arena in the 21st century. Basically, calling on patients to have a predominant and active role in the decisions that involve their health, how to safeguard it, and how to regain it should be *de rigueur* today.

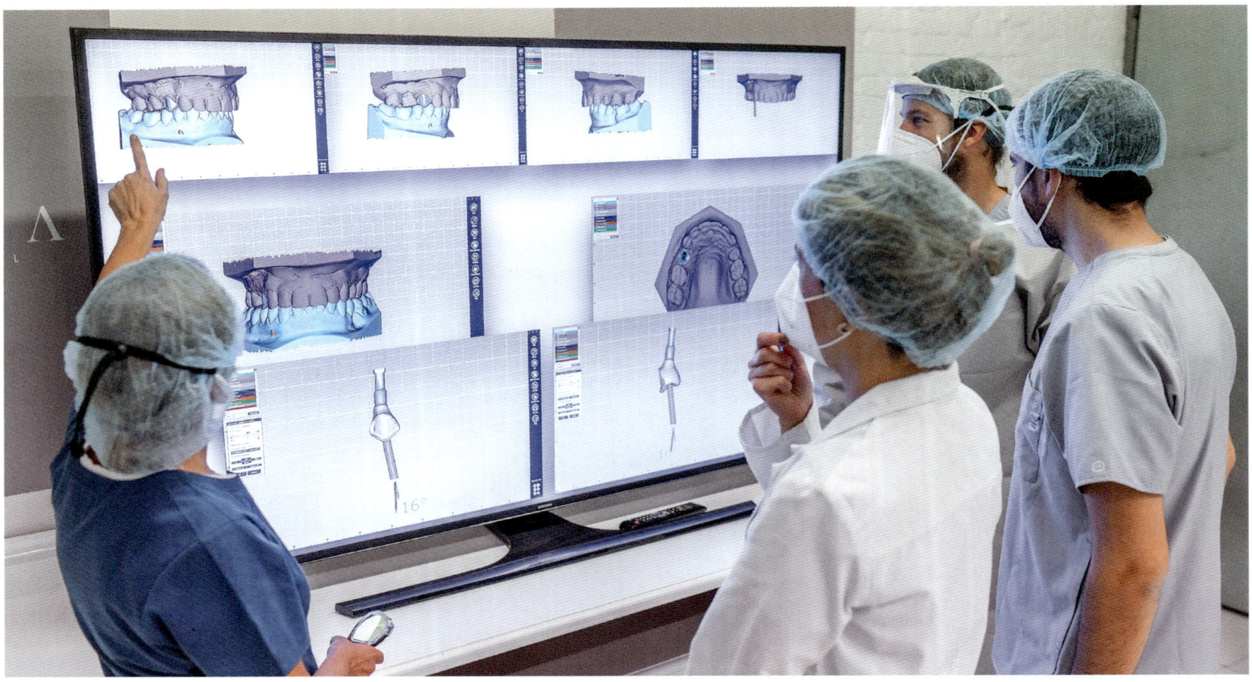

**Fig 10-41** Interaction among the TW team should be fluid, taking into consideration the multidisciplinary treatment approach that often is required by the TW patient. The joint venture formed by both parties, dentist and patient, begins with the open sharing of information that will lead to shared decision making and understanding of limitations and compromises.

## 9. Key Points: General Maintenance Guidelines for the Patient with TW

**Table 10-3** General maintenance guidelines for the patient with TW.

| | |
|---|---|
| Control of TW risk factors. | Check if new risks are in place (see appendix 1). |
| Whenever possible, determine if TW cause is still active or not. | Presence of hypersensitivity or absence of stains are normally indicators of activity. |
| Reevaluation of nutritional habits with a periodical 6-day diet diary.[57] | Changing lifestyle and dietary habits should not be taken for granted; therefore, periodical reevaluation and new coaching when needed are essential in the patient with TW. A saliva- stimulating oral care regimen is essential in the patient with TW. Erosion-protective oral care products are highly desirable. |
| Digital evaluation of the natural and restored dentition to detect signs of TW progression. | Natural dentition should be checked, both in cases where the patient has received TW treatment and in cases where the patient has chosen not to undergo TW treatment. Anatomical control and comparison over time, be it with analog stone cast models or by superimposing digital intraoral scans (eg, iTero TimeLapse, Align Technology or Primescan OraCheck, Dentsply Sirona). Photography and facial scans may also help in the monitoring of the patient with TW. |
| Clinical evaluation of efficient performance of anterior and canine guidance, be it on natural or restored dentition. | When anterior and canine guidance have been restored, reparations or repetitions have to be anticipated, and the patient should be informed accordingly. Monitoring the patient with incipient signs of TW who has chosen not to be treated yet is of paramount importance. |
| Clinical evaluation of the restored dentition to detect wear, fracture, or decementation. | Provided good bidirectional communication and confidence between the dentist and the patient has been established right from the start, new treatments, when needed, will be understood and tolerated by the patient with TW. |
| Clinical evaluation of protective nightguards. Determine if still in good function or if they require repair, remaking, or modification. | Although erosive wear appears in relation to an acidic challenge and not to clenching or bruxism the extensive restorative approach benefits from the use of protective nightguards.<br>When attrition is the cause of TW, especially if bruxism is diagnosed or suspected, a Michigan hard acrylic splint is ideal. |
| Saliva stimulation. | The use of a safe and effective saliva-stimulating regimen should be implemented. |

## References


1. Linden GJ, Herzberg MC; Working group 4 of the Joint EFP/AAP Workshop. Periodontitis and systemic diseases: A record of discussions of working group 4 of the Joint EFP/AAP Workshop on Periodontitis and Systemic Diseases. J Periodontol 2013;84(4 Suppl):S20–S23.
2. Loomans B, Opdam N, Attin T, et al. Severe tooth wear: European consensus statement on management guidelines. J Adhes Dent 2017;19(2):111–119.
3. Ireland RS, Jenner AM, Williams MJ, Tickle M. A clinical minimum data set for primary dental care. Br Dent J 2001;190:663–667.
4. Margaritis V, Mamai-Homata E, Koletsi-Kounari H, Polychronopoulou A. Evaluation of three different scoring systems for dental erosion: A comparative study in adolescents. J Dent 2011;39:88–93.
5. Olley RC, Wilson R, Bartlett D, Moazzez R. Validation of the Basic Erosive Wear Examination. Caries Res 2014;48(1):51–56.
6. Carvalho TS, Colon P, Ganss C, et al. Consensus report of the European Federation of Conservative Dentistry: Erosive tooth wear—Diagnosis and management. Clin Oral Investig 2015;19:1557–1561.
7. Lussi A. Dental erosion clinical diagnosis and case history taking. Eur J Oral Sci 1996; 104(2 Pt 2):191–198.
8. Seligman DA, Pullinger AG, Solberg WK. The prevalence of dental attrition and its association with factors of age, gender, occlusion, and TMJ symptomatology. J Dent Res 1988;67:1323–1333.
9. Mesko ME, Almeida RC, Porto JA, Koller CD, da Rosa WL, Boscato N. Should occlusal splints be a routine prescription for diagnosed bruxers undergoing implant therapy? Int J Prosthodont 2014;27:201–203.
10. van Rinsum C, Gerards S, Rutten G, Johannesma M, van de Goor I, Kremers S. The implementation of the coaching on lifestyle (CooL) intervention: Lessons learnt. BMC Health Serv Res 2019;19(1):667.
11. Carter S, Hartman Y, Holder S, Thijssen DH, Hopkins ND. Sedentary behavior and cardiovascular disease risk: Mediating mechanisms. Exerc Sport Sci Rev 2017;45(2):80–86.
12. Guilleminault L, Ouksel H, Belleguic C, et al. Personalised medicine in asthma: From curative to preventive medicine. Eur Respir Rev 2017;26(143):160010.
13. Peñalvo JL, Céspedes J, Fuster V. Sesame street: Changing cardiovascular risks for a lifetime. Semin Thorac Cardiovasc Surg 2012;24(4):238–240.
14. Holzmann SL, Dischl F, Schäfer H, Groh G, Hauner H, Holzapfel C. Digital gaming for nutritional education: A survey on preferences, motives, and needs of children and adolescents. JMIR Form Res 2019;3(1):e10284.
15. Lussi A, Jaeggi T, Zero D. The role of diet in the aetiology of dental erosion. Caries Res 2004;38)Suppl 1):34–44.
16. Lussi A, Hellwig E. Risk assessment and causal preventive measures. Monogr Oral Sci 2014;25:220–229.
17. Milosevic A, Lennon MA, Fear SC. Risk factors associated with tooth wear in teenagers: A case control study. Community Dent Health 1997;14(3):143–147.

18. Dugmore CR, Rock WP. A multifactorial analysis of factors associated with dental erosion. Br Dent J 2004;196(5):283–286.
19. Hede B, Determinants of oral health in a group of Danish alcoholics. Eur J Oral Sci 1996;104(4 Pt 1):403–408.
20. Staufenbiel I, Adam K, Deac A, Geurtsen W, Günay H. Influence of fruit consumption and fluoride application on the prevalence of caries and erosion in vegetarians—A controlled clinical trial. Eur J Clin Nutr 2015;69:1156–1160.
21. Centerwall BS, Armstrong CW, Funkhouser LS, Elzay RP. Erosion of dental enamel among competitive swimmers at a gas-chlorinated swimming pool. Am J Epidemiol 1986;123:641–647.
22. iegand A, Attin T. Occupational dental erosion from exposure to acids: A review. Occup Med (Lond) 2007;57(3):169–176.
23. Marro F, Jacquet W, Bottenberg P, Martens L. The influence of behavioural and socio-demographic risk indicators on erosive tooth wear in Flemish adolescents, Belgium. Caries Res 2018;52(1-2):119–128.
24. Rodriguez FR, Paganoni N, Weiger R, Walter C. Lower educational level is a risk factor for tooth loss—Analysis of a Swiss population (KREBS Project). Oral Health Prev Dent 2017;15(2):139–145.
25. Pretty IA, Gallagher MJ, Martin MV, Edgar WM, Higham SM. A study to assess the effects of a new detergent-free, olive oil formulation dentifrice in vitro and in vivo. J Dent 2003;31:327–332.
26. Rantanen I, Tenovuo J, Pienihäkkinen K, Söderling E. Effects of a betaine-containing toothpaste on subjective symptoms of dry mouth: A randomized clinical trial. J Contemp Dent Pract 2003;4(2):11–23.
27. Mejersjö C, Ovesson D, Mossberg B. Oral parafunctions, piercing and signs and symptoms of temporomandibular disorders in high school students. Acta Odontol Scand 2016;74(4):279–284.
28. Nilner M. Relationships between oral parafunctions and functional disturbances and diseases of the stomatognathic system among children aged 7-14 years. Acta Odontol Scand 1983;41(3):167–172.
29. Janson G, Oltramari-Navarro PV, de Oliveira RB, Quaglio CL, Sales-Peres SH, Tompson B. Tooth-wear patterns in subjects with Class II Division 1 malocclusion and normal occlusion. Am J Orthod Dentofacial Orthop 2010;137(1):14.e1–14.e7.
30. Jang SJ, Choi DS, Jang I, Jost-Brinkmann PG, Cha BK. Quantitative comparison of incisal tooth wear in patients receiving one-phase or two-phase treatment for skeletal Class III malocclusion with anterior crossbite. Angle Orthod 2018;88(2):151–156.
31. Kryger MH, Roth T, Dement WC. Principles and Practice of Sleep Medicine, ed 5. St Louis: Elsevier/Saunders, 2011.
32. Lavigne GJ, Rompré PH, Poirier G, Huard H, Kato T, Montplaisir JY. Rhythmic masticatory muscle activity during sleep in humans. J Dent Res 2001;80(2):443–448.
33. Lavigne GJ, Goulet JP, Zuconni M, Morrison F, Lobbezoo F. Sleep disorders and the dental patient: An overview. Oral Surg Oral Med Oral Pathol Oral Radiol Endod 1999;88:257–272.
34. Ranjitkar S, Kaidonis JA, Smales RJ. Gastroesophageal reflux disease and tooth erosion. Int J Dent 2012;2012:479850.
35. Kaidonis JA, Gratiaen J, Bhatia N, Richards LC, Townsend GC. Tooth wear prevention: A quantitative and qualitative in vitro study. Aust Dent J 2003;48(1):15–19.
36. Saeves R, Strøm F, Sandvik L, Nordgarden H. Gastro-oesophageal reflux—An important causative factor of severe tooth wear in Prader-Willi syndrome? Orphanet J Rare Dis 2018;13(1):64.
37. Levine MP. Universal prevention of eating disorders: A concept analysis. Eating Behav 2017;25:4–8.
38. Smink FR, van Hoeken D, Hoek HW. Epidemiology, course, and outcome of eating disorders. Curr Opin Psychiatry 2013;26:543–548.
39. Lie SØ, Rø Ø, Bang L. Is bullying and teasing associated with eating disorders? A systematic review and meta-analysis. Int J Eat Disord 2019;52:497–514.
40. Ship JA, McCutcheon JA, Spivakovsky S, Kerr AR. Safety and effectiveness of topical dry mouth products containing olive oil, betaine, and xylitol in reducing xerostomia for polypharmacy-induced dry mouth. J Oral Rehabil 2007;34:724–732.
41. Sreebny LM, Schwartz SS. A reference guide to drugs and dry mouth—2nd edition. Gerodontology 1997;14(1):33–47.
42. Bardow A, Nyvad B, Nauntofte B. Relationships between medication intake, complaints of dry mouth, salivary flow rate and composition, and the rate of tooth demineralization in situ. Arch Oral Biol 2001;46:413–423.
43. Martín M, Marín A, López M, et al. Products based on olive oil, betaine, and xylitol in the post-radiotherapy xerostomia. Rep Pract Oncol Radiother 2017;22(1):71–76.
44. Sreebny LM. Salivary flow in health and disease. Compend Suppl 1989;(13):S461– S469.
45. Davies BM, Gurland JB. Salivary secretion in depressive illness. J Psychosom Res 1961;5:269–271.
46. Bergdahl M, Bergdahl J. Low unstimulated salivary flow and subjective oral dryness: Association with medication, anxiety, depression, and stress. J Dent Res 2000;79:1652–1658.
47. Patel R, Shahane A. The epidemiology of Sjogren's syndrome. Clin Epidemiol 2014;6:247–255.
48. López-Pintor RM, Ramírez L, Serrano J, et al. Effects of Xerostom products on xerostomia in primary Sjogren's syndrome: A randomized clinical trial. Oral Dis 2019;25:772–780.
49. Souto-Souza D, Mourão PS, Barroso HH, et al. Is there an association between attention deficit hyperactivity disorder in children and adolescents and the occurrence of bruxism? A systematic review and meta-analysis. Sleep Med Rev 2020;53:101330.
50. Wang CW, Musumari PM, Techasrivichien T, et al. Overlap of traditional bullying and cyberbullying and correlates of bullying among Taiwanese adolescents: A cross-sectional study. BMC Public Health 2019;19(1):1756.
51. Donoghue C, Meltzer LJ. Sleep it off: Bullying and sleep disturbances in adolescents. J Adolesc 2018;68:87–93.
52. Hickner J. It's time to screen for bullying. J Fam Pract 2017;66(2):66.
53. Jackson DB, Vaughn MG, Salas-Wright CP. Poor nutrition and bullying behaviors: A comparison of deviant and non-deviant youth. J Adolesc 2017;57:69–73.
54. Jackson DB. Diet quality and bullying among a cross-national sample of youth. Prev Med 2017;105:359–365.
55. Goswami U, O'Toole S, Bernabé E. Asthma, long-term asthma control medication and tooth wear in American adolescents and young adults. J Asthma 2021;58:939–945.
56. Wiegand A, Gutsche M, Attin T. Effect of olive oil and an olive-oil-containing fluoridated mouthrinse on enamel and dentin erosion in vitro. Acta Odontol Scand 2007;65: 357–361.
57. Young WG. Tooth wear: Diet analysis and advice. Int Dent J 2005;55(2):68–72.
58. Magalhaes AC, Moraes SM, Rios D, Wiegand A, Buzalaf MA. The erosive potential of 1% citric acid supplemented by different minerals: An in vitro study. Oral Health Prev Dent 2010;8(1):41–45.
59. Attin T, Meyer K, Hellwig E, Buchalla W, Lennon AM. Effect of mineral supplements to citric acid on enamel erosion. Arch Oral Biol 2003;48:753–759.
60. Attin T, Weiss K, Becker K, Buchalla W, Wiegand A. Impact of modified acidic soft drinks on enamel erosion. Oral Dis 2005;11(1):7–12.
61. Barbour ME, Rees JS. The laboratory assessment of enamel erosion: A review. J Dent 2004;32:591–602.
62. Buzalaf MA, de Moraes Italiani F, Kato MT, Martinhon CC, Magalhães AC. Effect of iron on inhibition of acid demineralisation of bovine dental enamel in vitro. Arch Oral Biol 2006;51:844–848.
63. Kargul B, Caglar E, Lussi A. Erosive and buffering capacities of yogurt. Quintessence Int 2007;38:381–385.
64. Somaraj V, Shenoy RP, Panchmal GS, Jodalli PS, Sonde L, Nagaraj K. Effect of paneer and cheese consumption on salivary acidogenicity and calcium concentration: A comparative study. Oral Health Prev Dent 2018;16:169–174.
65. Gerber M, Hoffman R. The Mediterranean diet: Health, science and society. Br J Nutr 2015;113(Suppl 2):S4–S10.
66. Grosso G, Mistretta A, Frigiola A, et al. Mediterranean diet and cardiovascular risk factors: A systematic review. Crit Rev Food Sci Nutr 2014;54:593–610.
67. Widmer RJ, Flammer AJ, Lerman LO, Lerman A. The Mediterranean diet, its components, and cardiovascular disease. Am J Med 2015;128(3):229–238.
68. Kanzow P, Wegehaupt FJ, Attin T, Wiegand A. Etiology and pathogenesis of dental erosion. Quintessence Int 2016;47:275–278.
69. Zero DT. Etiology of dental erosion—Extrinsic factors. Eur J Oral Sci 1996;104 (2 Pt 2):162–177.
70. Chikte UM, Naidoo S, Kolze TJ, Grobler SR. Patterns of tooth surface loss among winemakers. SADJ 2005;60(9):370–374.
71. Dawson PE. Functional Occlusion: From TMJ to Smile Design. St Louis: Mosby, 2007.
72. Gracis S. Clinical considerations and rationale for the use of simplified instrumentation in occlusal rehabilitation. Part 2: Setting of the articulator and occlusal optimization. Int J Periodontics Restorative Dent 2003;23(2):139–145.
73. Kois J. Diagnostically driven interdisciplinary treatment planning. Seattle Study Club J 2002;6(4):28–34.
74. Levant E. An introduction to functional occlusion. J Prosthet Dent 1983;50:442–443.
75. Wiegand A, Schlueter N. The role of oral hygiene: Does toothbrushing harm? Monogr Oral Sci 2014;25:215–219.
76. Wiegand A, Kuhn M, Sener B, Roos M, Attin T. Abrasion of eroded dentin caused by toothpaste slurries of different abrasivity and toothbrushes of different filament diameter. J Dent 2009;37:480–484.
77. Wiegand A, Schwerzmann M, Sener B, et al. Impact of toothpaste slurry abrasivity and toothbrush filament stiffness on abrasion of eroded enamel—An in vitro study. Acta Odontol Scand 2008;66:231–235.
78. Bizhang M, Schmidt I, Chun YP, Arnold WH, Zimmer S. Toothbrush abrasivity in a long-term simulation on human dentin depends on brushing mode and bristle arrangement. PLoS One 2017;12(2):e0172060.

79. Wiegand A, Burkhard JP, Eggmann F, Attin T. Brushing force of manual and sonic toothbrushes affects dental hard tissue abrasion. Clin Oral Investig 2013;1:815–822.
80. Niemi ML, Sandholm L, Ainamo J. Frequency of gingival lesions after standardized brushing as related to stiffness of toothbrush and abrasiveness of dentifrice. J Clin Periodontol 1984;11:254–261.
81. Watanabe M, Nakatani E, Yoshikawa H, et al. Oral soft tissue disorders are associated with gastroesophageal reflux disease: Retrospective study. BMC Gastroenterol 2017;17(1):92.
82. Dawes C. What is the critical pH and why does a tooth dissolve in acid? J Can Dent Assoc, 2003;69:722–725.
83. Magalhães AC, Kato MT, Rios D, Wiegand A, Attin T, Buzalaf MA.The effect of an experimental 4% Tif4 varnish compared to NaF varnishes and 4% TiF4 solution on dental erosion in vitro. Caries Res 2008;42:269–274.
84. Magalhães AC, Stancari FH, Rios D, Buzalaf MA. Effect of an experimental 4% titanium tetrafluoride varnish on dental erosion by a soft drink. J Dent 2007;35:858–861.
85. Magalhães AC, Wiegand A, Rios D, Buzalaf MAR, Lussi A. Fluoride in dental erosion. Monogr Oral Sci 2011;22:158–170.
86. Magalhães AC, Wiegand A, Rios D, Honório HM, Buzalaf MA. Insights into preventive measures for dental erosion. J Appl Oral Sci 2009;17(2):75–86.
87. Wiegand A, Attin T. Influence of fluoride on the prevention of erosive lesions—A review. Oral Health Prev Dent 2003;1(4):245–253.
88. Villa A, Wolff A, Aframian D, et al. World Workshop on Oral Medicine VI: A systematic review of medication-induced salivary gland dysfunction: Prevalence, diagnosis, and treatment. Clin Oral Investig 2015;19:1563–1580.
89. Nakata T, Kitasako Y, Sadr A, Nakashima S, Tagami J. Effect of a calcium phosphate and fluoride paste on prevention of enamel demineralization. Dent Mater J 2018;37(1):65–70.
90. García-Godoy F, Hicks MJ. Maintaining the integrity of the enamel surface: The role of dental biofilm, saliva and preventive agents in enamel demineralization and remineralization. J Am Dent Assoc 2008;139(Suppl):25S–34S.
91. Sun Y, Li X, Deng Y, Sun JN, et al. Mode of action studies on the formation of enamel minerals from a novel toothpaste containing calcium silicate and sodium phosphate salts. J Dent 2014;42(Suppl 1):S30–S38.
92. Joiner A, Schäfer F, Naeeni MM, Gupta AK, Zero DT. Remineralisation effect of a dual-phase calcium silicate/phosphate gel combined with calcium silicate/phosphate toothpaste on acid-challenged enamel in situ. J Dent 2014;42(Suppl 1):S53–S59.
93. Aykut-Yetkiner A, Attin T, Wiegand A. Prevention of dentine erosion by brushing with anti-erosive toothpastes. J Dent 2014;42:856–861.
94. Robinson C, Hallsworth AS, Shore RC, Kirkham J. Effect of surface zone deproteinisation on the access of mineral ions into subsurface carious lesions of human enamel. Caries Res 1990;24:226–230.
95. Akal N, Over H, Olmez A, Bodur H. Effects of carbamide peroxide containing bleaching agents on the morphology and subsurface hardness of enamel. J Clin Pediatr Dent 2001;25:293–296.
96. Buchalla W, Attin T, Roth P, Hellwig E. Influence of olive oil emulsions on dentin demineralization in vitro. Caries Res 2003;37(2):100–107.
97. Featherstone JD, Rosenberg H. Lipid effect on the progress of artificial carious lesions in dental enamel. Caries Res, 1984;18(1):52–55.
98. Gómez-Moreno G, Aguilar-Salvatierra A, Guardia J, et al. The efficacy of a topical sialogogue spray containing 1% malic acid in patients with antidepressant-induced dry mouth: A double-blind, randomized clinical trial. Depress Anxiety 2013;30(2):137–142.
99. Furness S, Worthington HV, Bryan G, Birchenough S, McMillan R. Interventions for the management of dry mouth: Topical therapies. Cochrane Database Syst Rev 2011;(12):CD008934.
100. Aframian DJ, Mizrahi B, Granot I, Domb AJ. Evaluation of a mucoadhesive lipid-based bioerodable tablet compared with Biotene mouthwash for dry mouth relief—A pilot study. Quintessence Int 2010;41(3):e36–e42.
101. Iwabuchi H, Fujibayashi T, Yamane GY, Imai H, Nakao H. Relationship between hyposalivation and acute respiratory infection in dental outpatients. Gerontology 2012;58(3):205–211.
102. Thie NM, Kato T, Bader G, Montplaisir JY, Lavigne GJ. The significance of saliva during sleep and the relevance of oromotor movements. Sleep Med Rev 2002;6:213–227.
103. Ganss C, Young A, Lussi A. Tooth wear and erosion: Methodological issues in epidemiological and public health research and the future research agenda. Community Dent Health 2011;28(3):191–195.
104. Humphrey SP, Williamson RT. A review of saliva: Normal composition, flow, and function. J Prosthet Dent 2001;85(2):162–169.
105. Moss SJ. Clinical implications of recent advances in salivary research. J Esthet Dent 1995;7(5):197–203.
106. Tammes P, Purdy S, Salisbury C, et al. Can continuity of primary care decrease emergency care use? A nested case-control study. Lancet 2016;388(Suppl 2):S13.
107. Pereira Gray DJ, Sidaway-Lee K, White E, Thorne A, Evans PH. Continuity of care with doctors—A matter of life and death? A systematic review of continuity of care and mortality. BMJ Open 2018;8(6):e021161.
108. Glatzer W, Zapf W, Berger R. Lebensqualität in der Bundesrepublik: Objektive Lebensbedingungen und subjektives Wohlbefinden. Frankfurt: Campus-Verlag, 1984.
109. World Health Organization. WHOQOL-BREF: Introduction, administration, scoring and generic version of the assessment: Field trial version, December 1996. Geneva: World Health Organization, 1996.
110. Malden PE, Thomson WM, Jokovic A, Locker D. Changes in parent-assessed oral health-related quality of life among young children following dental treatment under general anaesthetic. Community Dent Oral Epidemiol 2008;36(2):108–117.
111. Schwartzmann L. Calidad de vida relacionada con la salud: Aspectos conceptuales. Ciencia y enfermería 2003;9(2):9–21.
112. Wilson IB, Cleary PD. Linking clinical variables with health-related quality of life. A conceptual model of patient outcomes. JAMA 1995;273(1):59–65.
113. Matsuyama Y, Aida J, Watt RG, et al. Dental status and compression of life expectancy with disability. J Dent Res 2017;96:1006–1013.
114. Matsuyama Y, Tsakos G, Listl S, Aida J, Watt RG. Impact of dental diseases on quality-adjusted life expectancy in US adults. J Dent Res 2019;98:510–516.
115. Bae KH, Kim HD, Jung SH, et al. Validation of the Korean version of the oral health impact profile among the Korean elderly. Community Dent Oral Epidemiol 2007;35(1):73–79.
116. Lopez R, Baelum V. Spanish version of the Oral Health Impact Profile (OHIP-Sp). BMC Oral Health 2006;6:11.
117. Oliveira BH, Nadanovsky P. Psychometric properties of the Brazilian version of the Oral Health Impact Profile-short form. Community Dent Oral Epidemiol 2005;33(4):307–314.
118. van der Meulen MJ, John MT, Naeije M, Lobbezoo F. The Dutch version of the Oral Health Impact Profile (OHIP-NL): Translation, reliability and construct validity. BMC Oral Health 2008;8:11.
119. Committee for Medicinal Products for Human Use. Reflection paper on the Regulatory Guidance for the Use of Health-Related Quality of Life (HRQL) Measures in the Evaluation of Medicinal Products. London: European Medicines Agency, 2005.
120. Truglio-Londrigan M, Slyer JT, Singleton JK, Worral P. A qualitative systematic review of internal and external influences on shared decision-making in all health care settings. JBI Libr Syst Rev 2012;10(58):4633–4646.
121. Rodriguez-Vilaboa B. Impacto del Desgaste Dental en la Calidad de Vida del paciente [thesis]. Madrid: University San Pablo CEU, 2017.

# APPENDIX 1 – Lifestyle and Health TW Questionaire

1. Can you attribute the signs of tooth wear that are present in your mouth to a single specific reason?

   ..........................................................................................................................................................................

   ..........................................................................................................................................................................

2. Do you clench or grind your teeth at night or during the day?

   ☐ YES ☐ NO ☐ CANNOT SAY/DON'T KNOW

3. Do you wake up with headaches or neck pain?

   ☐ YES ☐ NO ☐ CANNOT SAY/DON'T KNOW

4. Do you sleep with your mouth open?

   ☐ YES ☐ NO ☐ CANNOT SAY/DON'T KNOW

5. Do you snore at night?

   ☐ YES ☐ NO ☐ CANNOT SAY/DON'T KNOW

6. Do you suffer from sleep apnea?

   ☐ YES ☐ NO ☐ CANNOT SAY/DON'T KNOW

7. Do you sleep well at night?

   ☐ YES ☐ NO ☐ CANNOT SAY/DON'T KNOW

8. Do you use a nightguard or retainer to protect your teeth while you sleep?

   ☐ YES ☐ NO ☐ CANNOT SAY/DON'T KNOW

9. Do you need to take medication to help you sleep?

   ☐ YES ☐ NO ☐ CANNOT SAY/DON'T KNOW

10. Does your mouth feel dry?

    ☐ YES ☐ NO ☐ CANNOT SAY/DON'T KNOW

11. Does the amount of saliva in your mouth seem to be too little, too much, or you do not notice it?

    ☐ TOO LITTLE ☐ TOO MUCH ☐ DON'T NOTICE

12. Do you have any difficulty swallowing?

    ☐ YES ☐ NO ☐ CANNOT SAY/DON'T KNOW

13. Does your mouth feel dry when eating a meal?

    ☐ YES ☐ NO ☐ CANNOT SAY/DON'T KNOW

14. Do you sip liquids to aid in swallowing dry food?

    ☐ YES ☐ NO ☐ CANNOT SAY/DON'T KNOW

15. Do you bite your nails or skin on your fingers?

    ☐ YES ☐ NO ☐ CANNOT SAY/DON'T KNOW

16. Do you bite your lip?

    ☐ YES ☐ NO ☐ CANNOT SAY/DON'T KNOW

17. Do you have a habit of chewing objects such as pencils or pens?

    ☐ YES ☐ NO ☐ CANNOT SAY/DON'T KNOW

| | | |
|---|---|---|
| 18. Has a dentist ever told you that you brush your teeth too hard? | | |
| ☐ YES | ☐ NO | ☐ CANNOT SAY/DON'T KNOW |
| 19. Do you use a stiff toothbrush to brush your teeth? | | |
| ☐ YES | ☐ NO | ☐ CANNOT SAY/DON'T KNOW |
| 20. Do you follow a vegetarian or vegan diet? | | |
| ☐ YES | ☐ NO | ☐ CANNOT SAY/DON'T KNOW |
| 21. Do you use an electric toothbrush? | | |
| ☐ YES | ☐ NO | ☐ CANNOT SAY/DON'T KNOW |
| 22. What type of toothpaste do you use? ........................................ | | |
| 23. Do you eat a lot of citrus fruits? | | |
| ☐ YES | ☐ NO | |
| 24. Do you drink carbonated soft drinks such as cola? | | |
| ☐ YES | ☐ NO | |
| 25. How many soft drinks do you drink per day? ........................................ | | |
| 26. Do you use a straw to drink soft drinks? | | |
| ☐ YES | ☐ NO | |
| 27. Do you keep the soft drink in your mouth, savoring it before swallowing? | | |
| ☐ YES | ☐ NO | |
| 28. Do you drink fruit juices? | | |
| ☐ YES | ☐ NO | |
| 29. How many fruit juices do you drink per day? ........................................ | | |
| 30. Do you keep the fruit juice in your mouth, savoring it before swallowing? | | |
| ☐ YES | ☐ NO | |
| 31. Do you drink wine daily? | | |
| ☐ YES | ☐ NO | |
| 32. Do you hold the wine in your mouth, savoring it before swallowing? | | |
| ☐ YES | ☐ NO | |
| 33. Do you use lemon or vinegar in your salads? | | |
| ☐ NEVER | ☐ A LITTLE | ☐ A LOT |
| 34. Do you suffer from gastritis? | | |
| ☐ YES | ☐ NO | ☐ CANNOT SAY/DON'T KNOW |
| 35. Do you have a hiatal hernia? | | |
| ☐ YES | ☐ NO | ☐ CANNOT SAY/DON'T KNOW |
| 36. Do you suffer from heartburn? | | |
| ☐ YES | ☐ NO | ☐ CANNOT SAY/DON'T KNOW |
| 37. Do you suffer from gastroesophageal reflux? | | |
| ☐ YES | ☐ NO | ☐ CANNOT SAY/DON'T KNOW |

| | | |
|---|---|---|
| 38. How often do you drink alcohol? | | |
| ☐ NEVER | ☐ A LITTLE | ☐ A LOT |
| 39. Do you smoke? | | |
| ☐ YES | ☐ NO | |
| 40. Do you chew vitamin supplements with vitamin C or take vitamin C in effervescent tablets? | | |
| ☐ YES | ☐ NO | |
| 41. Do you chew aspirin with vitamin C? | | |
| ☐ YES | ☐ NO | |
| 42. Do you chew iron tablets? | | |
| ☐ YES | ☐ NO | |
| 43. Do you chew any other vitamin or mineral supplements? | | |
| ☐ YES | ☐ NO | |
| 44. Do you participate in sports or high-intensity physical exercise? | | |
| ☐ YES | ☐ NO | |
| → If yes, how many hours per week? ........................................ | | |
| 45. Do you drink sport drinks? | | |
| ☐ YES | ☐ NO | |
| → If yes, how many per day? ........................................ | | |
| 46. Do you swim in a chlorinated swimming pool? | | |
| ☐ YES | ☐ NO | |
| → If yes, how many hours per week? ........................................ | | |
| 47. Do you vomit frequently or easily? | | |
| ☐ YES | ☐ NO | ☐ CANNOT SAY/DON'T KNOW |
| 48. Do you suffer from, or have you previously suffered from, any form of eating disorder, such as: | | |
| → Anorexia? | | |
| ☐ YES | ☐ NO | ☐ CANNOT SAY/DON'T KNOW |
| → Bulimia? | | |
| ☐ YES | ☐ NO | ☐ CANNOT SAY/DON'T KNOW |
| 49. Do you suffer from any food intolerances or allergies? | | |
| ☐ YES | ☐ NO | ☐ CANNOT SAY/DON'T KNOW |
| 50. Are you taking any medication? | | |
| ☐ YES | ☐ NO | |
| → If yes, please list the medication(s) and how long you have been taking it/them: ........................................ | | |
| ........................................ | | |
| ........................................ | | |
| 51. Do you suffer from any illness? | | |
| ☐ YES | ☐ NO | |

| | | |
|---|---|---|
| 52. Please indicate if you suffer from the following illness or conditions: | | |
| – Diabetes | ☐ YES | ☐ NO |
| – Asthma | ☐ YES | ☐ NO |
| – ADHD | ☐ YES | ☐ NO |
| – Sleep apnea | ☐ YES | ☐ NO |
| – Eating disorders | ☐ YES | ☐ NO |
| – Gastroesophageal reflux | ☐ YES | ☐ NO |
| – Irritative chronic pharyngitis (coughing) | ☐ YES | ☐ NO |
| – Overweight | ☐ YES | ☐ NO |
| – Depression | ☐ YES | ☐ NO |
| – Anxiety | ☐ YES | ☐ NO |
| – Stress | ☐ YES | ☐ NO |
| 53. If patient is a child: Have you suffered bullying or cyberbulling? | ☐ YES | ☐ NO |
| 54. If patient is a woman in menopause: Do you feel that dryness in your genitourinary system disturbs your everyday life routines? | | |
| | ☐ YES | ☐ NO |
| 55. Have you ever received cancer treatment? | | |
| | ☐ YES | ☐ NO |
| → If yes, please indicate when: | ........................................ | |
| → Please indicate the type of cancer: | ........................................ | |
| → Did you receive chemotherapy or radiotherapy? | ☐ YES | ☐ NO |
| 56. What is the highest degree or level of education you have completed? | | |
| ☐ High School | ☐ Apprenticeship | ☐ University Degree |
| 57. Do you have any other habits that you think may be related to your tooth wear, apart from all those previously mentioned? | | |
| | ☐ YES | ☐ NO |
| → If yes, please share details: ........................................ | | |
| *Questionnaire adapted from the doctoral thesis: "The impact of tooth wear on the patient's quality of life," Dr Beatriz Rodríguez-Vilaboa, San Pablo CEU University, July 2017.* | | |

# APPENDIX 2 – Informed Consent for the Patient with Tooth Wear (To Be Adapted to Local-Regional Legal Status)

Having analyzed your case and thanks to your collaboration, we have been able to detect signs of varying types of tooth wear in your mouth.

As it has been explained to you, the origin of this tooth wear is multifactorial in the majority of cases.

Likewise, in the majority of cases, the tooth wear is progressive; therefore, if left untreated, it is expected that these signs of tooth wear will become progressively more significant over time.

Tooth wear can have consequences that include but are not limited to: shortening of the length of the teeth, dental fractures, hypersensitivity and/or pain, and even crown and/or root fractures that may require dental extraction.

By signing this document, you signify that you have received this information and that all of the below is true.

It has been explained to me that, in my case, it is recommended and advisable to proceed with the restoration of hard dental tissue in order to protect my teeth from the current tooth wear process and try to recover their anatomy and function with the use of specific restorative materials. The scientific literature has described the direct relationship between the correct anatomy (form, size, volume, and contour of the teeth) and ideal function.

I have been informed that orthodontic treatment may be required prior to my restorative treatment in order to provide the correct scenario for the restorations to be placed.

## Objectives/Benefits

1. My case is characterized as being a case of "premature or pathologic dental wear" as my mouth is presenting a loss of dental structure that cannot be attributed to the passing of time nor to the physiologic function of the mouth.
2. The main objective of this treatment is to restore the lost dental anatomy to the affected teeth, giving them the most appropriate form and size. In many cases, this will permit a more favorable relationship between the dental arches. This anatomy is necessary for function and also to help in the protection of the rest of the dentition from progressive and future wear.
3. In my case, special maintenance and preventive measures include periodic visits and monitoring; a mouthguard to protect from unwanted excessive forces; and diet, nutritional, and lifestyle counseling.
4. In my case, a saliva-stimulation regimen includes specific oral hygiene and topical measures as well as the recommendation to avoid harsh or abrasive hygiene products, either commercially available or homemade formulas, and aggressive tooth brushing.

## Information and Prior Warnings

1. The procedure could require local anesthetic, and I have been informed of the associated risks.
2. The tooth wear detected in my case is considered "premature" and does not correspond with my age, which means it cannot be considered as physiologic wear that occurs with age; rather it can only be explained in relation to other causes.
3. In the majority of cases, the origin of premature tooth wear is multifactorial: clenching, tooth grinding, exposure to excessive acidity of either extrinsic origin (food or drink) or intrinsic origin (stomach acid that refluxes into the oral cavity due to different health conditions), applying excessive force when brushing teeth or similar abrasion issues, or the combination of any of the above.
4. Aiming to be as conservative as possible and delaying as much as possible having to perform generalized conventional crown-type prostheses or fillings, rehabilitating the posterior sections with direct (done directly by the dentist at the dental chair) composite, indirect (done at the dental lab and delivered within a second appointment by the dentist) composite, or reinforced composite restorations has been proposed to me to replace the lost structure. A combination of direct and indirect restorations is usually done based on the grade of the tooth structure damage. These restorations are considered to be "long-lasting" temporary restorations. Their resistance to wear is similar to that of the tooth itself so that these materials will not wear the opposing teeth. When they no longer provide the required function or they have become worn

(depending on the case, this can be within a period of 3 to 5 years) they can be partially repaired or completely replaced.

5. In the anterior sector of the mouth, depending on the severity or location of the tooth wear, porcelain laminate veneers (or alternatively veneers made from other materials) might be used instead of direct composites. Depending on the objective of the treatment, it might be necessary to eliminate a certain amount of tooth structure, which is a fact that has been explained to me. This treatment procedure is compatible with preserving the maximum amount of the remaining dental structure while restoring the lost tooth structure, using what is today called *additive dentistry*.
6. Repairing or replacing these restorations cannot be ruled out over the course of the coming years given that the process and the causes of the original tooth wear can continue to remain active. The procedures listed above will generate a new cost estimate, separate to the initial treatment costs, and this estimate will be shared with the patient when these treatments are required.
7. The treatment recommended for me is based not just on years of experience but on results described by a multitude of working groups that have been collated in the scientific literature.
8. In some cases, an important objective of restorative work is to produce a "slight increase to the vertical dimension" (height) of the mouth to recuperate the correct height of the posterior sections and generate the required space to accommodate the necessary restorations in the anterior section of the mouth.
9. In addition to the planned treatment, I have been recommended to use retainers and/or nightguards as well as to continue modifying the habits and aspects of my diet that have been identified as causing or contributing to the tooth wear, as has been explained to me. The importance of this has been emphasized to me.
10. The treatment that has been proposed in my specific case to treat my tooth wear and to prevent it from continuing to progress, may consist of all or some of the following interventions:

- Diet counseling on my eating habits.
- Care protocol or specific dental hygiene.
- Use of retainers or nightguards.
- Orthodontic treatment.
- Direct or indirect composites.
- Indirect onlays. If my case is diagnosed as severe tooth wear, the need for conventional full-contour crowns, root canal treatment, or even implants cannot be ruled out.
- Porcelain laminate veneers.

I have understood the explanations that have been presented to me in clear and simple language, and the doctor who has been with me has allowed me to ask questions and has addressed all the doubts/concerns that I have raised. Therefore, I declare that I am satisfied with the information received, and I understand the scope and risks of the treatment.

Given the conditions above, I accept the proposed treatment.

| ______________________ | ______________________ | ______________________ |
|---|---|---|
| Patient/Guardian name (printed) | Patient/Guardian signature | Date |
| ______________________ | ______________________ | ______________________ |
| TW Team representative (printed) | TW Team representative signature | Date |

# FACING TOOTH WEAR

## FROM THE PATIENT'S PERSPECTIVE

Debora R. Vilaboa
Beatriz R. Vilaboa
Jose Manuel Reuss
Debora Reuss

QUINTESSENCE PUBLISHING

# WHAT IS TOOTH WEAR?



This supplement for patients is part of the book
TOOTH WEAR
THE QUINTESSENTIAL CHALLENGE

ISBN: 978-1-78698-120-2

QUINTESSENCE PUBLISHING DEUTSCHLAND

Quintessenz Verlags-GmbH
Ifenpfad 2–4
12107 Berlin
Germany
www.quintessence-publishing.com

Quintessence Publishing Co Ltd
Grafton Road, New Malden
Surrey KT3 3AB
United Kingdom
www.quintessence-publishing.com



Editing: Quintessence Publishing Co, Inc, Batavia, IL, USA
Layout, Production and Reproduction: Quintessenz Verlags-GmbH, Berlin, Germany

Printed and bound in Croatia by Grafički zavod Hrvatske d.o.o.

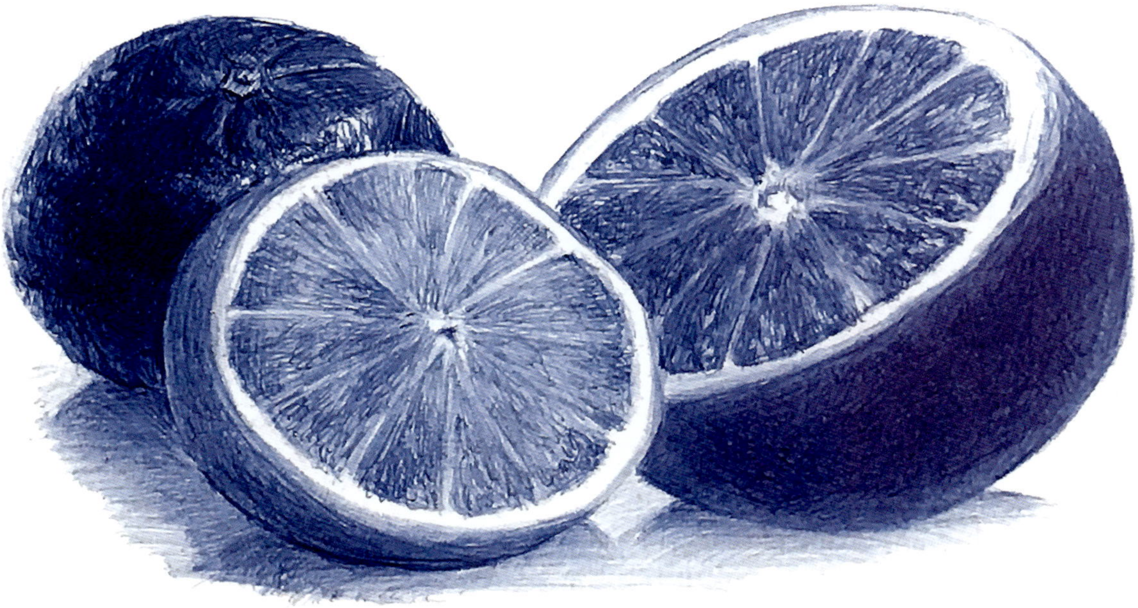

*The double-edged sword of modern life: a global world, global communications, and a fast and demanding lifestyle.*

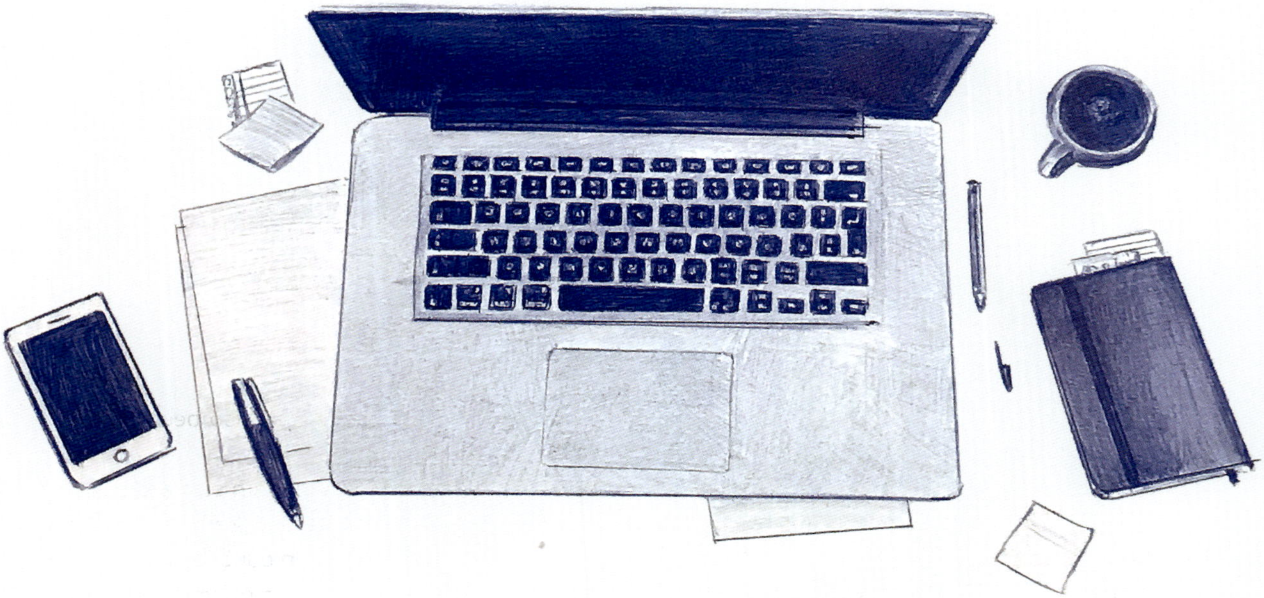

# WHAT IS TOOTH WEAR?

Tooth wear is an emerging condition in developed countries. Modern life, stress, and dietary trends of the Western world are behind contemporary tooth damage.

Soft drinks, fruit juices, highly acidic diets, stress, hyperconnectivity, sleep alterations, gastric reflux, food intolerances, eating disorders, dry mouth (caused by intake of medications and chronic diseases such as diabetes, hypertension, anxiety, and depression) all threaten tooth integrity. A simple questionnaire helps to determine true hyposalivation, one of the hidden causes that undermine tooth structure (Table 1).

Furthermore, with the mouth being the entrance of both the digestive and respiratory tracts, in addition to digestive alterations, respiratory conditions such as mouth breathing, asthma, and chronic pulmonary disease (amongst others) have also been linked to tooth wear.

Tooth wear is the loss of tooth structure starting primarily in the enamel—the external layer of the teeth and the hardest tissue in our body.

Tooth wear in most cases is progressive and can go undetected for a long period of time, exposing internal layers of the teeth such as dentin and even the pulp, eventually leading to pain and infection.

Tooth wear can be devastating if left untreated. The amount of tooth structure that is irreversibly lost will dictate the life cycle of the teeth and the amount of treatment required to restore the original anatomy. Therefore, the trend today is to tackle tooth wear in the initial stages or upon diagnosis.

**Table 1** Xerostomia Questionnaire.

| |
|---|
| 1. Does the amount of saliva in your mouth seem to be too little? |
| 2. Do you have any difficulty swallowing? |
| 3. Does your mouth feel dry when eating a meal? |
| 4. Do you sip liquids to aid in swallowing dry food? |
| **A positive answer to all four questions is associated with salivary gland malfunction.** |

## 1. Is All Tooth Wear the Same?

Tooth wear is a general term that includes several types of wear that differ according to the origin (Table 2).

**Table 2** Types of tooth wear, listed from lowest to highest wear factor.

| | |
|---|---|
| Abrasion | Physical wear of the tooth structure produced by foreign objects such as hard toothbrushes, fingernails, pens, or harsh foods (see Fig 1). |
| Attrition | Physical wear of the tooth structure produced by direct action between teeth such as bruxism, grinding, or clenching (see Fig 2). |
| Erosion | Chemical wear of the tooth structure produced by the action of acids from internal (eg, gastric reflux, vomiting) or external origin (eg, acidic foods, soft drinks, acidic medicaments) (see Fig 3). |

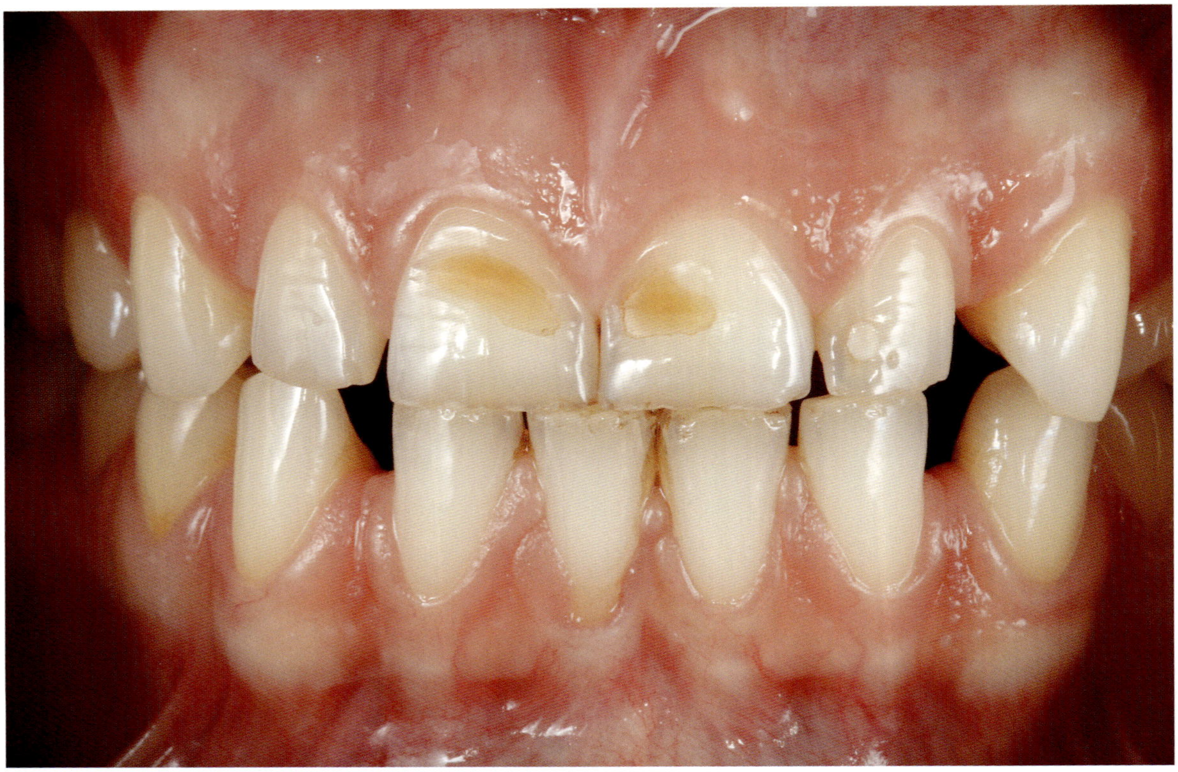

**Fig 1** Tooth wear caused by abrasion in this female patient in her 20s has led to exposure of the internal layer of dentin.

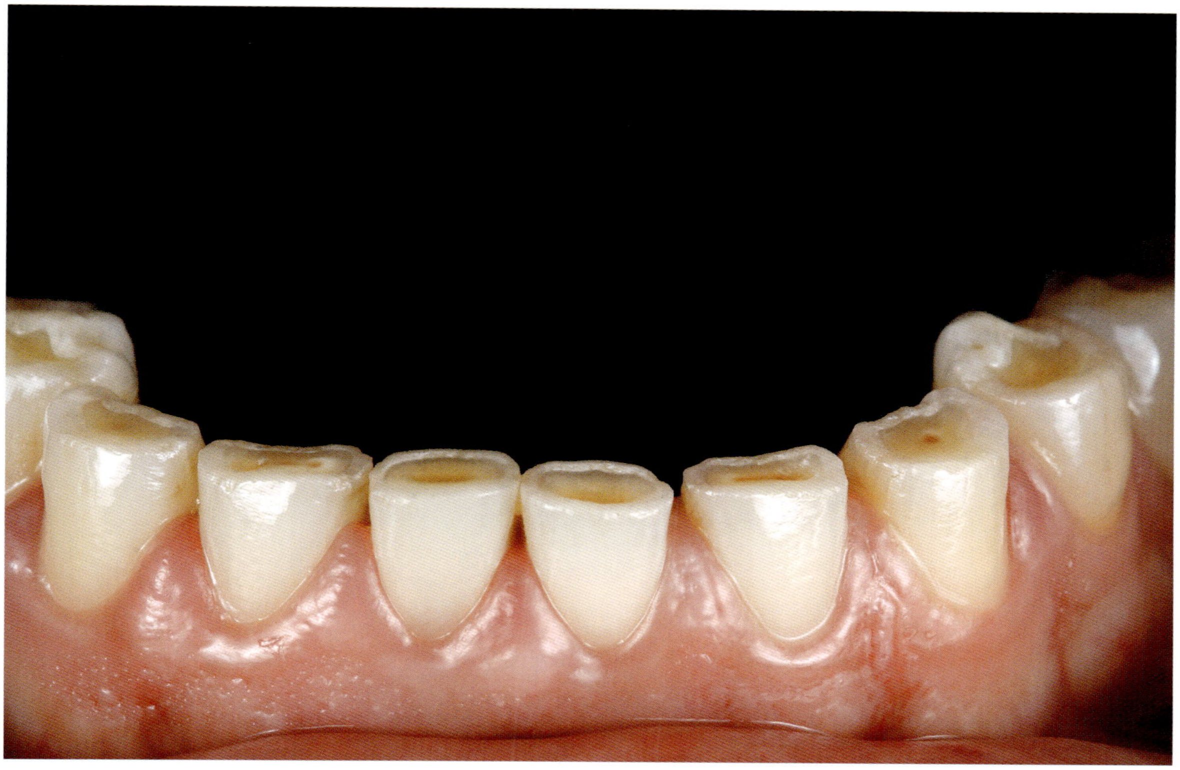

**Fig 2** Stress and a very fast-paced lifestyle are behind the severe wear produced by attrition in a 40-year-old male patient.

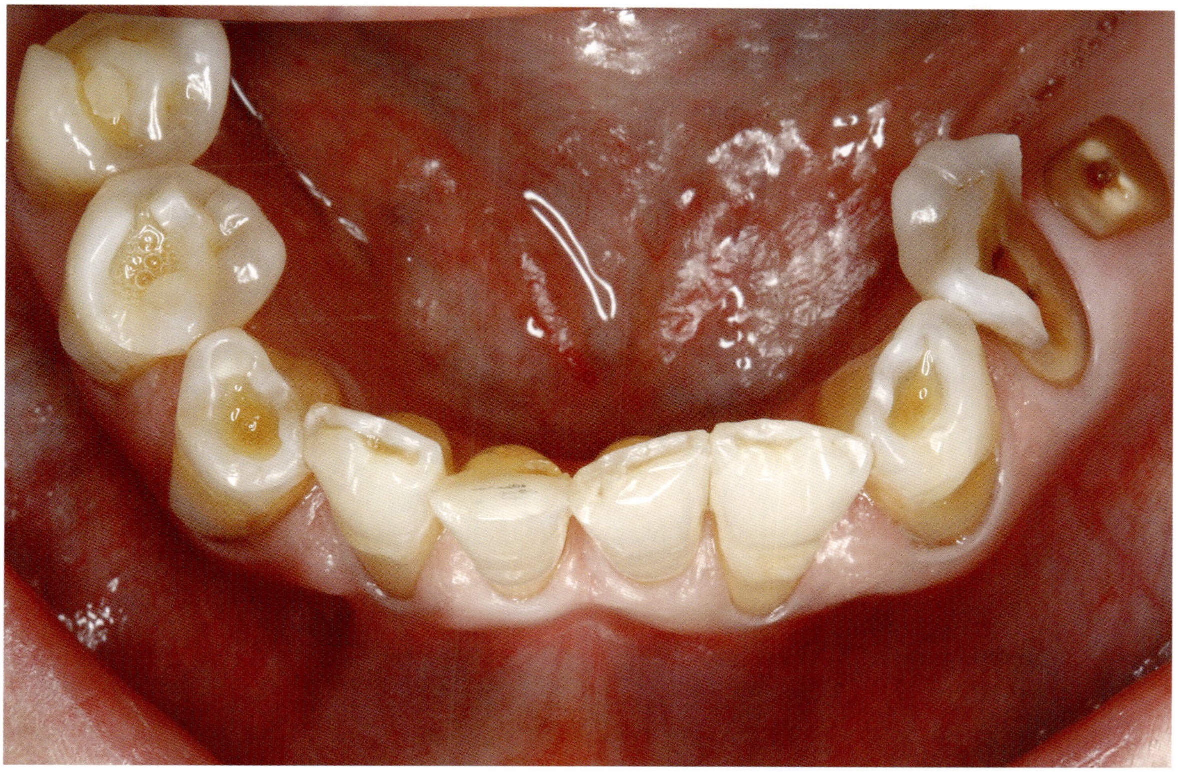

**Fig 3** Tooth wear in a 60-year-old female patient, presenting lesions of erosion, attrition, and abrasion. In the vast majority of cases, tooth wear is multifactorial, with chemical acid erosion being the major force leading to tooth wear today.

## 2. What Are the Signs and Symptoms of Tooth Wear?

Tooth wear may be asymptomatic for a long period of time, even decades, leading to further damage (Table 3 and Figs 4 to 14).

**Table 3** Signs and symptoms of tooth wear, graded according to severity.

| **Frequent signs and symptoms of tooth wear are:** | |
|---|---|
| Initial Tooth Wear | Loss of gloss of enamel, high retention of stains like lipstick, tea, coffee, etc |
| ↓ | Thinning of anterior teeth in the maxilla or mandible or both |
| | Tooth sensitivity |
| | Flattening of incisal edges and the tips of canines |
| | Shortening of teeth even to the extent they are not visible in the smile |
| | Mandibular teeth show more than maxillary teeth when talking or smiling |
| | Serrated "roller-coaster" smile line |
| | Transparent jellyfish-like borders of anterior teeth in the maxilla or mandible or both |
| | Posterior teeth show orange-brownish disk-like craters in the occlusal surfaces |
| | The necks of the teeth show notch-like defects, with or without gingival recession |
| | Flattening of the profile |
| | Wrinkling of lips and lower third of the face |
| | Persistent irritation of the corners of the mouth with blistering or bleeding |
| | Difficulty in speaking and/or chewing |
| | Repeated unexplained fractures |
| | Repeated restoration failure |
| Severe Tooth Wear | Pain, chronic infection, suppuration |

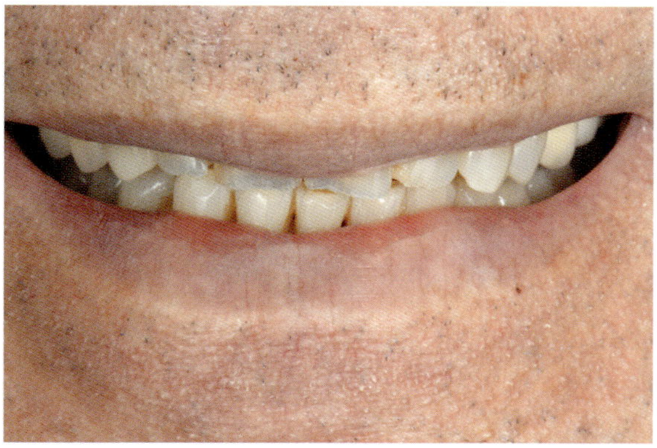

**Fig 4** Predominance of mandibular teeth during smile, typical of a worn dentition.

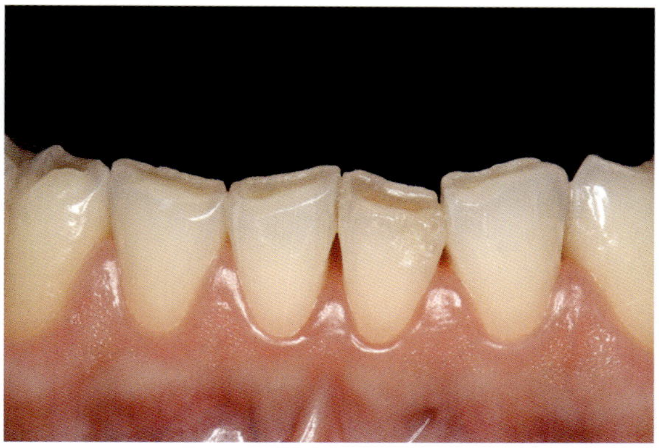

**Fig 5** The wear pattern has left a "roller-coaster" incisal line.

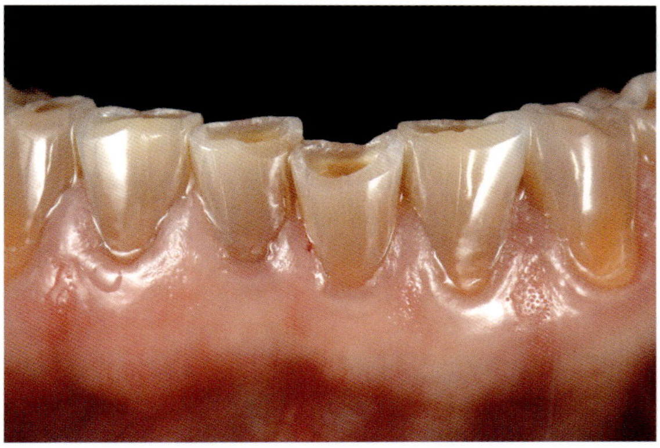

**Fig 6** Dramatic tooth structure loss in a young female patient suffering from multifactorial wear.

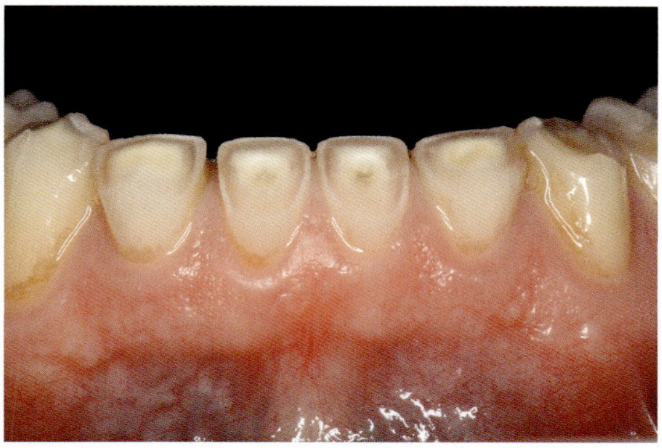

**Fig 7** Detail of advanced tooth wear that shows pulp transparency after loss of almost 50% of the tooth structure.

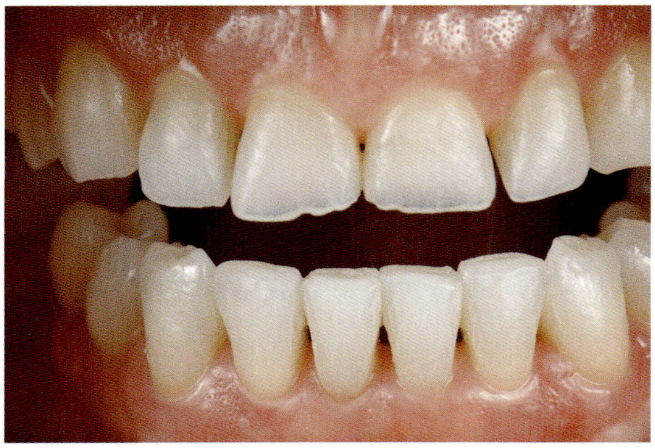

**Fig 8** Thinning of anterior teeth and shortening of the cusp tips of the canines in a young woman.

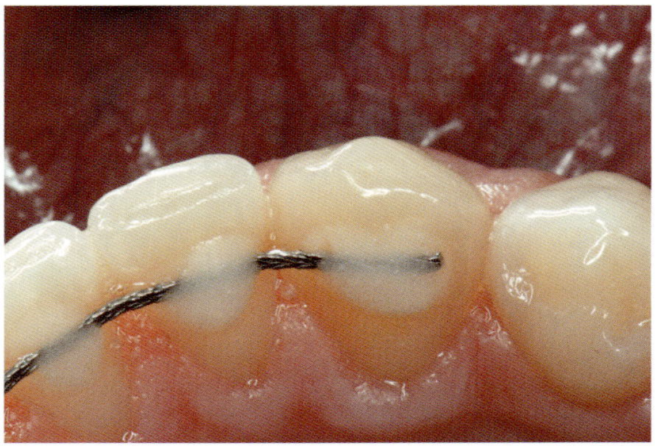

**Fig 9** Detail of the flattening of the cusp of a mandibular canine.

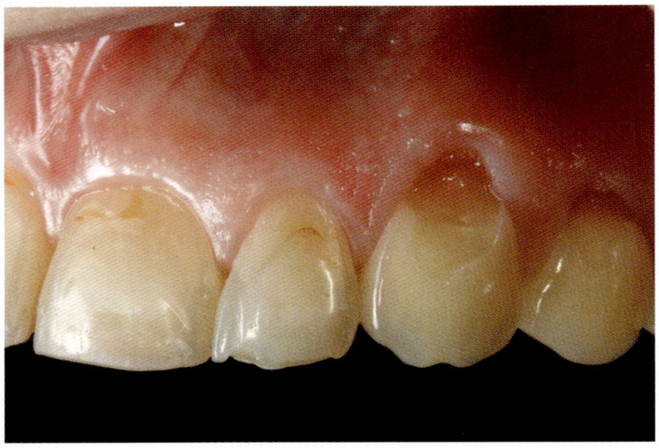

**Fig 10** Extensive loss of enamel and dentin in a patient with severe tooth wear with deep dentin exposure.

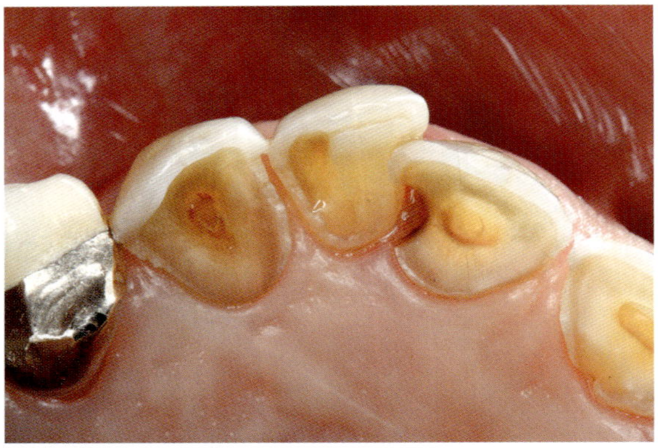

**Fig 11** Pulp exposure after dissolution of the palatal aspects of the anterior teeth.

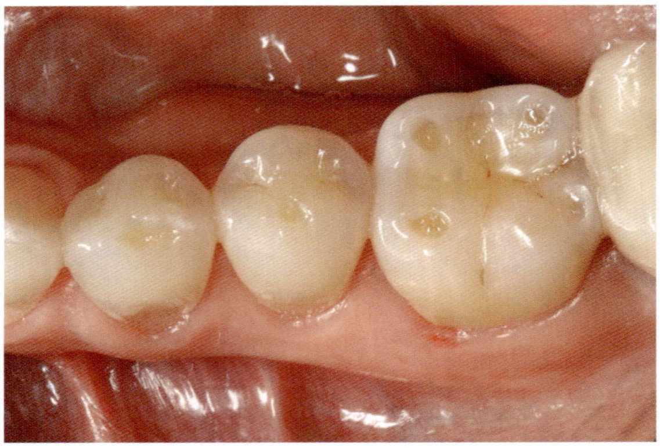

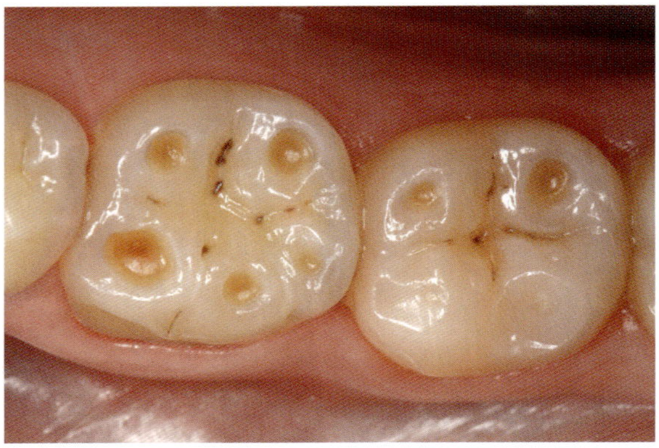

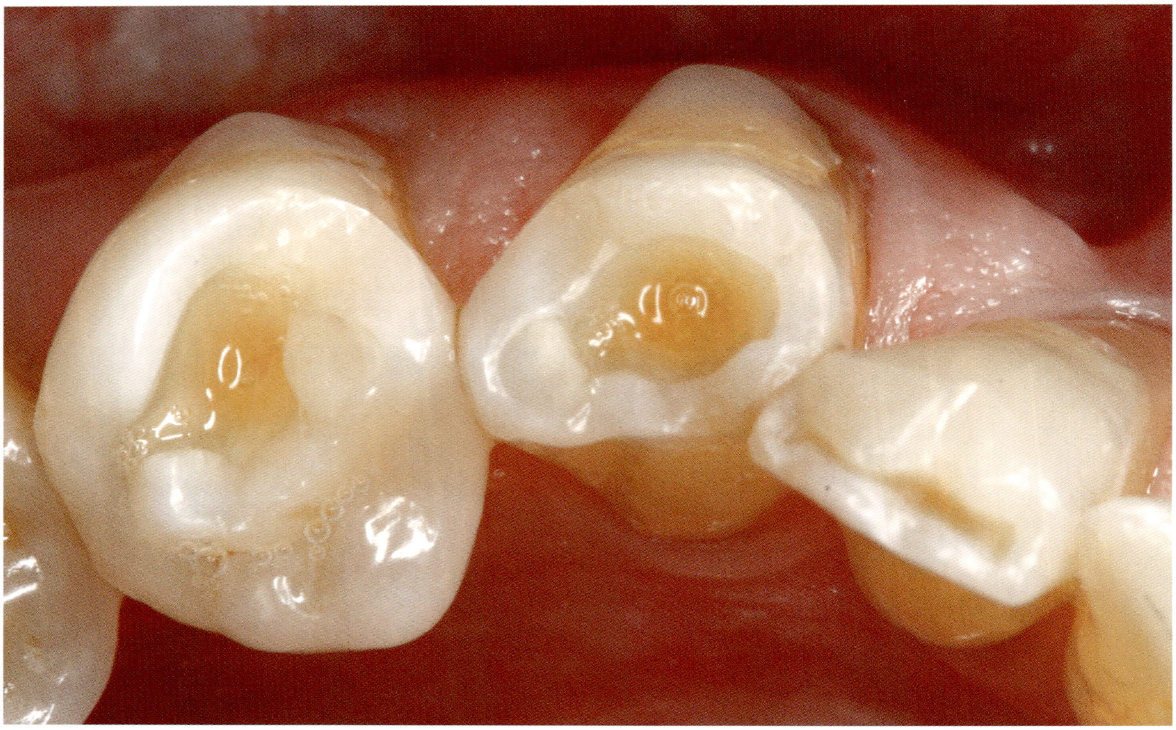

**Figs 12 to 14** Saucer-like lesions of different grades of tooth wear damage on the occlusal surfaces of teeth.

## 3. What Happens if I Wait?

Certain degrees of tooth wear are part of physiologic aging. However, retaining one's teeth has been linked to longer life expectancy with a healthier and better quality of life.

The rate at which tooth wear progresses is variable and can be rapid in some cases. Initial tooth wear may be localized and easily treated. Advanced tooth wear affects not only the mouth but may also have an impact on general health. It can affect appearance and self-esteem, causing early aging and leading to psychologic discomfort and even social incapacity.

While a preventive strategy is considered the ideal approach, there are complex risk factors involved in tooth wear that are difficult to eliminate overnight. A few of these are stress, polymedication, noncommunicable diseases, and in general all conditions that will cause reduced quality or quantity of saliva. Therefore, with tooth wear being a progressive condition (Figs 15 and 16), the general recommendation today is to treat the tooth wear patient as soon as possible and establish a routine to increase salivation.

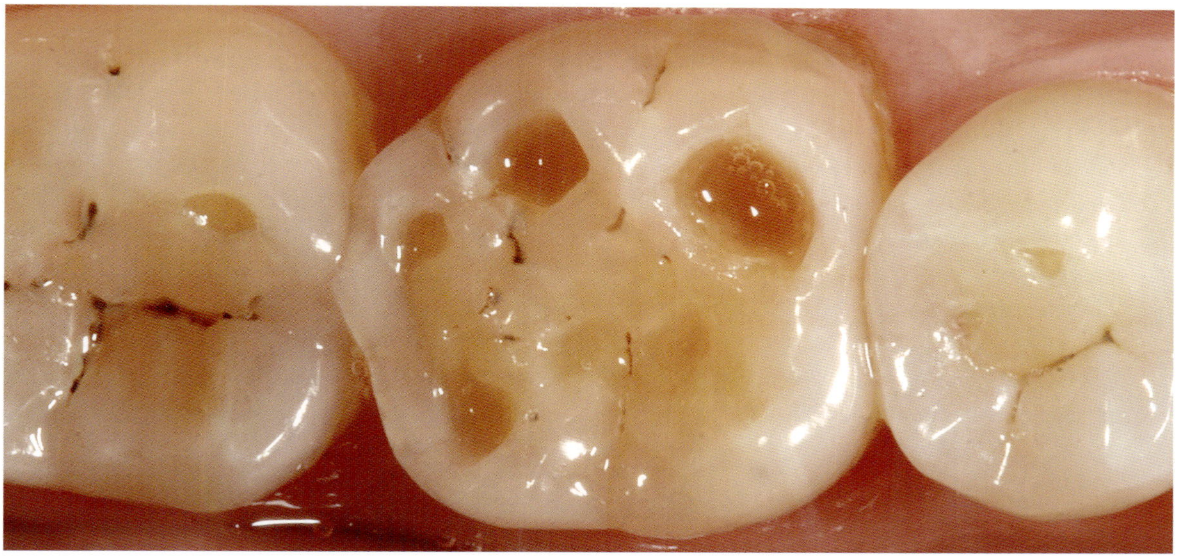

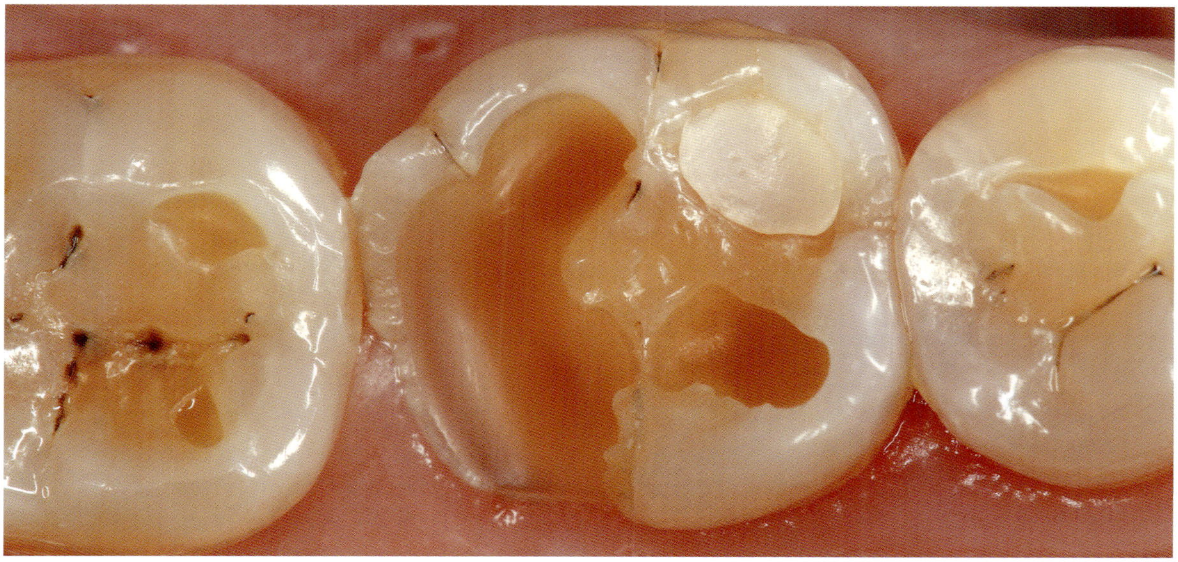

**Figs 15 and 16** Evolution of tooth wear over 8 years with exposed dentin as a result of prolonged exposure to an acidic environment. The patient was free of symptoms despite the unequivocal deep erosive lesions.

## 4. Can Tooth Wear Be Prevented?

Whenever possible, treatment strategies will include preventive measures in order to diminish or eradicate causative factors.

### Preventive Measures

Healthy and balanced dietary and lifestyle regimens may significantly aid in the effort to stop or reduce tooth wear progression. Dietary guidelines such as the following, which aim to reduce overall acid intake, are essential in those cases where acid erosion is the cause:

- Chewing fruit is preferable to drinking fruit juice.
- Soft drinks should be substituted with water.
- Never brush teeth immediately after drinking soda drinks or fruit juices.
- A balanced diet should include carbohydrates, proteins, and lipids, with the latter preferably coming from olive oil.
- Milk, cheese, and yogurt should be present in the diet.
- Chew slowly, allowing for healthy mastication and sufficient saliva production.
- Use a soft-bristled toothbrush and a nonabrasive remineralizing toothpaste with a neutral pH.
- Consult a physician if medications or conditions causing dry mouth are present.
- Apply tooth wear protection gels for dry mouth before bedtime.
- Move dinnertime earlier and take a walk before bedtime whenever possible.
- Where applicable, reduce alcohol and nicotine use and start a healthy diet and weight loss program.

### Treatment Measures

A minimally invasive approach is desirable whenever feasible. Direct simple composite restorations are many times an ideal option to restore posterior wear. Composite restorations provide the opportunity to restore wear lesions without the need to reduce any additional tooth structure and therefore oftentimes without the need for anesthesia. The need for repairs or further treatments in the future must be anticipated, which is why easily reparable techniques and materials should be used (Table 4 and Figs 17 to 22).

**Table 4** Recommended treatments.

| **Recommended treatments may include:** |
| --- |
| Orthodontic treatment to provide a better occlusal situation and/or the required space in order to restore the worn-out dentition. |
| Minor composite restorations to provide adequate protective anatomy that will stop or decelerate wear progression (restoring the tips of canines or incisal edges of anterior teeth). |
| Direct (performed chairside) or indirect (performed with the aid of a laboratory) restorations in order to recuperate the overall dental anatomy. |
| In cases of severe wear, the use of endodontic crowns or implants cannot be dismissed, which is why prompt intervention is recommended in cases of wear. |
| The use of occlusal splints is highly recommended in cases of tooth wear, although not all types of tooth wear can benefit from them. |

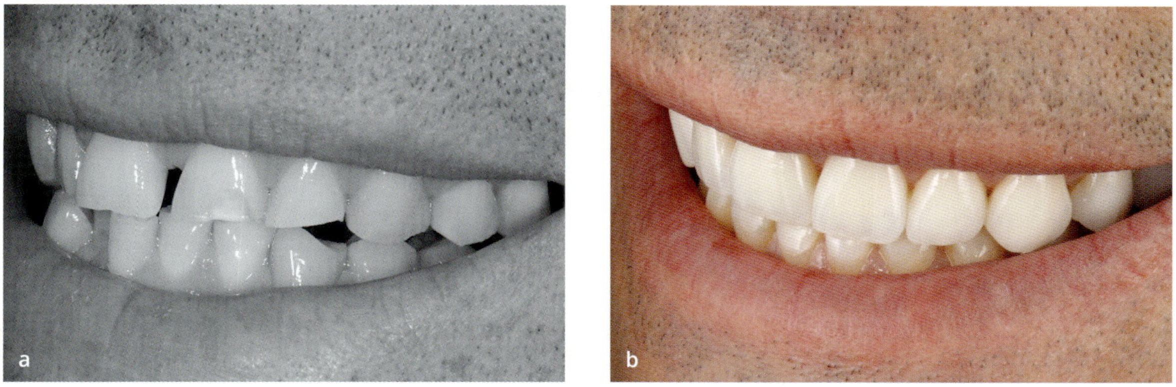

**Fig 17** Anterior wear can be restored with noninvasive porcelain laminate veneers, which provide excellent function and performance as well as optimal esthetic integration (a and b).

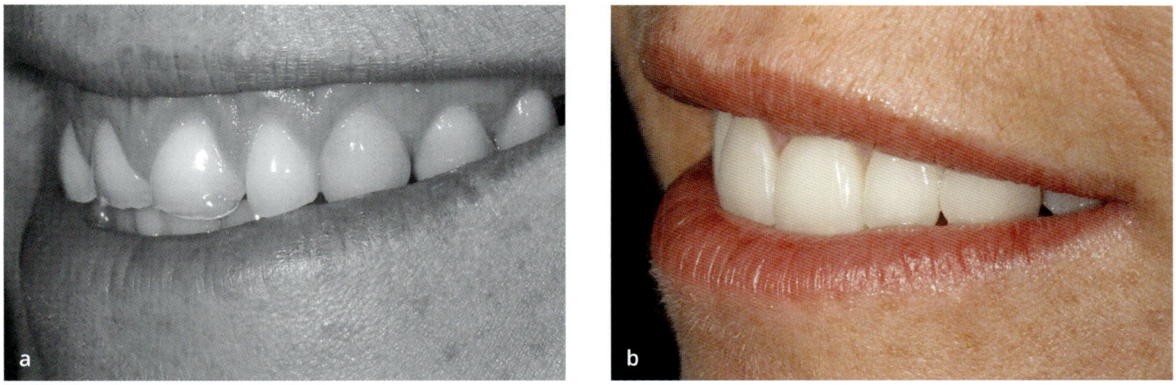

**Fig 18** Recuperating the optimal volume of tooth structure impacted by tooth wear provides a rejuvenated smile enhanced by improved lip support (a and b).

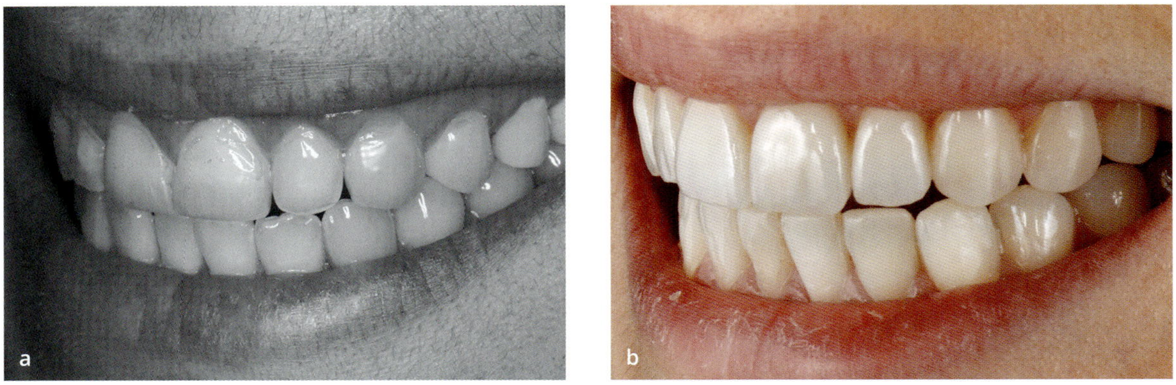

**Fig 19** Tooth wear may affect all surfaces of the teeth. The tooth wear team will recommend the optimal treatment approach depending on the case (a and b).

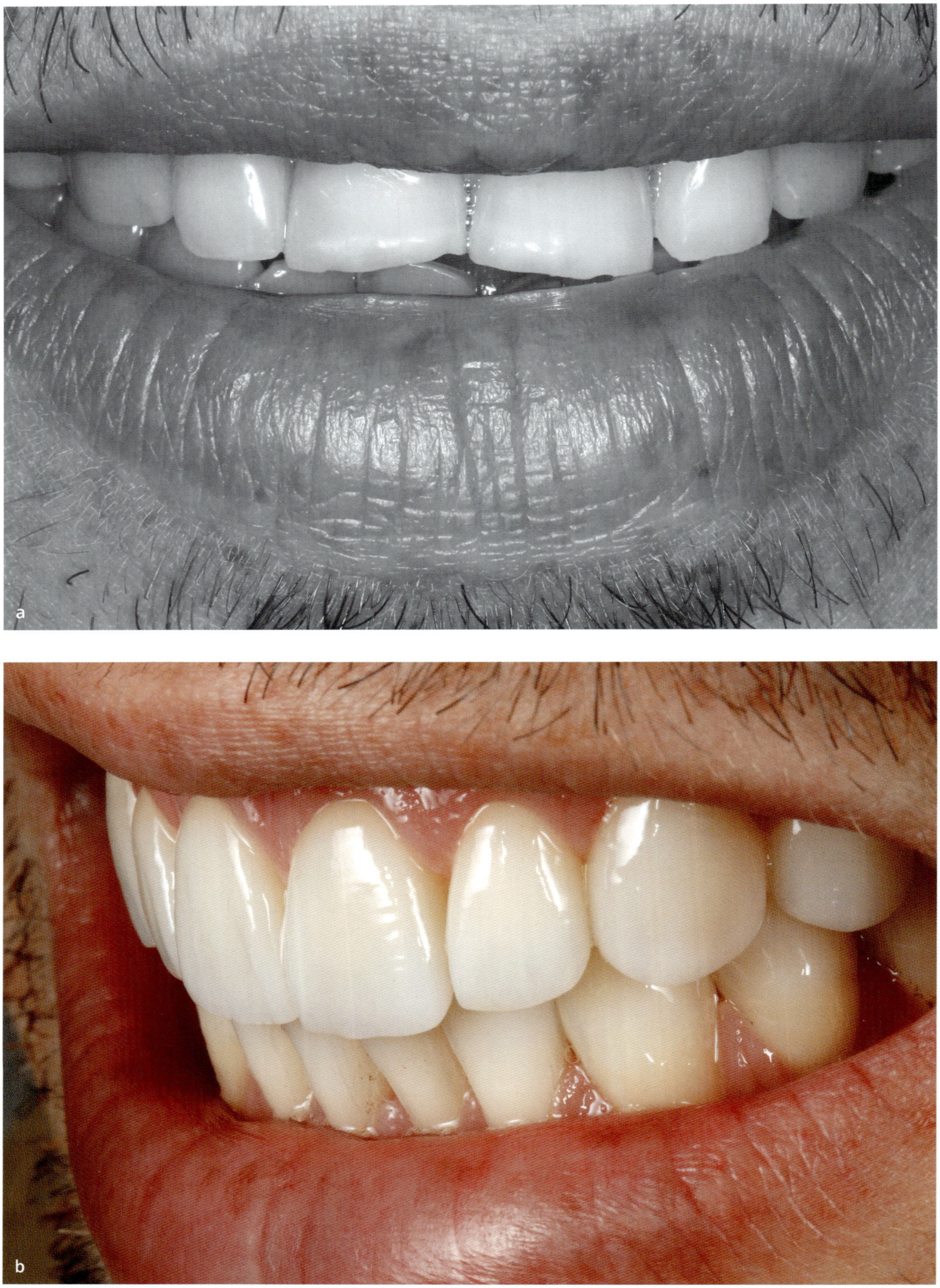


**Fig 20** It is not unusual to combine several types of treatment modalities in patients with tooth wear with the aim of saving the remaining tooth structure. Mimicking the beauty of natural enamel should be a priority in cases in which anterior teeth are affected by wear (a and b).

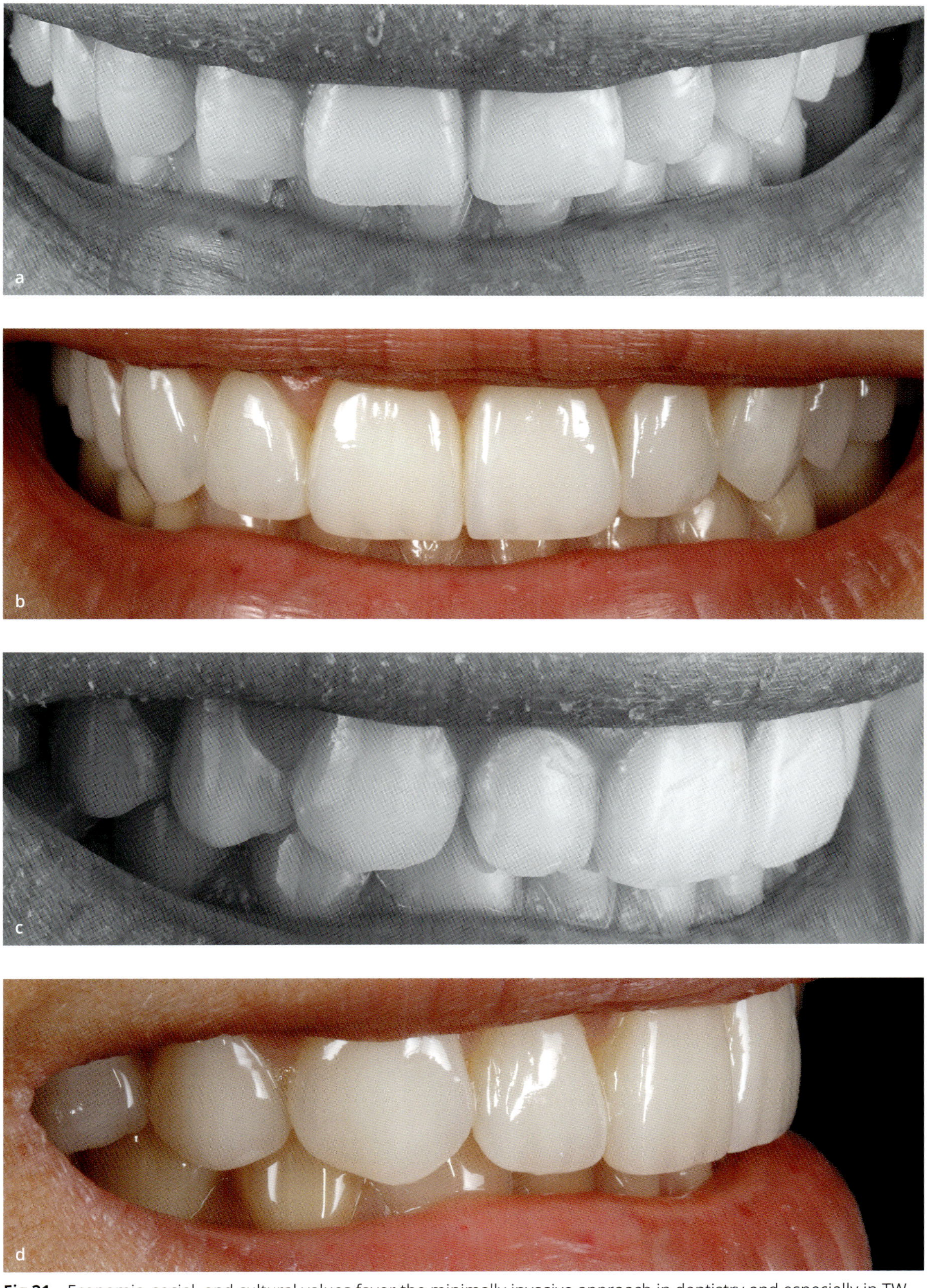


**Fig 21** Economic, social, and cultural values favor the minimally invasive approach in dentistry and especially in TW management (a to d).

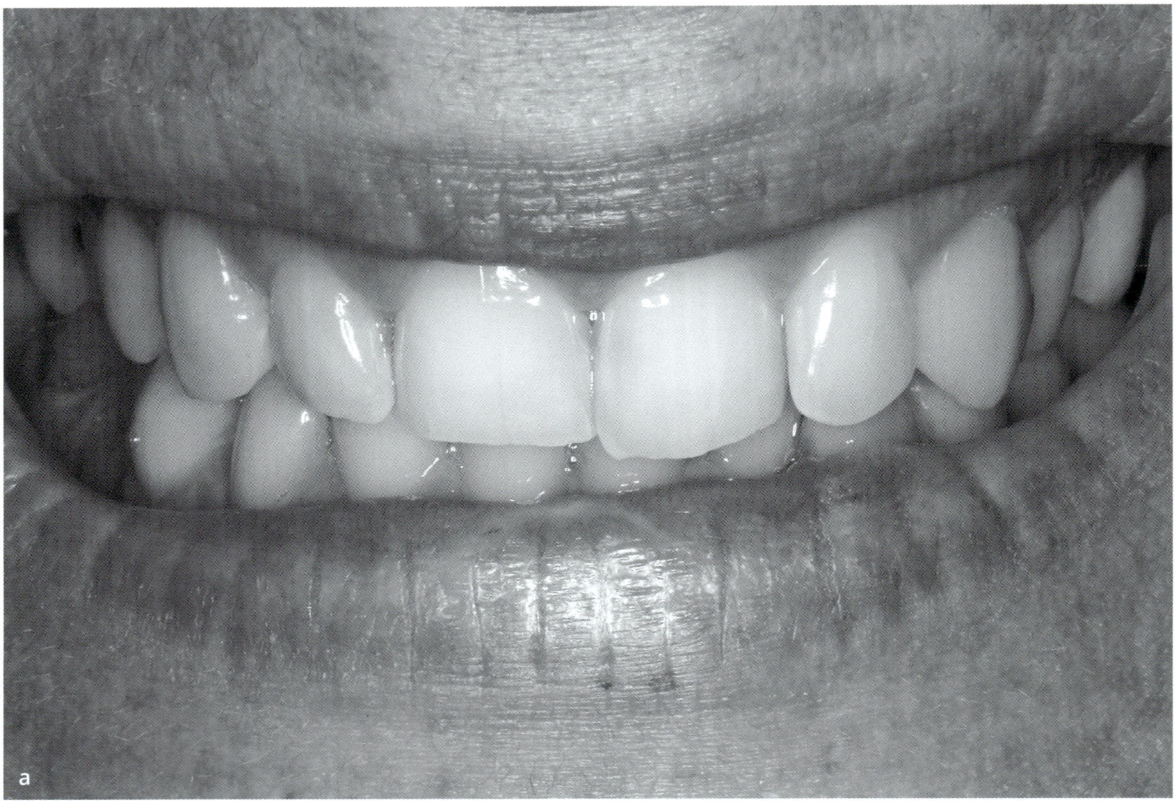

a

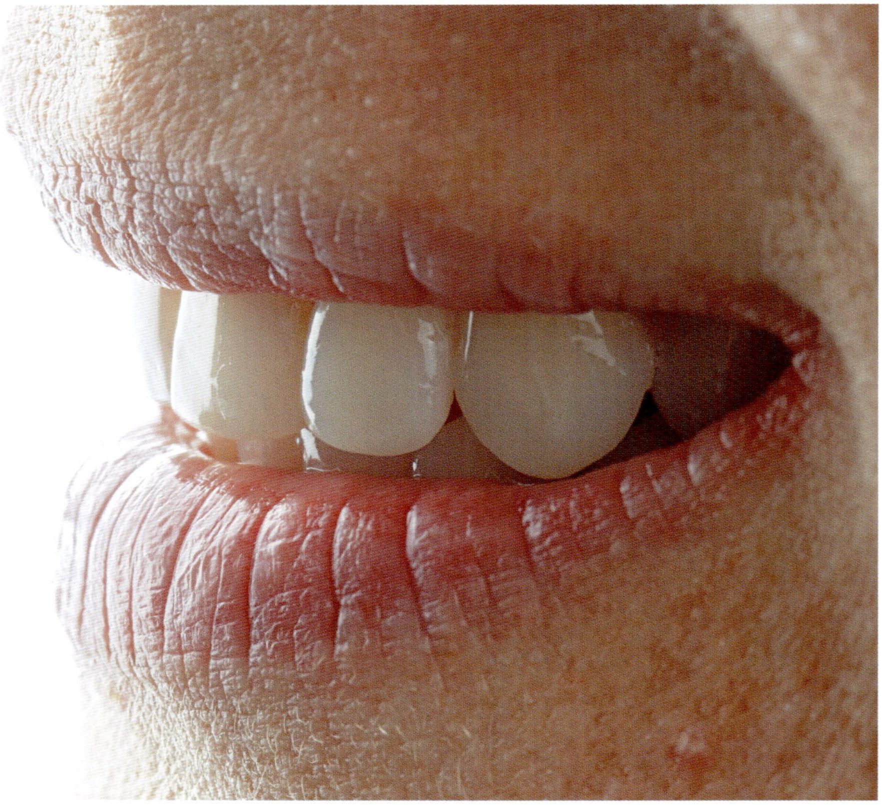

b

**Fig 22** Invisible orthodontic treatment and minor composite restorations have been performed in this young patient (a to c). The patient is wearing a soft, transparent nightguard to provide protection and assure orthodontic retention (d).

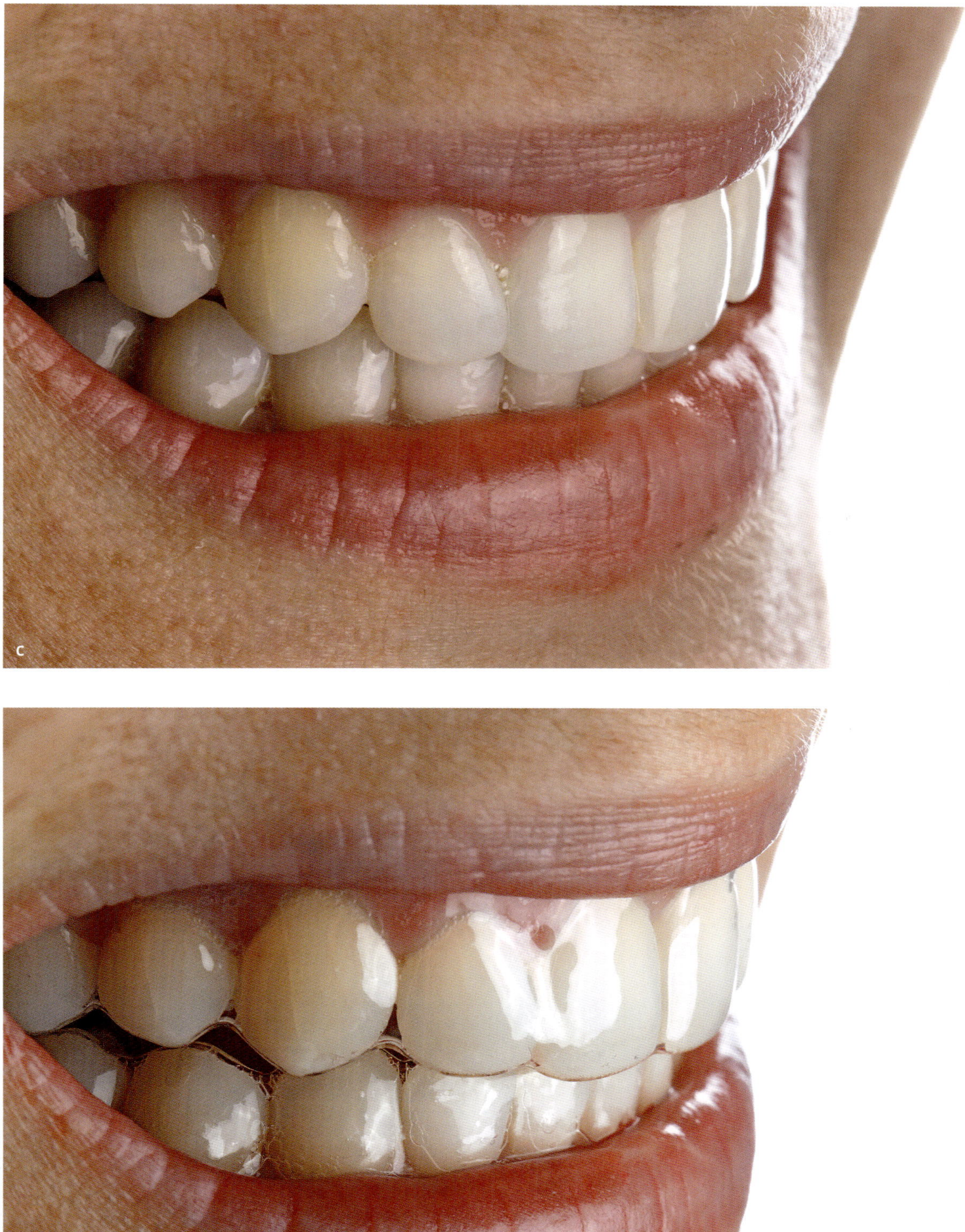
c
d

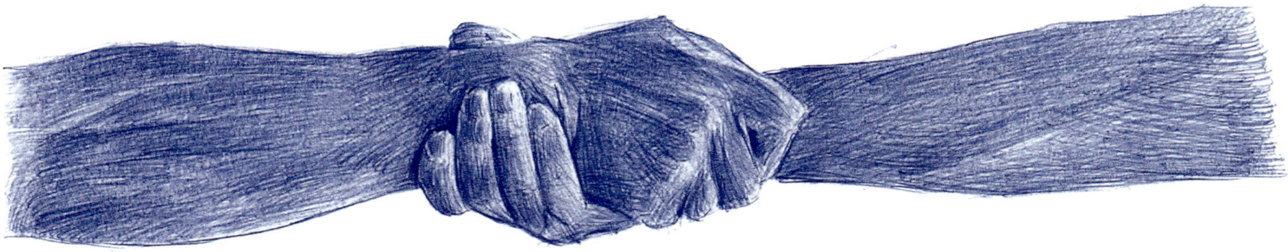

*A joint effort from both the patient and the dental team will enable a better prognosis for the worn dentition.*

This supplement for patients is part of the book
TOOTH WEAR
THE QUINTESSENTIAL CHALLENGE

ISBN: 978-1-78698-120-2

# Abbreviations

ACE – adverse childhood experience
ADHD – attention deficit hyperactivity disorder
AI – artificial intelligence
AN – anorexia nervosa
BEWE – Basic Erosive Wear Examination
BMI – body mass index
BN – bulimia nervosa
CAD/CAM – computer-aided design/computer-assisted manufacture
CBCT – cone beam computerized tomography
CEJ – cementoenamel junction
CTG – connective tissue graft
CPAP – continuous positive airway pressure
CR – centric relation
DME — deep margin elevation
EDs – eating disorders
EDNOS – eating disorders not otherwise specified
EFP – European Federation of Periodontology
EMA – European Medicines Agency
FCDP – fixed complete dental prosthesis
FDA – Food and Drug Administration
GER – gastroesophageal reflux
GERD – gastroesophageal reflux disease
GI – gastrointestinal
HPP – high-performance polymer
IDS – immediate dentin sealing
IoT – the internet of things
LOS – lower esophageal sphincter
MAD – mandibular advancement device
MIP – maximal intercuspal position
MISGD – medication-induced salivary gland dysfunction
NCCLs – non-carious cervical lesions
NCTSL – non-carious tooth surface loss
OSA – obstructive sleep apnea
PEEK – poly-ether-ether-ketone
PFM – porcelain-fused-to-metal
PICN – polymer-infiltrated ceramic network
PLVs – porcelain laminate veneers
PPIs – proton pump inhibitors
PPP – personalized preventive program
PREMs – patient-reported experience measures
PROMs – patient-reported outcome measures
PTFE – polytetrafluoroethylene
SARS-CoV-2 – severe acute respiratory syndrome coronavirus 2
SB – sleep bruxism
SGD – salivary gland dysfunction
SGH – salivary gland hypofunction
SSF – stimulated salivary flow
STL – stereolithography; also referred to as standard triangle language or standard tessellation language
TMJ – temporomandibular joint
TSL – tooth surface loss
TW – tooth wear
UOS – upper esophageal sphincter
USF – unstimulated salivary flow
VDO – vertical dimension of occlusion
WASS – Wear Aggravation Severity Scale
WECC – Wear Easy Clinical Classification
WHO – World Health Organization